Coronary Artery Stenosis

Coronary Artery Stenosis

K. Lance Gould, MD

Professor of Medicine
Department of Internal Medicine
Positron Diagnostic and Research Center
University of Texas Health Science Center
Houston, Texas

Elsevier
New York • Amsterdam • London

Cover Figure. A 3-D topographic map of myocardial perfusion during dipyridamole-hand-grip stress using rubidium-82. The inferior view is shown as if looking at the inferior-posterior wall of the heart with lateral (L) and septal (S) aspects of this posterior view labeled correspondingly. There is a severe septal and inferior apical defect in this view with a more moderate lateral perfusion defect. For other views and clinical information, see tomograms and polar maps of Figure 12-8, the other 3-D topographic views in Figure 20-1 and the clinical description of Case 1 in Chapter 20.

Elsevier Science Publishing Co., Inc.
655 Avenue of the Americas, New York, New York 10010

Sole distributors outside the United States and Canada:
Elsevier Science Publishers B.V.
P.O. Box 211, 1000 AE Amsterdam, The Netherlands

© 1991 by Elsevier Science Publishing Co., Inc.

This book has been registered with the Copyright Clearance Center, Inc.
For further information please contact the Copyright Clearance Center, Inc.
Salem, Massachusetts.

This book is printed on acid-free paper.

Library of Congress Cataloging-in-Publication Data

Gould, K. Lance.
    Coronary artery stenosis / K. Lance Gould.
       p.   cm.
    Includes bibliographical references.
    Includes index.
    ISBN 0-444-01544-2 (hardcover : alk. paper)
    1. Coronary artery stenosis—Pathophysiology. 2. Heart—
Tomography. I. Title.
    [DNLM: 1. Constriction, Pathologic—diagnosis. 2. Coronary
Circulation—physiology. 3. Coronary Disease—diagnosis. 4. Heart—
radiography. 5. Tomography, Emission-Computed. WG 300 G697c]
RC685.C58G68 1990
616.1′23—dc20
DNLM/DLC
for Library of Congress   90-3927
                                 CIP

Current printing (last digit):
10 9 8 7 6 5 4 3 2 1

Manufactured in the United States of America

To Lenja

Contents

Preface   ix

Acknowledgments   xi

Introduction   1

PART I:
ANATOMIC AND FUNCTIONAL CHARACTERISTICS OF CORONARY ARTERY STENOSES   5

1. Physiology of Coronary Circulation   7

2. Methods for Pressure-Flow Analysis and Arteriography   17

3. Interactions with the Distal Coronary Vascular Bed   31

4. Phasic Pressure-Flow and Fluid-Dynamic Analysis   41

5. Phasic Pressure-Flow and Arteriographic Geometry   53

6. Collapsing Stenoses   65

7. Coronary Flow Reserve   79

8. Quantitative Coronary Arteriography   93

9. Stenosis Flow Reserve by Quantitative Arteriography   109

10. Reversal by Risk Factor Modification   121

PART II:
POSITRON EMISSION TOMOGRAPHY OF THE HEART   137

11. Principles of Cardiac Positron Emission Tomography   139

12. PET Perfusion Imaging   143

13. Quantitation of PET Perfusion Images   159

14. Coronary Collateral Function Assessed by PET   169

15. Assessing Myocardial Infarction, Ischemia, and Viability   179

16. PET Compared to Other Imaging Modalities   197

17. Accuracy and Performance of the Positron Scanner   209

18. Economics of Cardiac PET   219

19. Radiation Burden, Facilities, and Regulatory Status   231

20. Case Studies with PET   233

References to Chapters 11–20   311

Index   319

Preface

This book describes the pressure flow characteristics, physiologic behavior, and quantitative geometry of coronary artery stenoses experimentally in vivo and clinically using the most advanced invasive arteriographic analysis and noninvasive perfusion-metabolic imaging available. It integrates essential concepts of coronary physiology, fluid dynamics, coronary flow reserve, quantitative coronary arteriography, myocardial metabolism, and PET imaging, including basic concepts, experimental validation, technology, clinical applications, and an atlas of cardiac PET as examples of applied clinical pathophysiology. The goal is synthesis of these diverse topics and their correlations leading to better understanding of coronary artery stenoses and more accurate, rational clinical decisions for optimal patient care that are also economical.

Rather than exhaustive literature review of the topic, each chapter provides only essential information in order to develop the sequence and interaction of the concepts into a cohesive theme on the functional and anatomic characteristics of coronary artery stenoses. Based on twenty years of physiologic and clinical research, the book develops the scientific basis for a new approach to the diagnosis and management of symptomatic or asymptomatic coronary atherosclerosis utilizing noninvasive positron emission tomography and invasive quantitative coronary arteriography.

The book has two sections. *Part I, Anatomic and Functional Characteristics of Coronary Artery Stenoses*, addresses the geometry and hemodynamic behavior of coronary artery narrowing. It is for the clinician, physiologist, cardiovascular scientist, or bioengineer interested in coronary pathophysiology and the scientific basis for effects of coronary artery stenoses in vivo and their diagnostic or quantitative assessment. This section develops the basic physical concepts of pressure and flow, the fluid dynamic equations characterizing stenoses, their physiologic consequences experimentally in vivo, coronary flow reserve, quantitative coronary arteriography, application of these concepts to man, and finally, changes in coronary artery stenoses during regression and/or progression of disease in humans.

Part II, Positron Emission Tomography of the Heart, applies the concepts of Part I to clinical cardiology and cardiovascular research. The principles of PET are described, as is the relation of technical imaging characteristics to physiologic measurements made or needed. This section is for the clinician, scientist, or physicist/engineer interested in cardiac imaging from either technical or biological points of view, or from the point of view of the relation between them. It is also a practical clinical text of cardiac PET for the cardiologist, radiologist, nuclear medicine specialist, or general internist who wants personally to carry out or refer his patients for the most advanced, accurate, noninvasive cardiac imaging currently available for assessing coronary heart disease.

The references for Part I and Part II are organized differently corresponding to different development of the integrated theme for each part. In Part I, which includes Chapters 1 through 10, references are listed after each chapter dealing with diverse aspects of coronary physiology, instrumentation, pressure-flow measurements, fluid dynamics, arteriography, and so forth. In Part II, which includes Chapters 11 through 20, references are listed in their entirety after the last chapter because the central theme throughout this part is cardiac PET.

K. Lance Gould, MD

Acknowledgments

The author would like to acknowledge the following: The Clayton Foundation for Research, particularly Mr. C. W. Wellen, current President, and Mr. M. T. Launius, former President, for the joint research program between The Clayton Foundation for Research and the University of Texas; Roger Bulger, MD, former President of the University of Texas Health Science Center at Houston, Frank Webber, MD, former Dean of the University of Texas Medical School at Houston, and John Poretto, Executive Vice-President for Administration and Finance, University of Texas Health Science Center at Houston, for their enlightened institutional leadership in support of innovation and excellence; the M. D. Anderson Foundation, the Houston Endowment Foundation, and the Enron Corporation for generous contributions to research; Barbara and Gerald Hines, Jean and John Joplin, Catherine and A. G. McNeese, Gail and Don Gross, Margaret and Ben Love, Nanette and Jerry Finger, Linda and Ken Lay, Judy and John Mixon, for their personal interest and encouragement; Thomas Andreoli, MD, for my appointment as Director of the Division of Cardiology at the University of Texas Medical School from which the scientific development, physical facilities, and clinical applications evolved for this book; Richard Kirkeeide, PhD, Nizar Mullani, Ross Hartz, Claire Finn, Ro Edens, Kathryn Rainbird, Richard Smalling, MD, PhD, Mary Haynie, RN, MBA, Mary Jane Hess, RN, Leonard Bolomey, Mark Franceschini, Yvonne Stuart, RT, Jackie Raymond, Dean Ornish, MD, Byron Williams, MD, Don Gordon, MD, Kirk Lipscomb, MD, Katharine Kelley, MD, and many others for their expertise, commitment, and talent as professional colleagues; Elizabeth B. Gould, who was my first professor and also my mother; Simon Dack, MD, for his insight and criticisms over many years in support of innovative scientific publications; and finally, the staff of Elsevier Science Publishing Co., Inc., for their editorial encouragement and patience in preparing this book.

David S. Hess, MD

Introduction

Coronary heart disease causes 1.5 million myocardial infarctions and 520,000 deaths per year, or one third to one half of deaths between the ages of 35 and 64 years in the United States (1,2). Up to 13% of middle-aged men in the general population have coronary atherosclerosis, most of it clinically silent (3,4). Silent ischemia is increasingly recognized in symptomatic and asymptomatic individuals (5–14). It has an unfavorable prognosis when occurring during exercise testing (7), in patients with recent unstable angina (8), or in asymptomatic patients with perfusion defects after dipyridamole (11–14). Up to 48% of asymptomatic subjects with silent ischemia have a cardiac event (angina pectoris, myocardial infarction, or sudden death) within 4 to 6 years (7,9). Forty to 60% of patients with sudden death or myocardial infarction present without previous symptoms (15–18). Therefore, silent coronary atherosclerosis remains a particular problem in cardiovascular medicine, because there are no warning symptoms until a major cardiac event occurs.

Risk factors do not accurately identify individuals with symptomatic or asymptomatic coronary artery disease. For example, of 40- to 55-year-old men with high cholesterol and blood pressure, two thirds remain well during the subsequent 25 years (19) whereas one third develop coronary heart disease. In asymptomatic males of this age group with risk factors, coronary arteriography shows disease in 15% to 35% (1,3,4,20,21) that is anatomically severe in 7% to 35% (1,21). Of middle-aged men without symptoms who have a positive ECG exercise test, only 30% to 43% have significant coronary artery disease by arteriography (1), and 5% to 46% (mean 25%) develop clinical disease over the next 13 to 25 years (1,19). Therefore, approximately two-thirds of men are resistant to clinical coronary artery disease despite having risk factors, while one-third develop it, often with only modestly elevated or normal cholesterol levels.

Although overwhelming epidemiologic evidence links coronary heart disease to smoking, serum cholesterol, hypertension, and family history, large trials of modest risk factor modification with mortality endpoints have been somewhat disappointing, failing to provide the expected definitive benefit on mortality, as subsequently reviewed. In contrast with these earlier, large clinical trials, three recent arteriographic studies—the CLAS study by Blankenhorn et al. (22), the LifeStyle Heart trial by Ornish et al. and Gould et al. (23,24), and the FATS trial by Brown et al. (25)—demonstrate that reversal of coronary artery stenosis in man is feasible.

However, marked life-style change (23,24) or lowering of serum cholesterol with multiple drugs (25) is necessary to prevent progression or to reverse the severity of coronary artery stenoses with reasonable certainty in individual patients. Such vigorous life style changes or drug interventions may not be appropriate for individuals with risk factors who do not have the disease. Those individuals who have coronary heart disease or a genetic predisposition to it may need more aggressive risk factor interventions than is indicated or possible for the general population or for individuals with modestly elevated cholesterol without coronary artery stenosis. Although community education programs are important, their target guidelines for diet or drug therapy are not likely to be as stringent as for a patient with documented coronary artery disease or a genetic predisposition toward it. Thus, the vigor of risk factor modification should justifiably increase with the probability or certainty of coronary artery disease.

Traditionally in medicine, the patient and physician wait until angina pectoris, myocardial infarction, arrhythmia, heart failure, or sudden death leads to medical or mechanical intervention. However, symptoms are usually late manifestations of advanced disease; at this point, therapy to reverse coronary artery stenosis is difficult and mechanical procedures are often necessary. As a guide to therapy, angina pectoris usually indicates severe coronary artery stenoses, does not predict sudden death or acute myocardial infarction, and can be improved or eliminated by medical therapy without affecting progression of disease. Furthermore, by the time angina pectoris develops, the optimal opportunity for reversal therapy early in the disease has passed. Consequently, diagnosing coronary artery stenosis and its severity at the mildest, earliest possible stage, particularly before symptoms, is important for instituting vigorous risk factor modification for reversal.

Percutaneous transluminal coronary angioplasty (PTCA) and thrombolytic therapy have profoundly changed our management of coronary artery disease. A formally diagnostic procedure, cardiac catheterization, has become a therapeutic intervention often substituting for cardiac surgery. Figure 1 shows the time trends of cardiac catheterization, PTCA, and bypass surgery in the United States (2). The increases are exponential, with a doubling time of 5 years for all procedures (Figure 2). The percent of diagnostic cardiac catheterizations going to mechanical intervention has increased from 30% to 60%, as shown in Figure 3. These increasing numbers in the face of declining incidence of coronary artery disease (26,27) suggest that criteria for mechanical intervention have changed in recent years. The changed criteria for mechanical intervention are not solely related to growth of PTCA, because bypass surgery has also recently increased at nearly the same rate.

1

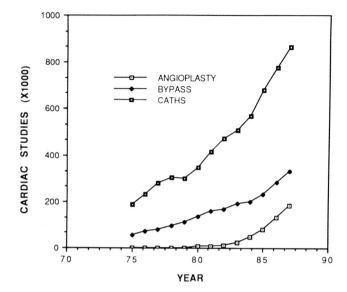

Fig. 1 Trends in cardiac catheterization, PTCA, and coronary artery bypass surgery.

Traditionally, mechanical intervention has been reserved for patients with angina pectoris or its equivalent that is refractory to medical therapy. With our current pharmacopeia of calcium channel and beta blockers, patients are uncommonly resistant to medical therapy, even with unstable angina. Those who are unstable usually go to emergent mechanical intervention. In early myocardial infarction, thrombolysis followed by mechanical intervention is the rule. The trend of more effective medical symptomatic therapy but increasing mechanical interventions suggests that therapeutic goals have appropriately extended beyond relief of cardiac

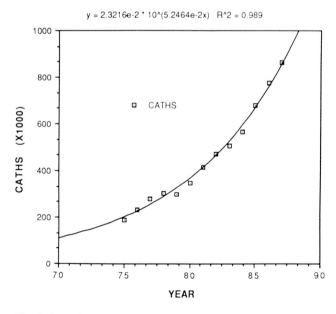

$$y = 2.3216e\text{-}2 \cdot 10\char94(5.2464e\text{-}2x) \quad R\char94 2 = 0.989$$

Fig. 2 Log plot of trends in cardiac catheterization, paralleled by PTCA and bypass surgery, with a recent doubling time of approximately 5 years for all three procedures.

symptoms on a widespread basis. Goals of cardiovascular therapy now include prevention of ischemia and myocardial infarction by earlier pharmacologic or mechanical reperfusion, salvage of myocardium during acute infarction, definitive restoration of coronary artery lumen, and prolonging life as well as its quality.

Although the goals of mechanical intervention are appropriately expanding, the clinical criteria for more frequent elective mechanical interventions in individual specific patients are frequently not clear. Quantitative coronary arteriography is not used widely, despite the recognized limitations of percent diameter stenosis by either caliper or visual estimates. Noninvasive thallium exercise testing has significant limitations for diagnosing or assessing severity of coronary artery disease or myocardial viability, as will be discussed in detail below. Accordingly, there is need for more accurate invasive quantitative coronary arteriography and noninvasive assessment of physiologic stenosis severity and of myocardial viability, equivalent to diagnostic cardiac catheterization in importance and reliability.

Thus, major questions for cardiovascular medicine are how to identify silent coronary artery disease in specific individuals, how to define its severity in either the symptomatic or asymptomatic patient, how to decide objectively among dietary, medical, and mechanical interventions, and how to assess the results, invasively and noninvasively. At the other end of the clinical spectrum, in patients with myocardial infarction, myocardial salvage by thrombolysis, PTCA, or bypass surgery require reliable measures of myocardial viability on which to base definitive mechanical interventions having significant risks.

Consequently, the goal of noninvasive myocardial perfusion or metabolic imaging is *accurately* to identify and assess severity of coronary artery stenosis and myocardial viability as a basis for choosing and following effects of interventions, including risk factor management, pharmacological agents, PTCA, thrombolysis, and bypass surgery. Accurate quantitation is particularly important in silent coronary artery disease as offering the only criteria for intervention to prevent sudden death or acute myocardial infarction.

Ideally, noninvasive cardiac imaging should provide sufficiently accurate functional information to determine the need for diagnostic catheterization as arteriographic confirmation for mechanical intervention based on the noninvasive test. Therefore, it should not only be a reliable guide to managing coronary artery disease in traditional cardiology practice based on symptoms, but should also provide the basis for vigorous medical or mechanical management of asymptomatic coronary atherosclerosis to prevent sudden death and myocardial infarction. Such accurate noninvasive evaluation by PET is not intended to replace cardiac catheterization but rather to identify individuals who really need it and to avoid unnecessary procedures in patients with either no coronary artery disease or only mild disease. Cardiac PET interfaces positively with invasive cardiology by making its application more efficient and selective even in the symptomatic patient.

Ideally, coronary arteriography should be carried out primarily for advanced coronary artery disease in patients being considered for mechanical intervention. Arteriograms should be quantitatively analyzed for the effects of percent narrowing, stenosis length, absolute cross-sectional area, shape, ec-

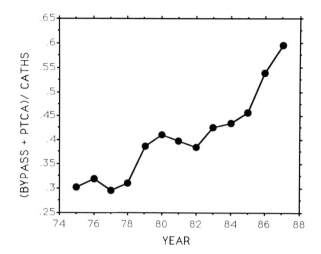

Fig. 3 Proportion of patients undergoing cardiac catheterization that subsequently go to PTCA or bypass surgery.

centricity, and diffuse disease on coronary flow capacity, without inter- and intraobserver variability characterizing visual estimates of percent stenosis. Because these multiple dimensions have cumulative hemodynamic effects and interact with one another, they have to be combined into a single clinically useful measure of anatomic severity that is independent of varying hemodynamic conditions such as pressure, heart rate, vasomotor tone, presence or absence of collaterals, and heart size. For this purpose, stenosis flow reserve by quantitative analysis of coronary arteriograms is well developed theoretically, validated by comparison with directly measured flow reserve experimentally, and proven clinically valuable by comparison with regional perfusion defects in patients, as described in subsequent chapters. Therefore, stenosis flow reserve by quantitative coronary arteriography is an optimal invasive "gold standard" for anatomically defining stenosis severity, for comparison to functional, metabolic, and perfusion imaging, for guiding mechanical intervention, and for assessing anatomically the effectiveness of medical and mechanical interventions.

Although reactive treatment triggered by symptoms appropriately remains central to cardiovascular medicine, advanced diagnostic and therapeutic technology provide opportunity for another major step in the evolution of cardiovascular medicine. Positron emission tomography has sufficient diagnostic power for a new therapeutic approach based on routine, economical noninvasive diagnosis and assessment of severity in symptomatic or asymptomatic individuals with intense dietary or medical treatment for reversal of coronary artery disease. Such therapy may not be appropriate for the general population or for individuals without known coronary artery stenosis. It is therefore targeted, individual-specific, preventive intervention. For severe silent disease identified by PET, coronary arteriography and mechanical intervention may be indicated to prevent myocardial infarction or sudden death.

In contrast with the traditional approach based on symptoms, this new approach is based on hemodynamic, functional, and anatomic characterization of stenoses and myo-

cardial viability with sufficient reliability in symptomatic or asymptomatic patients to justify medical or mechanical interventions having significant benefits and risks, or to avoid unnecessary ones.

REFERENCES

1. Guide to Clinical Preventive Services. Report of the U.S. Preventive Services Task Force. An assessment of the effectiveness of 169 interventions. ed. M. Fisher. Baltimore: Williams & Wilkins, 1989, pp. 3–11.
2. American Heart Association 1989 Heart Facts. Dallas: American Heart Association, 1988.
3. Olofsson BO, Bjerle P, Aberg T, Osterman G, Jacobsson KA. Prevalence of coronary artery disease in patients with valvular heart disease. Acta Med Scand 218:365–71, 1985.
4. Langou RA, Huang EK, Kelley MJ, Cohen LS. Predictive accuracy of coronary artery calcification and abnormal exercise test for coronary artery disease in asymptomatic men. Circulation 62(6):1196–203, 1980.
5. Campbell S, Barry J, Rebecca GS, Rocco MB, Nabel EG, Wayne RR, Selwyn AP. Active transient myocardial ischemia during daily life in asymptomatic patients with positive exercise tests and coronary artery disease. Am J Cardiol 57:1010–16, 1986.
6. Resnekov L. Silent myocardial ischemia: Therapeutic implications. Am J Med 79:30–34, 1985.
7. Fleg JL, Gerstenblith G, Zonderman AB, Becker LG, Weisfeldt ML, Costa PT, Lakatta EG. Prevalence and prognostic significance of exercise induced silent myocardial ischemia detected by thallium scintigraphy and electrocardiography in asymptomatic volunteers. Circulation 81:428–36, 1989.
8. Gottlieb SO, Weisfeldt ML, Ouyang P, Mellits ED, Gerstenblith G. Silent ischemia as a marker for early unfavorable outcomes in patients with unstable angina. N Engl J Med 314:1214–19, 1986.
9. Cohn PF. Clinical importance of silent myocardial ischemia in asymptomatic subjects. Circulation 81:691–93, 1989.
10. Cohn PF. Silent myocardial ischemia: Present status. Mod Concepts CV Dis 56:1–4, 1987.
11. Younis LT, Byers S, Shaw L, Barth G, Goodgold H, Chaitman BR. Prognostic importance of silent myocardial ischemia detected by intravenous dipyridamole thallium myocardial imaging in asymptomatic patients with coronary artery disease. J Am Coll Cardiol 14:1635–41, 1989.
12. Brown KA, O'Meara J, Chambers CE, Plante DA. Ability of dipyridamole-thallium-201 imaging one to four days after acute myocardial infarction to predict in-hospital and late recurrent myocardial ischemic events. Am J Cardiol 65:160- 67, 1990.
13. Hendel RC, Layden JJ, Leppo JA. Prognostic value of dipyridamole thallium scintigraphy for evaluation of ischemic heart disease. J Am Coll Cardiol 15:109–16, 1990.
14. Leppo J, Plaja J, Gionet M, Tumolo J, Paraskos JA, Cutler BS. Noninvasive evaluation of cardiac risk before elective vascular surgery. J Am Coll Cardiol 9:269–76, 1987.
15. Midwall J, Ambrose J, Pichard A, Abedin Z, Herman MV. Angina pectoris before and after myocardial infarction. Chest 81:681–86, 1982.
16. Reunanen A, Aromaa A, Pyörälä K, Punsar S, Maatela J, Knekt P. The Social Insurance Institution's coronary heart disease study: Baseline data and five-year mortality experience. Acta Med Scand Suppl 673:67–81, 1983.
17. Kannel WB, Abbott RD. Incidence and prognosis of unrecognized myocardial infarction. An update on the Framingham Study. N Engl J Med 311:1144–47, 1984.
18. Lown B. Sudden cardiac death: The major challenge confronting contemporary cardiology. Am J Cardiol 43:313–28, 1979.
19. Oliver MF. Strategies for preventing and screening for coronary heart disease. Br Heart J 54:1–5, 1985.
20. Uhl GS, Froelicher V. Screening for asymptomatic coronary artery disease. J Am Coll Cardiol 1:946–55, 1983.

21. Houck PD. Epidemiology of total cholesterol to HDL ratio in 11,669 Air Force personnel and coronary artery anatomy in 308 health aviators. J Am Coll Cardiol 11:222A, 1988.

22. Blankenhorn DH, Nessim SA, Johnson RL, Sanmarco ME, Azen SP, Cashin-Hemphill L. Beneficial effects of combined colestipolniacin therapy on coronary atherosclerosis and coronary venous bypass grafts. JAMA 257:3233–40, 1987.

23. Ornish DM, Scherwitz LW, Brown SE, Billings JH, Armstrong WT, Ports TA, McLanahan SM, Kirkeeide RL, Brand RJ, Gould KL. Can lifestyle changes reverse atherosclerosis? Circulation 78:Il-11, 1988.

24. Gould KL, Buchi M, Kirkeeide RL, Ornish D, Stein E, Brand R. Reversal of coronary artery stenosis with cholesterol lowering in man followed by arteriography and positron emission tomography (abstract). J Nucl Med 30:345, 1989.

25. Brown GB, Lin JT, Schaefer SM, Kaplan CA, Dodge HT, Albers JJ. Niacin or Lovastatin, combined with Colestipol regresses coronary atherosclerosis and prevents clinical events in men with elevated apolipoprotein B. Circulation 80:Il-266, 1989.

26. Levy RI, Moskowitz J. Cardiovascular research: Decades of progress, a decade of promise. Science 217:121–29, 1982.

27. Kuller LH, Traven ND, Rutan GH, Perper JA, Ives DG. Marked decline of coronary artery disease mortality in 35–44 year old white men in Allegheny County, Pennsylvania. Circulation 80:261–66, 1989.

Anatomic and Functional Characteristics of Coronary Artery Stenoses

Physiology of Coronary Circulation

The heart pumps blood to the body and to its own vascular bed over a wide range of pressure and work demands. Left ventricular contraction compresses the coronary vascular bed, inhibiting its perfusion. Therefore, pulsatility is necessary to store pressure energy in the compliant aorta and epicardial arteries during systole and to perfuse myocardium during diastole. The anatomy and physiology of the coronary microcirculation, macrocirculation, myocardial metabolism, and coronary endothelial behavior are integrated and adapted for this compression pump, generating the mechanical energy necessary for its own function. These anatomic, metabolic, and physiologic characteristics in turn determine the hemodynamic behavior of coronary artery stenosis in vivo, coronary flow reserve, the kinetics of radiotracers for perfusion and metabolic imaging, measurements of stenosis severity, the technical requirements of quantitative cardiac scanning, clinical manifestations of cardiac disease, and therapeutic interventions. Consequently, a brief review of coronary physiology is appropriate.

MYOCARDIAL METABOLISM AND OXYGEN CONSUMPTION

The primary source of energy for the resting working heart in the fasting state is oxidative metabolism of free fatty acids (FFA), which accounts for 70% to 90% of myocardial energy requirements in the presence of an adequate supply of oxygen (1–8). Free fatty acids are oxidized in the Krebs cycle, accounting for three-fourths of myocardial oxygen requirements of 8–10 cc O_2/min/100 g, with a fasting respiratory quotient of 0.74 (8). The balance of energy is provided by aerobic metabolism of glucose, lactate, and pyruvate. After fasting at rest, about 35% of radiolabeled glucose undergoes aerobic glycolysis by the Emder-Meyerhof pathway to pyruvate and is rapidly oxided, 15% is converted to lactate, and the remaining 50% is converted to myocardial glycogen (7,8). The proportion of glucose converted to glycogen rather than being oxidized may increase to 60% to 70%, particularly during repletion of glycogen stores after ischemia. Glutamate and ketones are also extracted by the heart but do not play a major role in energy balance in the presence of adequate oxygen.

The proportion of FFA, glucose, lactate, and pyruvate taken up by the heart depends on their plasma concentrations, hormonal regulation (particularly insulin as affected by dietary state), work demands, catechols, or disease such as diabetes mellitus. After a carbohydrate meal, increases in blood levels of insulin and glucose work synergistically to increase myocardial glucose uptake and to decrease serum FFA levels by inhibiting whole body lipolysis and myocardial uptake of FFA. After a carbohydrate meal, myocardial uptake of glucose and lactate account for virtually all concurrent oxygen uptake, with a respiratory quotient approaching 1.0. Aerobic metabolism of glucose produces 5.0 Kcal/L of oxygen compared to 4.7 for FFA and is therefore a more efficient fuel (8).

In animals and man there is an inverse relation between myocardial FFA and glucose uptake. Increased lipolysis and elevated FFA due to fasting or insulin antagonists such as catechols, cortisol, and glucagon inhibit myocardial glucose uptake. Decreased lipolysis and lowered FFA due to carbohydrate feeding, insulin, beta blockade, and nicotinic acid increase myocardial glucose uptake. With increased cardiac work in the absence of catechol stimulation (such as atrial pacing) myocardial glucose extraction is also increased. Treadmill exercise with its associated catechol increase is more complex, as discussed below.

With mild to moderate hypoxia or ischemia, myocardial FFA metabolism is suppressed, myocardial glycogen is broken down, and anaerobic glycolysis is stimulated by ischemic activation of phosphofructokinase. With severe ischemia, metabolic end products and intracellular acidosis inhibit glycolysis and glucose uptake.

Based on this metabolic behavior, cardiac PET of positron radiolabeled metabolic analogues are used to identify normal, ischemic, or necrotic myocardium for clinical purposes, as developed in detail in a subsequent chapter. However, some PET data will be presented here to clarify our understanding of myocardial metabolism in humans. The metabolic analog most widely used in clinical PET is F-18-fluoro-2-deoxyglucose (FDG). After intravenous injection, this radionuclide parallels glucose extraction by myocardium, where it is phosphorylated by hexokinase to FDG-6-phosphate. The phosphorylated FDG is trapped in myocardium since it is not metabolized further, dephosphorylated, or transported back out of the cell. FDG uptake on a PET scan therefore reflects the status of myocardial glucose uptake. It does not indicate whether glucose is subsequently converted to glycogen or broken down to pyruvate.

In fasted normals and fasted patients with stable chronic coronary artery disease, myocardial FDG uptake is low at rest, indicating a low level of glucose uptake. With exercise, myocardial perfusion increases except in the distribution of a flow limiting stenosis which becomes ischemic. FDG uptake in these ischemic areas *during* exercise probably follows flow delivery or distribution with greater increase in non-ischemic areas than ischemic areas (8), but due to the relatively low first-pass extraction of FDG this observation may depend on the duration of exercise. In the postexercise period after stress-induced ischemia and restoration of normal homogeneous resting flow, FDG injected intravenously after exercise is taken up intensely in the region that was formerly ischemic during stress; FDG uptake in normal non-ischemic areas during exercise is suppressed due to the combination of fasting and persisting circulating catechols in the absence of elevated work demands of exercise. The increased FDG uptake postexercise by previously ischemic myocardium may reflect either increased glucose metabolism or restoration of glycogen stores depleted by ischemia during exercise. This increased FDG uptake in areas of regional ischemia persists for many hours after the ischemic period during exercise. Postischemic FDG uptake does not imply persisting ischemic inhibition of FFA metabolism, which returns quickly after the ischemic period (5,6) with both glucose and FFA metabolism in postischemic myocardium.

In patients with unstable angina pectoris, FDG uptake is chronically elevated between episodes of clinical ischemia (8), consistent with the observation that conversion to anaerobic glycolysis during ischemia persists as aerobic glycolysis after the ischemia is over, perhaps up to 72 hours. The persistence of increased FDG uptake in areas previously ischemic for time periods longer than required for glycogen repletion suggests that ischemia causes enzyme induction for accelerated glucose uptake. This adaptation serves to maintain an energy source for cardiac work despite intermittent ischemia. It also allows convenient identification of ischemic myocardium during exercise for assessing severity of stenosis metabolically by PET imaging of FDG after exercise in the fasting state.

Myocardial FDG uptake is also used to distinguish between necrotic and underperfused viable myocardium, as described in detail in a subsequent chapter but summarized here to illustrate clinical application of myocardial metabolic behavior. After oral glucose loading at rest, hyperinsulinemia and hyperglycemia increase myocardial FDG uptake in normal or viable ischemic myocardium, but necrotic myocardium fails to take up FDG. Therefore, a defect on an FDG image under resting, glucose-loaded conditions identifies viable myocardium in an underperfused area (7). Under glucose-loaded conditions, maximum FDG uptake is stimulated by mild to moderate ischemia associated with reduction in perfusion down to 40% of normal (7). When perfusion is reduced further to 20% of normal, the more severe ischemia produces metabolic products of necrosis and intracellular acidosis that inhibits anaerobic glycolysis. Myocardium then does not take up FDG, indicating that it is necrotic (5–8).

CORONARY MICROCIRCULATION

Due to its constant workload, resting myocardial oxygen needs are high, 8–10 ml/min/100 g as compared to that for skeletal muscle of 0.15 cc/min/100 g (3,8). Table 1.1 shows the relative requirements for oxygen of the various types of work done by the heart (4). Volume work can be increased without a proportional increase in oxygen consumption. However, increased pressure work, contractility, or heart rate incurs a relatively greater proportional increase in myocardial oxygen consumption than does volume work.

With such high oxygen demands, even at rest, extraction of oxygen by the myocardial bed is high, 75%, as compared to systemic extraction, 25%, shown in Table 1.2 (1,3,9,10). Coronary sinus oxygen content, saturation, and PO2 are therefore much lower than for systemic venous blood even at rest, with relatively little oxygen left for myocardium to extract if work demands increase. Consequently, the coronary circulation meets elevated oxygen demands by increasing coronary blood flow since oxygen extraction cannot increase much further. Thus, there is a close correlation between metabolic demands and coronary blood flow, as shown in Figure 1.1 (11).

The anatomic structure of the coronary microcirculation is optimal for meeting its high oxygen demands, as summarized in Table 1.3 (3,4,12,13). At rest there are approximately 3500 capillaries per square mm of myocardium as compared to 400 capillaries per square mm in skeletal muscle. Approximately 50% to 70% of these myocardial capillaries are open at resting conditions with blood flowing through them. The capillaries throughout the myocardium are intermittently spontaneously closing or opening by contraction or relaxation of precapillary sphincters, with an average of 50% to 70% open in the left ventricle under resting conditions at any given moment. The mechanism and control of the continuously opening and closing of capillaries, called "winking," is unknown. Recruitment of capillaries refers to opening a larger proportion of the capillary bed to blood flow, as occurs with a fall in arterial PO2, ischemia, myocardial hypertrophy, in-

Table 1.1 Myocardial O_2 Consumption

6–8 cc/min/100 gm vs. 0.15 cc/min/100 gm Skeletal muscle	
Basal 20%	Volume work 15%
Electrical 1%	Pressure work 64%

For 50% ↑ in	MVO$_2$ ↑
Wall stress	25%
Contractility	45%
Pressure work	50%
Heart rate	50%
Volume work	4%

Table 1.2 Myocardial O_2 Extraction

	Vol. % Content	$_pO_2$	% Sat
Arteries	20	95	95%
Veins	16	40	40%
Cor. veins	5	20	20%
Myocardial extraction 75% vs. 20% systemically			

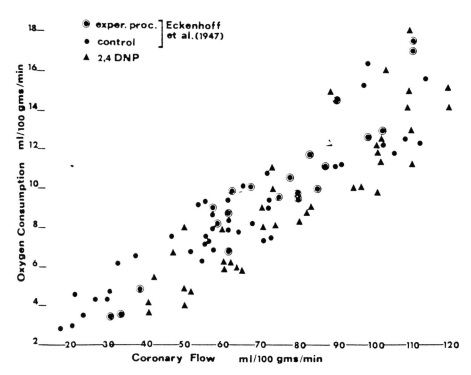

Fig. 1.1 Relation between coronary blood flow and myocardial oxygen consumption in the dog heart. Results from seven dogs. Experimental measurements were obtained when oxygen consumption was changed either by increasing blood volume, hemorrhage, intravenous administration of epinephrine, or intracoronary administration of 2, 4 dinitrophenol. Reproduced with permission from Eckenhoff JE, Hafkenschiel JH, Landmesser CM, 1947. (11).

creased oxygen demands, and pharmacologic coronary vasodilators.

At rest the coronary intercapillary distance averages 17 microns, decreasing to 11–14 microns with recruitment of additional capillaries. The normal myocardial cell diameter is 18 microns, increasing with hypertrophy to 30 microns with a one-to-one ratio of capillaries to myocardial cells. In resting normal skeletal muscle, by comparison, cell diameter is 50 microns, increasing to 90 microns for hypertrophied skeletal muscles. Because of the density of myocardial capillaries, the lower distance between capillaries, and the smaller diameter of myocardial cells, the relative capillary surface area for exchange of oxygen or other substrate in myocardium is 15 times that in skeletal muscle.

FACTORS INFLUENCING CORONARY BLOOD FLOW

The compressive effects and compensatory vascular bed changes during diastole are not uniformly distributed across the left ventricular wall. The subendocardium is affected most by these compressive forces, thereby making its perfusion relatively tenuous. Table 1.4 lists the differences between the subendocardium and subepicardium associated with or due to myocardial compression (3,4,9,14–21). Although resting perfusion is normally the same in the subepicardium and subendocardium, the subendocardium has greater oxygen consumption, lower venous oxygen saturation, lower $NAD:NADH^+$ ratios, lower ATP levels, and higher lactate levels. These differences between the subendocardium and the subepicardium are due to greater wall stress, greater oxygen consumption, and a lower perfusion pressure for the subendocardial myocardium—which, however, normally has a mean flow equal to that of the subepicardium. Consequently, there is a greater proportion of open, recruited capillaries, a lower coronary arteriolar resistance, and a lower coronary flow reserve in the subendocardium as compared to the epicardium. Therefore, the subendocardium is the part of the heart most likely to become underperfused if diastolic duration is short, diastolic perfusion pressure falls, or coronary blood flow is restricted. It is also the most susceptible to

Table 1.3 Myocardial Microcirculation

3,500 capillaries/mm^2 vs. 400/mm^2 skeletal muscle
50–70% Open at rest, ↑ with recruitment
Capillary diameters 4μ diastole, 3μ systole
Intercapillary distance 17μ rest, 11–14μ recruitment
Recruitment-opening of capillary reserves due to ↓pO_2, ischemia, hypertrophy, ↑ O_2 demands vasodilators
Normal heart cell diameter 18μ vs. 50μ skeletal muscle
Hypertrophied myocardial cell 30μ vs. 90μ skeletal muscle
Relative exchange survace 15× skeletal muscle

Table 1.4 Subendocardium vs. Subepicardium

Wall stress ↑	Tissue PO$_2$ ↓
MVO$_2$ ↑	Venous O$_2$ Sat ↓
Mean flow equal	ATP ↓
	Lactate ↑
Perfusion press ↓	Resistance ↓

More capillaries open (recruitment)
Less flow reserve due to used up reserves
Systolic endo flow lower due to compression
Diastolic endo flow higher due to lower resist
Mean endo flow equal epi flow

Table 1.5 Regulation of Coronary Blood Flow

Myocardial compression
Perfusion pressure (A_0 pressure, stenosis)
Metabolism (MVO_2 or O_2 demands)
Neural, parasympathetic and sympathetic
Endothelium

Table 1.7 Cardiovascular Neural Systems

Receptor	Site	Action
β_1	Myocardium	Increased contractility
	SA, AV node	Increased heart rate and conducton
β_2	Coronary arterioles	Vasodilation
	Large coronary arteries	Vasodilation
	Peripheral arterioles	Vasodilation
	Lungs	Bronchodilation
α	Large coronary arteries	Vasoconstriction
	Coronary arterioles	Vasoconstriction
	Peripheral arterioles	Vasoconstriction

inadequate oxygenation, because of its high myocardial oxygen demands.

The regulation of coronary blood flow is multifactorial. Table 1.5 lists the major influences on coronary blood flow. Metabolism and compression have already been mentioned. Other physiologic control systems for coronary flow are now reviewed.

NEURAL REGULATION OF CORONARY BLOOD FLOW

The sensory afferent neural system and mechanisms for perception of myocardial pain are not well defined. Some normal subjects, particularly diabetics, have no cardiac pain and therefore may have a defective anginal warning system (22). Experimentally, mechanical stretch of the myocardium as well as metabolic products of ischemia stimulate afferent sympathetic and/or afferent vagal fibers which participate in a number of complex reflexes involved in the autonomic manifestations of cardiac pain. These include vagal mediated bradycardia, hypotension, sweating, and nausea, or pain-induced, sympathetic-mediated, reflex hypertension (23–28).

The efferent neural system consists of parasympathetic and sympathetic subsystems in opposing balance (29–43). As shown in Table 1.6, the direct primary effect of parasympathetic or vagal stimulation (31–35) is coronary artery vasodilation with increased coronary flow, slowing of the heart rate, and fall in blood pressure. The dominant secondary effect is a decrease in coronary blood flow due to decreased metabolic demands associated with a fall in heart rate and blood pressure. The net result is a fall in coronary blood flow, due to the metabolic-mediated control mechanism overriding the direct neural effects of parasympathetic stimulation. These indirect effects explain the diagnostic and therapeutic test of carotid sinus massage during chest pain. After carotid sinus massage, angina typically disappears in association with slowing of the heart rate. Vagal parasympathetic fibers

also mediate the carotid reflex and the Bezold-Jarisch reflex, both of which are blocked by atropine.

The adrenergic sympathetic system involves beta and alpha receptors as listed in Table 1.7 (29,30,36–43). The $beta_1$ receptor mediates increased myocardial contractility, increased heart rate, and increased conduction of the SA node, AV node, and His-Purkinje system. The $beta_2$ receptor mediates vasodilation of the coronary arterioles, large epicardial coronary arteries, systemic peripheral muscular arteries, and bronchial dilation of bronchial smooth muscle. The alpha receptor mediates vasoconstriction of coronary arterioles, large epicardial coronary arteries, systemic peripheral muscular arteries, and peripheral arterioles, as well.

In experimental animals and man there is a chronic, adrenergic, alpha-mediated coronary constrictor tone which may modify metabolically mediated coronary vasostimuli (37–40). Figure 1.2 demonstrates that alpha blockade results in a higher coronary flow for any given myocardial oxygen demand, due to unopposed $beta_2$ activity causing coronary vasodilation (39). Beta blockade causes coronary and peripheral artery vasoconstriction due to an unbalanced alpha-mediated vasoconstriction. However, as indicated previously, there are secondary metabolic effects that override these direct neural effects, as outlined in Table 6.

Understanding the opposing direct and indirect effects of neural control is important to clinical physiology. For example, the primary neural effect of direct vagal stimulation is to cause coronary vasodilation and an increase in coronary blood flow. However, the heart rate and blood pressure fall associated with vagal stimulation cause decreased metabolic demands and a secondary vasoconstriction in response to diminished oxygen needs. Thus, the net effect of parasym-

Table 1.6 Neural Control Coronary Blood Flow

Parasympathetic	1° Neural	2° Metabolism
Vagal stimulation CSP vagotonic Bezold-Jarish reflex	Vasodilation flow ↑	HR, BP ↓, vasoconstrict, flow ↓
Sympathetic		
Alpha stimulation	Vasoconstriction flow ↓	BP ↑, vasodilation, flow ↑
Beta stimulation	Vasodilation flow ↑ (β_2)	HR, contractility ↑ dilation, flow ↑ (β_1)
Stellectomy relieves chronic alpha constrictor tone		
Metabolism	Overrides neural control but alpha constriction limits vasodilation	

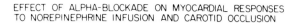

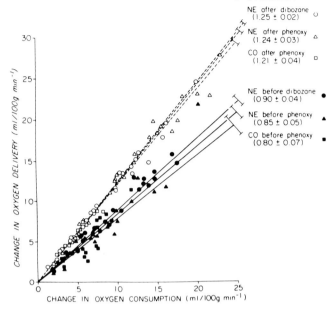

Fig. 1.2 Changes in myocardial oxygen delivery in relation to changes in myocardial oxygen consumption produced by intracoronary norepinephrine infusion (NE) and carotid occlusion (CO) before (solid symbols) and after (open symbols) α-receptor blockade. Lines represent the average response slope (change in oxygen delivery/change in oxygen consumption—not regression lines) for each set of experimental conditions. In all cases, response slopes before alpha-receptor blockade were significantly less than those recorded after alpha-receptor blockade (P < 0.001). For a given increase in oxygen consumption, oxygen delivery increased approximately 30% less before alpha-receptor blockade than after it. The restricted increase in oxygen delivery before alpha-blockade is evident throughout the range of changes in oxygen consumptions investigated. Bars represent ± SE of the mean response slopes (n = 4 for dibozane experiments, n = 8 for phenoxybenzamine experiments). Reproduced with permission from Mohrman DE, Feigel EO, 1978. (39).

pathetic stimulation is a fall in coronary blood flow, due to the overriding effects of lowered metabolism opposite to the primary vasodilatory neural effect.

The primary neural effect of sympathetic alpha stimulation is coronary vasoconstriction with a fall in coronary flow. However, there is a secondary increase in blood pressure and associated metabolic demands after sympathetic stimulation, resulting in metabolically induced coronary vasodilation and an increase in coronary flow. Therefore, the net result of alpha stimulation is a metabolically mediated increase in coronary flow that overrides the direct vasoconstrictive effect. The primary neural effect of sympathetic beta stimulation is coronary vasodilation with an increase in coronary flow mediated by the beta$_2$ receptor. Simultaneously, there is an increase in heart rate and contractility, resulting in increased metabolic demands with coronary vasodilation and increase in coronary flow that is mediated by the beta$_1$ receptor. Therefore, the primary neural and the secondary

metabolic stimuli of beta activation both lead to coronary vasodilation and an increase in coronary flow.

In summary, metabolically mediated control mechanisms override neural control, but neural mechanisms do modify coronary flow response to metabolic needs. There is a chronic alpha constriction that limits coronary vasodilation. Sympathetic stellectomy, particularly on the left side, or alpha blockade relieves the chronic alpha constrictor tone and results in greater coronary flow for any given metabolic stimulus.

CORONARY ENDOTHELIUM

Coronary vascular smooth muscle is strongly modulated by local vasoactive substances secreted by the layer of squamous cells lining arteries and arterioles in direct contact with blood, particularly platelets. Since it interfaces between vascular smooth muscle and blood, the role of endothelium is defined by blood–endothelial interactions that release vasodilator or vasoconstrictor substances, which further inhibit or promote platelet aggregation in a feedback cycle. Although many different vasoactive substances have been identified, the current most important for this brief overview (44–50) include prostacyclin (PGI$_2$), endothelium-derived relaxing factor (EDRF), and endothelial contracting factor (EDCF) or endothelin (50). PGI$_2$ and EDRF are potent coronary vasodilators and synergistically inhibit platelet aggregation. They are produced constantly under normal conditions with synthesis and release, increasing above baseline after a variety of stimuli. Stimuli for endothelial release of EDRF include low oxygen tension, thrombin, prostacyclin, acetylcholine, increased flow velocity or shear forces, and platelet products, particularly serotonin and ADP or ATP.

With intact normal endothelium, baseline production of EDRF and PGI$_2$ in response to one or more of these stimuli inhibits platelet aggregation and maintains normal vasomotor tone by producing a balance of vasocontractor and vasodilator substances, as in Figure 1.3. (46). Increased coronary flow due to metabolic demands is augmented by shear-induced vasodilation, which also regulates flow distribution throughout the coronary vascular tree. Basal EDRF release may be augmented by dietary fish oil or may be impaired by either acute or chronic endothelial injury (46).

With dysfunctional, denuded, or regenerating endothelium, as in Figure 1.4 (46), prostacyclin and EDRF production are impaired, with consequent platelet aggregation and loss of vasodilator balance. Previously listed stimuli causing vasodilation in the presence of normal endothelium may cause vasoconstriction with absent or defective endothelium, and may propagate platelet aggregation. Platelet aggregation releases serotonin and thromboxane A$_2$, which in turn cause more vasoconstriction and more platelet aggregation. Balloon angioplasty denudes endothelium and therefore may cause vasospasm and complete or partial thrombosis (sludging). Hypercholesterolemia reduces production of EDRF, as does localized coronary atheroma, probably explaining clinical coronary artery spasm in the absence of severe stenosis. Impairment of EDRF and prostacyclin production with progressive platelet aggregation and release of serotonin and thromboxane A$_2$ may lead to unstable angina or nontrans-

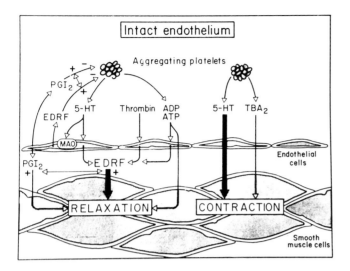

Fig. 1.3 Illustration of current concepts of endothelium-derived factors and their modulation of vascular smooth muscle contraction. Endothelium-derived relaxing factor (EDRF), a powerful vasodilator of the underlying smooth muscle, increases cyclic GMP (cGMP) levels through activation of soluble guanylate cyclase. The chemical nature of EDRF may be simply nitric oxide or a complex containing it. Prostacyclin (PGI$_2$) is another vasodilator released from the endothelium whose effects depend on elevation of cyclic AMP (cAMP) through activation of adenylate cyclase. EDRF and prostacyclin act synergistically to relax vascular smooth muscle and inhibit platelet aggregation. The endothelial cells also secrete a hyperpolarizing factor (EDHF). The exact nature of EDHF is unknown; it most likely is a metabolite of arachidonic acid, presumably an epoxide or lipoxide. At least two endothelium-derived contracting factors exist; one is indomethacin-insensitive (EDCF$_1$), and the other is indomethacin-sensitive (EDCF$_2$). Recent data suggest that EDCF$_1$ may be endothelin, and EDCF$_2$ may be superoxide anions, although this remains to be proved. EDHF has a vasodilator effect and may contribute in part to the initial portion of endothelium-dependent relaxations. Key: ACh, acetylcholine; 5-HT, 5-hydroxytryptamine, serotonin; ADP, adenosine diphosphate; AA, arachidonic acid; +, synergism or facilitation; −, inhibition; ?, exact nature unknown; M, muscarinic receptor; S, serotonergic receptor; P, purinergic receptor; T, thrombin receptor; V, vasopressinergic receptor. Reproduced with permission from Van Houtte PM, Shimokawa H, 1989. (46).

mural or transmural myocardial infarction (47). These unstable syndromes are experimentally prevented by serotonin or thromboxane A$_2$ inhibitors or antagonists (47).

Recurrent endothelial injury with platelet aggregation also releases platelet-derived growth factor (PDGF), causing intimal and smooth muscle cell proliferation (51). The interaction of cholesterol, macrophages, and proliferating smooth muscle cells may convert a fatty streak to the fibrotic-cholesterol laden lesions of atherosclerosis. These fibrous plaques may become fissured or ulcerated in association with loss of endothelial function and acute unstable syndromes or progressive stenosis.

With regression of atherosclerosis, endothelium-dependent coronary vasodilation is restored to some extent (49), despite remaining intimal fibrosis, diffuse narrowing, and re-

stricted flow reserve (52,53). As discussed in detail in a subsequent chapter on reversal of coronary artery stenosis, angina pectoris in patients on reversal protocols decreases markedly within months after therapy, before anatomic improvement of stenosis severity could have occurred. This observation is consistent with that of improved endothelial function accompanying lowered cholesterol and an endothelial-mediated increase in coronary flow.

Thus, in recent years endothelial function has been recognized as a dominant factor in the acute and chronic regulation of coronary blood flow. Pharmacologic or genetic manipulation of endothelial function is feasible with major clinical implications (47).

AUTOREGULATION

Although the various individual factors affecting coronary blood flow have been well described, the integrated mechanisms for the control of coronary flow in vivo are not well understood. The phenomenon of autoregulation, Figure 1.5, (54) is a basic concept in coronary physiology illustrating this point. Perfusion pressure is plotted on the vertical axis with coronary blood flow on the horizontal axis, in an animal preparation in which coronary perfusion was independently controlled. If coronary perfusion pressure is increased with constant workload, coronary blood flow initially increases correspondingly but then regulates back down to near-con-

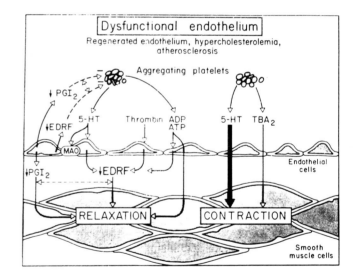

Fig. 1.4 Illustration of endothelium-dependent responses under pathologic conditions. The endothelium is dysfunctional in a regenerated state, in hypercholesterolemia, and in atherosclerosis, releasing less endothelium-derived relaxing factor (EDRF), whereas the ability of the smooth muscle to contract is unaltered. As a result, the contractions predominate. In atherosclerosis, the production of both EDRF and prostacyclin (PGI$_2$) is reduced, and their synergistic actions against aggregating platelets may not occur. Key: 5-HT, 5-hydroxytryptamine, serotonin; ADP, adenosine diphosphate; ATP, adenosine triphosphate; TBA$_2$, thromboxane A$_2$; MAO, monoamine oxidase; −, inhibition; +, synergism. Reproduced with permission from Van Houtte PM, Shimokawa H, 1989. (46).

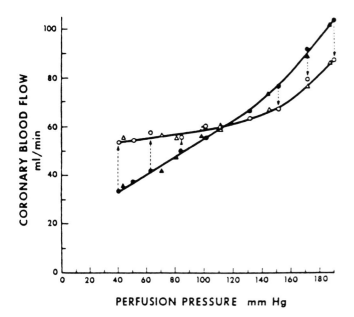

Fig. 1.5 Autoregulation of coronary blood flow in the beating dog heart. The point where the curves cross represents the control steady-state pressure and flow. A sudden, sustained change in perfusion pressure caused an abrupt change in flow represented by the filled symbols (transient flow). The open symbols represent the steady-state flows obtained at each perfusion pressure. The points represented by triangles were obtained after blockade of cardiac prostaglandin synthesis with indomethacin. Reproduced with permission from Rubio K, Berne KM, 1975. (58).

trol levels despite the persisting elevation in perfusion pressure. This adaptive change of flow back toward normal is indicated by the dashed small arrows of Figure 5. Similarly, with a fall in perfusion pressure, coronary blood flow initially falls. However, there is autoregulatory coronary vasodilation with an increase in coronary flow back to the control level, despite the decrease in perfusion pressure. There are limits to altered perfusion pressure beyond which autoregulation fails to maintain flow within the normal range. While the phenomenon of autoregulation is an essential physiologic and clinical observation, the mechanisms which mediate the changes in blood flow are unknown.

REACTIVE HYPEREMIA

A final physiologic observation germane to this chapter is that of reactive hyperemia (55,56), Figure 1.6 (57). Upon release of a temporary coronary artery occlusion of any duration, even fractions of a second, there is an immediate rapid rise in coronary blood flow out of proportion to the oxygen debt incurred during the temporary occlusion. Correspondingly, the volume of blood repaid after the occlusion is typically three to five times the volume deficit during the temporary occlusion. At peak flow during reactive hyperemia, myocardial AV oxygen difference narrows, indicating that the myocardium extracts less oxygen than under control resting flow conditions before reactive hyperemia. Therefore, adequate

oxygen is available to the myocardium but is not extracted during the elevated flow after release of the occlusion.

By contrast, if perfusion is temporarily maintained with deoxygenated blood in lieu of total occlusion of comparable duration, the increase in coronary blood flow following termination of deoxygenated perfusion is just adequate to repay the oxygen debt incurred during the deoxygenated perfusion (57). Thus, some factor other than lack of oxygen during occlusion stimulates coronary flow out of proportion to or unrelated to oxygen needs. Release of the metabolite adenosine, formerly hypothesized to be important in the metabolic regulation of coronary blood flow (58), has now been discounted as a mediator of increased coronary blood flow (59–68) following temporary occlusion, increased metabolic demands, or hypoxia.

One potential explanation for reactive hyperemia is that high shear forces associated with sudden restoration of flow after occlusion may stimulate EDRF release, which causes further vasodilation and prolongation of higher coronary flow than expected on the basis of the oxygen debt of brief occlusion. Other evidence favors oxygen tension as a direct coronary arteriolar vasoregulator either by direct relaxation of vascular smooth muscle (67,68) or as mediated by endothelium.

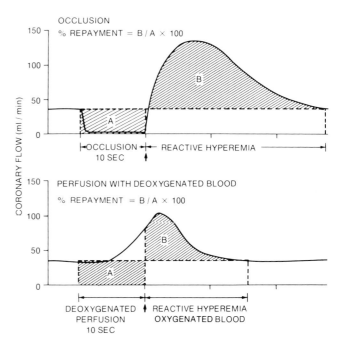

Fig. 1.6 Schematic diagram of data analysis. Mean coronary flow was recorded. Coronary perfusion pressure during deoxygenated perfusion was the same as during the control period. In the top panel, → indicates the release of occlusion, and in the lower panel, → indicates where perfusion with deoxygenated blood was switched back to oxygenated perfusion from the dog. Area B in both panels is hyperemia with oxygenated blood from the dog's subclavian artery. In each case, the volume of oxygenated hyperemia is compared with the preceding volume of flow at control levels during which there was no oxygen available to the myocardium.

The most reasonable synthesis of the many influences on coronary flow is that no single factor or mechanism regulates coronary flow in all or even a specific circumstance, such as metabolic demand or reactive hyperemia. A changing balance of interacting, cumulative, nonlinear control mechanisms appears to regulate coronary flow, including perfusion pressure, systolic compression, neural regulation, metabolic demand, and endothelium.

REFERENCES

1. Burton AC. Physiology and Biophysics of the Circulation. Chicago: Yearbook Medical Pub., 1965, pp. 151.
2. Gibbs CL. Cardiac energetics. Physiologic Reviews 58:174, 1978.
3. Feigl EO. The coronary circulation. Chapter 16 in Physiology and Biophysics II (ed. 20), ed. Ruch TC, Patton HD; Philadelphia, Saunders, 1974, p. 254.
4. Klocke FJ, Mates RE, Copley DP, Orlick AE, et al. Physiology of the coronary circulation in health and coronary disease. Chapter 1 in Progress in Cardiology (ed. 5), ed. Yu PN, Goodwin JF; Philadelphia, Lea & Febiger, 1976.
5. Liedtke AJ. Alterations of carbohydrate and lipid metabolism in the acute ischemic heart. Prog CV Disease 23:321–36, 1981.
6. Liedtke JA, DeMaison L, Eggleston AM, Cohen LM, Nellis SH. Changes in substrate metabolism and effects of excess fatty acids in reperfused myocardium. Circ Res 62:535–42, 1988.
7. Schelbert HR, Buxton D. Insights into coronary artery disease gained from metabolic imaging. Circ 78:496–505, 1988.
8. Camici P, Ferranni E, Opie LH. Myocardial metabolism in ischemic heart disease: Basic principles and application to imaging by positron emission tomography. Prog CV Disease 32:217–38, 1989.
9. Weiss HR, Neubauer JA, Lipp JA, Sinha AK. Quantitative determinations of regional O_2 consumption in the dog heart. Circ Res 42:394–401, 1978.
10. Weiss HR, Sinha AK: Regional O_2 saturation of small arteries and veins in canine myocardium. Circ Res 42:119–261, 1978.
11. Eckenhoff JE, Hafkenschiel JH, Landmesser CM, Harmel M, et al. Cardiac oxygen metabolism and control of the coronary circulation. Am J Physiol 149:634–639, 1947.
12. Henquell L, Honig CR. Intercapillary distance and capillary reserve in right and left ventricles: significance for control of tissue PO_2. Microvascular Res 12:35–41, 1976.
13. Honig CR. Modern Cardiovascular Physiology. Boston: Little, Brown & Co., 1981.
14. Griggs DM, Tchokoev VV, Chien CC. Transmural differences in ventricular substrate levels due to coronary constriction. Am J Physiol 222:705–09, 1972.
15. Kirk ES, Honig CR. Nonuniform distribution of blood flow and gradients of O_2 tension within the heart. Am J Physiol 207:661–68, 1964.
16. Allison TB, Holsinger JW. Transmural metabolic gradients in normal dog LV. effect of pacing. Am J Physiol (Heart, Circ) 233:H217–21, 1977.
17. Hoffman JIE, Buckberg GD. Transmural myocardial perfusion. Chapter 3 in Progress in Cardiology, ed 5, Ed. Yu PN, Goodwin JF, Lea and Febiger, Philadelphia, 1976.
18. Hoffman JIE. Determinants and prediction of transmural myocardial perfusion. Circ 58:381–391, 1978.
19. Hoffman JIE. Transmural myocardial perfusion. Prog CV Dis 29:429–64, 1987.
20. Gertz EW, Wisneski JA, Neese R, Houser A, Korte R, Bristow D. Myocardial lactate extraction: multidetermined metabolic function. Circ 61:256–261, 1980.
21. Apstein CS, Gravindo F, Hood Jr WB, et al. Limitations of lactate production as an index of myocardial ischemia. Circ 60:877–888, 1979.
22. Cohn PF. Silent myocardial ischemia in patients with a defective anginal warning system. Am J Cardiol 226:1094, 1974.
23. Uchida Y, Murao S. Excitation of afferent cardiac sympathetic nerve fibers during coronary occlusion. Am J Physiol 226:1094–1099, 1974.
24. Bishop VS, Peterson DF. The circulatory influences of vagal afferents at rest and during coronary occlusion in conscious dogs. Circ Res 43:840–847, 1978.
25. Malliani A, Recordati G, Schwartz PJ. Nervous activity of afferent cardiac sympathetic fibers with atrial and ventricular endings. J Physiol 229:457–469, 1973.
26. Brown A: Excitation of afferent cardiac sympathetic nerve fibers during myocardial ischemia. J Physiol 190:35, 1967.
27. Peterson DF, Bove AM. Pressor reflexes produced by stimulation of afferent fibers in cardiac sympathetic nerves of the cat. Circ Res 28:605–610, 1971.
28. Lathers CM et al. Role of the adrenergic nervous system in arrhythmia produced by acute coronary occlusion. In Pathophysiology and Therapeutics of Myocardial Ischemia, ed. Lefer AM, Kelliher GJ, Rovetto MJ; New York, Spectrum Publ., 1976.
29. Ross G. Adrenergic responses of the coronary vessels. Circ Res 39:461–65, 1976.
30. Koelle GB: Neurohumoral transmission and the autonomic nervous system. Chapter 21 in The Pharmacologic Basis of Therapeutics (ed. 5), ed Goodman, LS, Gilman, A; New York, Macmillan Publ. Co., 1975.
31. Feigl EO. Carotid sinus reflex control of coronary blood flow. Circ Res 23:223, 1968.
32. Feigl EO. Reflex parasympathetic coronary vasodilation elicited from cardiac receptors in the dog. Circ Res 37:175–82, 1975.
33. Vatner SF, Franklin D, VanCitters RL, Braunwald E. Effects of carotid sinus nerve stimulation on the coronary circulation of the conscious dog. Circ Res 27:11–21, 1970.
34. Young MA, Knight DR, Vatner SF. Autonomic control of large coronary arteries and resistance vessels. Prog CV Dis 30:211–34, 1987.
35. Feigl EO. Reflex parasympathetic coronary vasodilation elicited from cardiac receptors in the dog. Circ Res 37:175–82, 1975.
36. Gross GJ, Feigl EO. Analysis of coronary vascular beta receptors in situ. Am J Physiol 228:1909–1913, 1975.
37. Feigl EO. Control of myocardial oxygen tension by sympathetic coronary vasoconstriction in the dog. Circ Res 37:88–95, 1975.
38. Powell JR, Feigl EO. Carotid sinus reflex coronary vasoconstriction during controlled myocardial oxygen distribution in dog. Circ Res 44:44–51, 1979.
39. Mohrman DE, Feigel EO. Competition between sympathetic vasoconstriction and metabolic vasodilation in the canine coronary circulation. Circ Res 42:79–86, 1978.
40. Swartz PJ, Stone HL. Tonic influence of the sympathetic nervous system on myocardial reactive hyperemia and coronary blood flow distribution in dogs. Circ Res 41:51–58, 1977.
41. Belloni FL. Review: The local control of coronary blood flow. Cardiovasc Res 13:63, 1979.
42. Linden RJ. Reflexes from the heart. Prog CV Disease 18:201, 1975.
43. Vatner SF et al. Coronary dynamics in unrestrained conscious baboons. Am J Physiol 221:1396, 1971.
44. Furchgott RF. Role of endothelium in responses of vascular smooth muscle. Circ Res 53:557–73, 1983.
45. Bassenge E, Busse R. Endothelial modulation of coronary tone. Prog CV Disease 30:349–80, 1988.
46. Van Houtte PM, Shimokawa H. Endothelium derived relaxing factor and coronary vasospasm. Circulation 80:1–9, 1989.
47. Willerson JT, Golino P, Eidt J, Campbell WB, Buja LM. Specific platelet mediators and unstable coronary artery lesions. Circulation 80:198–205, 1989.
48. Freiman PC, Mitchell GG, Heistad DD, Armstrong ML, Harrison DG. Atherosclerosis impairs endothelium dependent vascular relaxation to acetylcholine and thrombin in primates. Circ Res 58:783–89, 1986.
49. Harrison DG, Armstrong ML, Freiman PL, Heistad DD. Restoration of endothelium-dependent relaxation by dietary treatment of atherosclerosis. J Clin Invest 80:1808–11, 1987.
50. Yanagisawa M, Kurihara H, Kimura S, Tomobe Y, Kobayashi M,

Mitsui Y, Yazaki Y, Goto K, Masaki T. A novel potent vasoconstrictor peptide produced by vascular endothelial cells. Nature 332:411–15, 1988.

51. Ross R. The pathogenesis of atherosclerosis—An update. N Eng J Med 314:488–500, 1986.

52. Armstrong ML, Heistad DD, Marcus ML, Piegors DJ, Abboud FM. Hemodynamic sequelae of regression in experimental atherosclerosis. J Clin Invest 71:104–14, 1983.

53. Small DM. Progression and regression of atherosclerotic lesions. Arteriosclerosis 8:103–29, 1988.

54. Mosher P, Ross J, McFate P, Shaw RF. Control of coronary blood flow by an autoregulatory mechanism. Circ Res 14:250–58, 1964.

55. Eikens E, Wilchem DE. Reactive hyperemia in the dog heart. Circ Res 35:702–11, 1974.

56. Schwartz GG, McHale PA, Greenfield JC. Hyperemic response of the coronary circulation to brief diastolic occlusion in the conscious dog. Circ Res 50:28–37, 1982.

57. Kelley KO, Gould KL. Coronary reactive hyperemia after brief occlusion and after deoxygenated perfusion. Cardiov Res 15:615–22, 1981.

58. Rubio K, Berne KM. Regulation of coronary blood flow. Prog CV Disease 18:105–21, 1975.

59. Dole WP, Montville WJ, Bishop VS. Dependency of myocardial reactive hyperemia on coronary artery pressure in the dog. Am J Physiol H709–15, 1981.

60. Gewirtz H, Brautigan DL, Olsson R, Brown P, Most AS. Role of adenosine in the maintenance of coronary vasodilation distal to a severe coronary artery stenosis. Circ Res 53:42–51, 1983.

61. Downing SE, Chen V. Dissociation of adenosine from metabolic regulation of coronary flow in the lamb. Am J Physiol 251:H40–46, 1986.

62. Gewirtz H, Olsson RA, Most AS. Role of adenosine in mediating the coronary vasodilative response to acute hypoxia. Cardiov Res 21:81–89, 1987.

63. Dole WP, Yamada N, Bishop VS, Olsson RA. Role of adenosine in coronary blood flow regulation after reductions in perfusion pressure. Circ Res 56:517–24, 1985.

64. Hanley FL, Grattan MT, Stevens MB, Hoffman JIE. Role of adenosine in coronary autoregulation. Am J Physiol 250:H558–66, 1986.

65. Edlund A, Sollevi A, Wennmalm A. The role of adenosine and prostacyclin in coronary flow regulation in healthy man. Acta Physiol Scand 135:39–46, 1989.

66. Decking VKM, Juengling E, Kammermeier H. Interstitial transudate concentration of adenosine and inosine in rat and guinea pig hearts. Am J Physiol 23:H1125–32, 1988.

67. Dole WP, Nuno DW: Myocardial oxygen tension determines the degree and pressure range of coronary autoregulation. Circ Res 59:202–15, 1986.

68. Downey HF, Crystal GJ, Bockman EL, Bashour FA. Nonischemic myocardial hypoxia: coronary dilation without increased tissue adenosine. Am J Physiol 243:H512–16, 1982.

2

Methods for Pressure-Flow Analysis and Arteriography

The fluid dynamic characteristics of stenoses have been extensively examined by in vitro models (1–10). The effects of narrowing on flow in peripheral arteries (1,3,5) and in the coronary arteries have been studied in anesthetized animals and in awake animals by flowmeters and microsphere techniques. However, experimental techniques described here were the first reported (11–17) for performing coronary arteriography and for determining the pressure flow characteristics of controlled, variable coronary stenoses in intact, unanesthetized, chronically instrumented animals. This chapter describes the surgical methods and instrument manufacture for studying coronary artery stenoses in intact animals without the disturbing effects of anesthesia and thoracotomy (18–21).

SURGICAL CHRONIC INSTRUMENTATION

Labrador or field hounds, which weigh 28 to 35 kg, are the optimal size for coronary instrumentation. The animals were treated preoperatively with dipyridamole, 100 mg, and with aspirin, 600 mg, given orally daily for two days before surgery and with 1 g sodium methicillin given intravenously 1 h before anesthesia with 400 to 600 mg sodium thiopental intravenously. Respirations were controlled through a cuffed endotracheal tube with a Harvard volume respirator or with a Metamatic veterinary anesthesia-respirator (Ohio Medical Products). Anesthesia was maintained with methoxyflurane anesthetic gas delivered through a calibrated vaporizing bottle in line with the respirator. Expiratory volume was monitored with a Drager volumeter and vented to wall suction. Supplemental oxygen, 2 L/min, was delivered with anesthetic gas. Under sterile conditions, a left thoracotomy was made, and the left circumflex coronary artery was dissected free. A snugly fitting Doppler flow transducer was placed around the proximal circumflex coronary artery so that the piezoelectric ceramic chips faced upstream. A saline-filled, circumferential balloon constrictor was tied into place 2 to 3 mm distally. A small, tapered polyvinylchloride catheter described subsequently was inserted into the lumen of the distal main circumflex coronary artery and was sutured into place with 6-0 silk passed through a cuff on the catheter. Similar catheters were implanted into the proximal circumflex artery, aortic root, left atrium, and pulmonary artery and sutured to the epicardium and chest wall.

PROXIMAL CORONARY CATHETER IMPLANTATION

The catheter for injecting contrast medium into the proximal circumflex for arteriography was implanted differently after manufacture, as follows. A 10-cm section of the small Tygon tubing 0.025 inch ID × 0.04 inch OD, described subsequently, was heated in oil and drawn to a fine diameter, frozen on dry ice, cut with bevel, and inserted through a disposable 21-gauge needle, 1.5 cm long, with hub cut off. The tubing was then pulled through the needle until the larger part of the drawn tubing jammed into the proximal cut-off end of the needle. Excess tubing at the point of the needle was cut off, and the needle was bent into a curve. The opposite end of this section of tubing was then cut to 5 cm and welded with cyclohexanone to a 60-cm section of larger Tygon tubing, 0.04 inch, described subsequently. A Tygon cuff was attached for securing to the arterial wall. At insertion, the curved needle was passed into and out of the proximal circumflex artery at its origin, as described by Herd and Barger (19). The distal end of this catheter was pulled until the cuff abutted the arterial adventitia and was then cut off 3–4 mm beyond the cuff; since it was cut under tension, the cut end recoiled back into the coronary artery. This catheter was then 2–3 mm long in the artery and at least 5–8 mm proximal to the flow probe. For the proximal catheter, this technique was used because the pulmonary artery interferes with the straight-needle technique used on the distal circumflex artery as described below.

DISTAL CORONARY CATHETER IMPLANTATION

Catheters for distal coronary implantation were made of Tygon microbore tubing, custom-ordered to 0.025 inch ID × 0.04 inch OD (formulation S-54-HL for medical use, Norton Plastics Co.). Tubing was dipped in oil heated to 140°C, drawn to a taper, cooled on dry ice and cut to fit snugly over a 25-gauge needle. A 2- to 3-cm section of this small tapered tubing was welded with cyclohexanone to a 25-inch section of larger tubing, 0.04 inch ID × 0.15 inch OD. A 4-inch, 25-gauge needle was inserted through the tubings until the tip projected 1 mm beyond the tip of the tapered small catheter. A slanted, 1-mm-long Tygon cuff was welded onto the small tubing 3 mm from the tapered end for coronary catheters. For aortic, left atrial, and pulmonary artery catheters this cuff was 1.5 cm from the tip. The tip was further smoothed by inserting a 25-gauge rod into the tubing for support, freezing the tip of the catheter in liquid nitrogen, and sanding the cut-off end of the tapered section.

At insertion, the needle and catheter were thrust through the arterial wall with a twisting motion up to the cuff and secured to the adventitia of the artery with a 6-0 silk suture previously passed through the Tygon cuff. The needle was then withdrawn, and the tubing was flushed with saline, clamped with a rubber-shod hemostat, wiped dry with a gauze sponge and welded with cyclohexanone to a 60 cm section of the larger tubing for exiting from the chest. After 1 min drying time, this joint was strong enough to withstand aortic pressure. Blood was then aspirated to remove any residual cyclohexanone, and the catheter was flushed and filled with heparin. There was no bleeding site with this technique, since there was no arteriotomy nor exit hole in the artery.

Catheters were flushed daily, filled with heparin, and stoppered with obturators made from 19-gauge needles cut off at the tip and filled with Silastic. A more recent improvement is to weld a teflon tip cut from a standard 22-gauge Gelco

intravenous catheter to the Tygon tubing. The proximal end of the teflon tip is etched with Chemgrip etch (Norton Plastics, L93-3M686R), inserted into the PVC tubing, and bonded with Duro superglue. The teflon tip slides through the arterial wall around the needle more easily than the sanded Tygon. However, the Tygon tip may either clot off or malfunction more often than the PVC tip.

All catheters and wires were sutured to the epicardium and to the chest wall; they were tunneled under the skin with a bronchoscopy forceps and exited individually 2 cm apart through 2-mm stab wounds in the skin over the back. The intercostal muscle layer was closed with interrupted, everting, mattress Dexon sutures with careful control of bleeding, particularly due to the effects of dipyridamole and aspirin. Closure was completed with two more deep layers of continuous Dexon suture, one subcutaneous, and a buried cutaneous Dexon suture.

The technique of implanting arterial catheters described by Herd and Barger (19) has been extremely useful for physiological studies of the coronary arteries in awake, unsedated animals. It is particularly applicable for measuring pressure in coronary arteries distal to a constrictor. A disadvantage of the technique is the exit site where a curved needle and attached tubing have been passed into and out of the arterial lumen. After the implanted tubing is cut at the exit site, a bleeding point is left which frequently must be repaired. The straight needle method described here avoids this problem, since there is no exit hole in the artery. The exit site repair is easily accomplished on the proximal left circumflex, but it is difficult for the distal left circumflex artery, owing to limited surgical exposure. For the distal left circumflex catheter the straight needle technique is more appropriate, whereas for the proximal left circumflex catheter the Herd–Barger method is better.

Figure 2.1 shows the surgical exposure and placement of the Doppler transducer, constrictor, and catheters (14). In large dogs with a sufficiently long left circumflex coronary artery, a proximal coronary catheter was implanted instead of the aortic catheter shown in Figure 2.1 (14).

POSTOPERATIVE COURSE

Postoperatively, blood gases, electrolytes, hematocrit, and the electrocardiogram were monitored daily for one week. In many dogs, a stable, unifocal, ventricular tachycardia at rates of 100–150 beats/min appeared on the second or third postoperative day with no evidence of myocardial injury observed by electrocardiogram or at subsequent postmortem examinations after experiments were completed. This ventricular tachycardia usually responded to one dose of intravenous or intramuscular diphenylhydantoin, 500 mg, and phenobarbital, 130 mg (22), without recurrence, although occasionally a second dose on the following day was necessary. Procainamide, quinidine, propranolol, and lidocaine were less effective in treating the postoperative ventricular tachycardia of these dogs. Dipyridamole and aspirin were continued in preoperative doses for 10 days after surgery to prevent formation of platelet clots on the catheters in the postoperative period. After 10 days, these drugs were discontinued without ill effects or malfunction of the catheters.

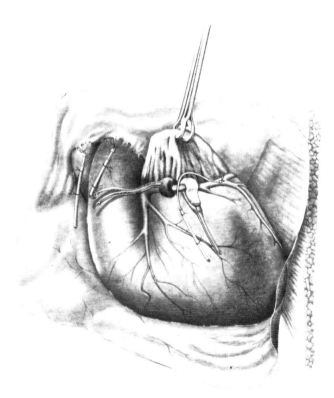

Fig. 2.1 Surgical preparation as viewed through a left thoracotomy with Doppler transducer proximally, constrictor, and catheters. Reproduced with permission from Gould KL, Lee D, Lovgren K, 1978. (14).

Mortality within the first 14 days of surgery averaged 15% from technical surgical problems usually associated with small coronary arteries of 1.5–2.0 mm in diameter that are too small for the coronary catheters. Postoperatively, these small coronary arteries may occlude at the site of catheter insertion. This problem can be avoided by selecting dogs weighing 28 kg or more. Pneumothorax and empyema are problems that can be avoided by meticulous sterile surgical technique.

Within two weeks of surgery, dogs were active, eating, and trained to lie on an angiography table for up to 2 h. The animals demonstrated considerable variability in basal levels of coronary flow in response to external stimuli such as sudden noises, being petted, tail wagging, or strangers in the room. Average resting coronary flow velocity was 23 ± 8 cm/s under standard conditions after 10 min of quiet rest in a darkened room.

The average life span of the surgical survivors was 68.9 ± 39.7 days, with an average of 58.4 ± 36.6 days per dog for data gathering in which all implanted devices functioned properly. Of the surgical survivors, 50% eventually died or were sacrificed at one to three months after surgery because of instrument or catheter malfunction, 20% died of late ventricular tachycardia and fibrillation, 20% died of hemorrhage at the site where the aortic catheter pulled out, and the balance died of miscellaneous causes. The cumulative functioning life span of Doppler transducers implanted (and reimplanted) in dogs averaged 112 ± 56 days per transducer with a range of 50–214 days.

ACUTE EXPERIMENTS

For acute open-chest experiments in anesthetized dogs, an appropriately sized, perivascular electromagnetic flow transducer (Zepeda) was implanted. A variable snare-type occluder was placed distal to the flow transducer. It consisted of a 2–3-mm wide band of umbilical tape passed around the artery, through a stiff tubing, and attached to a machinist's micrometer. The snare could be closed by small, precise amounts according to the 0.01 mm micrometer scale. Approximately 1 cm distal to the constrictor, a small (1 mm OD by 1.5 inches long), teflon, end-hole catheter (Bardic 1968-T) was inserted 2 mm into the coronary lumen and sutured to adventia. This catheter in the circumflex coronary artery was used for injecting vasodilators distally into the coronary artery and for recording coronary pressure distal to the constrictor. Alternately, in acute open-chest preparations, just distal to the flow transducer a concentric coronary stenosis was produced by constricting the artery with 0.5-cm-long drilled plastic half blocks of varying internal diameters. A steel ball, 3.18 mm in diameter, was sutured to the epicardium just adjacent to the stenosis as a size reference.

CORONARY ARTERIOGRAPHY

Coronary arteriograms were obtained by injecting radiopaque contrast medium (Renografin-76) into the proximal coronary catheter while triggering exposure of a single-spot film from the ECG at mid-diastole or by cine angiography. The cut film

injection/x-ray sequence was automated and precisely controlled using a timing circuit triggered by the R wave from the ECG. The contrast medium was injected using a thermodilution injector (OMP Lab, Inc.) modified to inject from an energized solenoid, triggered from the ECG. The injector was powered with compressed air regulated to inject the contrast medium through the catheter at a flow rate not exceeding the dog's coronary arterial flow.

With this system, less than 2 mL of contrast medium produced adequate filling for visualization of the stenotic region as well as proximal and distal normal sections of the circumflex artery. A Viamonte Hobbs programmable power injector triggered off the ECG was also used for later studies. The x-rays were taken with a General Electric Maxiray 100 tube with a 0.3-mm focal spot, a $6\frac{1}{2}$ degree target angle and a 26-inch tube-to-film distance. Exposures were at $\frac{1}{60}$ or $\frac{1}{30}$ s, 200 mA, at 90–116 kV using Ultra Detail, Cronex 4, DuPont 3 x-ray film and either Ultra Detail phosphor Radelain cassettes or Kodak X-Omatic cassettes with regular intensifying screens. The cut film system had a resolution of 11 line pairs/mm or 215 line pairs/inch, compared to 2–3 line pairs/mm for cine film. Quantitative analysis of coronary arteriograms is described in a subsequent chapter.

ECG standard lead II, mean and instantaneous phasic flow, proximal and distal coronary pressure, and differential coronary pressure were recorded on an Electronics for Medicine DR 12 with a direct writer and on a Honeywell 7600 tape recorder for analog-to-digital computer conversion and subsequent analysis.

EXPERIMENTAL PROCEDURE

Dogs were trained to lie quietly on a table for up to 2 h, and experiments were begun two weeks postoperatively when resting heart rates had fallen to 60–80 beats/min and resting aortic pressure was 65–85 mm Hg. The dogs were positioned on their right side for biplane x-rays. Some of the dogs were lightly sedated with xylazine (1 mg/kg i.m.) to facilitate a stable position during the x-rays. During a 5-min rest period, initial flow and pressure calibrations were made and baseline control recordings made of the ECG, phasic coronary flow or flow velocity, aortic, coronary, and differential pressures between the distal coronary and proximal or aortic catheters. The coronary flow response was recorded after a 10-s occlusion or after a dose of 0.4–0.8 mL papaverine in a concentration of 2.0 mg/mL in saline injected through the coronary catheter. The coronary constrictor was then inflated with saline under pressures of up to 1,000 mm Hg (20 lb/inch²), depending on the severity of stenosis desired. The expansion pressure was held constant at the chosen level by a water-sealed ball valve in line with an automatic pressure regulator attached to a compressed air source.

The stenosis was allowed to stabilize for 20–30 min. Four sets of data were obtained to characterize the pressure-flow relation of each stenosis.

CORONARY ARTERIOGRAMS AT REST

Orthogonal biplane arteriograms were taken during baseline flow conditions in the left anterior oblique and left posterior oblique view. Alternatively, when only a single plane system was available, the two separate orthogonal arteriograms were taken sequentially, separated by at least 3 min, such that flow and heart rate had returned to baseline values before the second arteriogram was taken. In preliminary studies, repeated arteriograms in the same plane demonstrated return of all dimensions to control baseline at 3 min.

MEASURED PRESSURE-FLOW DATA AT REST

The pressure and flow velocity transducers were recalibrated and baseline control recordings were made of the ECG, coronary flow velocity, and proximal, distal, and differential coronary pressures.

MEASURED PRESSURE-FLOW DATA AT VASODILATION

A dose of 0.4–0.8 mL of papaverine in a concentration of 2.0 mg/mL was injected as a bolus through the distal coronary catheter to produce a transient increase in flow while phasic pressures and flow velocity were recorded. Transducer calibrations were verified at the end of data collection.

CORONARY ARTERIOGRAMS AT VASODILATION

The same dose of papaverine was injected again and arteriograms were taken at 10 s and 60 s after the injection. The dog was repositioned for the opposing orthogonal view and the same hyperemia arteriogram sequence was repeated. Arteriograms were developed with the stenosis still in place and were repeated if cut films were of poor quality. The entire experiment lasted 1 h. Data were obtained over a wide range of coronary constrictions for each dog during repeated studies over four to six weeks.

PRESSURE AND PRESSURE GRADIENT MEASUREMENTS

Arterial pressures were measured with BioTec BT-70 or Ailtech MS-10 external pressure transducers. Differential pressure between aortic or proximal coronary artery pressure and coronary pressure distal to the stenosis was measured with a differential pressure transducer (LX1701D, National Semiconductor Corp., Santa Clara, Calif.), mounted in a plastic manifold to which the standard non-differential external pressure transducers were also attached. Needle obturators, stopcocks, and plastic parts were all filled by immersion under sterile saline in a vacuum changer, which was then evacuated under high vacuum to remove minute air bubbles and maximize frequency response. Sterile saline debubbled in the vacuum chamber was used for flushing connections between catheters and pressure gauges. For each experiment, pressure calibrations were recorded with 100 mm Hg pressure applied to the aortic, coronary, and differential transducers at the beginning, middle, and end of each study.

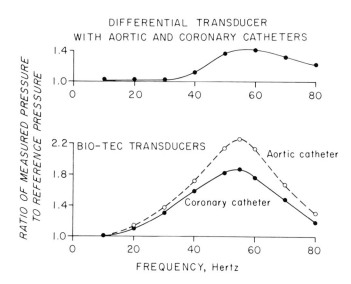

Fig. 2.2 Frequency responses of catheter-manometer systems used to record aortic pressure, coronary pressures, and differential pressure or gradient across the stenosis. Frequency of input sine wave pressure is on horizontal axis. In upper panel, vertical axis shows response of differential pressure transducer to a sine wave pressure applied simultaneously to the two catheters used to record pressure proximal and distal to the stenosis. In lower panel, vertical axis shows the ratio of measured pressure to reference pressure for the Bio Tec pressure transducer on a catheter. Reproduced with permission from Gould KL, Lee D, Lovgren K, 1978. (14).

The pressure and differential pressures recording systems were tested for frequency response with a sine wave pressure generator. Sine wave pressure of 20 mm Hg amplitude applied simultaneously to two coronary catheters (or one coronary and one aortic catheter) attached to the differential gauge produced no resonant differential pressure (± 5% of reference input pressures) until 30 Hz, shown in the upper panel of Figure 2.2 (14). At higher frequencies the slightly different hydraulic characteristics of the two catheters caused resonance that was recorded as an undamped pressure differential. The Bio Tec single, external transducer-catheter system was flat (±5%) to 15 Hz and had natural resonant frequencies of 55 Hz, shown in the lower panel of Figure 2.2. Catheters filled with contrast medium were critically damped with no distinct resonant frequency and were flat (±5%) to 15–20 Hz. The frequency responses in Figure 2.2 were from the catheters used for chronic implantation (14). An analysis of pressure recording and frequency response is detailed at the end of this chapter as background for understanding these high-fidelity pressure recordings essential for studying the pressure-flow characteristics of stenoses.

CORONARY CONSTRICTORS

Coronary constrictors were made by wrapping a 2.5-cm section of Silastic tubing (0.058 × 0.077 inch) around a 4-mm diameter steel rod and bonding a stiff radiolucent backing (strips of x-ray film) over the tubing with self-leveling Silastic RTV734. Dow Corning Primer 1200 was used on the strips to bond the Silastic to them. After curing, the tubing with backing was peeled off the steel rod. One end of the tubing was sealed with RTV and the other end bonded to a 50-cm-long, thick-walled, Silastic actuator tubing (OD, 0.095 inches; ID, 0.030 inches) for exiting from the chest. The constrictor was evacuated under high vacuum and filled with debubbled saline before each experiment. To produce coronary stenoses, the constrictor was inflated with saline under pressures up to 1,000 mm Hg (20 lb/inch^2) depending on the severity of stenosis desired. The expansion pressure was held constant at the chosen level by a water-sealed ball valve in line with a sensitive automatic pressure regulator attached to a compressed air source.

Silastic rubber is sufficiently porous that air, saline, and oil leak or "sweat" through the rubber out of the system, thereby reducing the severity of the stenosis if the cuff is inflated once and the actuator tubing clamped. For example, a cuff inflated with air once and clamped will leak enough air through the rubber to lose the stenosis in 15–60 min, depending on the thickness of the rubber, size of the occluder, and initial inflation pressure. Inflation with water slows this rate of cuff deflation and prolongs the loss of constriction to several hours, again depending on the mechanical characteristics of the cuff. Mercury, also a satisfactory inflation medium, is not radiolucent and therefore prevents coronary arteriography. Oil is unsatisfactory because it "sweats" through the porous walls of the actuator tubing and constrictor cuff into surrounding tissue. Thus, saline is the most useful inflation liquid, but it requires constant inflation pressure.

Although constant inflation pressure produced constant cuff inflation, it did not produce stable coronary stenoses in vivo after initial constrictor inflation. During the first 30 min after inflation of the constrictor in chronically instrumented animals, the stenosis tended to become less severe despite constant inflation pressure. This early stenosis drift was most likely due to squeezing fluid out of the tissue that grew between the arterial wall and the constrictor. After 30–60 min of adjustment, the stenosis remained stable at whatever severity was selected. The initial drift in the stenosis severity despite constant inflation pressure could be marked. Application of a new, more severe stenosis during an experiment required a repeated, although abbreviated, drift period. After the two-week postoperative recovery period, a stenosis of any selected severity could be approximately reproduced by selecting the same inflation pressure after the 30-min period of stenosis drift.

DOPPLER MANUFACTURE FLOW VELOCITY TRANSDUCER

Doppler flow velocity transducers were made from 3.5 mm × 4.5 LTZ-2 lead titanate-zirconate piezoceramic soldered to stainless steel coaxial cable (9AS633-ISS, 38AWG, Cooner Sales Co.) and mounted with epoxy in previously cast epoxy half-rings with air backing. Two half-rings were cemented together, and a slit was cut for insertion onto the artery. The piezoceramic chips made a 45-degree angle to the direction of flow. The transducer was then coated with parylene C by

vapor phase deposition (Nova Tran Corp.) in order to insulate the piezoceramic, wire, and epoxy against body fluids. The parylene-coated wire and wire-epoxy junction was pulled through Silastic tubing, which was then filled with RTV734 Silastic as a protective coating against mechanical abrasion. A finished transducer had external dimensions of 6 × 6 × 6 mm and an internal diameter of 3.8 mm, and weighed 0.6 g.

A continuous wave-directional Doppler (L and M Electronics, Daly City, Calif.) was used with these transducers to measure instantaneous mean cross-sectional flow velocity. Each transducer was calibrated on shrink tubing (OD, 3.54 mm; ID, 3.0 mm) immersed in a water bath at 37°C, through which dog blood flowed under constant pressure. Volume flow, F, was measured with a graduated cylinder and stopwatch. Mean cross-sectional velocity, V, was calculated from the equation V = F/A, where A is the cross-sectional area of the lumen of the shrink tubing. The voltage output of the Doppler was measured with a digital voltmeter for at least 15 points over a range of flow from 0 to 156 cm/s, and the calibration factor was calculated as cm/s per volt output.

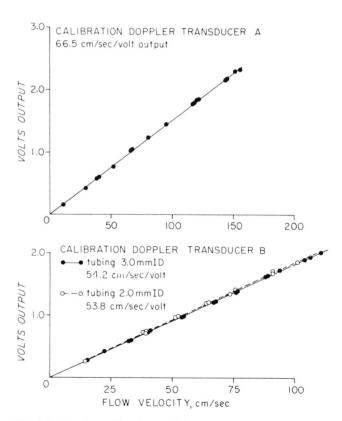

Fig. 2.3 Doppler calibration and flow response. Flow velocity through the transducer is plotted on the horizontal axis, and the corresponding voltage output response of the Doppler is plotted on the vertical axis (upper panel). Calibration of a Doppler transducer on a 3-mm ID tubing (solid line, lower panel) was the same as on a 2-mm ID tubing (dashed line, lower panel). Velocity calibrations were therefore independent of vessel size. Flow velocity scale of lower panel is expanded to demonstrate two separate calibration lines. Reproduced with permission from Gould KL, Lee D, Lovgren K, 1978. (14).

The L and M Doppler with these transducers is linear from zero velocity to the maximum measured velocity of 156 cm/s (600 mL/min through a 3-mm ID tube), with maximum Doppler shifts up to 12 kilocycles. The calibration factor, expressed in cm/s per volt output of the Doppler, was constant over this range, and for any given transducer was the same for a 3.8-mm ID transducer on large tubing (OD, 3.54 mm; ID, 3 mm) as on small tubing (OD, 2.4 mm; ID, 2 mm). Figure 2.3 shows a typical calibration and response of a Doppler flow velocity transducer (14). As shown in the upper panel of Figure 2.3, the Doppler system was linear to two or three times the maximum flow velocity recorded during reactive hyperemia (14). These in-vitro calibration factors were the same as those obtained by postmortem blood perfusion of the circumflex coronary artery with the Doppler transducer encased around it.

For experiments the Doppler was operated at 8–9 MHz and was tuned to maximum signal-to-noise ratio in vivo and in vitro. Signal-to-noise ratios of 50:1 to 100:1 were obtained by measuring the audio output of the Doppler on an RMS (root-mean-square) voltmeter during flow (at 7.5 kilocycle shift) and with no flow. At peak flow, during both in-vivo and in-vitro calibrations, signal voltage at the audio output of the L and M Doppler was typically 3–4 V; electronic "noise" with no flow, or during complete occlusion of the artery, was 0.03–0.04 V, and threshold voltage of the frequency detector was 0.1 V. Each transducer was tuned by varying the driving frequency to the transmitting piezoelectric crystal until maximum signal-to-noise ratios were obtained.

Doppler instruments typically have stable baseline, and occlusive zero equals electronic zero baseline (23). On the other hand, for physiological studies requiring volume flow, Doppler velocity measurements must be multiplied by the cross-sectional area of the artery in order to obtain volume flow in mL/min. Determination of the arterial cross-sectional area in this model required arteriography.

DATA ANALYSIS

Data were processed either manually or automatically as follows. Phasic recordings of differential pressure and flow velocity obtained at 100 mm/s paper speed on photographic paper were manually traced on a Grafpen GP-2 ultrasonic digitizing tablet or automatically digitized from ECG, pressure, pressure gradient, and flow velocity from a Honeywell model 7600 half-inch magnetic tape recorder. With an appropriately designed electronic interface, cardiac cycles could be selected from the tape storage and fed through analog-to-digital converters into a PDP-8E computer or later to a VAX 11/780 computer for automatic digitizing.

For each stenosis, the relation of instantaneous differential pressure to instantaneous flow velocity was determined for each of four to six heart cycles for flow levels ranging from resting control to peak flow during pharmacologic vasodilation. Analog voltage recordings of phasic flow velocity and phasic differential pressure (stenosis pressure gradient) from the diastolic portion of the selected cardiac cycles were converted to digital signals at 100 samples/s with the PDP-8E computer. Data were processed by a digital filter equivalent to a low-pass filter flat to 15 Hz and with linear rolloff from 15 to 30 Hz (− 40 db down at 30 Hz with no phase shift).

During each cardiac cycle, the pressure gradient and flow velocity were correlated by a quadratic equation that has the general form $\Delta P = FV + SV^2$, where ΔP = pressure loss (mm Hg), V = coronary flow velocity (cm/s), F = the coefficient of pressure loss due to viscous friction, and S = the coefficient of pressure loss due to flow separation or localized turbulence downstream from the stenosis (15–17) as discussed in a subsequent chapter. For single heart cycles, we determined the constants F and S, which best fit this general equation to the experimental data by computer, using a general-purpose, curve-fitting algorithm previously described (15–17). The computer output consisted of the coefficients F and S, the mean velocity, the average velocity, and the mean and phasic differential pressure for each heart cycle, as well as a graph of the experimental values for the differential pressure versus flow velocity and the calculated best-fit curve for each heart cycle.

The quadratic relations between ΔP and V for several single cardiac cycles at different flows for each stenosis were used to establish a composite relation for ΔP and V over the entire range of flows for that stenosis. Five beats were selected, one at rest and four over a range of increased flow during vasodilation. Flow velocity was then converted to volume flow by multiplying flow velocity by the cross-sectional area of the vessel at the site of the Doppler flow probe. This cross-sectional area was determined from orthogonal arteriograms taken in each experiment. The cross-sectional area of the artery at the site of the velocity transducer from the rest x-ray was multiplied three times flow velocity data for the rest heart cycle and the cross-sectional area of the artery at the velocity transducer from the vasodilated x-ray was mul-

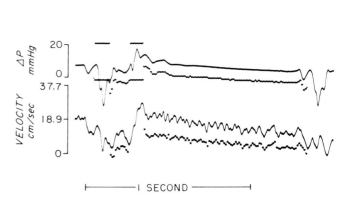

Fig. 2.4 Coronary flow velocity and pressure gradient across a stenosis, as originally recorded on photographic paper (solid continuous line) and by computer reconstruction (digital or stepped line). Vertical scales apply to original recordings only. Computer-reconstructed tracings are displaced downward so that they will not overlay the original recordings in the illustration. Reproduced with permission from Gould KL, Lee D, Lovgren K, 1978. (14).

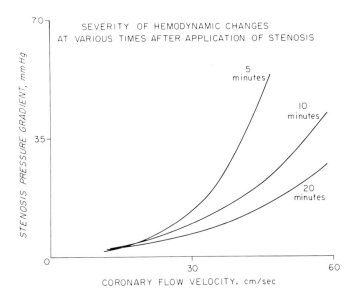

SEVERITY OF HEMODYNAMIC CHANGES
AT VARIOUS TIMES AFTER APPLICATION OF STENOSIS

Fig. 2.5 Stenosis drift from a greater to a less severe constriction the first 30 min after application of a constant inflation pressure. Each curve shows pressure gradient-flow velocity relation over a wide range of coronary flow velocities induced by coronary vasodilators. At the various time intervals shown, pressure-flow curves moved downward and rightward, indicating a lower pressure gradient for any given flow velocity and therefore a less severe stenosis. Reproduced with permission from Gould KL, Lee D, Lovgren K, 1978. (14).

tiplied times flow velocity data for the heart cycles at high flow after vasodilators.

We demonstrated by sequential arteriograms that this arterial cross-sectional area was relatively constant after injection of the vasodilator for the 60-s period of data collection. For each stenosis, the pressure gradient and flow-volume data from the five heart cycles was combined into a single composite ΔP-Q relation. The combined data was curvilinear and did not fit a simple quadratic relationship, owing to changing stenosis geometry during vasodilation, as discussed later (15–17). Therefore, a general-purpose, curve-fitting algorithm was used to derive a cubic equation that best fit the composite data in the form $\Delta P = aQ + bQ^2 + cQ^3$. This cubic equation was used to calculate the average single pressure gradient at any particular flow rate for that stenosis. The pressure gradient for different stenoses in different experiments could then be compared for the same flow rates (15–17).

Figure 2.4 shows tracings of coronary flow velocity and pressure gradient across a coronary stenosis at resting control conditions (14). The dashed tracings are computer-regenerated from digitized data stored in the computer, in order to demonstrate the fidelity of regenerated digitized data compared to original recordings. Electively controlled blanking pulses, shown by the short, straight, horizontal segments of the computer-regenerated traces in early and late systole, were introduced in order to selectively sample any part of the cardiac cycle. These blanking pulses were used for editing

out periods of early systolic deceleration of coronary flow and late systolic acceleration of coronary flow (15–17) in which the pressure-flow relation was determined by inertial forces rather than severity of the stenosis (5,6), as detailed in a subsequent chapter. The "noise" in the flow velocity trace is typical and inherent in Doppler recordings even with the high-quality linear instruments used here.

Figure 2.5 shows computer-generated graphs relating the pressure gradient due to stenosis of a coronary artery and the flow velocity through the artery. The steeper, more curved relationship indicates more severe stenosis. This figure also illustrates the drift in severity of a coronary stenosis within the first 30 min after inflation of the constrictor at a constant inflation pressure in an awake, chronically instrumented animal. The early stenosis drift is evidenced in Figure 2.5 by a less steep pressure-flow relation with time. The stenosis severity stabilized after 30–60 min so that experiments could be carried out.

ARTERIAL PRESSURE ANALYSIS

Since they are important for analyzing pressure flow characteristic of stenoses, pressure, and pressure recording systems are briefly reviewed here.

The force of cardiac contraction is transmitted to the arterial system as pressure, which maintains patency of blood vessels and perfusion of capillaries. The term "pressure" is derived from the Latin verb *premere,* meaning "to act on with steady force or weight." It is defined as the static force per unit area exerted by a column of fluid according to the equation $P = h \times d \times a$, where h and d are the height and density of the column of fluid, a is the acceleration of gravity, and P is pressure. In physics or engineering, the units of pressure are expressed in absolute units of the cgs (centimeter-gram-second) system as $cm \times g/cm^3 \times cm/s^2$. This expression reduces to $g/s^2 - cm$ or $g - cm/s^2 - cm^2$ or $dynes/cm^2$, where the dyne is the unit of force. However, for the cardiovascular system, these units are simplified to the height in millimeters of a standard reference fluid—mercury, by convention—with the density of mercury, d, and the acceleration of gravity, a, omitted, since they are constants.

In physiology, the units of pressure are then expressed as mm Hg. Mercury is used as a standard fluid because of its high density, thereby permitting measurement of arterial pressure with a relatively short tube. The relation between mm Hg and cgs units can be calculated as follows: 1 mm Hg $= (0.1 \, cm)(13.6 \, g/cm^3)(980 \, cm/s^2)$, where 0.1 cm is 1 mm height of the column, 13.6 g/cm^3 is the density of mercury, and 980 cm/s^2 is the acceleration due to gravity. One mm Hg, therefore, equals 1,333 $dynes/cm^2$ or 0.019 $lb/inch^2$; 52 mm Hg equals 1 $lb/inch^2$.

As an alternative, the unit "centimeter of saline" is also used for low pressures, such as venous pressure. In absolute units, 1 cm saline would be equal to $(1.0 \, cm)(1.04 \, g/cm^3)(980 \, cm/s^2)$, where 1.04 g/cm^3 is the density of saline. Therefore, 1 cm saline equals 1,019 $dynes/cm^2$ of pressure. Similarly, the units of pressure could be expressed as centimeters of blood (density 1.055 g/cm^3) and 1 mm Hg calculated to equal to 1.29 cm of blood.

ZERO REFERENCE FOR ARTERIAL PRESSURE

Arterial pressures are measured relative to a reference point outside the body arbitrarily defined as zero and chosen as the level of the mid-right atrium, Figure 2.6 (24). Actual or absolute pressure at this level outside the body is not actually zero but atmospheric pressure, or approximately 760 mm Hg. Therefore, an arterial pressure of 95 mm Hg means that the pressure is 95 mm Hg above atmospheric pressure. The reference point of zero of a catheter-external pressure manometer system is determined by the position of the manometer relative to the atria. If the external manometer is 12.9 cm below the level of the artria, the manometer will record the pressure at the tip of the catheter plus the pressure produced by a column of blood 12.9 cm high, equivalent to 10 mm Hg.

It is important to understand the relation of body position to the zero reference point when measuring arterial pressure. Different pressures will be recorded with the external manometer located at the level of the atria, as compared to having the transducer at the level of the head or feet, as illustrated in Figure 2.6. In the supine position, arterial pressures measured at the head, feet, and aortic root relative to the zero reference at the atria are all equal. In the standing position, arterial pressure at the level of the head, feet, and aortic root relative to the zero reference at the atrial level are also equal.

However, the arterial pressure at the level of the feet relative to a zero reference also at the level of the feet is increased by that amount of pressure produced by the column

of blood between the atria and the feet. This pressure is termed the transmural pressure and is the pressure "seen" or sustained by the arterial wall. It is equal to the standard intra-arterial pressure (referenced to the atria) plus the pressure produced by the column of blood above the feet. At the level of the head, the transmural pressure relative to a zero reference also at the level of the head is equal to the standard arterial pressure relative to an atrial zero reference, minus the pressure due to the column of blood between the head and atria.

The force or pressure generated by the heart is described by the standard intra-arterial or aortic pressure with zero reference at the atria. The transmural force or pressure on the arterial wall is described by the arterial pressure plus (for anatomic sites below the heart) or minus (for anatomic sites above the heart) the pressure due to the column of blood between the atria and the anatomic site at which the transmural pressure is being determined. Blood pressure measurements by sphygmomanometer are the measure of transmural pressure and are therefore affected by the position of the limb on which the blood pressure cuff is placed. A cuff-measured blood pressure on an arm raised overhead in a standing patient will be lower than in a standing patient with the arm at the level of the atria, even though actual intra-arterial pressure is constant.

Similarly, pulmonary capillary wedge pressure referenced to an external zero at atrial level is constant in all positions, whether the patient is sitting, standing, or supine. However, transcapillary pressure referenced to zero at any lung level between diaphragm and lung apex is higher in supine and lower in upright positions. Because pulmonary alveolar fluid transudate is determined by the transcapillary pressure, it is greater when the patient is supine, associated with dyspnea, and is less in the upright position. However, pulmonary wedge pressure referenced to zero at the atria is constant for supine and upright positions. There is a little-recognized paradox between constant positional pulmonary wedge pressure referenced to zero at the atria and supine dyspnea of pulmonary edema. The explanation is that pulmonary edema and dyspnea are not directly related to pulmonary wedge pressure referenced to zero at the atria but, strictly speaking, are related to transcapillary pressure related to zero at various vertical points of the lung. However, for uniform standardization clinically, pulmonary wedge pressures are referenced to zero at the atrial level.

TIME CHANGING PRESSURE

Pressure per se is a force per unit area and is by definition static, involving no motion, fluid displacement, distance, or time increment. However, in cardiovascular systems, pressure fluctuates periodically with cardiac contraction. A pressure-recording apparatus must, therefore, have not only static accuracy but also dynamic accuracy for recording pressure at each instant in time during rapid fluctuations of pressure. The dynamic responses of fluid-filled catheter-manometer systems have been previously described in mathematical and experimental detail (24–29). A brief review of wave form analysis is appropriate here in order to understand how to measure and optimize dynamic accuracy and how to rec-

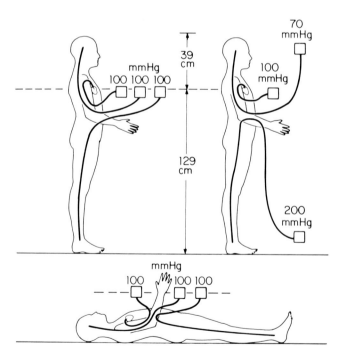

Fig. 2.6 Zero reference for intra-arterial pressure in the left atrium regardless of body position. Transmural pressure across the arterial wall referenced to zero at sites in the head or legs is dependent on body position. Reproduced with permission from Gould KL, 1980. (24).

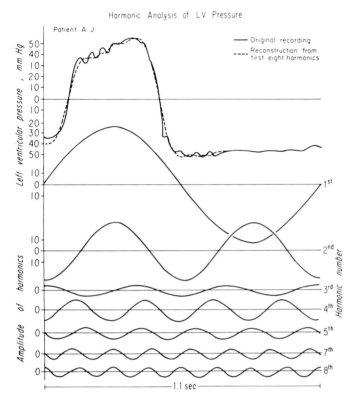

Fig. 2.7 Harmonic analysis of a left ventricular pressure wave, which is the most difficult pressure form in the body to record accurately. Reproduced with permission from Gould KL, 1980. (24).

the harmonic is the maximum displacement of the sine wave above or below the midline zero reference. The phase shift defines the beginning of a harmonic sine wave in time relative to the basic cycle or first harmonic. When the harmonics are added up, the various deflections above or below zero reference accumulate to produce the positive wave during systole and cancel each other during diastole.

Poor dynamic accuracy or distortion of pressure waves by fluid-filled catheter-manometer systems may be understood in terms of the failure to record faithfully the amplitude and phase shifts of all essential harmonics of the pressure wave. Exaggeration of some harmonics by pressure resonance or oscillation in the fluid-filled catheter, failure to record some harmonics due to damping, or changes in the phase of some harmonics but not others will distort the recorded pressure wave form. There are mathematical equations corresponding to the sine waves of the harmonic analysis conceptually illustrated in Figure 2.7 (24–29). However, in practice, it is not necessary to utilize sine wave equations in the analysis of dynamic accuracy of a given catheter-manometer system, and details will not be given here.

In general, at least 20 harmonics are required to reconstitute exactly a left ventricular pressure wave, particularly the rate of rise or upstroke, dp/dt, of the pressure trace (30–35). The exact number of harmonics changes with the heart rate, as discussed subsequently (33,34). Only eight to 10 harmonics are required to reconstitute an approximation of the left ventricular pressure with the correct peak systolic pressure. Other details, such as the rate of pressure rise and abrupt fluctuations in pressure, cannot be reconstituted with the first eight harmonics, illustrated in Figure 2.7 and Figure

ognize "bad" or "good" pressure recordings during clinical or experimental studies.

Cardiac contraction generates a transient pulse of force which passes along the aorta and arteries as a pressure wave. This pressure wave may be described and analyzed mathematically as the sum of a series of theoretical sine wave pressures which, when added together, reconstitute or equal the original wave form, Figure 2.7 (24). Each of these theoretical sine waves is called a harmonic and is characterized by harmonic number, amplitude, and phase shift. The process of determining the number and characteristics of the harmonics necessary to reproduce the original wave form when added together is called harmonic or Fourier analysis. Figure 2.7 illustrates an example. At the top is a recording of a left ventricular pressure wave. For purposes of analysis, the zero pressure baseline has been moved up so that the pressure wave can be described in terms of pressures above and below zero: for example, a wave −40 to +50 mm Hg rather than the conventional terms of 0 to 90 mm Hg. The pressure wave can then be defined by a series of sine wave pressures shown below the left ventricular pressure trace.

The harmonic number is the number of complete sine waves falling within the time period of the original cycle, in this case 1.1 s. The first harmonic has one complete sine wave within this period. The second harmonic has two complete sine waves within this period, and so forth. The amplitude of

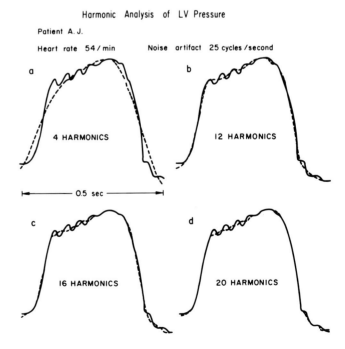

Fig. 2.8 Accuracy of reconstructing a left ventricular pressure wave form using different harmonics. Reproduced with permission from Gould KL, 1980. (24).

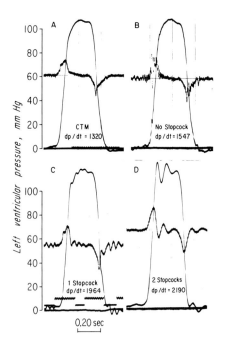

Fig. 2.9 Patterns of good and poor recordings of left ventricular pressure. Reproduced with permission from Gould KL, Trenholme S, Kennedy JW, 1973. (35).

FREQUENCY RESPONSES OF CATHETER MANOMETER SYSTEMS

These concepts of harmonic analysis may be related functionally to a catheter-manometer system by testing its dynamic accuracy with a device that generates sine wave pressures at any selectable frequency. A number of different types of sine wave pressure generators have been described and are commercially available. The device consists of a fluid-filled chamber, into which the tip of a catheter is inserted and sealed. The pressure in the chamber fluctuates in a sine wave pattern with waves of 20–30 mm Hg amplitude at variably controlled frequencies. This pressure is recorded by a reference pressure transducer attached directly to the chamber. Thus, two pressures are recorded: the standard or reference pressure and the pressure through the catheter attached to a second or test transducer.

Figure 2.10 (24) shows an example of testing a catheter-manometer system with a sine wave pressure generator. At the top is the electrical driving signal. At the bottom is the reference sine wave pressure in the test chamber having an amplitude of 20 mm Hg. In the middle is the pressure recorded through the catheter-manometer system being tested. The numbers at the bottom of each panel indicate the frequency of the pressure waves or cycles per second, also termed Hertz, where 1 Hz equals 1 c/s. For frequency of pressure waves up to 20 Hz, the catheter-manometer system recorded the pressure waves fairly accurately. However, at 50 Hz, the catheter pressure was distorted—that is, it was amplified to approximately 45 mm Hg, even though the pressure waves in the chamber were actually 20 mm Hg in amplitude. At 103 Hz, the pressure waves recorded through the catheter were 150 mm Hg in amplitude, as compared to 20 mm Hg in the reference chamber. Thus, the catheter-manometer system distorted or amplified the actual pressure waves to 7.5 times the actual amplitude of the pressure waves in the test chamber.

Such distortion is due to underdamping. That frequency at which maximum amplification occurs is called the resonant frequency. A catheter-manometer system is said to have a uniform or flat response up to the frequency that produces a 5% increase in pressure wave amplitude. In this example, the catheter-manometer system had a flat response to approximately 20 Hz and a resonant frequency of 103 Hz. The

2.8 (24). If only four harmonics are used, the reconstituted pressure wave is grossly distorted, as shown in Figure 2.8A. Therefore, a catheter-manometer recording system that fails to record higher harmonics produces a distorted pressure wave, as shown.

Most fluid-filled catheter-manometer systems are underdamped, with the result that the column of fluid in the catheter oscillates or resonates at one or several of the higher harmonics. The harmonic at which resonance occurs, therefore, becomes accentuated and its amplitude becomes artifactually large. The reconstituted pressure is therefore distorted, as shown in Figure 2.9D (35), with parts of the recorded pressure wave being greater than the actual or real undistorted pressure wave.

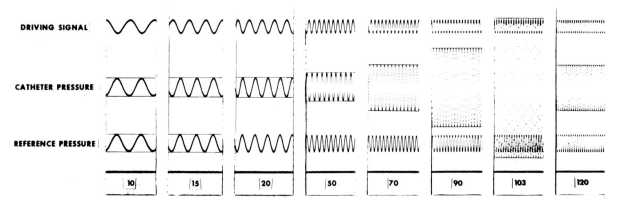

Fig. 2.10 Measuring frequency responses of catheter-manometer systems. Reproduced with permission from Gould KL, 1980. (24).

frequency to which the system has a flat, uniform response (within ± 5% overshoot) is usually about 20% of the resonant frequency for most clinical—that is, underdamped—catheters. In this illustration, the resonant frequency was 103 Hz and the system should be flat to 20% × 103 Hz, or 21 Hz, as compared to 20 Hz observed experimentally.

It is incorrect to view the sine wave pressures in the test chamber described above as physical analogues of the sine waves in the harmonic analysis described earlier. Harmonics are conceptual, mathematical expressions describing a wave form regardless of the period or duration of the pressure wave cycle in real time. At a heart rate of 60 beats/min, or 1 beat/s, the period of the first harmonic is 1 s. At a rate of 120 beats/min, or 2/s, the period of the first harmonic is 0.5 s. At a heart rate of 30, the period of the first harmonic is 2 s. Although not analogous, the number of harmonics, or theoretical mathematical sine waves, necessary to faithfully reconstitute a pressure wave is related to the empirically determined frequency response of a catheter-manometer system depending on the heart rate (34).

For example, let us assume that 15 harmonics are required for approximate reproduction of a given left ventricular pressure wave. At a heart rate of 60 or 1 beat/s, the period of the first harmonic is 1 s and the 15th harmonic would have 15 cycles within this 1-s period. A catheter-manometer system would, therefore, have to have a uniform or flat response to 15 Hz in order to faithfully record the pressure wave at a heart rate of 60. At a heart rate of 120 or 2 beats/s, the period of the first harmonic is 0.5 s and the 15th harmonic would have 15 cycles within this 0.5-s period, or 30 cycles within a 1-s period. A catheter-manometer system would have to have a flat response to 30 Hz to faithfully record the pressure wave at a heart rate of 120. Knopp et al. (33) have shown experimentally that the number of harmonics required to faithfully reproduce a pressure wave increases with heart rate, as would be theoretically expected.

SLOW AND FAST CATHETER MANOMETER SYSTEMS

The results of testing a catheter-manometer system on a sine wave pressure generator may be displayed as a graph, illustrated in Figure 2.11 (24). The horizontal axis shows the frequency in Hz of the generator pressure. The vertical axis shows the ratio of the amplitude of the catheter-manometer pressure wave to the amplitude of the reference pressure wave. An amplitude ratio of 1.0 indicates no error or overshoot. An amplitude ratio of 2.0 indicates that the catheter-manometer pressure wave has an amplitude two times as large as the actual amplitude of the reference pressure wave. An amplitude ratio of 1.05 indicates an overshoot of ±5% and is conventionally defined as the limit of acceptable error for a catheter system. A "fast" system has a frequency response curve to the right side of the graph, such as the transseptal catheter. It faithfully records pressure waves up to 25 Hz. A "slow" system falls to the left side of the graph, such as a 7F Gensini with one stopcock; it faithfully records pressure waves up to only 10 Hz. In addition, this slower system is more damped than the others, as indicated by a lower peak amplitude ratio of 6.0 compared to 13.0 for the faster systems.

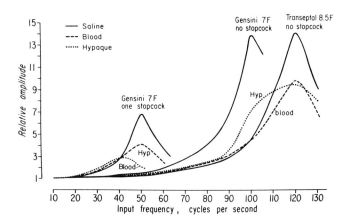

Fig. 2.11 Frequency response characteristics of catheter-manometer systems. Reproduced with permission from Gould KL, 1980. (24).

All the catheters in Figure 2.11 are underdamped. A critically damped system (not shown) would have no peak amplitude ratio; it would be flat to some input frequency, and thereafter its response would fall off to less than 1.0. Standard 8 French Gensini and 8.5 French transseptal catheters without intervening stopcocks have natural frequencies of 115–120 Hz and are flat to 20–25 Hz. One stopcock decreases uniform amplitude response to 12–15 Hz. In these relatively large catheters, blood or hypaque increased damping slightly—that is, it lowered the height of the resonance peak, but did not change the frequency at which peak resonance occurred.

CLINICAL IMPLICATIONS OF CATHETER FREQUENCY RESPONSES

Virtually everyone who has studied frequency responses of catheters has found that consistent, reproducible clinical recordings or frequency response testing requires repeated careful flushing of the catheter-manometer system with boiled or deaerated sterile saline (25,27–29,35,35–43). For example, Futamura (40) has quantified the progressive improvement in frequency response with successive flushing up to 5 flushes in sequence. Thereafter, frequency responses remained stable. Similarly, elimination of stopcocks and connector tubing is important for obtaining good frequency responses.

In clinical practice in the cath lab, there are three types of pressure wave distortions, all visually recognizable. Clinical catheter-manometer systems are either underdamped and slow, underdamped and fast, or overdamped. Examples are illustrated in Figure 2.9 (24). The pressure recording in Figure 2.9A is an ideal reference left ventricular pressure trace, recorded by catheter-tip micromanometer and therefore unaffected by catheter-induced distortion. Pressure in Figure 2.9B is a recording through an underdamped, fast catheter-manometer system. There is considerable high-frequency resonance, or "hash," due to underdamping, but the system has a flat dynamic response to 20–25 Hz and a resonant frequency of greater than 100 Hz. Therefore, the recording contains accurate pressure information, and the basic wave form is correct. The high-frequency hash is visually unattractive but does not deform the pressure wave. It can be removed by filtering the signal through an electronic analog filter or a frequency-limited galvanometer recorder, or through digital computer filtering.

Pressure in Figure 2.9C is a recording through an underdamped, moderately slow catheter-manometer system flat to 10–13 Hz with a resonant frequency of 40–50 Hz, in which the pressure wave is somewhat distorted but clinically useful for measuring peak systolic and end-diastolic pressure. Pressure in Figure 2.9D is a grossly distorted recording through an underdamped, very slow catheter-manometer system flat to 3–5 Hz with a resonant frequency of 13–17 Hz. It is so distorted that the pressure information and basic wave form have been lost. No type of processing can extract a correct pressure wave from this recording. The cause of such distortion is one or several of the following: improper flushing of the system, two or more stopcocks or multiple manifold connectors in the system, or long, soft extender tubings between the catheter and the transducer.

Maximum dp/dt, or rate of pressure rise, is very sensitive to catheter-induced distortion of the pressure wave. Underdamping causes pressure overshoot at any given instant on the rising pressure trace and therefore results in an erroneously high dp/dt, as shown in Figure 2.9. Even the fast system in 2.9B has enough artifactual effect to give a dp/dt that is 17% too high, as compared to the reference or true value determined by catheter-tip manometer. In 2.9D, the dp/dt is 66% higher than the true value.

Pressure recordings obtained by catheter-manometer systems are technically good only if the system is fast—that is, flat to 20–25 Hz—and if the pressure waves look like those shown in Figure 2.9A. Technically acceptable tracings for recording peak systolic, end-diastolic, and the approximate pressure wave can be obtained with a system flat to about 15 Hz; the pressure waves look like those in Figure 2.9C. A slower system producing recordings like those of Figure 2.9D is not technically acceptable for clinical measurements.

Most standard clinical catheters 125 cm long or less and 7 French or greater in diameter, if properly flushed with sterile deaerated saline and with no more than a single stopcock between the transducer and catheter, will produce adequate pressure recordings for qualitative evaluation of the wave form and quantitative measurement of systolic or diastolic pressure.

For good clinical pressure tracings, the following procedure is optimal. Initially record pressure with only one three-way large-bore stopcock in the system flushed as follows with sterile, deaerated saline (e.g., Abbott). Pour saline gently into a basin and draw into a syringe, preferably plastic, without creating bubbles. Attach the filled syringe to the side arm of the stopcock and flush back through the stopcock, being careful to flush out all bubbles. Attach the transducer to the stopcock while flushing gently. If the transducer with a plastic dome is used, the entire dome should be flushed through. Then turn the stopcock so as to flush forward through the male end. Remove any other stopcocks from the catheter, let it bleed backward, and attach to the male end of the flushed stopcock with the syringe in place on the side arm. Aspirate blood into the syringe and then flush forward.

While flushing, turn the stopcock through to record pressure. Remove the syringe, turn the stopcock to air to establish zero baseline, then turn the stopcock to pressure for recording. If optimized high-fidelity recordings are desired, then record a second pressure after removing all stopcocks and attaching the bleeding catheter directly to the gauge. Zero reference is recorded while the gauge is being held waiting for the back bleeding to wash out all saline. After recording three to four heartbeats, quickly reintroduce a stopcock, aspirate a syringe of blood, and flush the system with saline in order to avoid blood clotting in the catheter. Any other routine such as a continuous flush-through system is acceptable as long as the basic requirements are met: that is, careful repeated flushing and no more than one stopcock in line between the catheter and transducer.

Peripheral artery (e.g., brachial, radial) systolic pressures are greater than central aortic systolic pressures, because the peripheral artery itself acts like an underdamped catheter, causing overshoot as the pressure wave is transmitted distally (42). Thus, some overshoot in peripheral arteries may not indicate a poor recording system but may be a physiologic in-vivo phenomenon. However, even peripheral artery pressures do not have the undulations seen in the tracing of Figure 2.9D.

The catheter-manometer system for recording coronary pressure gradients across stenoses for data presented here was flat to 30 Hz, as shown in Figure 2.2. It is therefore a high-fidelity system suitable for quantifying pressure data.

REFERENCES

1. Berguer R, Hwang NHC. Critical arterial stenosis: a theoretical and experimental solution. Ann Surg 180:39–50, 1974.
2. Karayannacos PE, Talukder N, Nerem RM, Roshon S, Vasko JS. The role of multiple non-critical arterial stenoses in the pathogenesis of ischemia. J Thoracic Cardiovascular Surg 73:458–69, 1977.
3. May AG, DeWeese JA, Rob CG. Hemodynamic effects of arterial stenosis. Surgery 53:513–24, 1963.
4. Young DF, Cholvin NR, Kirkeeide RL, Roth AC. Hemodynamics of arterial stenoses at elevated flow rates. Circulation Res 41:99–107, 1977.
5. Young DF, Cholvin NR, Roth AC. Pressure drop across artificially induced stenoses in the femoral arteries of dogs. Circulation Res 36:735–43, 1975.
6. Young DF, Tsai FY. Flow characteristics in models of arterial stenosis. I. Steady flow. J Biomech 6:395–410, 1973.
7. Young DF, Tsai FY. Flow characteristics in models of arterial stenosis. II. Unsteady flow. J Biomech 6:547–559, 1973.
8. Binder RC. Fluid Mechanics (ed. 5). Englewood Cliffs, N.J.: Prentice-Hall, 1973.
9. Daily JW, Harleman DRF. Fluid Dynamics. Reading, Mass.: Addison-Wesley, 1966, p. 316.
10. Daugherty RL, Ingerson AC. Fluid Mechanics with Engineering Applications. New York: McGraw Hill, 1954, p. 195.
11. Gould KL, Lipscomb K. Effects of coronary stenoses on coronary flow reserve and resistance. Am J Cardiol 34:48–55, 1974.
12. Lipscomb K, Gould KL. Mechanism of the effect of coronary artery stenosis on coronary flow in the dog. Am Heart J 89:60–67, 1975.
13. Gould KL, Lipscomb K, Calvert C. Compensatory changes of the distal coronary vascular bed during progressive coronary constriction. Circulation 51:1085–94, 1975.
14. Gould KL, Lee D, Lovgren K. Techniques for arteriography and hydraulic analysis of coronary stenoses in unsedated dogs. Am J Physiol 235:H350–56, 1978.

15. Gould KL. Pressure-flow characteristics of coronary stenoses in unsedated dogs at rest and during coronary vasodilation. Circ Res 43:245–53, 1978.
16. Gould KL, Kelley KO. Experimental validation of quantitative coronary arteriography for determining pressure-flow characteristics of coronary stenoses. Circ 66:930–37, 1982.
17. Gould KL, Kelley KO. Physiologic significance of coronary flow velocity and changing stenosis geometry during coronary vasodilation in awake dogs. Circ Res 50:695–704, 1982.
18. Herd JA. Overall regulation of the circulation. Ann Rev Physiol 32:289–312, 1970.
19. Herd JA, Barger AC. Simplified technique for chronic catheterization of blood vessels. J Appl Physiol 19:791–92, 1964.
20. Leshin SJ, Mullens CV, Templeton GH, Mitchell JH. Dimensional analysis of ventricular function: effects of anesthesia and thoracotomy. Am J Physiol 222:540–45, 1972.
21. Rushmer RF. Shrinkage of the heart in anesthetized thoracotomized dogs. Circulation Res 2:22–27, 1954.
22. Harris SA, Kokernot RH. Effects of diphenylhydantoin sodium and phenobarbital sodium upon ectopic ventricular tachycardia in acute myocardial infarction. Am J Physiol 163:505–16, 1950.
23. Vatner SF, Franklin D, Van Citters RL. Simultaneous comparison and calibration of the Doppler and electromagnetic flowmeters. J Appl Physiol 29:907–10, 1970.
24. Gould KL. Intraarterial Pressure in Methods in Angiology. ed. M. Werstraete. Belgium: BF Commandeur Pub., 1980.
25. Fry DL. Physiologic recording by modern instruments with particular reference to pressure recording. Physiol Rev 40:753–88, 1960.
26. Attinger EO, Anne A, McDonald DA. Use of Fourier series for the analysis of biological systems. Biophys J 6:291–304, 1966.
27. Yanof HM, Rosen AL, McDonald NM, McDonald DA. A critical study of the response of manometers to forced oscillations. Phy Med Biol 8:407–22, 1963.
28. Yanof HM. Biomedical Electronics. Philadelphia: Davis Pub., 1965, p 265–84.
29. Fry DL, Noble FW, Mallos AJ. An evaluation of modern pressure recording systems. Circ Res 5:40–46, 1957.
30. Gleason WL, Braunwald E. Studies on the first derivative of the ventricular pressure pulse in man. J Clin Invest 41:80–91, 1962.
31. Wallace AG, Skinner NS, Mitchell HJ. Hemodynamic determinants of the maximal rate of rise of the left ventricular pressure. Amer J Physiol 205:30–36, 1963.
32. Patel DJ, Mason DT, Ross J, Braunwald E. Harmonic analysis of pressure pulses obtained from the heart and great vessels of man. Amer Heart J 69:785–94, 1965.
33. Knopp TJ, Rahimtoola SH, Swan HJC. The first derivative of ventricular pressure recorded by means of conventional cardiac catheter. Cardiovas Res 4:398–404, 1970.
34. Gersh BJ, Hahn CEW, Prys-Roberts C. Physical criteria for measurement of left ventricular pressure and its first derivative. Cardiovas Res 5:32–40, 1971.
35. Gould KL, Trenholme S, Kennedy JW. In vivo comparison of catheter manometer systems with the catheter tip micromanometer. J Appl Physiol 34:263–67, 1973.
36. Cronvich JA, Burch GE. Frequency characteristics of some pressure transducer systems. Amer Heart J 77:792–97, 1969.
37. Shapiro GG, Krovetz LJ. Damped and undamped frequency responses of underdamped catheter manometer systems. Amer Heart J 80:226–36, 1970.
38. Scruggs V, Pietras RJ, Rosen KM. Frequency response of fluid filled catheter micromanometer systems used for measurement of left ventricular pressure. Amer Heart J 89:619–24, 1975.
39. Falsetti HL, Mates RE, Carroll RJ, Gupta RL, Bell AC. Analysis and correction of pressure wave distortion in fluid filled catheter systems. Circulation 44:165–72, 1974.
40. Futamura Y. Correction of distortions of pressure waves obtained with catheter-manometer systems. Jap Heart J 18:664–78, 1977.
41. Krovetz LJ, Jennings, RB, Golgbloom SD. Limitation of correction of frequency dependent artefact in pressure recordings using harmonic analysis. Circulation 50:992–97, 1974.
42. Rowell LB, Brengelmann GL, Blackmon JR, Bruce RA, Murray JA. Disparities between aortic and peripheral pulse pressures induced by upright exercise and vasomotor changes in man. Circulation 32:954–64, 1968.
43. Dear HD, Spear AF. Accurate method for measuring dp/dt with cardiac catheters and external transducers. J Appl Physiol 30:897–99, 1971.

CHAPTER

3

Interactions with the Distal Coronary Vascular Bed

The pressure-flow characteristics of coronary artery stenosis in vivo are largely determined by interaction with, and hemodynamic behavior of, the distal coronary vascular bed. As illustrated in Figure 3.1, resting coronary artery flow and regional flow distribution (solid line) remain normal despite progressive, relatively severe coronary artery narrowing (1–4). However, free flow in an open-ended tube in vitro (dashed line) is linearly related to the cross-sectional area of any narrowing. The difference between these hemodynamic characteristics of any given fixed stenosis is due to the presence of the distal coronary vascular bed and varies with its resistance to flow, as determined by coronary arteriolar vasomotor tone.

It is commonly but erroneously thought that resting coronary flow remains normal despite progressively severe coronary stenosis because of compensating distal arteriolar vasodilation. The correct explanation is found in the relation between resting coronary vascular tone, or resistance, and the resistance of the proximal coronary stenosis in series with the vascular bed. Resting flow in a model artery (top of Fig. 3.1) is determined by the total pressure gradient, ΔP, divided by the sum of resistances in series, the stenosis resistance, R_s, and the coronary vascular bed resistance, R_b, of Figure 3.1. Normal resting coronary vascular resistance is very high, four to five times its minimum resistance in the maximally vasodilated state. Since flow is determined by resistances in series, the proximal stenosis has to be fairly severe before its resistance approximates that of resting coronary vascular bed resistance and begins to reduce resting flow. Therefore, up to about 65% to 75% diameter narrowing, progressive coronary stenosis has no effect on resting coronary flow and causes no distal compensatory vasodilation.

Thus, the coronary vascular system is normally a low-flow, high-resistance system at rest, teleologically suited to meet increased work demands by increasing flow. Consequently, resting coronary flow is an insensitive, poor measure of stenosis severity. Similarly, symptoms of restricted coronary blood flow, angina pectoris, appear late in the pathophysiologic course of coronary atherosclerosis, after severe stenoses have developed. The normal, high resting coronary vascular resistance makes coronary atherosclerosis a clinically silent disease until it is anatomically severe and advanced. This normal high resting coronary vascular resis-

tance therefore requires some measure of stenosis severity other than resting flow for scientific and medical quantitation.

Since the hemodynamic characteristics of a fixed coronary stenosis in vivo are determined by the behavior of the distal coronary vascular bed, some form of compartmental analysis is necessary whereby the stenosis is analyzed sep-

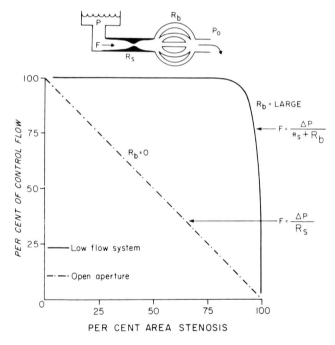

Fig. 3.1 Explanation for maintenance of normal resting flow during progressive arterial narrowing. Flow through the artery is determined by the total pressure drop divided by the sum of resistances in series, the stenosis resistance (R_s), and the distal bed resistance (R_b). Normally, at rest, the distal bed resistance is high, such that the stenosis must be fairly severe before its resistance approximates that of the distal vascular bed and begins to affect flow. The dashed line represents an open tube in which progressive narrowing causes a linear decrease in flow, since there is no distal resistance.

31

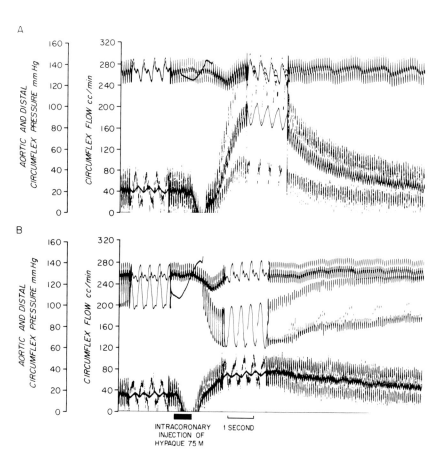

Fig. 3.2 Recordings of coronary flow and proximal and distal coronary pressures in a normal coronary artery (A) and in a stenotic coronary artery (B). In panel A, superimposed aortic and distal coronary pressure are in the upper recordings. In the lower recordings are superimposed mean and phasic coronary flow. In panel B, aortic pressure, distal coronary pressure, and superimposed mean and phasic coronary flow recordings are displayed from top to bottom. At rest, coronary blood flow is normal in both the normal and stenotic arteries; but the stenosis caused a resting pressure gradient of approximately 30 mm Hg between the aorta and the distal coronary artery. Following a vasodilatory stimulus (injection of Hypaque), mean coronary flow in the normal artery increased by four to five times its resting level. In the stenotic artery, flow increased to only twice its resting value, with a marked increase in the stenosis pressure gradient and a fall in distal coronary pressure. Reproduced with permission from Lipscomb K, Gould KL, 1975. (3).

arately from the distal vascular bed. The most common physiologic and fluid-dynamic compartmental approach uses stenosis resistance and distal bed resistance separately to describe stenosis severity and its interaction with the distal coronary bed. Determining resistance requires measurements of the pressure gradient across the stenosis and vascular bed and flow through each over a range of coronary flows.

Figure 3.2 shows experimentally measured coronary flow, aortic pressure, and coronary pressure distal to a constrictor on the left circumflex coronary artery (3). In the absence of a stenosis, coronary flow increases four- to fivefold after a pharmacologic flow stimulus such as intravenous dipyridamole or intracoronary papaverine, or the contrast media Hypaque 75 M, in this instance. Pressure gradient from aorta to coronary at rest and peak flow is small in the absence of coronary narrowing. With a coronary artery stenosis that does not reduce resting flow, there is a resting 25 mm Hg gradient. After the flow stimulus, coronary flow increases by only two times baseline, or half the normal response, with a marked increase in the pressure gradient across the stenosis of approximately 60 mm Hg.

Figure 3.3 graphs the mean stenosis pressure gradient against the mean coronary flow for three progressively severe stenoses (4). Mean pressure-flow relations for progressively severe stenoses are linear, with a steeper slope corresponding

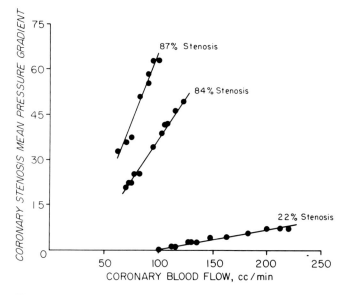

Fig. 3.3 Characteristic regression lines relating pressure gradient across a coronary stenosis to flow through it. Stenoses of 22%, 84%, and 87% diameter narrowing are illustrated. Correlation coefficients (r) for these relations are above 0.99. Reproduced with permission from Gould KL, Lipscomb K, Calvert C, 1975. (4).

to more severe narrowing. The mean correlation coefficient for regression equations relating mean pressure gradient to mean coronary blood flow was 0.98 for 157 stenoses studied. All regression lines intercepted the flow axis at a positive flow for a zero pressure gradient. This positive flow intercept indicates that there is some low level of flow through the stenosis at which the pressure gradient across the stenosis is negligible.

DEFINING SEVERITY OF CORONARY ARTERY STENOSIS

A method of hemodynamically characterizing severity of coronary artery stenoses is important to the systematic or statistical evaluation of their effects in vivo. For a geometrically fixed stenosis, pressure gradients across stenoses are variable, depending on flow, as shown in Figure 3.2 (3) and Figure 3.3 (4), and cannot be used alone to quantify the effects of stenoses. Calculated stenosis resistance was therefore evaluated as a means of characterizing stenoses hemodynamically. For each of the experimental pressure flow points in Figure 3.3 for each stenosis, stenosis resistance was calculated as pressure gradient divided by flow for that point on the graph of Figure 3.3. Each of the resulting resistance values are graphed as a function of flow in Figure 3.4 (4). For an anatomically fixed stenosis, stenosis resistance varied over a wide range, depending on flow. For example, the resistance

of the 22% stenosis was 0.8 mm Hg/cc per min at resting flow but was 3.7 mm Hg/cc per min at peak flow. Thus, there was no single resistance value characterizing the anatomically fixed stenosis. Consequently, calculated resistance was not useful experimentally for describing stenosis severity.

Computer-derived curves best fitting the experimental data shown in Figure 3.4 indicate that resistance was a hyperbolic function of flow. For these studies, length and absolute cross-sectional area of the coronary arteries were the same for each progressive stenosis. Consequently, percent narrowing was used as an approximate geometric measure of stenosis severity for comparison to their mean pressure-flow characteristics in these controlled experimental preparations, where other stenosis dimensions were constant.

Although derived from experimental observations of pressure and flow, the increased calculated stenosis resistance found with increasing flow (or decreased distal coronary bed resistance) is misleading as a measure of stenosis severity due to the way stenosis resistance is calculated from mean pressure and mean coronary flows. This increased stenosis resistance does not imply more severe geometric stenosis but is an artifact arising from the definition of stenosis resistance as follows: $R_s = G/Q$, where R_s is stenosis resistance, G is the mean reduction in pressure or gradient across the constriction, and Q is mean flow through it. This experimental relation between the mean stenosis pressure gradient and mean coronary flow is linear, with the regression line intercepting the flow axis at zero gradient, indicating that at some positive mean flow values there is no measurable mean pressure gradient. This relation can therefore be expressed as the equation $G = a + bQ$, where a is the flow or X-axis intercept at zero gradient and b is the slope of the regression line relating the pressure gradient, G, to the flow, Q—that is, the change in gradient per unit change in flow, $\Delta G/\Delta Q$. Substitution of this equation for G in the previous equation for calculated stenosis resistance gives the final expression:

$$R_s = G/Q = b + a/Q = \Delta G/\Delta Q + a/Q.$$

This equation shows that stenosis resistance calculated from mean pressure and mean flow values is a hyperbolic function of flow. As flow increases from low values, R_s increases nonlinearly and is not a fixed constant at all flows, because of the last term of the equation, a/Q. This observation has been confirmed experimentally, with stenosis resistance increasing nonlinearly as flow increased from low or resting values (4). Thus, by definition, stenosis resistance calculated from mean values of pressure and flow is dependent on flow despite constant, fixed stenosis geometry and is therefore an unsatisfactory measure of stenosis severity.

Since calculation of stenosis resistance was of limited value, the mean pressure gradient-flow relation during hyperemia was used to quantify the hemodynamic severity of stenoses for purposes of correlating them with compensatory changes of the distal coronary vascular bed. The linear relation for each stenosis shown in Figure 3.3 is characterized by a constant slope, $\Delta G/\Delta F$, which increases with increasing severity of narrowing. This slope is expressed as mm Hg change of mean pressure gradient for each cc per min change in mean coronary flow. For example, the 84% stenosis characterized hemodynamically in this manner was 0.56 mm Hg

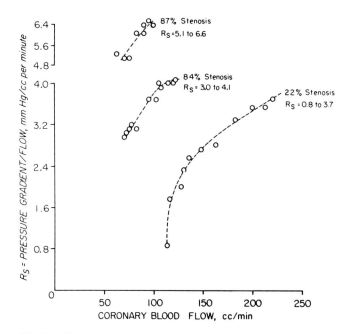

Fig. 3.4 Relation of stenosis resistance (R_s), calculated as absolute resting pressure gradient/flow, to flow through the stenosis. The curves best fitting the experimental data points are hyperbolas. The ranges of values obtained for an anatomically fixed stenosis at resting (lowest value) and at maximal flow (highest value) are shown. Reproduced with permission from Gould KL, Lipscomb K, Calvert C, 1975. (4).

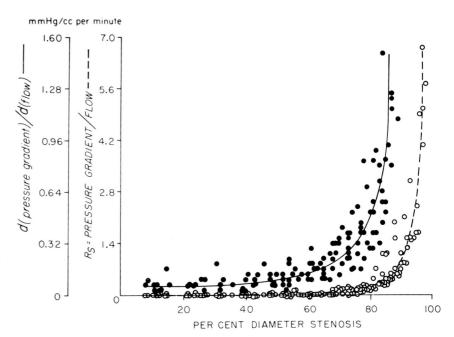

Fig. 3.5 Relation of percent diameter stenosis to the slope of the gradient-flow regression line during hyperemia (solid line) and to resistance (absolute pressure gradient/flow) at resting flow (dashed line). Reproduced with permission from Gould KL, Lipscomb K, Calvert C, 1975. (4).

change for each cc per minute change in flow at resting as well as at maximum flow. Thus, the characterization of stenoses as change in mm Hg pressure gradient per change in mL of flow from the slope of the $\Delta G/\Delta Q$ relation was empirically independent of flow over the range observed, whereas stenosis resistance defined as absolute pressure gradient divided by absolute flow, $\Delta G/Q$, was dependent on flow.

The usefulness of characterizing stenoses by the slope of the pressure gradient-flow relation during hyperemia is demonstrated in Figure 3.5 (4). Percent diameter stenosis is graphed against the slope of the mean pressure gradient-flow relation, or d(gradient)/d(flow), and against stenosis resistance (absolute gradient/flow) at resting flow. The slope of the gradient-flow relation during hyperemia increased at rela-

tively modest anatomic stenoses, indicating altered gradient-flow characteristics. In contrast, stenosis resistance defined as absolute resting gradient/flow remained normal, since there was no resting gradient for those stenoses despite altered gradient-flow relation during hyperemia. These results indicate that the slope of the gradient-flow relation is more sensitive than resistance values in detecting and characterizing the effects of subcritical coronary stenoses.

Since small changes in arterial diameter have major hemodynamic consequences for stenoses above 60%, the increased sensitivity of this method for hemodynamically characterizing a stenosis becomes more apparent if plotted against pressure gradient across the stenoses, as in Figure 3.6 (4). Stenoses of progressively increased severity to 85%

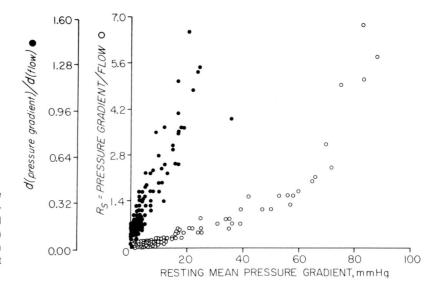

Fig. 3.6 Relation of pressure gradient across the stenosis to the slope of the gradient-flow regression line during hyperemia (closed circles) and to resistance (absolute pressure gradient/flow) at resting flow (open circles). Reproduced with permission from Gould KL, Lipscomb K, Calvert C, 1975. (4).

Table 3.1 Coronary Pressure Flow Responses during Hyperemia in the Presence of 92% ± 3% Diameter Stenosis of Circumflex Artery

	Flow, cc/min	Cor. pressure mm Hg	Gradient mm Hg	Cor. pressure/flow
Rest, no stenosis	49 ± 8	110 ± 12	0	2.37 ± 0.71
Rest, stenosis	37 ± 14	53 ± 20	57 ± 17	1.46 ± 0.25
Hyperemia, stenosis	46 ± 22	38 ± 11	69 ± 7	0.91 ± 0.23
% Δ, hypermia	+18 ± 20	−25 ± 12	+35 ± 53	−37 ± 16

Cor. = coronary; ± one standard deviation; % Δ is the mean of changes in individual experiments; + = increase; − = decrease.

Source: Adapted with permission from Gould KL, Lipscomb K, Calvert C, 1975. (4).

narrowing demonstrated resting pressure gradients and large increases in the slope of the gradient-flow relation, whereas stenosis resistance defined as absolute gradient/flow showed relatively little change.

COMPENSATORY DISTAL CORONARY VASODILATION IN RESPONSE TO PROXIMAL CORONARY STENOSES

Table 3.1 (4) shows the coronary pressure flow responses during hyperemia in the presence of stenoses averaging 92% ± 3% diameter narrowing, which reduced coronary flow to 74% ± 20% of normal control values. Following the flow stimulus of intracoronary contrast media in the presence of these severe stenoses, coronary flow increased by 18% over resting levels in association with a 25% further decrease in coronary pressure distal to the stenosis and a 37% further decrease in coronary vascular resistance (P < 0.001). This response indicates that in addition to vasodilation already present in compensation for the severe stenoses, a pharmacologic arteriolar vasodilator causes further vasodilation of the coronary bed. Mean vascular resistance (distal/pressure flow) was also calculated in order to compare with severity of stenosis.

Figure 3.7 (4) shows the compensatory changes of the distal coronary vascular bed in response to progressive proximal stenosis of coronary arteries. With progressive coronary artery constriction, the slope of the gradient-flow relation of the stenosis did not increase significantly until approximately 60% diameter reduction. Thus, resting coronary flow is not altered by constrictions up to 60%, since the stenosis resistance is essentially negligible compared to distal bed resistance; in effect, there is simply no hydraulic resistance to flow

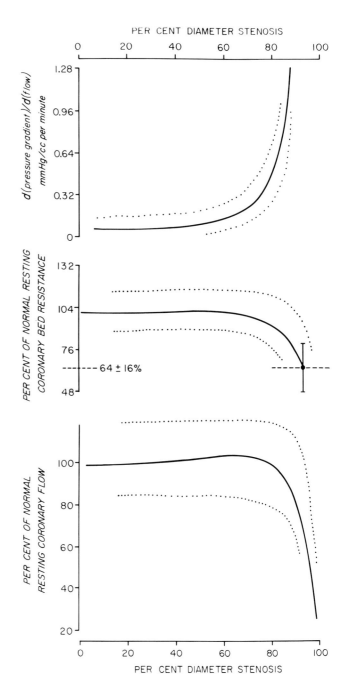

Fig. 3.7 Relation of percent stenosis to resting coronary flow, distal vascular bed resistance, and the slope of the gradient-flow relation during hyperemia. Coronary flow is expressed as percent of normal, control, resting coronary flow. Distal coronary vascular bed resistance is expressed as percent of resting, distal vascular bed resistance in the absence of stenoses. In compensation for progressive coronary constriction, distal vascular bed resistance reached a minimum of 64% ± 16% of control values. Reproduced with permission from Gould KL, Lipscomb K, Calvert C, 1975. (4).

at resting flow levels. For coronary narrowing between 60% and 85%, the pressure gradient-flow slope characterizing the stenosis increased significantly and a resting gradient appeared. However, resting coronary flow remained normal because of compensatory decrease in coronary vascular bed resistance. For narrowing greater than approximately 85% diameter stenosis, there was no further compensatory decrease in vascular bed resistance, and resting flow fell precipitously with further coronary constriction.

Since small geometric changes of severe stenoses have major hemodynamic effects, the compensatory changes of the distal vascular bed become more apparent if plotted against resting pressure gradient, as shown in Figure 3.8 (4). In effect, this figure expands that part of the previous figure for stenoses above 85%. It shows that when resting coronary flow was reduced to 74% ± 20% of normal control values by stenoses, calculated coronary vascular resistance was 1.46 ± 0.25 mm Hg/cc per min, or 64% ± 16% of the normal control resting value of 2.37 ± 0.71 mm Hg/cc per min. Intracoronary injection of contrast media resulted in further vasodilation (Table 3.1) and an additional further decrease in vascular resistance down to 0.91 ± 0.23 mm Hg/cc per min, or 40% ± 11% of normal resting values. With further narrowing, the distal bed did not compensate with further vasodilation. Distal coronary bed resistance may actually increase if coronary pressure approaches the critical closing pressure of the vasculature distal to the stenosis. Minimum vascular resistance during hyperemia in the absence of stenosis was 0.53 ± 0.11 mm Hg/cc per min or 23% ± 4% of resting control values.

Thus, there is vasodilator reserve remaining, even when total coronary artery blood flow is reduced by proximal stenoses. Despite relatively severe stenoses, resting coronary flow remains normal, because at resting flow levels stenoses of up to 60% diameter narrowing do not cause a pressure gradient or offer measurable resistance to resting flows. At rest there is no pressure-flow abnormality for which the distal vascular bed needs to compensate. Compensatory changes of the distal coronary vascular bed develop only for stenoses above 60% diameter narrowing and are relatively ineffective for stenoses above 85%. Vasodilatory reserve is still present despite stenoses that reduce resting coronary flow (4). This observation has been subsequently confirmed by Canty et al. (5), with additional information on transmural flow distribution, discussed below.

These data explain why resting coronary flow remains normal with progressive coronary artery stenosis until very severe narrowing is reached. It is a common misconception that compensatory distal coronary vasodilation maintains resting flow with progressive narrowing, shown here not to play a major role. The correct explanation is that at resting conditions, resistance of the non-stenotic coronary vascular bed is so high at 2.37 mm Hg/cc flow that a severe stenosis has to be present before its resistance approaches this value. From Figure 3.5, measured stenosis resistance (open circles) approaches 2.37 mm Hg/cc flow only at approximately 85% to 90% diameter narrowing. At resting conditions, compensatory distal coronary vasodilation does not begin until a significant resting stenosis pressure gradient develops at approximately 60% to 70% diameter narrowing, as in Figures 3.5, 3.6, and 3.7.

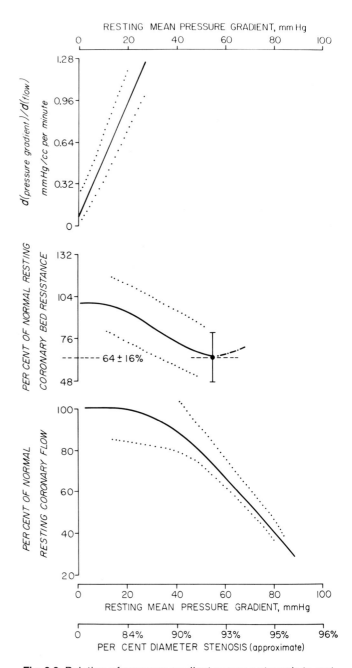

Fig. 3.8 Relation of pressure gradient across a stenosis to resting coronary flow, distal vascular bed resistance, and the slope of the gradient-flow relation during hyperemia. Vertical axes are identical to those of Figure 3.7. Reproduced with permission from Gould KL, Lipscomb K, Calvert C, 1975. (4).

With progressive narrowing beyond this point, compensatory vasodilation begins to occur. Additional flow demands, as with exercise, may increase flow somewhat but also cause a proportionately greater pressure gradient and fall in perfusion pressure distal to the stenosis. This fall in coronary pressure distal to a flow-limiting stenosis after increased flow demands may cause subendocardial ischemia and angina pectoris, particularly with the tachycardia of exercise.

PHYSIOLOGIC CONSEQUENCES OF DECREASED CORONARY PERFUSION PRESSURE DISTAL TO A CORONARY ARTERY STENOSIS

Experimentally, at a fixed heart rate of 60, decreased coronary perfusion pressure reduces perfusion uniformly in subendocardium and subepicardium (5). No selective underperfusion of subendocardium is observed as perfusion pressure falls, until reaching a distal coronary perfusion pressure of 25 mm Hg. At pressures above this level, pharmacologic vasodilator reserve remains uniform transmurally in both subepicardium and subendocardium. At pressures below 25 mm Hg, pharmacologic vasodilation does not increase subendocardial flow further while epicardial flow reserve remains. Therefore, in the absence of tachycardia, endocardial vasodilator reserve persists to pressures of 25–35 mm Hg and maintains normal subendocardial perfusion. At lower pressures, subendocardial vasodilator reserve is exhausted before epicardial vasodilator reserve (5).

Tachycardia and shortened diastolic flow period impair subendocardial flow for a given distal coronary perfusion pressure. Downey et al. (6) and Bellamy et al. (7) have demonstrated that reactive hyperemia after temporary coronary occlusion occurs first in the subepicardium, with a delay in reactive hyperemia of the subendocardium, as shown in Figure 3.9. Therefore, after systolic compression empties the vascular bed, the surge of diastolic flow reaches the subepicardium first, with a delay in early diastolic flow reaching the subendocardium.

The degree of delay in the early diastolic flow surge after systolic compression depends on coronary perfusion pressure. At normal perfusion pressure, this delay is not significant enough to impair subendocardial flow, even with short diastolic duration of tachycardia. However, with low perfusion pressure, the time required to perfuse the subendocardium after systolic compression is longer than diastole during tachycardia, thereby causing subendocardial ischemia.

This delayed subendocardial diastolic perfusion after systolic compression explains the susceptibility of subendocardium to ischemia. Neither tachycardia alone nor lowered coronary perfusion pressure distal to a stenosis alone (down to 25 mm Hg) will reduce subendocardial flow (5). However, tachycardia with increased flow demands arising from exercise and lowered perfusion pressure distal to a flow-limiting stenosis impairs diastolic perfusion of subendocardium. Since the subepicardium is not subject to the same compressive systolic forces or to delay in diastolic perfusion, its perfusion is not as tenuous as for the subendocardium.

Any factors that delay subendocardial diastolic perfusion after systolic compression are likely to contribute to subendocardial ischemia during tachycardia. In addition to coronary artery stenosis, left ventricular hypertrophy, delayed left ventricular diastolic relaxation, elevated left ventricular end diastolic pressure, and excess coronary arteriolar tone all may contribute to delayed subendocardial diastolic perfusion after systolic compression. These factors added together in some circumstances combined with tachycardia may cause subendocardial ischemia. However, coronary artery stenosis is the severest limitation to rapid subendocardial perfusion after systole, since the stenosis prevents or damps out the rapid diastolic flow increase that is present normally, as discussed in detail in the next chapter.

Although the antianginal mechanism of beta blockade is considered to be reduced demands by lowering heart rate and contractile force, an important unrecognized benefit is prevention of shortened diastole associated with tachycardia, thereby improving subendocardial perfusion despite lowered coronary perfusion pressure distal to a stenosis during exercise. Drugs that lower heart rate alone may act as antianginal agents by improving subendocardial perfusion by prolonging diastolic myocardial perfusion, in addition to lowering oxygen demands.

MEAN PRESSURE-FLOW CHARACTERISTICS OF SEQUENTIAL CORONARY ARTERY STENOSES

Examples of mean pressure-flow relations for each of two stenoses in series are shown in Figure 3.10 (2). The slope of each regression line (R) is indicated beside each line. Figure 3.10A illustrates the separate individual regression lines of two coronary stenoses (R_p, proximal, and R_d, distal) in series. The slope of total mean pressure-flow relation (R_t) across both stenoses was calculated from normalized flow and total pressure gradient. It is equal to the sum of the slopes of the mean pressure-flow relation of the proximal (R_p) and distal (R_d) stenosis separately. Figure 3.10B illustrates the same pressure-flow relations and slopes with a relatively greater distal constriction. The slope of the regression line characterizing this greater distal stenosis is much steeper than before, indicating a greater gradient for a given flow level. For these stenoses of different severities, the slope of the mean pressure-flow relation for the total pressure gradient across both stenoses is equal to the sum of slopes for each stenosis separately. One hundred twenty-five pairs of stenoses in se-

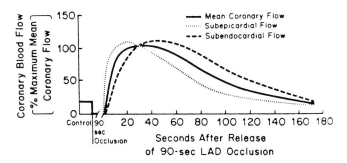

Fig. 3.9 Coronary flow as a percent of maximal flow versus time during reactive hyperemia. The increases in flow occur earlier in subepicardial than subendocardial layers. Reproduced with permission from Downey HF, Crystal GJ, Bashour FA, 1983. (6).

ries were experimentally analyzed, with all behaving in this manner (2).

In these studies, the slope of the mean pressure-flow relation of the anatomically fixed proximal stenosis was observed to decrease slightly as the distal stenosis became more severe, illustrated in Figure 3.11 for two stenoses in series; the proximal constriction was anatomically fixed at 75% narrowing, while the distal constriction was progressively increased (2). As the slope of the mean pressure-flow relation of the distal stenosis increased from less than 1 up to 42, the pressure-flow slope of the fixed proximal stenosis decreased from approximately 10 to five. This modest decrease to half the initial slope was a relatively small change compared with the increase of greater than 40 times for the distal stenosis.

On the average, the resistance of the anatomically fixed

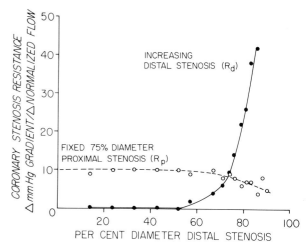

Fig. 3.11 Relation of the coronary stenosis gradient-flow slope for a fixed proximal 75%-diameter stenosis to percent diameter narrowing of a progressive distal stenosis. As distal constriction increases, distal stenosis gradient-flow slope (R_d) increases; however, the gradient-flow slope of the anatomically fixed proximal 75%-diameter stenosis (R_p) decreases slightly in comparison with the large increase in severity of the distal stenosis. Reproduced with permission from Lipscomb K, Gould KL, 1975. (2).

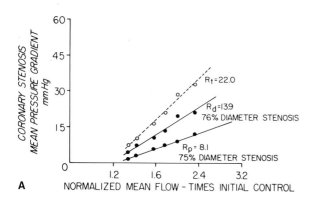

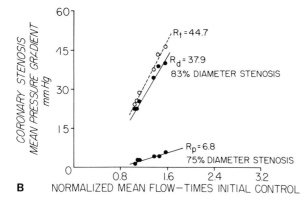

Fig. 3.10 (**A**) Representative regression lines relating normalized mean circumflex coronary flow to the stenosis gradient across a proximal (R_p) and distal (R_d) stenosis separately and to the total gradient across both stenoses together (R_t). The slope of each regression line is given beside the line. Numerical values of proximal stenosis gradient-flow slope (R_p), distal stenosis slope (R_d), and total slope of both together (R_t) are shown. Total gradient-flow slope, R_t, calculated separately from the total pressure gradient-flow relations, always equals the sum of the slopes for each individual stenosis. Gradient-flow slopes for two moderately severe, relatively similar stenoses are shown as well as their sum total slope. (**B**) Relations are as described in **A**; however, the distal stenosis is much greater than the proximal one. Total gradient-flow slope is still equal to the sum of each individual slope in series. Reproduced with permission from Lipscomb K, Gould KL, 1975. (2).

proximal stenosis decreased to 0.6 times its initial value as the distal stenosis increased by an average of 34 times. This relatively minor decrease in the resistance of the fixed proximal lesion after the addition of a more severe distal stenosis is probably due to the distal stenosis eliminating exit turbulence downstream from a proximal stenosis, as observed in vitro (8). Elimination of downstream turbulence and the kinetic energy loss associated with it would theoretically reduce the energy loss, and therefore pressure loss, across the proximal stenosis for a given flow level. This decreased pressure gradient for any given flow value would be reflected as a slightly decreased resistance, even if the proximal stenosis were anatomically fixed.

LIMITATIONS OF MEAN PRESSURE-FLOW DATA

Analysis of mean pressure-flow data has provided considerable insight into the hemodynamic behavior of coronary stenoses and its interaction with the coronary vascular bed. However, mean pressure-flow analysis raises a major conceptual difficulty in describing stenosis severity. The mean pressure gradient-flow relation for coronary artery stenoses in vivo are uniformly linear, with high linear correlation coefficients of 0.98 to 0.99 in many hundreds of stenoses over a wide range of flows, stenosis severities, and sequential stenoses in series (1–4). However, according to basic fluid-dynamic principles derived in vitro, the pressure loss across a narrowed tube is related to flow by a quadratic equation containing terms for viscous pressure loss related linearly to flow and inertial pressure loss related to flow raised to the second power. Classical, proven fluid-dynamic equations therefore indicate that the pressure gradient-flow relation characterizing a stenosis should be curvilinear, with proportionately increasing pressure loss as flow increases due to a term dependent on flow squared. This apparent fundamental disagreement between fluid-dynamic equations for stenotic tubes in vitro and the pressure gradient-flow relation based on measured mean data in vivo was not initially clear (1–4) but has now been explained, as reviewed in the next chapter.

REFERENCES

1. Gould KL, Lipscomb K, Hamilton GW. A physiologic basis for assessing critical coronary stenosis. Am J Cardiol 33:87–94, 1974.
2. Gould KL, Lipscomb K. Effects of coronary stenoses on coronary flow reserve and resistance. Am J Cardiol 34:48–54, 1974.
3. Lipscomb K, Gould KL. Mechanism of the effect of coronary artery stenosis on coronary flow in the dog. Am Heart J 89:60–67, 1975.
4. Gould KL, Lipscomb K, Calvert C. Compensatory changes of the distal coronary vascular bed during progressive coronary constriction. Circulation 51:1085–94, 1975.
5. Canty JM, Klocke FJ. Reduced myocardial perfusion in the presence of pharmacologic vasodilator reserve. Circulation 71:370–77, 1985.
6. Downey HF, Crystal GJ, Bashour FA. Asynchronous transmural perfusion during coronary reactive hyperemia. Cardiovas Res 17:200–06, 1983.
7. Bellamy RF, Lowensohn HS, Olsson RA. Factors determining delayed peak flow in canine myocardial reactive hyperemia. Cardiovas Res 13:147–51, 1979.
8. Robbins SL, Bentov I. The kinetics of viscous flow in a model vessel. Lab Invest 16:864–74, 1967.

4

Phasic Pressure-Flow and Fluid-Dynamic Analysis

BASIC FLUID-DYNAMIC PRINCIPLES

According to fluid-dynamic equations for flow in rigid tubes (1–15), the energy or pressure losses across a coronary artery stenosis occur primarily because of two geometric characteristics: narrowness of the arterial lumen, and its abrupt expansion at the distal end as it opens into the normal-sized artery. Along the narrowed lumen of the stenosis, viscous friction is generated by the layers of blood sliding against each other and against the endothelium of the artery. This same phenomenon occurs in all arteries (normal or abnormal), but because it is inversely related to the fourth power of the lumen diameter, the energy loss due to viscous friction is great in the narrowed, diseased artery. The pressure loss accompanying viscous friction is also directly proportional to the length of the narrowing, the viscosity of blood, and the flow through the stenosis.

Flow of blood out of the stenotic lumen and into the distal normal-sized artery is analogous to flow of water from a narrow chute of rapids into a wide river. As flow emerges from the narrowing, inertia or momentum keeps it moving forward, not allowing it to expand immediately with the enlarged flow channel. The bulk of the flow therefore separates from the channel boundaries and mixes violently with the surrounding slow-moving blood, thereby forming eddies, localized turbulence and jets, all of which dissipate energy. The energy lost in this abrupt expansion is therefore termed an inertial loss and increases with the square of blood flow. Expansion loss depends primarily on kinetic energy of flow at the point of flow separation (at, or just distal to, the minimal stenotic area section), which is inversely related to the minimal stenotic area squared when expressed in terms of the volumetric flow rate, Q. There is a minor inertial loss at the entrance to a stenosis, but it is small enough to ignore in vivo.

Inertial energy loss due to pulsatility of coronary blood flow appears to contribute little to the more important exit inertial pressure losses across moderately stenotic coronary arteries, for several reasons. Rapid changes in coronary flow are confined to the brief periods of isovolumetric contraction and relaxation. During the remainder of diastole, time-dependent changes in flow are much smaller, and instantaneous pressure losses are dominated by the viscous and expansion

components. Even modestly severe coronary artery stenoses dampen the coronary flow waveform, thereby reducing its pulsatile shape. Thus, for purposes of analyzing the instantaneous diastolic pressure drop across significant coronary stenoses, blood flow can be considered as quasi-steady (1,3,4,9,14).

The total pressure drop across a stenosis is the sum of viscous and expansion losses, expressed in the general form of a quadratic equation relating pressure gradient, ΔP, across a stenosis to the volumetric flow, Q, through it as follows:

$$\Delta P = fQ + sQ^2$$

where f is the constant of pressure loss due to the viscous friction and s is the constant describing inertial pressure loss due to expansion and separation of flow profile (11–13). At resting conditions with relatively low coronary flow, the first term, due to viscous friction, accounts for the greatest proportion of total pressure loss. However, at high-flow conditions, the second term accounts for a greater proportion of the total pressure loss, because the effect of this expansion term increases as the square of blood flow.

Based on hydraulic studies of flow through pipes with narrowed segments and abrupt expansion in vitro, flow from the proximal portion of the stenoses to its minimal area is laminar and fully developed, thereby implying that flow velocities are parabolically distributed across the lumen in this segment. At the minimal area section, or slightly distal to it, the flow separates and thereafter behaves as a one-dimensional flow through an abrupt expansion in a pipe (in which the velocity profiles are everywhere flat). The constants f and s are then related to stenosis geometry as follows:

$$f = \frac{8\pi\mu L}{A_s^2} \quad \text{and} \quad s = \frac{P}{2}\left(\frac{1}{A_s} - \frac{1}{A_n}\right)^2$$

where ΔP is pressure loss across the stenosis, μ is absolute blood viscosity, L is stenosis length, A_n is the cross-sectional area of the normal artery, A_s is the cross-sectional area of the stenotic segment, Q is volume flow, and P is blood density. The critical dimensions are stenosis length raised to the first power, and diameter of the stenotic segment and of the normal artery raised to the fourth power. Since the stenosis diameter affects flow by a fourth-power term, a small change in stenosis diameter may cause a profound effect on pressure or flow, whereas length has a proportionately lesser effect. For tapering stenoses, the length-cross-section area effects are integrated.

If these geometric dimensions are known or measured on coronary arteriograms, the functional or hemodynamic characteristics of the stenosis may be predicted by substituting the geometric dimensions into these equations. The result is a specific quadratic equation, with known values of f and s characteristic of a given stenosis describing the relation of the pressure gradient to flow. A graphic plot of ΔP on the vertical axis and Q on the horizontal axis for the quadratic equation above would show the pressure gradient-flow relation curving upward over the range of pressures and flows of one diastole at resting control conditions.

This equation may also be written for flow velocity rather than volume flow. The velocity and flow equations are compared below, where the terms are as before, V is flow velocity, and F and S are friction and separation coefficients, respectively, for the velocity equation (11–13).

$$\Delta P = \frac{8\pi\mu L}{A_s}\left(\frac{A_n}{A_s}\right)V + \frac{P}{2}\left(\frac{A_n}{A_s} - 1\right)^2 V^2$$

or

$$\Delta P = FV + SV^2 \tag{1}$$

$$\Delta P = \frac{8\pi\mu L}{A_s}\left(\frac{1}{A_s}\right)Q + \frac{P}{2}\left(\frac{1}{A_s} - \frac{1}{A_n}\right)^2 Q^2$$

or

$$\Delta P = fQ + sQ^2 \tag{2}$$

In the flow equation (Equation 2), $1/A_n$ is much smaller than $1/A_s$ for stenoses of modest to severe degree. Therefore, A_n, or the normal size of the artery, has little influence on severity of stenosis in the flow equation, and changes in the normal arterial diameter due to vasomotion have little effect on resulting pressure gradient–flow relation describing stenosis severity by the flow equation. Thus, stenotic severity in the flow equation depends primarily on the absolute diameter of the stenotic segment, not on relative percent stenosis, and also accounts for the modest effects of normal artery diameter.

Severity of stenosis in the velocity equation (Equation 1) is highly dependent on relative percent stenosis as well as on absolute stenosis diameter. There is no term in the equation for lumen area of the normal arterial segment other than as the reciprocal of percent narrowing (A_n/A_s). Since cross-sectional lumen area of the normal arterial segment, A_n, times flow velocity, V, equals volume flow, Q, an increase in A_n due to vasodilation for a constant flow results in a fall in flow velocity, V. For constant coronary blood flow and fixed segmental stenosis, vasodilation of the normal arterial segment causes flow velocity to decrease for any given pressure gradient. This lower flow velocity for any pressure gradient makes the pressure gradient–velocity characteristics for the stenosis steeper. Therefore, the pressure gradient–velocity relation becomes steeper or worsens with vasodilation of the normal part of the artery in the presence of a fixed stenotic segment with constant flow and pressure gradient. Describing

stenosis severity by a pressure gradient–flow velocity relation may therefore suggest worsening stenosis during vasodilation of the normal segment of artery on either side of a fixed stenosis for which the gradient-volume flow relation is little changed. The consequences of this observation are surprising and explain why percent diameter narrowing so poorly describes functional severity of stenoses, as discussed subsequently.

Both equations show that the pressure gradient across a stenosis increases sharply and in a progressive curvilinear fashion with increases in coronary flow. Therefore, the effects of a stenosis will be least at resting coronary flow and greatest at high flows. The question now arises, do these theoretical quadratic pressure–flow relations fit those measured experimentally in vivo?

ANALYSIS OF PHASIC PRESSURE-FLOW DATA AT RESTING CONDITIONS

In chronically instrumented awake dogs with intact coronary control mechanisms, the relation of coronary flow or flow velocity to the pressure drop across coronary artery stenoses of varying severity has been described (11–13).

Coronary flow velocity or flow and stenosis pressure gradient show characteristic phasic patterns, illustrated in Figure 4.1. In early systole, distal left circumflex coronary pressure rose slightly before aortic root pressure, thereby producing a sudden momentary pressure reversal, with coronary pressure being higher than aortic pressure. Immediately thereafter, coronary flow velocity fell with the typical early systolic phasic pattern due to systolic myocardial compression of the coronary capillary bed. In the presence of a stenosis, this momentary, early systolic drop or reversal of aorta to coronary pressure gradient always preceded the systolic deceleration of coronary flow. In late systole and very early diastole, as myocardial compression ended, coronary flow increased rapidly during a phase of flow acceleration. In midsystole and throughout diastole, these sudden decelerative and accelerative changes in flow were absent.

During progressive coronary constriction under resting conditions, diastolic flow *decreased* and systolic flow *increased* until the characteristic phasic pattern of coronary flow was damped out with mean coronary flow still normal, as in Figure 4.1. Further coronary constriction caused a fall in mean flow. When mean flow was reduced to half or less of control values, the phasic pattern of coronary flow resembled the aortic pressure pattern, with systolic flow being higher than diastolic flow.

Figure 4.2A shows the primary pressure gradient–flow velocity recordings and Figure 4.2B shows a typical example of the relation between coronary flow velocity and the pressure gradient for a stenosis under resting conditions (11). Throughout diastole and midsystole, the relation followed a curve of the general form $\Delta P = FV + SV^2$. During systolic flow deceleration, the pressure gradient was proportionately lower than flow, compared to the rest of the cardiac cycle, because systole increased pressure in the coronary artery by direct compression of the coronary vascular bed. An early systolic decrease in the pressure gradient preceded the sys-

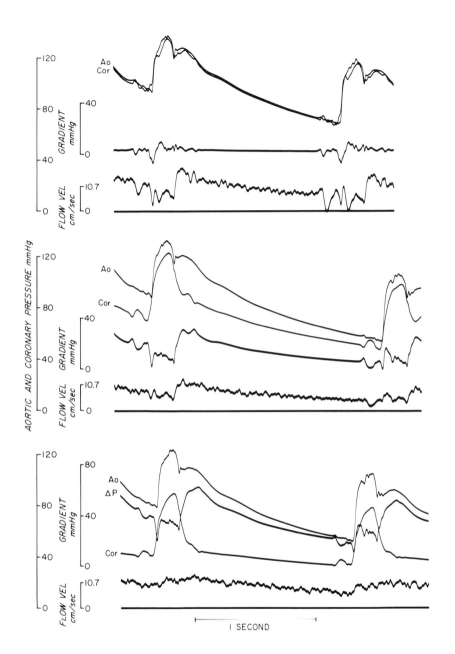

Fig. 4.1 Recordings of coronary flow velocity, aortic pressure, and coronary pressure distal to progressive stenosis of the left circumflex coronary artery at resting, baseline flow conditions. For the upper panel there was a mild coronary artery narrowing. The middle and lower panels show progressively severe coronary artery stenoses.

tolic fall in flow, and the gradient even became negative or reversed momentarily (coronary pressure greater than aortic root pressure), thereby producing a downward-directed "tail" (dotted lines) at the lower, left end of the gradient-flow velocity relation. During diastolic flow acceleration, the pressure gradient increased before flow increased and was therefore proportionately larger than flow, compared to the rest of the cardiac cycle. This increase in the pressure gradient in early diastole preceded the increase in flow until reaching peak values of flow at the upper, right end of the gradient-flow graph. Consequently, the acceleration phase appeared as an open "loop" (dashed lines) extending from late systole at the lower left to early diastole at the upper right of the gradient-flow graph.

The flow deceleration tail and acceleration loop were due to the inertia of coronary blood flow and were therefore more dependent on strength of contraction, heart rate, and epicardial artery compliance than on severity of stenosis. The purely fluid-dynamic character of the stenosis—that is, the pressure gradient–flow velocity relation characteristic of the stenosis without the extraneous effects of deceleration and acceleration—is shown in Figure 4.2C. Here the data points during decelerative and accelerative phases of coronary flow during the cardiac cycle have been manually edited out and discarded.

The distortion of the pressure gradient–flow velocity relation by these inertial factors was marked for short cardiac cycles (tachycardia) having a narrow range of pressure and velocity data. The pressure gradient–flow velocity relation was so distorted by flow acceleration with pressure gradient

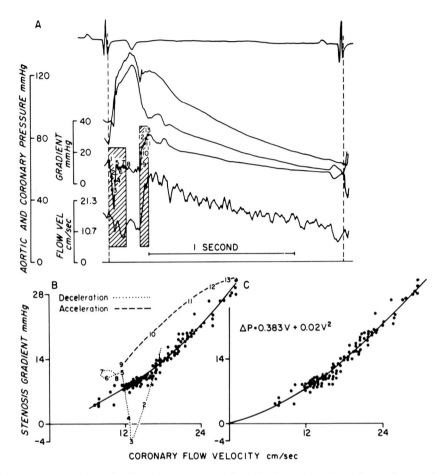

Fig. 4.2 Relation between coronary flow velocity and pressure gradient due to a stenosis under resting control conditions. Panel A shows the original pressure and velocity recordings. Panel B shows the relation between the pressure gradient, ΔP, on the vertical axis and flow velocity, V, on the horizontal axis. The numbered points on the gradient-velocity relation correspond to the numbered points on the original recordings and illustrate the effects of early systolic deceleration and late systolic acceleration of flow (shaded areas). Panel C shows the gradient-velocity relation after the effects of deceleration and acceleration, which were unrelated to the severity of the stenosis, had been discarded. The passive diastolic relation is characterized by a quadratic equation. The first, or linear, term gives the pressure loss due to viscous friction, and the second, or nonlinear, term gives the pressure loss due to flow separation. In the example shown, the coefficient of friction loss is 0.383 and the coefficient of separation loss is 0.02, both characteristic of moderate stenoses. Reproduced with permission from Gould KL, 1978. (11).

reversal during early systole and flow deceleration with pressure gradient augmentation during early diastole that mean pressure flow measurements did not fit the characteristic quadratic curvilinear pressure flow relation expected from the fluid-dynamic equations for stenosis geometry.

Therefore, analysis of stenosis severity from phasic-pressure flow recordings in vivo required the passive diastolic pressure gradient–velocity relation with elimination of the accelerative phase of early diastole and decelerative phase of systole. When only postaccelerative diastolic data were used, the pressure-flow characteristics of coronary artery stenoses under resting, control conditions in unsedated dogs were described by a quadratic equation containing a linear term describing the pressure loss due to viscous friction and a nonlinear term describing the pressure loss due to flow separation at the distal end of the stenosis. The findings, therefore, demonstrate the validity of applying in-vitro fluid-

dynamic equations to the awake animal under resting conditions during the diastolic phase of coronary flow.

PHASIC RESTING PRESSURE-FLOW CHANGES WITH PROGRESSIVE CORONARY ARTERY STENOSIS

The pattern of systolic flow deceleration and diastolic flow acceleration changed with progressive stenosis. With mild to moderate stenoses, the phasic form of the pressure gradient and the phasic form of coronary flow changed differently. In the presence of coronary artery stenosis, systolic compression produced a rise in distal coronary pressure before aortic pressure, with a momentary reversal or decrease in the stenosis pressure gradient and a subsequent deceleration or fall in coronary flow, all unrelated to stenosis severity. This ob-

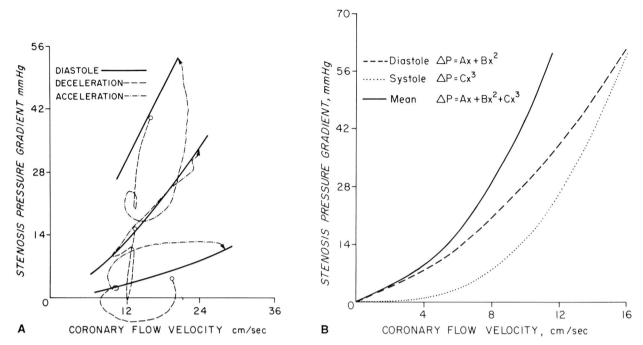

Fig. 4.3 (**A**) Pressure gradient–velocity relation of three cardiac cycles: one at resting baseline coronary flow, one at maximum coronary flow, and one at an intermediate range of coronary flow after intracoronary papaverine. The altered pressure gradient–velocity relation during systolic deceleration and early diastolic acceleration of coronary blood flow are also indicated (broken lines). Reproduced with permission from Gould KL, 1982. (15). (**B**) Pressure-flow relation of systole, diastole, and their sum, or mean pressure-flow relation, of a fixed coronary artery stenosis.

servation again suggests that pressure energy was momentarily transmitted directly to the coronary circulation during early systole, independent of, and without being transmitted from, the aorta through the stenosis to the distal coronary artery. This systolic change in pressure gradient was therefore not related to flow through the artery, to stenosis severity, or to the geometric characteristics of the stenosis.

In the presence of coronary artery stenosis, at end systole and early diastole, myocardial relaxation again resulted in a sudden fall in distal coronary pressure before the diastolic fall in aortic pressure. There was a corresponding increase in aortic- to coronary-pressure gradient, followed by acceleration of coronary flow, also independent of stenosis severity. These inertial effects of deceleration and acceleration were independent of the geometric characteristic of the stenosis for mild to moderate stenoses; they appeared to be affected by heart rate, the vigor of myocardial contraction, compliance of the epicardial coronary arteries, and the rate of myocardial relaxation at end systole. With more severe stenoses, the characteristic phasic pattern of coronary flow was damped out due to systolic flow increasing and diastolic flow decreasing; however, the phasic changes in pressure gradient due to systolic compression and diastolic relaxation remained the same for mild to moderate stenosis as without stenosis. Therefore, the pressure gradient during systole for a given flow was less than the pressure gradient during diastole for the same coronary flow. Consequently, during systole the gradient-flow relation was shifted downward, indicating a lower pressure gradient for a given flow in systole as compared to diastole. With still more severe constriction, mean coronary flow fell. The pattern of flow then followed that of aortic pressure, with the greatest flow occurring during systole and lowest flow during diastole.

For a fixed stenosis, systolic flow deceleration and diastolic flow acceleration changed as flow increased, shown in Figure 4.3A (15). The systolic pressure gradient during systolic flow deceleration was always less than the passive diastolic gradient, regardless of whether coronary flow was high or low. The pressure gradient during diastolic acceleration was higher than the rest of diastole for mild stenoses, due to the sudden flow increase after systolic compression. For severe stenoses, it was lower than the rest of the diastolic gradient, owing to damping of diastolic flow increase after systole. The mean pressure gradient–flow velocity relation for diastole and systole are graphed separately over a range of flows in Figure 4.3B. These effects of myocardial contraction and relaxation on the fluid dynamics of a stenosis are unique to the coronary circulation and do not apply to systemic arteries.

LIMITATIONS OF APPLYING FLUID-DYNAMIC EQUATIONS TO CORONARY ARTERIES IN VIVO

The application of traditional fluid-dynamic equations over a range of coronary flows in vivo is complicated by several physiologic characteristics of the coronary circulation not accounted for by in-vitro rigid tube models, or by plastic plug stenoses in vivo or in anesthetized preparations. The first characteristic is systolic flow deceleration and diastolic flow acceleration, discussed above. The second complication is caused by active vasomotor change of large epicardial coronary arteries on either side of a fixed stenotic segment of the artery, which alters its geometry and fluid-dynamic severity. Epicardial coronary arteries are vasoactive (16–19), depending on the extent of diffuse disease in the arterial wall, on the technique for measuring diameter changes, and on the stimulus for epicardial vasodilation. With relatively severe stenoses, a small increase in percent-diameter narrowing produces marked hemodynamic effects. Similarly, a small increase in divergence angle from only 10° to 30° will markedly increase flow separation, whereas greater changes of more acute angles, such as from 40° to 90°, have little additional effect (20–22). Thus, even a modest increase in percent-diameter narrowing and increased divergence angle resulting from normal artery vasodilation adjacent to a fixed stenosis may have significant hemodynamic effect. The third limitation is in the use of flow velocity rather than volume flow. As the normal segment of epicardial coronary artery vasodilates, the

flow velocity falls for a constant flow and pressure gradient across a fixed stenosis. Therefore, the phasic pressure gradient–flow velocity relation may become steeper, implying more severe stenosis, while the volume flow–pressure gradient relation of biological importance is little changed. The fourth limitation is due to flexible arterial wall segments at the narrowest part of a stenosis, which may collapse at high flows, as discussed in detail subsequently.

In man, coronary artery vasodilation makes the relative percent stenosis of coronary lesions appear worse on angiograms than it does before vasodilation (23). Vasoconstriction and dilation of the narrowest segment of coronary arteries also occurs in man, with significant hemodynamic consequences (14–18). Therefore, the hemodynamic changes observed in intact, awake dogs are pertinent to patients with coronary disease. A coronary artery stenosis may vary geometrically over a period of minutes, and its pressure gradient–flow or flow-velocity relations may also change dynamically, depending on the physiological characteristics of the rest of the artery. Since coronary arteries and stenoses are not fixed, pipe-like tubes, these limitations and the applicability of traditional fluid-dynamic equations in vivo need

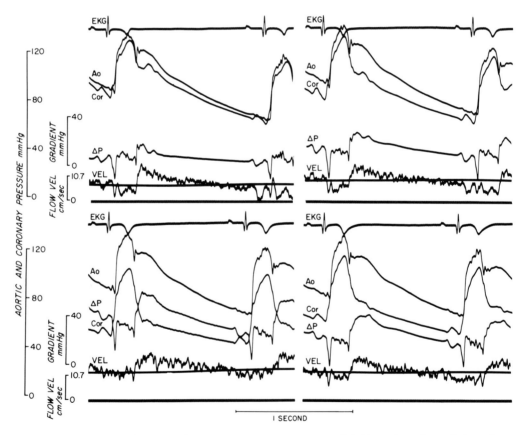

Fig. 4.4 Recordings of coronary flow velocity, aortic pressure, coronary pressure distal to a stenosis, and stenosis pressure gradient (ΔP) under resting baseline conditions (upper left) and during coronary vasodilation at onset (upper right), at peak (lower left), and after peak vasodilation (lower right). During vasodilation, flow velocity increased, the phasic pattern of coronary flow became damped, and the pressure gradient, ΔP (aortic pressure minus distal coronary pressure) increased. Momentary gradient reversal, with coronary pressure higher than aortic pressure, characteristically occurred in early systole. Reproduced with permission from Gould KL, 1978. (11).

to be examined over a range of coronary blood flows and differing states of vasomotion, as described below and in subsequent chapters.

PHASIC PRESSURE-FLOW CHARACTERISTICS OF CORONARY STENOSES AT HIGH FLOW CONDITIONS

Figure 4.4 shows pressure and flow velocity recordings in the presence of a mild, fixed coronary stenosis under control, baseline conditions and during the increased flow produced by selective coronary arteriolar vasodilation after intracoronary papaverine (11). Under resting, baseline conditions (upper left panel), the pressure gradient was small and coronary flow velocity showed its characteristic phasic pattern. During coronary vasodilation following intracoronary injection of papaverine, the gradient became more severe as flow increased. As mean coronary flow increased (upper right panel), systolic flow increased proportionally more than diastolic flow until phasic variation was damped out at peak mean flow for a fixed constant stenosis (lower left panel). As the response to vasodilatory stimulus subsided and flow fell

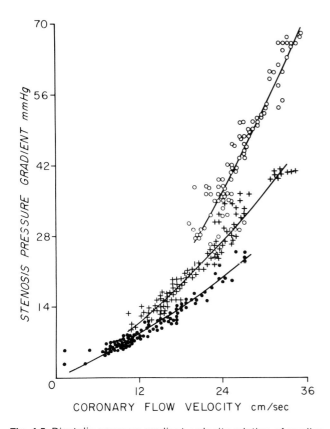

Fig. 4.5 Diastolic pressure gradient–velocity relation of cardiac cycles at resting control flow (solid circles), at peak vasodilation (open circles), and at an intermediate stage of vasodilation (crosses) with an anatomically constant, fixed stenosis. Reproduced with permission from Gould KL, 1978. (11).

towards baseline, the phasic flow changes returned to the resting pattern (lower right panel).

Figure 4.5 shows the pressure gradient–flow velocity relation for each of a series of cardiac cycles ranging from resting coronary flow up to maximum flow for one fixed stenosis in one dog. During the transient flow increase after intracoronary papaverine, this relation became steeper than at rest. In other words, the anatomically fixed stenosis became hemodynamically more severe during vasodilation, with markedly greater pressure loss at any given flow velocity, than would be predicted by the resting equation.

One reason for this worsening of the pressure gradient–flow velocity characteristics of the anatomically fixed stenosis is that the normal coronary artery just distal to the stenosis dilated and became larger while the stenotic segment remained fixed. Therefore, the relative percent stenosis and the exit angle became more severe during vasodilation of the normal segment of the artery. Relative stenosis and exit angle are major determinants of the separation coefficient, S. Therefore, with vasodilation and an increase in coronary flow, the relative stenosis became more severe, the separation coefficient became larger, and the gradient-velocity curve became steeper. This point is shown conceptually in the schema of Figure 4.6. In addition to being worse by virtue of a higher percent stenosis, vasodilation of adjacent normal artery also caused flow velocity to decrease for a given volume flow and gradient, thereby making the gradient flow–velocity reaction proportionately steeper than would be due simply to worsening percent stenosis and exit pressure losses.

The effect of vasodilating normal arterial segments on the gradient-flow characteristics of a stenosis was observed in all of the 100 stenoses studied for all of the vasodilator agents tested, including intravenous dipyridamole and intracoronary contrast medium, papaverine, or adenosine triphosphate. For all 100 stenoses, the average value of the separation coefficient, S, at rest was 0.009 ± 0.015, whereas the average peak value of S during vasodilation was 0.02 ± 0.02, a significant difference ($P < 0.001$). The relatively wide standard deviation is caused by averaging values for mild, moderate, and severe stenoses together.

As a consequence of these experiments, we were the first to report proximal epicardial coronary artery vasodilation in response to increase in coronary flow induced by distal intracoronary injection of arteriolar vasodilators or reactive hyperemia (13). This observation was subsequently confirmed by Hintze (24) and shown by Furchgott (25) and Van Houte (26) to be mediated by shear-induced release of endothelial relaxing factor (EDRF), now thought to be nitric oxide (24).

Figure 4.7 illustrates the consistency of worsening pressure gradient–flow velocity relations at high coronary flows after intracoronary papaverine or dipyridamole (11) in six examples of 100 stenoses studied. The heavy solid line of each data set is a best empirical fit of all diastolic pressure-flow data from resting to maximum flows lumped together.

These observations indicate that no single diastolic cardiac cycle characterized all of the pressure gradient-flow velocity relations observed over the entire range of flows during coronary vasodilation. Even though the narrowest stenotic segment was fixed and constant, the overall functional geometry of the stenosis in vivo was dynamic, due to vasodilation of the epicardial coronary artery adjacent to the fixed

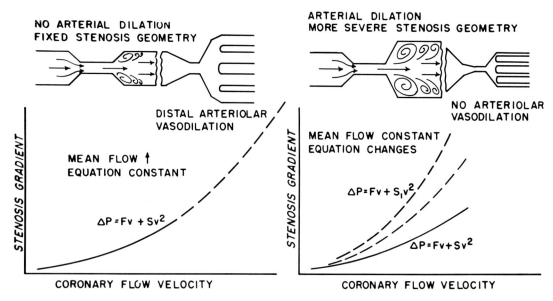

Fig. 4.6 Hypothetical scheme showing conceptually the effects of distal arteriolar vasodilation and the effects of proximal, epicardial artery vasodilatation on the geometry of the stenosis and on the gradient-velocity relation. With arteriolar vasodilation alone, stenosis geometry would remain constant and the pressure gradient, ΔP, would increase proportionately with velocity, V, according to the quadratic equation shown. With large epicardial artery vasodilation, the relative percent stenosis would become worse, since the stenotic segment would remain fixed while the adjacent normal segment of artery became larger. The angle of divergence would also become greater. Consequently, greater pressure loss due to flow separation would occur, the gradient velocity curve would become steeper, and the separation coefficient would increase from S to S_1. Reproduced with permission from Gould KL, 1978. (11).

stenotic segment. These dynamic changes in stenosis geometry were systematically related to vasodilation and therefore to the increase in coronary flow; the geometric effect of vasodilation on hemodynamic severity could be accounted for by obtaining arteriograms during maximum coronary flow, as subsequently discussed.

Figure 4.8 illustrates, for a stenosis in one dog, the extent to which the pressure gradient–velocity relation at resting coronary flow failed to predict the pressure gradient at peak flow during coronary vasodilation (11). For all 100 stenoses in all dogs, at peak flow the pressure gradient expected on the basis of the resting gradient–velocity relationship only was 64% ± 14% (P < 0.001) of the actual higher pressure gradient measured experimentally. Over and above the pressure loss due to friction and flow separation at rest, the additional pressure loss at high flows associated with altered stenosis geometry and proportionately reduced flow velocity due to larger arterial lumen area during vasodilation accounted for 36% ± 15% (P < 0.001) of the total pressure gradient at peak flow. The wide standard deviations are due

primarily to averaging data from mild, moderate, and severe stenoses together.

With progressive stenosis, there was a family of pressure gradient–flow velocity curves and equations in which the coefficients of friction (F), separation (S), and augmented separation during dilation (D) became progressively more severe for each stenosis applied. Figure 4.9A shows, for one experiment, the family of curves ranging from no stenosis (lowest curve) to a very severe stenosis (upper curve) that reduced mean resting coronary flow to 85% of control. The friction coefficient (first term) and the separation coefficients (second term) of each equation increased steadily with progressive stenosis.

The vasodilation coefficient, or third term, which indicated the effect of normal segment vasodilation, was negligible or zero with mild arterial narrowing but became larger during progressive constriction, up to very severe stenosis that reduced resting coronary flow and damped the phasic flow pattern. At that point, the third term again became negligible, since, with stenosis severe enough to reduce resting

Fig. 4.7 Examples from each dog of the gradient-velocity relation of cardiac cycles at resting control flow (solid circles), at peak vasodilation (open circles), and at an intermediate flow (crosses). The light lines show the relationship for individual cardiac diastoles. The heavy lines show the composite relationship according to a cubic equation including a term for the excess pressure gradient due to worsening percent stenosis: $\Delta P = FV + SV^2 + DV^3$. The specific values for the coefficients F, S, and D are given for each example. Only one composite curve is shown for each dog. Multiple curves were obtained over a range of stenosis severity for each dog but are not shown because of redundancy and space limitations. Reproduced with permission from Gould KL, 1978. (11).

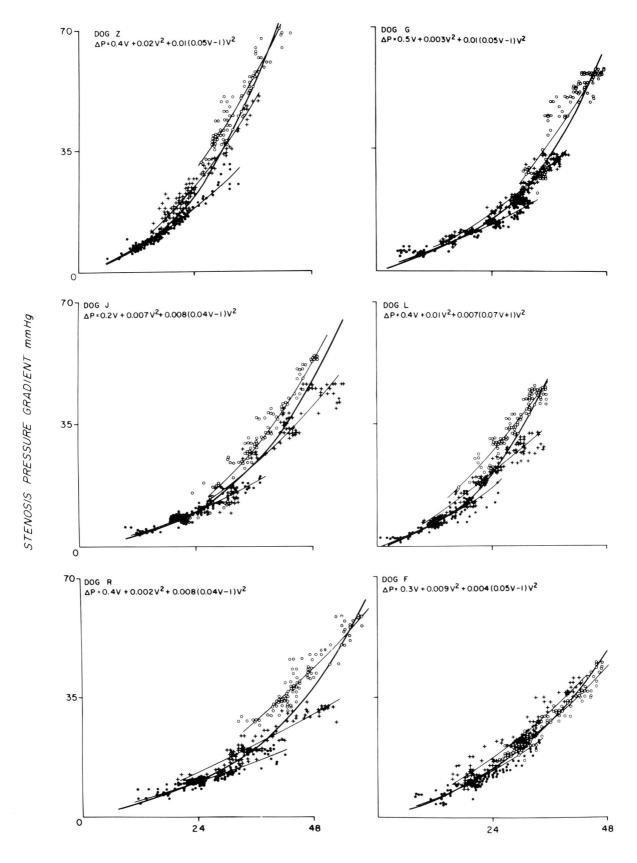

DOG Z
$\Delta P = 0.4V + 0.02V^2 + 0.01(0.05V-1)V^2$

DOG G
$\Delta P = 0.5V + 0.003V^2 + 0.01(0.05V-1)V^2$

DOG J
$\Delta P = 0.2V + 0.007V^2 + 0.008(0.04V-1)V^2$

DOG L
$\Delta P = 0.4V + 0.01V^2 + 0.007(0.07V+1)V^2$

DOG R
$\Delta P = 0.4V + 0.002V^2 + 0.008(0.04V-1)V^2$

DOG F
$\Delta P = 0.3V + 0.009V^2 + 0.004(0.05V-1)V^2$

STENOSIS PRESSURE GRADIENT mmHg

CORONARY FLOW VELOCITY cm/sec

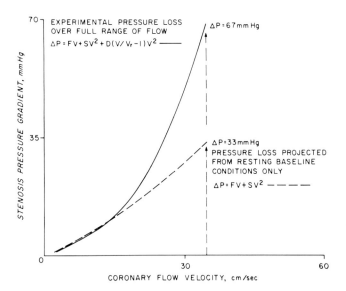

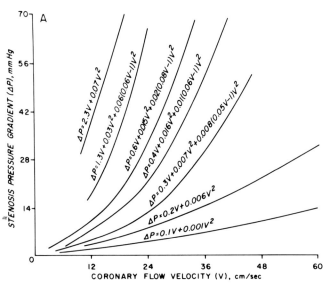

Fig. 4.8 Measured pressure gradient–velocity relation at resting coronary flow (lower dashed line) projected to high coronary flows (vertical dashed line), compared to the experimentally measured gradient-velocity relation during coronary vasodilation (solid line) for one stenosis in a dog. For this example, the equation for the gradient-velocity relationship at resting coronary flow (lower dashed line) was $\Delta P = 0.58\ V + 0.01\ V^2$ and failed to predict the experimentally observed pressure gradient (ΔP) at peak flow. The experimentally determined equation for the gradient-velocity relationship over the entire range of flow during coronary vasodilation was $\Delta P = 0.58\ V + 0.01\ V^2 + 0.017(0.07\ V\text{-}1)V^2$, owing to worsening percent stenosis. Reproduced with permission from Gould KL, 1978. (11).

blood flow, phasic patterns were damped out and coronary flow increased little or not at all after vasodilation. With such severe stenoses, flow or flow velocity uncouples or is no longer related to pressure gradient but is determined by aortic pressure alone, as discussed in the chapter on collapsing stenosis.

To analyze statistically all stenoses from all dogs together, the continuous spectrum of curves ranging from no stenosis up to stenosis that reduced resting flow were divided into arbitrary categories shown in Figure 4.9B as mild, moderate, and severe stenoses. For each of these categories, Table 4.1 shows average values of the coefficients of friction (F), of separation (S), and of augmented worsening of the pressure gradient–flow velocity relation during vasodilation (D). There is a progressive increase in pressure losses due to each of these factors as stenoses become more severe. The last column shows the projected pressure gradient (ΔP) expected at peak velocity during coronary vasodilation on the basis of the resting gradient-velocity relation, without including augmented separation losses during geometric changes with large artery vasodilation. This projected ΔP is expressed as a percent of the observed ΔP. On the average, at peak flow, the projected ΔP from the resting gradient-velocity equation alone was only 61.8% $\pm$ 14.3% of the observed ΔP for the mild stenoses. The balance, or 39.2% of the observed ΔP, was

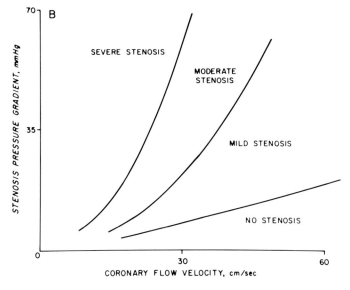

Fig. 4.9 Panel A shows composite pressure gradient–velocity relation for one dog of seven separate stenoses, ranging from no constriction up to severe constriction. Panel B shows an arbitrary classification of pressure gradient–velocity curves into categories of mild, moderate, and severe stenoses for statistical analysis shown in Tables 4.1 and 4.2. Reproduced with permission from Gould KL, 1978. (11).

due to augmented separation pressure loss and lower flow velocity associated with altered normal diameter during coronary vasodilation. Table 4.2 shows values of resting flow velocity and pressure gradient as well as peak flow velocity and pressure gradient following coronary vasodilators. Also shown are values of the separation coefficient, S, at rest and after vasodilators. The $\pm$ sign indicates $\pm$ one standard deviation. P values show significance of differences between resting and peak values.

For all stenoses in all dogs, the relative proportions of

Table 4.1 Average Hydraulic Coefficients by Stenosis Severity

	Friction, F	Coefficients separation, S	Dilation, D	Projected ΔP* (% of observed ΔP)
No stenosis	0.193 ± 0.067	0.0013 ± 0.0029	0.00076 ± 0.00138	99.5 ± 1.8
Mild stenosis	0.272 ± 0.172	0.0049 ± 0.0032†	0.0071 ± 0.0043‡	61.8 ± 14.3‡
Moderate stenosis	0.549 ± 0.217‡	0.014 ± 0.011‡	0.0167 ± 0.0099‡	64.6 ± 14.2‡
Severe stenosis	1.33 ± 0.77‡	0.0353 ± 0.0258‡	0.0315 ± 0.0319†	84.3 ± 11.3‡

Values are expressed as mean ± 1 SD.

*ΔP (pressure gradient) expected at peak velocity on basis of the rest equation.

† $P < 0.005$ compared to no stenosis by unpaired t-test.

‡ $P < 0.001$ compared to no stenosis by unpaired t-test.

Source: Adapted with permission from Gould KL, 1978. Reference 11.

Table 4.2 Changes in Presure-Flow Characteristics of Stenoses after Coronary Vasodilators

	Mean velocity (cm/sec)		Pressure gradient (mm Hg)		Separation coefficient, S	
	Rest	Peak	Rest	Peak	Rest	Peak
No stenosis	22 ± 8	54 ± 20 *	4 ± 2	11 ± 4 *	0.0013 ± 0.0029	0.0028 ± 0.0038 $P < 0.005$
Mild stenosis	28 ± 8	46 ± 9 *	11 ± 4	46 ± 11 *	0.0049 ± 0.0032	0.0118 ± 0.0066 *
Moderate stenosis	22 ± 6	31 ± 6 *	17 ± 8	60 ± 11 *	0.014 ± 0.011	0.0296 ± 0.0374 $P < 0.025$
Severe stenosis	15 ± 4	21 ± 5 $P < 0.005$	32 ± 9	63 ± 2 *	0.035 ± 0.0258	0.0437 ± 0.0264 NS†
All stenosis	25 ± 8	38 ± 2 *	13 ± 9	47 ± 19 *	0.0112 ± 0.014	0.0213 ± 0.026 *

Values are expressed as mean ± 1 SD.

* $P < 0.001$ for comparison of resting with peak values by paired t-test.

† NS = not significant.

Source: Adapted with permission from Gould KL, 1978. Reference 11.

pressure losses due to viscous friction and to flow separation were different at resting flows as compared to peak coronary flows. At resting flows, the first term of the equation, describing pressure loss due to viscous friction, accounted for 65% ± 23% of the total resting pressure gradient ($P < 0.001$), and the second term, due to flow separation, accounted for 35% ± 23% of total pressure loss ($P < 0.001$). At peak flows during coronary vasodilation, the viscous loss, or first term, decreased to 33% ± 17% of total peak pressure gradient ($P < 0.001$), whereas total separation losses, or the second and third terms together, increased to 67% ± 17% of the total ($P < 0.001$).

The question remaining is, how much of the excess steepness in the observed pressure gradient–flow velocity relation at high flows over that for a stenosis at resting flow is due to additional separation pressure loss caused by greater percent narrowing? How much is due to decreased flow velocity caused by vasodilation of normal adjacent arterial segments? The answers to these questions in the next chapter raise some basic issues about how functional stenoses severity should be described.

REFERENCES

1. Young DF. Fluid mechanics of arterial stenosis. J Biomech Eng 101:157–75, 1979.
2. Young DF, Tsai FY. Flow characteristics in models of arterial stenoses. I. Steady flow. J Biomech 6:395–410, 1973.
3. Young DF, Tsai FY. Flow characteristics in models of arterial stenoses. II. Unsteady flow. J Biomech 6:547–59, 1973.
4. Young DF, Cholvin NR, Roth AC. Pressure drop across artificially induced stenoses in the femoral arteries of dogs. Circ Res 36:735–43, 1975.
5. Young DF, Cholvin NR, Kirkeeide RL, Roth AC. Hemodynamics of arterial stenoses at elevated flow rates. Circ Res 41:99–107, 1977.
6. Seeley BD, Young DF. Effect of geometry on pressure losses across models of arterial stenoses. J Biomech 9:439–48, 1976.
7. Talukder N, Karayannacos PE, Nerem RM, Vasko JS. An experimental study of the fluid dynamics of multiple noncritical stenoses. J Biochem Eng 74–82, 1977.
8. Brown BG, Bolson E, Frimer M, Dodge HT. Quantitative coronary arteriography. Estimation of dimensions, hemodynamic resistance, and atheroma mass of coronary artery lesions using the arteriogram and digital computation. Circulation 55:329–37, 1977.
9. Mates RE, Gupta RL, Bell AC, Klocke FJ. Fluid dynamics of coronary artery stenosis. Circ Res 42:152–62, 1978.

10. Lipscomb K, Hooten S. Effect of stenotic dimensions and blood flow on the hemodynamic significance of model coronary arterial stenoses. Am J Cardiol 42:781–92, 1978.
11. Gould KL. Pressure-flow characteristics of coronary stenoses in unsedated dogs at rest and during coronary vasodilation. Circ Res 43:242–53, 1978.
12. Gould KL, Kelley KO, Bolson EL. Experimental validation of quantitative coronary arteriography for determining pressure-flow characteristics of coronary stenosis. Circulation 66:930–37, 1982.
13. Gould KL, Kelley KO. Physiological significance of coronary flow velocity and changing stenosis geometry during coronary vasodilation in awake dogs. Circ Res 50:695–704, 1982.
14. Cassanova RA, Giddens DP. Disorder distal to modeled stenoses in steady and pulsatile flow. J Biomech 11:441–53, 1978.
15. Gould KL. Hemodynamics of Coronary Stenoses in Coronary Artery Disease. Ed. A.P. Santamore, AA Bove. Urban and Schwarzenberg Pub., 1982.
16. Brown BG, Bolson E, Peterson RB, Pierce CD, Dodge HT. The mechanisms of nitroglycerin action: Stenosis vasodilation as a major component of the drug response. Circulation 64:1089–100, 1981.
17. Brown BG, Bolson EL, Dodge HT. Arteriographic assessment of coronary atherosclerosis. Review of current methods, their limitations, and clinical applications. Arteriosclerosis 2:2–15, 1982.
18. Brown BG, Lee AB, Bolson EL, Dodge HT. Reflex constriction of significant coronary stenosis as a mechanism contribution to ischemic left ventricular dysfunction during isometric exercise. Circulation 70:18–24, 1984.
19. Brown GB. Response of normal and decreased epicardial coronary arteries to vasoactive drugs: Quantitative arteriographic studies. Am J Cardiol 56:23E–29E, 1985.
20. Daugherty RL, Ingersol AC. Fluid Mechanics with Engineering Applications. New York: McGraw Hill, 1954, p. 195.
21. Daily JW, Harleman DRF. Fluid Dynamics. Reading, Mass.: Addison-Wesley, 1966, p. 316.
22. Binder RC. Fluid Mechanics (ed. 5). Englewood Cliffs, N.J.: Prentice-Hall, 1973.
23. Feldman R, Pepine C, Curry RC, Conti R. A case against the routine use of glyceryltrinitrate before coronary angiography. British Heart J 40:992–97, 1978.
24. Hintze TH, Vatner SF. Reactive dilation of large coronary arteries in conscious dogs. Circ Res 54:50–57, 1984.
25. Furchgott RF. Role of endothelium in responses of vascular smooth muscle. Circ Res 53:557–73, 1983.
26. Houte PM, Shimokawa H. Endothelium derived relaxing factor and coronary vasospasm. Circulation 80:1–9, 1989.
27. Gould KL, Lee D, Lovgren K. Techniques for arteriography and hydraulic analysis of coronary stenoses in unsedated dogs. Am J Physiol 235:H350–56, 1978.
28. Vatner SF, Franklin D, Van Citters RL. Simultaneous comparison and calibration of the Doppler and electromagnetic flowmeters. J Appl Physiol 29:907–10, 1970.
29. Gould KL. Dynamic coronary stenosis. Am J Cardiol 45:286–92, 1980.
30. Gould KL. Quantification of coronary artery stenosis in vivo. Circ Res 57:341–53, 1985.
31. Gould KL. Percent coronary stenosis: Battered gold standard, pernicious relic, or clinical practicality? J Am Coll Cardiol 11:886–88, 1988.
32. Gould KL, Goldstein RA, Mullani NA, Kirkeeide R, Wong G, Smalling R, Fuentes F, Nishikawa A, Matthews W. Noninvasive assessment of coronary stenoses by myocardial perfusion imaging during pharmacologic coronary vasodilation. VIII. Clinical feasibility of positron cardiac imaging without a cyclotron using generator-produced rubidium-82. J Am Coll Cardiol 7:775–89, 1986.
33. Marcus ML, Skorton DJ, Johnson MR, Collins SM, Harrison DG, Kerber RE. Visual estimates of percent diameter coronary stenosis: "A battered gold standard." J Am Coll Cardiol 41:882–85, 1988.
34. White CW, Wright CB, Doty DB, Hiratza LF, Eastham CL, Harrison DG, Marcus ML. Does visual interpretation of the coronary arteriogram predict the physiologic importance of a coronary stenosis? N Engl J Med 310:819–24, 1984.
35. Wilson RF, Laughlin DE, Ackell PH, Chilian WM, Holida MO, Hartley CJ, Armstron ML, Marcus ML, White CW. Transluminal, subselective measurement of coronary artery blood flow velocity and vasodilator reserve in man. Circulation 72:82–92, 1985.
36. Gould KL, Lipscomb K, Hamilton GW. Physiologic basis for assessing critical coronary stenosis: Instantaneous flow response and regional distribution during coronary hyperemia as measures of coronary flow reserve. Am J Cardiol 33:87–94, 1974.

5

Phasic Pressure-Flow
and Arteriographic Geometry

The worsening diastolic pressure gradient–flow velocity characteristics of coronary artery stenosis at high flows described in the last chapter were hypothesized as due to dynamically changing stenosis geometry. This hypothesis has been confirmed by quantitative coronary arteriography obtained at rest and at high flows after intracoronary injection of papaverine, as reviewed here (1,2). Although quantitative coronary arteriography is reviewed in detail in a subsequent chapter, results are presented here to complete the logical development of pressure-flow characteristics of coronary artery stenoses.

Stenosis geometry from coronary arteriograms taken during vasodilation (Fig. 5.1A) (3) changed in comparison to the arteriograms taken at rest in chronically instrumented awake dogs (1–4). To study effects of geometric changes early in the course of coronary vasodilation, a subset of 28 stenoses was studied by orthogonal arteriograms taken at 10 s after distal intracoronary injection of papaverine during maximum coronary flow. Arteriograms were also taken at 60 s after papaverine, when coronary flow had fallen toward baseline (Table 5.1) (2). During maximum coronary flow 10 s after intracoronary papaverine, there was a small but statistically significant reduction in minimum stenosis lumen area from 0.39 ± 0.15 mm^2 at rest to 0.36 ± 0.16 mm^2 (P = 0.002). Normal segments of the vessel on either side of the stenotic segment increased somewhat in size during early vasodilation but showed greatest vasodilation at 60 s after papaverine, when coronary flow had begun to return toward baseline. Therefore, there was a time lag in the large epicardial artery vasodilation of approximately 50 s after peak coronary flow due to arteriolar vasodilation. The small decrease in the minimum stenosis area during early vasodilation was probably due to passive collapse in the stenotic segment by the Bernoulli effect when flow velocities were high, as detailed in a subsequent chapter.

Mean data for a total of 51 stenoses in Table 5.2 were obtained at rest and during vasodilation from arteriograms taken 60 s after distal intracoronary injection of papaverine, when epicardial arterial vasodilation appeared maximal (2). At this point, flow velocity was lower than the peak levels immediately following intracoronary injection of papaverine, and the partial passive collapse of the narrowest segment of

the stenosis had nearly disappeared. For all 51 stenoses studied at 60 s after papaverine, there was no significant change from control in the minimal cross-sectional area at the site of the constriction, the mean value at rest being 0.40 ± 0.16 mm^2 and at vasodilation being 0.40 ± 0.02 mm^2, although early in the course of vasodilation there was a transient decrease in this dimension at 10 s after papaverine.

There were significant changes in size of the normal vessel on either side of the stenosis. During vasodilation at 60 s after intracoronary papaverine, the cross-sectional area of the proximal portion of the vessel increased from 4.98 ± 2.09 to 5.87 ± 2.67 mm^2, and distal vessel cross-sectional area increased from 4.44 ± 1.07 to 4.97 ± 1.27 mm^2. These changes in the area of the normal artery resulted in an increase in percent diameter stenosis from 68% to 71% $\pm$ 5% and in percent area stenosis from 90.7% $\pm$ 4.0% to 92.1% $\pm$ 3.1%. Although small, all of these changes were significant (P < 0.001). The large standard deviations for all mean values in this study are due to averaging together the data from mild, moderate, and severe stenoses.

Based on the equation in Figure 5.1B for viscous and separation pressure losses, these geometric changes during coronary vasodilation caused a 22% increase in the coefficient of pressure loss due to separation or disturbed flow, but no change in the viscous coefficient, as shown in Table 5.3 (2). As coronary flow increased, the pressure gradient also increased, as expected from the quadratic relation of pressure gradient to volume flow. As shown in Table 5.4, the relative proportion of pressure losses due to viscous friction and separation also changed as coronary flow increased. Using the resting arteriographic geometry and a resting coronary flow of 0.25 mL/s (15 mL/min), the arteriographically predicted viscous losses accounted for 67% and the separation losses accounted for 33% of the total pressure gradient across the stenosis. Using arteriographic geometry after coronary vasodilators at higher coronary flows of 1 mL/s (60 mL/min), the arteriographically predicted viscous losses accounted for 32% and the separation losses accounted for 68% of the total pressure gradient across the stenosis. Thus, at higher flows the separation losses became greater than viscous losses.

Figure 5.2 graphs the changes in these relative proportions over a range of coronary flows using the mean values

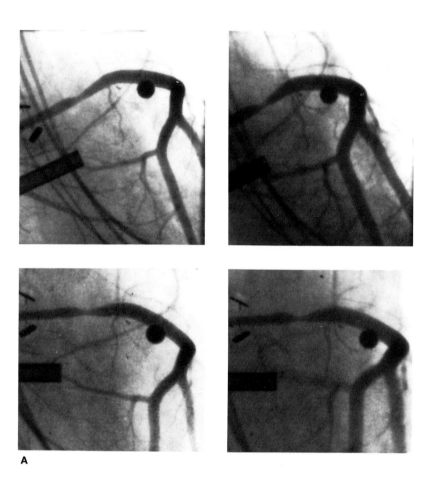

A

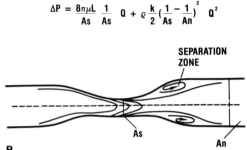

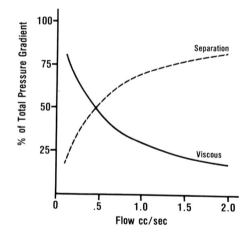

B

Fig. 5.1 (**A**) Coronary arteriogram of a "fixed" coronary stenosis recorded during resting coronary flows (left panel) and 3 min later during peak vasodilation (right panel) in the same view, without moving the dog. The radioopaque sphere is a stainless steel ball, 3.18 mm in diameter, sewed into position adjacent to the artery at the time of surgery. The radioopaque bar is a second marker. The small radioopaque chips are piezoelectric crystals of the Doppler flow velocity transducer. The small lead wires visible connecting the conducting cable to the crystals are 0.003 in in diameter and indicate the excellent resolution of the arteriogram. The percent narrowing is worse with vasodilation of normal arterial segments on either side of the stenosis. Reproduced with permission from Gould KL. (3). (**B**) Fluid-dynamic equations for viscous and separation pressure losses.

for f and s from Table 5.4 (2). These arteriographically predicted proportions are approximately the same as those of viscous and turbulent losses previously determined from pressure-flow measurements alone, without arteriographic geometry.

For these arteriographic studies, the pressure gradient was measured and volume blood flow was determined at the time of arteriography as the product of flow velocity and cross-sectional lumen area of the artery in the Doppler velocity transducer. The pressure gradient across the stenosis increased at elevated coronary blood flow, for two reasons. The first is the expected increase in pressure gradient due to the quadratic pressure gradient–volume flow (ΔP-Q) relation. The second is the increase in the separation coefficient at higher blood flows due to worsening percent stenosis as compared to resting levels. The previously noted decreased velocity with normal artery vasodilation was eliminated by determining volume flow as the product of flow velocity and normal lumen area.

In order to analyze the additional pressure losses for any given flow due to altered geometry after vasodilators, it is necessary to calculate the pressure gradient from arteriographic geometry at rest and after vasodilators but using the same coronary blood flow. At high flows of 1 mL/s, the pressure gradient predicted from resting arteriographic geometry was 47 ± 41 mm Hg, whereas the pressure gradient predicted from arteriographic geometry at vasodilation, also at a flow

Relative Contribution of Viscous Friction and Exit Separation to Total Pressure Gradient

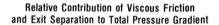

Fig. 5.2 Graphic plot of the relative proportion of pressure losses caused by viscous friction and by separation or disturbed flow to total pressure gradient as a function of coronary blood flow. At resting control conditions, viscous friction accounted for two-thirds or more of the total pressure loss, with separation losses accounting for one-third or less. At high coronary blood flows, this proportion was reversed. Reproduced with permission from Gould KL, Kelley KO, 1982. (2).

Table 5.1 Early Changes in Stenosis Geometry after Vasodilation

28 Stenoses	Rest		Vasodilation		
			Early		Late
Min X-Sect area mm^2	0.39 ± 0.15		0.36 ± 0.16		0.38 ± 0.22
		$P = 0.002$		NS	
Prox X-Sect area mm^2	5.70 ± 2.51		6.24 ± 3.07		6.90 ± 3.09
		$P = 0.002$		$P = <0.001$	
Dist X-Sect area mm^2	4.32 ± 1.28		4.82 ± 1.58		4.99 ± 1.51
		$P = 0.008$		$P = 0.049$	
Probe X-Sect area mm^2	2.68 ± 1.0		3.18 ± 1.2		3.39 ± 1.0
		$P <0.001$		$P = 0.056$	
% Diameter stenosis	67 ± 8		70 ± 5		71 ± 5
		$P <0.001$		NS	
% Area stenosis	90 ± 5		92 ± 3		92 ± 3
		$P <0.001$		NS	
Viscous coefficient (f)	17 ± 13		22 ± 24		20 ± 20
		NS		NS	
Turb coefficient (s)	35 ± 37		49 ± 69		49 ± 56
		NS		NS	

Results are expressed as mean ± SD.

Source: Adapted with permission from Gould KL, Kelley KO, 1982. Reference 2.

Table 5.2 Changes in Stenosis Geometry after Coronary Vasodilation

51 Stenoses	Rest	Vasodilation	% Change	Significance
Min X-Sect area mm^2	0.40 ± 0.16	0.40 ± 0.20	−3 ± 18	NS
Prox X-Sect area mm^2	4.98 ± 2.09	5.87 ± 2.67	16 ± 14	<0.001
Dist X-Sect area mm^2	4.44 ± 1.07	4.97 ± 1.27	12 ± 18	<0.001
Probe X-Sect area mm^2	2.37 ± 0.9	3.00 ± 1.0	32 ± 32	<0.001
% Diameter stenosis	68 ± 7	71 ± 5	4 ± 7	<0.001
% Area stenosis	90.7 ± 4.0	92.1 ± 3.1	2 ± 3	<0.001
Divergence angle°	31 ± 11	33 ± 10	7 ± 19	NS

Results are expressed as mean ± SD.

Source: Adapted with permission from Gould KL, Kelley KO, 1982. Reference 2.

Table 5.3 Hemodynamic Effects of Altered Stenosis Geometry after Vasodilation

X ray geometry	Flow (mL/sec)	Pressure gradient (mm Hg)			% Contribution	
		Viscous	Separation	Total	Viscous	Separation
Rest x-ray	0.25	3.6 ± 2.7	2.0 ± 1.9	5.7 ± 4.5	67 ± 8	33 ± 8
Vasodilation x-ray	1.0	16.5 ± 16.5	41.8 ± 45.3	58.2 ± 60.7	32 ± 8	68 ± 8

Results are expressed as mean ± SD; $n = 51$.

Source: Adapted with permission from Gould KL, Kelley KO, 1982. Reference 2.

Table 5.4 Hemodynamic Effects of Altered Stenosis Geometry after Vasodilation

51 Stenoses	Rest	Vasodilation	% Change	Significance
Viscous coefficient (f)	14.5 ± 10.7	16.5 ± 16.5	4 ± 30	NS
Separation coefficient (s)	32.5 ± 30.7	41.8 ± 45.3	22 ± 47	0.001

Where $\Delta P = fQ + sQ^2$; Q = flow ml/sec; units f = mm Hg/ml per sec; s = mm Hg/ml^2 per sec^2. Results are expressed as mean ± SD.

Source: Adapted with permission from Gould KL, Kelley KO, 1982. Reference 2.

of 1 mL/s, was 58 ± 61 mm Hg, or a 16% ± 39% difference (P < 0.002). Thus, with coronary vasodilation and worsening stenosis severity, the arteriographically predicted pressure gradient at 1 mL/s was 16% higher than it would have been had there been no geometric changes of the stenosis during high coronary flow.

In the previous chapter the pressure gradient at maximum flow, using the measured pressure gradient–flow *velocity* relation, was 36% higher than expected on the basis of resting gradient velocity relation, compared to a 16% difference for the gradient–*volume flow* relation. Thus, about 44% (16%/36%) of the excess pressure gradient at high flows over that expected on the basis of the resting pressure flow relation is due to real, physiologically significant, worsening stenosis severity caused by worsening percent diameter stenosis and separation losses. The balance of 56% is basically an artifact, caused by measuring flow velocity that shifts the gradient–flow *velocity* relation further leftward than the more physiologically relevant gradient–*volume flow* relation.

ACCURACY OF ARTERIOGRAPHICALLY PREDICTED VERSUS MEASURED GRADIENT-FLOW RELATION

The gradient-flow relation based on changing arteriographic geometry was graphically correlated with the corresponding measured pressure gradient–flow relation for each stenosis. The instantaneous pressure gradient–flow relation, ΔP-Q, measured during diastole for a single heart cycle, was curvilinear and fit a quadratic relation, $\Delta P = fQ + sQ^2$, where ΔP equals pressure gradient (mm Hg), Q is flow (mL/min), f

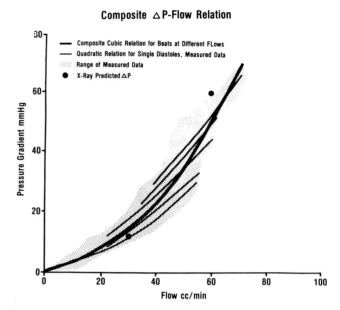

Fig. 5.4 Composite pressure gradient–flow relations of cardiac diastoles through a range of coronary blood flows, from resting up to higher flows after coronary vasodilation. The light solid lines represent the pressure gradient–flow relation of individual cardiac diastoles, and the heavy solid line represents the composite equation fitting the data over the entire range of flow. The shaded area indicates the range of primary data, and the dark solid circles indicate the x-ray-predicted pressure gradient–flow characteristics at rest (the lower solid circle) and after coronary vasodilators (upper solid circle). Reproduced with permission from Gould KL, Kelley KO, Bolson EL, 1982. (1).

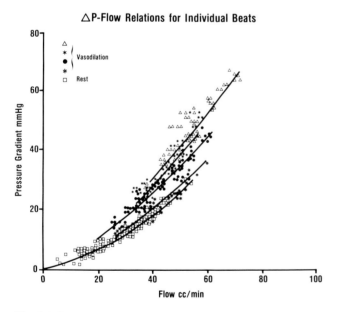

Fig. 5.3 Pressure gradient–flow relation of cardiac diastoles at resting control flow (open squares), at peak vasodilation (open triangles), and at intermediate stages of vasodilation (stars and solid circles). Reproduced with permission from Gould KL, Kelley KO, Bolson EL, 1982. (1).

is the coefficient of viscous friction loss, and s equals the coefficient of separation loss, determined by curve-fitting to the measured pressure flow data (not from arteriograms). For a given stenosis, the quadratic relation changed as flow increased during vasodilation. The coefficients f and s for the quadratic relation for measured pressure flow data became greater at higher flow levels, indicating an increase in the true severity of the stenosis. Thus, for each stenosis, there was a family of curves describing the measured ΔP-Q relation over a range of flow from rest to vasodilation (Fig. 5.3). The combined data for heart cycles at several flow rates for a given stenosis did not fit a simple composite quadratic relationship, owing to changing stenosis geometry at high flows, as previously described (1). Therefore, a cubic equation was fit to the combined data in the form $\Delta P = aQ + bQ^2 + cQ^3$ so that, with the coefficients for the best-fit cubic equation, the average pressure gradient at any flow for that stenosis could be calculated on the basis of measured phasic pressure flow data for comparison to those predicted by stenosis geometry from the arteriogram taken during maximum flow after intracoronary papaverine. This average experimental pressure gradient for a given flow was a single value within the range of actual data points measured during the experiment, for comparison to the arteriographically predicted pressure gradient at the same flow. A sample of this analysis is shown in Figure 5.4 (1).

The ΔP-Q relation and total pressure gradient at a given flow for each stenosis were also predicted from arteriographic geometry and dimensions of the stenosis at resting conditions. Since vasodilation caused a change in stenosis dimensions, a second ΔP-Q relationship for each stenosis was obtained from a second set of orthogonal arteriograms taken during vasodilation. The pressure gradient–flow relation from the measured pressure-flow data and from the arteriographic analysis at rest and at vasodilation were graphed together. Figure 5.5 shows examples from four experiments (1). There was good agreement between ΔP-Q relations derived from arteriograms at rest and during vasodilation with those derived from direct experimental pressure-flow measurements.

At elevated coronary flows of 45, 60, 75, and 90 mL/min, the measured pressure gradient and the pressure gradient predicted from arteriograms at the same flow were similarly correlated. Over the entire range of flow using combined resting and high-flow data, the regression line correlating arteriogram with directly measured pressure gradients was ΔP (arteriogram) = 1.11 ΔP (measured) + 0.75, with r equaling 0.95. One standard deviation for the regression line was ± 9.4 mm Hg, and 95% confidence intervals for individual arteriographic predicted values was ± 18.5 mm Hg; that is, 95%

of the arteriographically predicted values fell within ± 18.5 mm Hg of measured values (Fig. 5.6) (1).

There was no significant difference in the mean values for the measured pressure gradient at rest, 10.1 ± 7.7 mm Hg, and the arteriographically predicted pressure gradient at rest, 10.9 ± 5.6 mm Hg (Table 5.5) (1). At high flows after papaverine, there was a slight but significant (P < 0.001) difference between the mean values of the measured pressure gradient, 48.2 ± 23.1 mm Hg, and the arteriographically predicted pressure gradient, 55.8 ± 28.8 mm Hg, at the same flow. Thus, on the average, the arteriograms slightly overestimated the pressure gradient during vasodilation as compared to measured values, probably related to visually identifying borders of the arterial lumen used at the time these experiments were carried out (the later, automated method is described in subsequent chapters). The mean value for the difference between the arteriographically predicted and the measured pressure gradient was 3.9 ± 4.3 mm Hg at rest and 11.9 ± 10.5 mm Hg during vasodilation after papaverine.

These data in intact, instrumented dogs validate the applicability of classic fluid-dynamic equations to tapering stenoses for single diastolic periods in vasoactive, flexible coronary arteries in vivo using quantitative coronary arteriog-

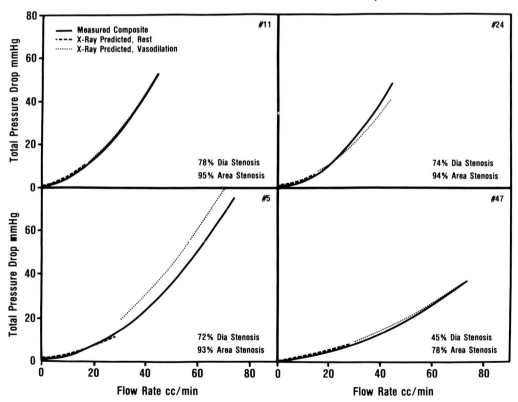

Pressure Gradient-Flow Relationship

Fig. 5.5 Relations of diastolic pressure gradient and coronary blood flow for mild to severe coronary stenoses. With an increase in coronary blood flow, the stenosis pressure gradient increases. The arteriographically predicted pressure gradient–flow relations (dashed lines indicate rest geometry, dotted lines indicate vasodilated geometry) are compared to those directly measured by implanted catheter and flowmeters in a dog model of coronary stenosis (solid lines). The steeper curves are associated with the more severe stenoses. [Dia = diameter.] Reproduced with permission from Gould KL, Kelley KO, Bolson EL, 1982. (1).

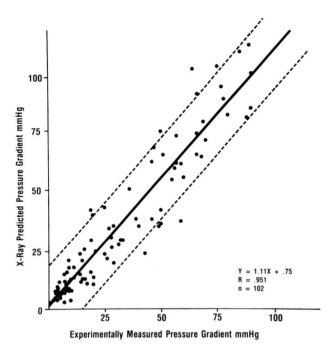

$$Y = 1.11X + .75$$
$$R = .951$$
$$n = 102$$

Fig. 5.6 Correlation of arteriographically predicted pressure gradient and measured pressure gradient for the entire range of coronary blood flows after coronary vasodilators. The dashed lines indicate 95% confidence limits; that is, 95% of the predicted x-ray values fall within ± 18.5 mm Hg of experimentally measured values. Reproduced with permission from Gould KL, Kelley KO, Bolson EL, 1982. (1).

raphy for predicting hemodynamic severity of coronary artery stenoses from arteriographic geometry alone. However, simultaneous phasic pressure gradient–volume flow measurements in diastole must be used for comparison to arteriograms obtained at the same flows and state of vasodilation of large epicardial arteries as those during which the direct pressure flow measurements were made.

For rigid tubes of in-vitro models, the stenosis geometry remains constant over the full range of pressure-flow measurements. Therefore, all of the data fit a single characteristic pressure-flow equation over the full range of flows. For invivo arteries, the stenosis is constant only for the range of flows in a single diastolic period. Over the full range of cor-

onary flows, all experimental stenoses changed geometry, becoming worse at high flows. Consequently, there is no single quadratic equation, no single pressure gradient–flow relation that characterizes the stenosis over the full range of flows in vivo. Therefore, although traditional fluid-dynamic equations apply to stenoses during a single diastole, they do not apply over the full range of flows in vivo in the same way that they apply to rigid tubes in vitro. A corollary is that mean pressure gradient–flow measurements do not follow traditional fluid-dynamic equations characterizing stenoses, owing to the effects of systolic deceleration, diastolic acceleration, and changing geometry over the range of coronary flows in vivo.

COMPARISON OF THE PRESSURE GRADIENT-VOLUME FLOW RELATION TO THE PRESSURE GRADIENT-FLOW VELOCITY RELATION

Quantitative arteriography predicts only the pressure-flow relation characteristic of stenosis severity. It cannot predict an actual pressure gradient in clinical circumstances, because absolute coronary flow is unknown. However, even measuring coronary flow at rest would not be very useful, because resting pressure gradients are small until very severe stenoses are present, as shown previously. The severity of a coronary artery stenosis can be characterized adequately by direct pressure-flow measurements only by increasing flow to maximum levels by a potent arteriolar vasodilator, such as dipyridamole, papaverine, or adenosine. However, by making pressure-flow measurements over a range of flows, the geometry of the artery and stenosis are altered. This altered stenosis geometry affects the pressure gradient–volume flow (ΔP-Q) relation or the pressure gradient–flow velocity (ΔP-V) relation to a greater or lesser extent, depending on the degree of vasodilation of the normal arterial segment on either side of the stenosis and/or collapse of the narrowest segment, if it has flexible walls.

Tables 5.1 and 5.2 show the changes in the arterial cross-sectional area within the Doppler transducer for 51 stenoses studied by two sequential x-rays at resting conditions and maximum flow (3). There was an average 32% ± 32% increase in vessel area at the flow probe during maximal vasodilation, 2.37 ± 0.9 mm^2 at rest to 3.0 ± 1.0 mm^2 after distal coronary vasodilators (P < 0.001). The standard deviations are wide owing to varying arterial size. The mean cross-sectional area of the artery at the Doppler transducer for a subset of 28 separate stenoses x-rayed sequentially three times was 2.68 ± 1.0 mm^2 at rest flow, 3.18 ± 1.2 mm^2 at peak flow 10 s after intracoronary papaverine, and 3.39 ± 1.0 mm^2 during maximal epicardial arterial vasodilation 60 s after papaverine. These increases in arterial cross-sectional area during elevated flow after distal intracoronary injection of papaverine were significant, with P < 0.001 by paired *t*-test analysis.

Because of the increased arterial diameter in the Doppler transducer during elevated coronary flow, the relative increase in flow velocity was proportionately less than the relative increase in volume flow. The percent increase in flow and percent increase in flow velocity during vasodilation is shown in Figure 5.7 (2). For this schematic, the velocity mea-

Table 5.5 Measured and x-ray-predicted Pressure Gradient (*n* = 51)

	Measured (mm Hg)	X-ray (mm Hg)	P	Mean difference in ΔP (mm Hg), x-ray minus measured
Rest	10.1 ± 7.7	10.9 ± 5.6	NS	3.9 ± 4.3
Vasodilators	48.2 ± 23.1	55.8 ± 28.8	<0.001	11.9 ± 10.5

Values are mean ± SD.

Source: Adapted with permission from Gould KL, Kelley KO, Bolson EL, 1982. Reference 1.

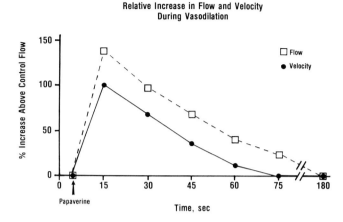

Fig. 5.7 Relative increase in coronary volume flow and flow velocity following injection of papaverine in the distal intracoronary catheter. The horizontal axis shows time after injection, and the vertical axis shows percent increase above control values. Reproduced with permission from Gould KL, Kelley KO, 1982. (2).

surements were taken at six different flow rates for a single stenosis; volume flow during vasodilation was then calculated using the mean increase in vessel area for 28 stenoses at peak flow and during vasodilation. The increase in velocity is always 30% to 40% less than the increase in volume flow. The duration of flow elevation is also correspondingly shorter when flow velocity is used as a measure of flow change, because when flow velocity has returned to baseline control, volume flow remains somewhat elevated because the arterial diameter is still larger than at baseline control.

This difference between the volume-flow measurement and the flow-velocity measurement during vasodilation is plotted in Figure 5.8 as the percent error in relative flow change if flow velocity is recorded by a Doppler transducer as a measure of relative flow change on the assumption that arterial diameter remains constant, when in fact arterial diameter enlarges (2). Velocity measurements during flow elevation after papaverine significantly underestimate the true increase in volume flow. The magnitude of volume-flow in-

crease after vasodilators is obtained only with accurate measurements of the changes in vessel area at the transducer and multiplication by flow velocity in order to obtain volume flow.

We observed a systematic, consistent increase in the coronary arterial cross-sectional area within the chronically implanted parylene-coated Doppler velocity transducer during coronary flow elevation (2). These observations were made in repeated experiments 10–60 days postoperatively, when the transducer was encased with soft connective tissue. If we had assumed a constant arterial cross-sectional area, as virtually all previous studies in the literature have done, then recordings of coronary flow velocity as measures of relative changes in coronary flow would have been in error by up to 40%.

The phasic flow response of a Doppler velocity transducer has been previously studied in comparison to an electromagnetic flowmeter implanted with it side-by-side on the femoral artery by Vatner et al. (5). Both flowmeters had similar phasic output and linear response over physiological flow rates. This previous study did not compare relative percent changes in flow by both electromagnetic and Doppler flowmeters but reported only linear flowmeter signal outputs as perfusion through an artery was increased from 0.3 to 12 cm³/s for calibration purposes (5). These investigators also made the observation that the implanted transducers were firmly attached to the vessel by fibrosis. They concluded, therefore, that changes in arterial diameter within the transducer would be negligible, but no measurements of arterial diameter were made.

In our study, arterial area measured in vivo changed significantly within the transducer from rest flow to high flow states. We conclude that Doppler velocity meters made of parylene-coated epoxy may not accurately measure relative changes in volume flow unless arterial cross-sectional area is also measured (4,5). The results of Vatner (5) do not conflict with our own conclusion, since he demonstrated simply that his instruments were linear as flow increased under conditions where there was no change in arterial dimensions. Although he did not measure arterial diameter in the Doppler transducer, it may have been fixed in his experimental preparation with his type of implanted Doppler transducer. Our results show that with our type of linear Doppler velocity transducer in unanesthetized animals for studying the detailed hemodynamics of coronary stenoses, significant coronary vasodilation occurs in the transducer, the consequence of which is that flow velocity does not parallel volume flow. Consequently, we conclude that the Doppler velocity transducer cannot be used to accurately measure changes in volume flow in the absence of direct measurement of vessel cross-sectional area within the Doppler transducer during each different flow state. However, the changing normal arterial diameter with changing flow more closely parallels actual events in animals in vivo and in man.

The increase in arterial cross-sectional area inside our chronically implanted Doppler transducer during coronary vasodilation has significant impact on assessing stenosis severity in terms of either the pressure gradient–velocity relation or the pressure gradient–volume flow relation. In this study, each stenosis was characterized according to classical fluid-dynamic equations, in which viscous friction losses are described by a first-power term and pressure losses due to

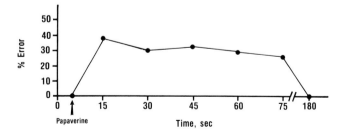

Fig. 5.8 Percent error in relative coronary flow change, if flow velocity is recorded by Doppler velocity meter as a measure of volume flow based on the erroneous assumption that arterial diameter remains constant. Reproduced with permission from Gould KL, Kelley KO, 1982. (2).

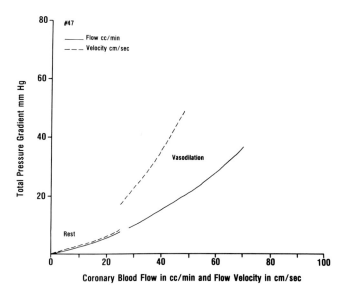

Fig. 5.9 Relation of stenosis pressure gradient to coronary volume flow and flow velocity at rest and during coronary vasodilation. The gradient-volume flow relation is a continuous quadratic curve, whereas the gradient-velocity relation "breaks" with a steeper slope, indicating a more geometrically severe stenosis. Reproduced with permission from Gould KL, Kelley KO, 1982. (2).

exit losses are described by a second-power term. At rest and elevated flows, a quadratic equation that best fit the phasic pressure gradient and flow-velocity data was therefore obtained during the diastolic portion of a single heart cycle, in order to obtain a gradient–flow velocity relation to characterize stenosis severity. The simultaneous pressure gradient–volume flow relation for the same stenosis was then derived by multiplying the area of the vessel at the Doppler transducer by each value of flow velocity, thereby obtaining volume flow.

An example of flow velocity and flow analysis applied to the same stenosis is shown in Figure 5.9 (2). At resting flow, the quadratic relation for the pressure gradient–velocity relation and for the pressure gradient–flow relation are identical. During vasodilation, there is a major change in the pressure gradient–velocity relation as indicated by a steeper curve in the velocity-pressure relation at high flows. This steeper curve shows that, for a given flow velocity, the pressure gradient is greater, thereby suggesting worsened stenosis severity. Quantitatively, the separation coefficient, S, of the velocity equation is worse. In contrast, the pressure gradient–volume flow relation for this stenosis did not change during vasodilation, indicating no more additional pressure losses at higher flows than would be expected on the basis of the resting pressure gradient–flow relation. The data at high flows is a continuous extension of the data at rest flow and thereby indicates no change in stenosis severity.

A more typical comparative example for most stenoses is graphed in Figure 5.10 (2). In this example, flow and flow-velocity equations differ at rest flow in addition to a steeper gradient-velocity relation at high flows, suggesting increased stenosis severity. The pressure gradient–volume flow relation

is somewhat steeper, consistent with some worsening stenosis severity, but the change in the gradient–volume flow relation is not as great as for the gradient-velocity relation. The pressure gradient–velocity relation typically indicates marked worsening of stenosis at high flows, whereas the pressure gradient–volume flow relation usually indicates mild worsening of stenosis at high flows. Whether the ΔP-Q or the ΔP-V relation best describes what is important physiologically for stenoses in vivo depends on one's choice of definitions for describing stenosis severity hemodynamically.

In our study, the ΔP-V relation for a given stenosis after vasodilation is steeper, with a sharper upward break, than the simultaneous ΔP-Q relation, thereby indicating greater stenosis severity at high coronary flows than is suggested by the ΔP-Q relation. We have identified the reason for the difference between the ΔP-V and ΔP-Q relations as due to the increase in the cross-sectional area of the normal coronary artery within the Doppler transducer following vasodilators. Thus, for a given increase in volume flow, there is a proportionately smaller increase in flow velocity measured at the Doppler transducer, since the diameter of the artery within the transducer increased. Figures 5.9 and 5.10 illustrate the major differences between describing stenosis severity by the ΔP-Q relation and describing it by the ΔP-V relation. Even though fluid-dynamic equations in terms of ΔP, Q, and V are mathematically equivalent and also equivalent for in-vitro rigid tube systems used in fluid-dynamic experiments, different conclusions result from their application to vasoactive arteries in vivo.

The problem therefore becomes one of a "philosophical"

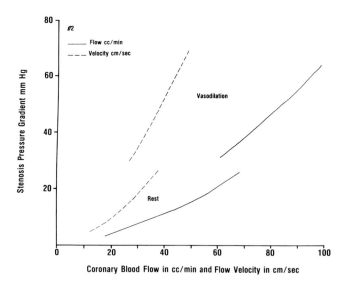

Fig. 5.10 Relation of stenosis pressure gradient to coronary volume flow and to flow velocity. The relations are as described in the previous figure, except that both relations (both solid and dashed lines) demonstrate steeper slopes after vasodilation. The gradient–velocity relation shows a much more prominent increase in slope, however, illustrating that it is more sensitive to vasodilation on either side of the stenotic segment. Reproduced with permission from Gould KL, Kelley KO, 1982. (2).

choice of which reference system, the ΔP-V or the ΔP-Q relation, should be used for defining severity of stenosis (6). Should one use flow velocity with relative percent stenosis as the dominant term, or volume flow with absolute stenosis diameter as the dominant term? These equations do not give the same answers for vasoactive arteries of different sizes in vivo. It is therefore appropriate to outline the pros and cons of these alternatives.

PRESSURE GRADIENT–FLOW VELOCITY RELATION

Changes in flow velocity do not reflect proportionately the changes in volume flow to the distal vascular bed during coronary vasodilation, since the cross-sectional area of the normal artery also increases significantly. If changes in the cross-sectional area of the coronary artery are not accounted for, measurements of the changes in flow velocity will differ by up to 40% from changes in volume flow, thereby causing the ΔP-V relation to be steeper than the ΔP-Q relation during elevated coronary flows.

Thus, the ΔP-V relation becomes steeper for two reasons: (a) the artery on either side of the stenotic segment vasodilates and percent stenosis increases, and (b) flow velocity does not increase proportionately with volume flow, owing to increased cross-sectional area of the normal artery adjacent to the stenosis. The dominant geometric influence on the ΔP-V relation is relative percent stenosis squared. Other terms include absolute stenosis lumen area and length. There is no term in the velocity equation for normal lumen area to account for changing normal diameter. Therefore, as the normal artery vasodilates, flow velocity becomes less for a constant volume flow and pressure gradient, and percent stenosis and the ΔP-V relation worsens (becomes steeper), suggesting a worse stenosis. However, this apparent worsening of the ΔP-V relation is of little importance to myocardium, since volume flow for a given pressure is much less affected. The ΔP-V relation for describing stenosis severity in vivo varies with changes in diameter of the normal artery that do not impair flow for a given pressure and do not have physiologic consequences. Since percent stenosis is the dominant term in the ΔP-V relation, this observation explains why percent diameter stenosis and the ΔP-V relation as descriptors of stenosis severity are imprecise both in principle and experimentally, and do not correlate well with physiologic effects until very severe narrowing has developed (1–3,7–11).

In an artery that does not change size during high coronary flow, such as the human left main or proximal left anterior descending or left circumflex coronary arteries, changes in flow velocity may faithfully reflect the changes in volume arterial flow (12). Therefore, coronary flow reserve measured by a Doppler tip catheter at one of these sites is accurate. Similarly, flow velocity in an implanted Doppler transducer that causes sufficient scarring to prevent vasomotion within its ultrasound beam will also reflect volume flow. However, flow velocity in a normally vasoactive artery as measured by our Doppler transducers (5), or by pressure gradient–flow velocity equations in principle, do not accurately reflect physiologic stenosis severity if normal diameter changes.

Having concluded that the pressure gradient–flow velocity relation is not optimal for vasoactive coronary arteries that undergo change from normal diameters, it would be appropriate to outline its major advantage and why percent stenosis has served as a rough clinical guide to severity over the years.

Mean cross-sectional flow velocities in different-sized arteries throughout the body at resting conditions tend to be fairly uniform within a relatively narrow range of 20 to 40 cm/s. By comparison, volume flow ranges from very small in a small artery to 6,000 mL/min in the aorta. Measurement of flow velocity therefore normalizes for normal arterial size or size of vascular bed. Percent narrowing also normalizes for different arterial sizes. Therefore, for comparing severity of stenoses in different-sized arteries throughout the body or between individuals under fixed resting stable conditions, gradient velocity equations and percent stenosis serve as a rough guide.

To illustrate this point, Figure 5.11, upper panel, shows the hypothetical gradient-velocity relation (that is, a graphic plot of the velocity equation) for stenoses of equal physiologic severity in a large and a small artery (6). Physiologic severity in this example is defined for both the large and small artery as the capacity to increase flow four times over resting

VELOCITY EQUATIONS - ADVANTAGES

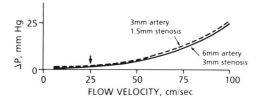

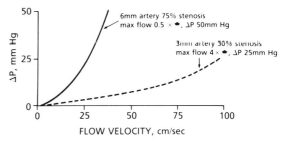

Fig. 5.11 Upper panel, relation of pressure gradient (ΔP) and arterial flow velocity for physiologically equal stenoses (50% diameter) in a small artery with a diameter of 3 mm (dashed line) and in a large artery with a diameter of 6 mm (solid line). The arrow indicates the normal value for coronary flow velocity at rest (25 cm/s). Lower panel, similar relation for physiologically unequal stenoses of 1.5 mm absolute diameter in the small (dashed line) and the large (solid line) artery. Reproduced with permission from Gould KL, 1980. (6).

values with a maximal pressure gradient of 25 mm Hg. The curve for the small artery is the same as that for the large artery, indicating equal hydraulic severity. The lower panel of Figure 5.11 shows the gradient-velocity relation for stenoses of unequal physiologic severity but of equal absolute stenosis diameter, 1.5 mm. The more severe physiologic lesion is associated with a capacity to increase flow by only 0.5, or 50%, with a 50 mm Hg maximal gradient; it has a steeper gradient-velocity curve than that of the milder physiologic lesion, regardless of arterial size. Thus, by using velocity measurements (or equations), physiologically equal lesions in arteries of different sizes appear hydraulically equal and physiologically unequal lesions appear hydraulically unequal.

Based on this logic, the author formerly favored pressure gradient–flow velocity relations for describing stenosis severity, as is the prevalent viewpoint in fluid-dynamic engineering. However, the experimental results described in these chapters document the limitations of the pressure gradient–flow velocity relation for precisely defining stenosis severity in vasoactive arteries in vivo.

PRESSURE GRADIENT-VOLUME FLOW RELATIONSHIP

The ΔP-Q relation for a given stenosis at rest flow changes only slightly at high flow during vasodilation of the normal artery on either side of the stenotic segment. With ΔP-Q analysis, the slight worsening of percent stenosis due to altered stenosis geometry at high flows caused only a 16% increase in pressure gradient over that expected in the absence of vasodilation of the normal arterial segments. This degree of worsening is physiologically "real," in the sense that for a flow of 60 cc/min the stenosis gradient is 16% greater and distal coronary pressure is 16% lower than it would have been in the absence of vasodilation of the normal segment of the coronary artery. Since the ΔP-Q equation contains a term for normal lumen area, vasomotor changes of normal segments are accounted for. The dominant geometric influence in the ΔP-Q relation is absolute stenosis diameter, not relative percent narrowing. Thus, the ΔP-Q relation becomes only slightly steeper with vasodilation and more accurately describes hemodynamic characteristics of biological importance in vivo.

Although the ΔP-Q relation reflects stenosis severity during vasomotion of the normal artery, it has significant disadvantages. There is no normalization of the absolute cross-sectional lumen area of the stenosis to the normal area of the artery in the ΔP-Q relation—that is, no percent stenosis term. Since a small artery transports less volume flow in mL/min for any given pressure, the ΔP-Q relation will appear much steeper and hence appear worse for a smaller vessel when compared to a large vessel with the same percent stenosis having the same physiological consequences on distal organ function by virtue of equal percent stenosis. The ΔP-Q relation is therefore inappropriate for comparing severity of stenosis in different-sized arteries. For example, an absolute stenosis diameter of 2 mm in a coronary artery normally 3 mm in diameter is not a physiologically severe stenosis, but a stenosis of 2 mm diameter in an aorta that is normally 15 mm in diameter is a physiologically severe stenosis. Thus,

we can interpret the significance of the geometric severity in the gradient-flow equation only if we know what the normal flow volume for a specific coronary vascular bed size is. Expressing flow in units of cc/min/g instead of cc/min does not solve the normalization problem, because one then needs to know the size of the vascular bed, or what the volume flow should be for a given artery and its distal bed size. Hemodynamic effects of a stenosis are related to the total flow through the artery in mL/min, not mL/min/g.

For discussion purposes, to clarify this disadvantage of the ΔP-Q relation as a descriptor of stenosis severity, let us define functional stenosis severity as before in terms of the capacity to increase flow over baseline. For discussion purposes, let us assume the capacity for increasing flow (flow reserve) is four times resting flow and is not reduced by a 50% diameter stenosis, with peak pressure gradient across a 50% stenosis at maximum flow of 25 mm Hg, as observed experimentally. Now consider two different-sized coronary arteries of 6 mm and 3 mm in diameter, each with a 50% stenosis, reducing the absolute lumina to 3 mm and 1.5 mm in diameter at the narrowest part.

Figure 5.12 shows the gradient-flow relation for stenoses of equal physiologic severity, as just defined (flow reserve of

FLOW EQUATIONS - DISADVANTAGES

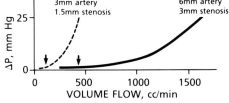

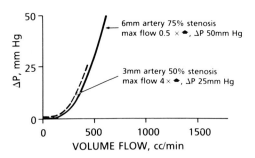

Fig. 5.12 Upper panel, relation of pressure gradient (ΔP) and arterial volume flow for physiologically equal stenoses in a small (dashed line) and a large (solid line) artery. The arrows on the horizontal axis represent normal volume flow at rest in each of these two arteries, corresponding to a flow velocity at rest of 25 cm/s. Lower panel, similar relation for physiologically unequal stenoses of 1.5 mm absolute diameter in the small (dashed line) and large (solid line) artery. Reproduced with permission from Gould KL, 1980. (6).

4, 25 mm Hg peak gradient, and 50% diameter stenosis) in the small and large artery (6). The gradient-flow relation for the small artery is steeper and leftward, indicating less flow for the same gradient; by this graph the small artery appears to have a hydraulically more severe lesion than the larger artery, when in fact the two stenoses are physiologically the same with the same flow reserve of four times baseline. Thus, stenoses of equal physiologic severity in two arteries of different sizes appear unequal hydraulically if analyzed in terms of volume-flow equations.

The lower panel of Figure 5.12 shows the gradient-flow relation for stenoses of unequal physiologic severity but of equal absolute stenosis diameter, 1.5 mm. The more severe physiologic lesion, which is associated with a capacity to increase flow by only 0.5, or 50% over baseline and a 50 mm Hg maximal gradient, has a gradient-flow curve that is the same as for a physiologically milder lesion in the smaller artery characterized by a flow capacity of four times baseline with a 25 mm Hg gradient. Thus, physiologically unequal lesions in two different arteries appear hydraulically equal if analyzed in terms of volume flow equations.

Because of these disadvantages of the gradient-flow equations, the author formerly favored the use of flow-velocity measurements and equations and concluded that relative percent stenosis is more important than absolute stenosis minimal lumen area, a point of view held by most clinicians, perhaps without knowing the reason for it. However, the ΔP-V and percent narrowing are not precise measures of stenosis severity in vasoactive coronary arteries in vivo, as described here, although for different-size arteries or different distal vascular bed sizes they are better than ΔP-Q equations.

CONCLUSION

Thus, both ΔP-Q and ΔP-V fluid-dynamic equations have advantages and disadvantages for assessing vasoactive coronary arteries of different sizes in vivo. The pressure gradient–flow velocity equation normalizes for size of artery or vascular bed but fails to account for vasomotion changing the size of the normal artery. The pressure gradient–volume flow equation accounts for vasomotion of the normal artery but fails to normalize for artery or vascular bed size.

However, the disadvantages of the ΔP-Q equation for describing stenosis severity can be resolved by expressing flow as a multiple of normal resting flow rather than using absolute units of cc/min or cc/min/g, thereby normalizing for the size of the artery and size of the distal vascular bed. Based on the logic and data presented in these chapters, the author concludes that the ΔP-Q relation whereby flow is expressed as a ratio to baseline more correctly describes functional stenosis severity than the ΔP-V relation. Traditional fluid-dynamic equations using the ΔP-V relation adequately describe events in stenotic rigid tubes. However, for vasoactive coronary arteries in vivo that dynamically change in size, pressure-velocity equations are imprecise descriptors of stenosis severity, both in principle and experimentally. The additional term for normal cross-sectional area that must be included in the velocity equation to account for vasomotion of the normal artery, makes it a pressure-flow equation. As considered intuitively, the myocardium depends on volume flow, not flow velocity. Consequently, a useful measure of stenosis

severity must reflect pressure gradient–normalized volume flow behavior.

Therefore, the optimal way of describing coronary stenosis severity that is most applicable in vivo to vasoactive arteries of changing size is a pressure gradient–flow equation, with normalized flow expressed as a ratio to resting flow. Such equations lead to the concepts of coronary flow reserve and stenosis flow reserve described in detail in subsequent chapters. Coronary flow reserve is a single, clinically useful expression accounting for all geometric dimensions of a stenosis that describes its functional severity normalized for arterial or vascular bed size. Stenosis flow reserve, as subsequently described, also normalizes for other physiologic variables of aortic pressure, heart rate, and vasomotor tone. Although the phenomenon of coronary flow reserve in stenotic coronary arteries was discovered empirically by the author (13), subsequent experimental data relating functional and geometric characteristics of coronary artery stenosis in vivo, as reviewed here, provide strong theoretical basis, experimental validation, and clinical demonstration that it is a fundamental descriptor of stenosis severity in coronary arteries.

REFERENCES

1. Gould KL, Kelley KO, Bolson EL. Experimental validation of quantitative coronary arteriography for determining pressure-flow characteristics of coronary stenosis. Circulation 66:930–37, 1982.
2. Gould KL, Kelley KO. Physiological significance of coronary flow velocity and changing stenosis geometry during coronary vasodilation in awake dogs. Circ Res 50:695–704, 1982.
3. Gould KL. Pressure-flow characteristics of coronary stenoses in unsedated dogs at rest and during coronary vasodilation. Circ Res 43:242–53, 1978.
4. Gould KL, Lee D, Lovgren K. Techniques for arteriography and hydraulic analysis of coronary stenoses in unsedated dogs. Am J Physiol 235:H350–56, 1978.
5. Vatner SF, Franklin D, Van Citters RL. Simultaneous comparison and calibration of the Doppler and electromagnetic flowmeters. J Appl Physiol 29:907–10, 1970.
6. Gould KL. Dynamic coronary stenosis. Am J Cardiol 45:286–92, 1980.
7. Gould KL. Quantification of coronary artery stenosis in vivo. Circ Res 57:341–53, 1985.
8. Gould KL. Percent coronary stenosis: Battered gold standard, pernicious relic, or clinical practicality? J Am Coll Cardiol 11:886–88, 1988.
9. Gould KL, Goldstein RA, Mullani NA, Kirkeeide R, Wong G, Smalling R, Fuentes F, Nishikawa A, Matthews W. Noninvasive assessment of coronary stenoses by myocardial perfusion imaging during pharmacologic coronary vasodilation. VIII. Clinical feasibility of positron cardiac imaging without a cyclotron using generator-produced rubidium-82. J Am Coll Cardiol 7:775–89, 1986.
10. Marcus ML, Skorton DJ, Johnson MR, Collins SM, Harrison DG, Kerber RE. Visual estimates of percent diameter coronary stenosis: "A battered gold standard." J Am Coll Cardiol 41:882–85, 1988.
11. White CW, Wright CB, Doty DB, Hiratza LF, Eastham CL, Harrison DG, Marcus ML. Does visual interpretation of the coronary arteriogram predict the physiologic importance of a coronary stenosis? N Engl J Med 310:819–24, 1984.
12. Wilson RF, Laughlin DE, Ackell PH, Chilian WM, Holida MO, Hartley CJ, Armstrong ML, Marcus ML, White CW. Transluminal, subselective measurement of coronary artery blood flow velocity and vasodilator reserve in man. Circulation 72:82–92, 1985.
13. Gould KL, Lipscomb K, Hamilton GW. Physiologic basis for assessing critical coronary stenosis: Instantaneous flow response and regional distribution during coronary hyperemia as measures of coronary flow reserve. Am J Cardiol 33:87–94, 1974.

CHAPTER

6

Collapsing Stenoses

Within the spectrum of previously described dynamic behavior of coronary artery stenoses (1–6), two basic alternative pressure-flow phenomena were observed having physiologic and clinical significance. In the first of these alternatives, distal coronary arteriolar vasodilation caused a rise in coronary blood flow associated with an increase in stenosis pressure gradient, according to conventional fluid-dynamic equations (1–9), applicable to single diastoles either with or without worsening due to normal artery vasodilation (1–3). In the second alternative, previously described for critically severe, flexible-walled stenosis in open-chest dogs (10–18), coronary flow dramatically fell after distal coronary arteriolar vasodilation with a corresponding large increase in calculated stenosis resistance. For this latter phenomenon, the conventional pressure-flow relation for stenoses appeared to break down completely and no longer described the pressure-flow events even for single diastoles.

In experimental animals, a variety of coronary vasodilator stimuli in the presence of severe stenoses caused this phenomenon, including vasodilator drugs (15), exercise (12), and pacing (17), which was reversible by coronary vasoconstrictors (16,17). Benchtop model experiments showed that this fall in coronary blood flow after vasodilation in the presence of severe stenoses occurred only in flexible-walled tubes or coronary arteries and was not seen in stiff-walled, rigid stenoses (13,14). These observations are of potential clinical relevance because, in the presence of a severe stenosis with part of its lumen wall normally flexible, normal physiologic stimuli for distal coronary vasodilation may lead to a profound fall in distal coronary pressure and coronary flow.

The chapter provides an explanation for these observations and demonstrates quantitatively in intact animals that a severe stenosis of a flexible-walled, epicardial coronary artery may behave as a pressure-dependent flow resistor that resembles a Starling resistor in vivo within the range of pressures and flows observed experimentally. For such stenoses, flow becomes independent of or decoupled from the stenosis pressure gradient. Therefore, conventional fluid-dynamic equations do not describe the hemodynamic behavior of these severe stenoses.

BACKGROUND REVIEW OF THE STARLING RESISTOR

Starling (19) in 1912 described the characteristics of flow in collapsible tubes, using a model now called the Starling Resistor and analyzed subsequently by many investigators, including Holt (20,21), Rodbard (22), Conrad (23), Shapiro (24), and Lyon (25).

For a fairly severe stenosis of 85% diameter narrowing, the total energy content in the proximal coronary artery consists of a large amount of potential or pressure energy and low flow velocity or low kinetic energy. In the stenotic segment, however, by Bernoulli's principle, the flow velocity or kinetic energy is high, and potential or pressure energy is low, associated with a fall in intraluminal pressure to below 20–30 mm Hg in the stenotic segment. Thus, at resting control conditions in the stenotic segment, the pressure energy is converted to kinetic energy, with resulting loss of distending pressure in the lumen of the stenotic segment.

With distal coronary vasodilation, the pressure difference across the stenosis rises markedly for such severe narrowing, and distal coronary pressure, as well as intraluminal pressure in the stenotic segment, correspondingly falls further (1–3,26). Since intraluminal pressure in the stenotic segment was low even before distal coronary arteriolar vasodilation, it may fall below the external pressure, owing to vasomotor tone or arterial elasticity, acting to collapse a narrow segment of the artery. When the intraluminal pressure becomes less than the external collapsing pressure, the flexible stenotic segment partially collapses.

A number of previous studies (20–25) have shown that in this circumstance, flow is no longer related to or proportional to the pressure difference across the stenosis but is proportional to the difference between aortic pressure and the external collapsing pressure acting on the artery. Consequently, as the intraluminal pressure distal to the stenosis falls further with coronary vasodilation, the pressure difference across the stenosis increases, but coronary flow fails to increase, since at that point it is related to the difference between aortic and external collapsing pressure and not to the pressure difference across the stenosis.

With the collapsing stenosis phenomenon, stenosis resistance calculated as the pressure difference across the stenosis, divided by coronary blood flow, increased markedly. However, calculated resistance in these circumstances is meaningless, because flow is unrelated and not dependent on the pressure difference across the stenosis but is related primarily to aortic pressure. The concept of resistance, defined as pressure divided by flow, describes steady-state flow relations in rigid tubes but does not apply to non-steady flow phenomenon in collapsible tubes, an observation made by many previous investigators (20–25), particularly Conrad (23). The use of calculated resistance to describe the characteristics of stenoses in partially collapsing arteries is conceptually incorrect and does not describe the physical phenomenon that actually occurs (20–25).

Collapsing stenoses are characterized by transition from fluid-dynamic behavior in which flow is proportional to the stenosis pressure gradient to fluid-dynamic behavior associated with collapsible tubes, in which flow is not proportional or related to the stenosis pressure gradient. It has been considered to be a sudden, all-or-nothing change occurring when the intraluminal distending pressure in the stenotic segment becomes less than the external collapsing pressure acting on the artery (20–25). This transitional change in collapsible tubes is a different phenomenon from the gradual, incremental changes in structural stenosis geometry, which can be quantitatively measured after coronary vasodilation of the normal coronary artery on either side of the stenotic segment, as previously described (1–6,26).

In these circumstances, the stenosis geometry is not worse in a primary, fixed, measurable, structural sense causing greater pressure difference but rather is dynamically collapsing as a consequence of fluctuating changes in transmural pressure of the stenotic segment. The altered geometry is a passive change in a flexible arterial wall partially collapsing because of reduced distending or transmural pressure characteristic of high-velocity flow in collapsible tubes.

Severely stenotic flexible-walled stenoses are unstable and flutter between partial collapse and patency at a frequency depending upon flow (20–25), an observation that can be explained as follows. With the fall in intraluminal pressure, the walls of the flexible stenotic segment tend to collapse, thereby causing a higher local flow velocity, a further drop in the intraluminal distending pressure, and consequently progressive collapse of the stenotic segment. When the arterial segment is almost collapsed by this process, flow ceases, kinetic-energy content of the system falls to zero, and the total pressure head or energy content of the system becomes available as intraluminal distending pressure. The restoration of distending pressure opens the flexible segment, flow begins again, and pressure energy is again converted to kinetic energy, with a subsequent fall in intraluminal distending pressure, causing collapse again.

This cycle of conversion between kinetic and pressure energy with corresponding collapse and opening of the stenotic segment causes a fluttering of the arterial walls, fluctuations in distal coronary pressure, and intermittent, fluctuating coronary flow. It is important to recognize that mean coronary flow does not drop to zero since the flexible, collapsing segment is partially open for half of the time during these cyclic changes. As long as aortic pressure remains higher than the external collapsing pressure acting on the artery, mean coronary flow will remain above zero, although at a low level.

THEORETICAL BACKGROUND FOR EXPERIMENTAL MEASUREMENTS

The hemodynamic severity of fixed stenoses is described conventionally in terms of the relation between flow, or flow velocity V, through the stenosis and the pressure fall or gradient, ΔP, across it (1–3,7–9). This ΔP-Q relation in conventional fluid-dynamic terms for rigid tubes is described by a quadratic equation, $\Delta P = FV + SV^2$, where ΔP is the pressure gradient across the stenosis, V is flow velocity, F is the coefficient of pressure loss due to viscous friction, and S is the coefficient of pressure loss due to flow separation (1–3). Both F and S are determined by the geometry of the stenosis. The left panel of Figure 6.1 illustrates a generalized graphic plot of the form of this conventional quadratic equation for a rigid stenosis. The reason for using flow velocity is addressed subsequently.

The general quadratic equation above applies to stenotic but flexible-walled coronary arteries as long as the intraluminal distending pressure is greater than the external pressure or vasomotor tone tending to collapse the artery, labeled P_e in Figure 6.1. If intraluminal pressure falls below P_e in the presence of a flexible-wall stenosis, then the stenotic segment tends to collapse and a completely new pressure-flow relation develops, as shown in the right panel of Figure 6.1.

Several investigators have previously shown that flow through a Starling resistor is related to the difference between the proximal intraluminal driving pressure, P_1, and the external pressure, P_e, tending to collapse the flexible conduit (9–29). This principle can be written as a linear equation as follows: $P_1 - P_e = AV$, where P_1 is the proximal driving pressure, P_e is the external collapsing pressure, V is flow velocity, and A is a constant describing the slope of the linear relation between $P_1 - P_e$ and V. This equation indicates that flow velocity, V, is related to the difference between aortic pressure and the external pressure tending to collapse the artery. Flow then becomes unrelated or decoupled from the distal coronary pressure and therefore from the stenosis pressure gradient, $P_1 - P_2$. This new pressure-flow behavior described by the above linear equation is, by definition, an adequate and necessary operational description of a Starling resistor (21,23,28,29).

In live, intact animals there is no technique currently known for measuring intraluminal pressure in the narrowed segment of an arterial stenosis. Neither is it possible to measure directly external pressure, P_e, since it depends on the complex cumulative effects of intrathoracic or intrapericardial pressure, arterial vasomotor tone, and elasticity of the arterial wall at the site of the stenosis as well as on the elasticity and fit of the circumferential inflatable stenosing device. Thus, although the intrathoracic or pericardial pressure around the coronary artery may be negative, vasomotor tone, tissue pressure, and the external compression of the inflatable cuff make the arterial collapse pressure positive. These factors also make it virtually impossible to measure directly

FLEXIBLE WALL CORONARY STENOSIS

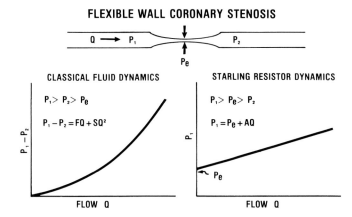

Fig. 6.1 Schematic showing pressure-flow relations described by the conventional quadratic equation for a rigid stenosis model (left panel) and described by the linear equation of a pressure-gradient decoupled model characteristic of a flexible-walled stenosis or a Starling resistor (right panel). When the intraluminal distending pressure in the stenotic segment is greater than the net pressure, P_e, or force comprised of vasomotor tone and external compression of the artery, even a flexible-wall coronary artery will behave as a rigid tube according to the conventional quadratic equation. Such stenoses are characterized by a curvilinear relation between pressure gradient across the stenosis and coronary flow in the form of the quadratic equation, as shown in the left panel. However, a severely stenotic artery with a flexible arterial wall will behave as a pressure-gradient decoupled system or a Starling resistor when the intraluminal distending pressure falls below those elastic, vasomotor, or external compressing forces tending to collapse the artery. Stenoses behaving like a Starling resistor demonstrate a linear relation between proximal coronary driving pressure and flow independent of distal coronary pressure, P_2, as demonstrated in the right panel.

the net force or pressure acting to collapse the arterial stenosis.

Consequently, the fluid dynamics of a Starling resistor in vivo have previously been operationally described for other parts of the vascular system by indirect measurements, namely the relation between proximal *driving pressure* and flow as opposed to the relation between *pressure gradient* across the stenosis (or vascular bed) and flow through it. Previous studies have demonstrated that the behavior of a Starling resistor is characterized by flow being independent of or decoupled from the pressure gradient across a vascular bed (30,31). Similarly, for a coronary artery stenosis behaving like a Starling resistor, coronary flow is decoupled from the pressure gradient across the stenosis and from distal coronary pressure, as well as from distal vasodilation (28,29). Coronary flow in that case becomes related to aortic pressure only. The linear equation above then describes an empirical model for the hemodynamic behavior of a stenosis which, for convenience, is called the pressure-gradient decoupled model and which, within the range of measured data, behaves as a Starling resistor. It is important to note that the linear equation is here used to describe relations among empirical data within the range of measured data, and particularly the

uniqueness of fit of a model to experimental data. Its use does not imply linearity beyond the range of measured data.

Therefore, if the measured pressure-flow characteristics of a coronary arterial stenosis are curvilinear following the quadratic equation $P_1 - P_2 = FV + SV^2$, the stenosis then empirically fits the conventional form of fluid-dynamic equations for rigid stenoses. However, if the pressure-flow characteristics of a coronary stenosis fit the linear equation $P_1 - P_e = AV$, then the stenosis behaves like a pressure-gradient decoupled system, or a Starling resistor, over the range of experimental observations. By measuring experimentally the pressure-flow characteristics of a given stenosis, we therefore can determine empirically whether it behaves according to conventional quadratic equations for rigid stenoses or behaves as a pressure-gradient decoupled system characteristic of a Starling resistor. By analyzing the uniqueness of the fit of experimental pressure-flow data to either the rigid stenosis model ($\Delta P = FV + SV^2$) or the pressure-gradient decoupled model ($P_1 = P_e + AV$), we can determine in vivo whether the coronary stenosis is behaving as a collapsing flexible-walled stenosis or not.

As described below, a series of experimental coronary stenoses were analyzed for uniqueness of fit of experimental pressure-flow data to the rigid stenosis model ($\Delta P = FV + SV^2$) and to the pressure-gradient decoupled model ($P_1 = P_e + AV$) in order to determine whether a coronary stenosis behaves in vivo as a rigid stenosis or as a flexible-walled stenosis resembling a Starling resistor.

In this study, flow velocity, V, was used because the zero baseline for Doppler transducers is very stable without drift, allowing recordings of low flow levels associated with severe stenosis. Electromagnetic zero baseline is unstable enough to be a problem technically. Furthermore, conversion of velocity recordings to volume flow requires coronary arteriography to obtain the arterial lumen area at the Doppler transducer. However, injection of contrast media changes flow, flow velocity, and pressure in the artery, thereby changing the unstable configuration of flexible-walled stenosis, whose shape is highly variable depending on pressure and flow. The injection of contrast media tends to open the collapsed stenosis, due to the higher injection pressure and to the viscosity of contrast media, which slows flow velocity.

Arteriography therefore changes the geometry of what it is intended to measure. Accordingly, in this analysis, arteriography was used to determine severity of the stenoses at resting conditions but not to study the collapsing stenosis phenomenon. The collapsing stenosis phenomenon can be studied only by continuous pressure–flow velocity measurements, since the electromagnetic flowmeter is a problem for establishing stable zero baselines for low flows observed with these severe stenoses. Although flow-velocity measurements have the quantitative limitations described in previous chapters, the endpoint here is a qualitative, major, large, sudden breakdown of the pressure–flow velocity relation of a stenosis to a totally different aortic pressure–flow velocity relation.

Two forms of analysis were used for all data from all stenoses in this study. In the first case, the stenosis was analyzed by determining the r value and standard error of estimate (SEE) of the best-fitting, conventional quadratic equation to the measured pressure difference across the stenosis (proximal pressure-distal pressure) and blood flow velocity as described by the relation $\Delta P = FV + SV^2$, where V and ΔP are coronary flow velocity and pressure gradient across the stenosis. In the curve-fitting process, F and S were allowed to change at rest and after intracoronary vasodilators to whatever values produced the curve best fitting all the recorded pressure-flow data over the entire range of flow. In the second case, the same data for that stenosis were also analyzed by determining the r value and SEE of the best-fitting linear equation to the measured pressure-flow data as described by the equation $P_1 = P_e + AV$, where V is flow velocity and P_1 is proximal coronary, or aortic, pressure. P_e is the net pressure or force due to vasomotor tone and external collapsing pressure acting on the artery, which cannot be directly measured but is simply determined as the vertical axis intercept of the linear equation $P_1 = P_e + AV$. In this equation describing behavior of a Starling resistor, flow velocity through the stenosis is independent of stenosis pressure gradient and independent of distal coronary pressure.

Thus, the data measured experimentally were fit to these two equations, with a correlation coefficient obtained for each in order to determine which equation best fit the data for each stenosis. Coefficients F, S, and A were found from "least squares" regression analyses, as described previously (1,2,15,31). The correlation coefficient (r) and standard error of the estimate (SEE) for the regression equation were used to quantify the uniqueness of each model to the data and were computed by the relations:

$$r = \sqrt{\frac{\Sigma(Y_i - \hat{Y}_i)^2}{\Sigma(Y_i - Y_{avg})^2}}$$

$$SEE = \sqrt{\frac{\Sigma(Y_i - \hat{Y}_i)^2}{(N - 2)}}$$

where $\hat{Y}_i = a + bX_i$ with a and b being the contacts of the regression equation relating Y_i and X_i. For the Starling model, $y = P_1$, $x = Q$, $a = Pe$, and $b = A$. For the quadratic model, $y = \Delta P$, $X = Q$, $a = F$, and $b = S$. Y_i and X_i are the individual data coordinates for proximal pressure and velocity or pressure gradient and velocity, Y_{avg} is the average y value of the data ensemble, N is the number of data points applied to the regression analysis, and Y_i is the value predicted by either the linear or quadratic regression analysis on a given velocity value (33). The standard error of the estimate depends on the sum of squared residuals divided by the degrees of freedom for the polynomial, where the residuals are the $Y_i - y$

difference between the actual data point and predicted data point. Thus, the r value and SEE are indicators of the goodness of fit of the regression to the data and of the variation in the data around the fitted curve.

The 13 stenoses studied were ranked on the basis of increasing severity; stenoses 1 through 7 were relatively mild and characterized by a pressure–flow velocity relation that best fit the quadratic equation for a rigid stenosis, $\Delta P = FV + SV^2$. Stenoses 8 through 13 were more severe, and the pressure–flow relation for these best fit the linear equation for a pressure-gradient decoupled stenosis, $P_1 = P_e + AV$, consistent with behavior of a Starling resistor. Thus, the values of r and SEE were used to separate the stenoses into two subsets. The other data for the two groups were then compared using a non-paired t-test for the difference of means (33). All values in the tables are expressed as mean ± one standard deviation for the group, except where indicated as the SEE.

For any given stenosis, if the r values were higher and the SEEs lower for the quadratic equation with variable F and S, that stenosis would follow conventional fluid-dynamic relations and the Starling concept would be disproved for that stenosis. However, if the r values were higher and the SEEs were lower for the linear Starling equation, that stenosis would be adequately described by the Starling model and the conventional fluid-dynamic relations would not be applicable.

EXPERIMENTAL OBSERVATIONS

Pressure gradient $(P_1 - P_2)$ and flow velocity were plotted for several diastoles from resting coronary flow to elevated flow for each stenosis in order to obtain the best-fitting quadratic equation for all stenoses, as shown in the left part of Figure 6.2, stenoses 1 through 7. In this analysis, an increase in stenosis severity is indicated by an increase in the steepness of the quadratic curve. For stenoses 1–7, the correlation coefficients for fitting quadratic equations to the measured data were all above r = 0.8, with a mean r value of 0.937 ± .051. In these figures, the number of measured data points, n, for each curve fit, the r value, and the standard error of estimate are shown. There are so many data points for each analysis that they may appear as continuous lines in each pressure–flow velocity graph.

For the more severe stenoses, 8 through 13, the experimentally measured pressure gradient-flow velocity data did

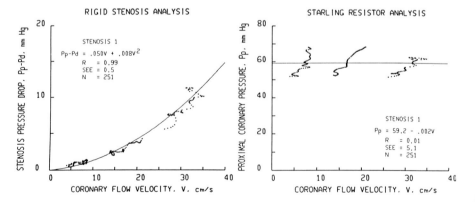

Fig. 6.2 Plots of the measured pressure-flow data for each stenosis. The left panels show the best-fit quadratic equation for a rigid stenosis. The right panels show the best-fit linear equation for a pressure-gradient decoupled model. P_p is proximal coronary pressure and P_d is coronary pressure distal to the stenosis. For example, for the first stenosis shown, the conventional quadratic equation fits the data with a

Legend continued on next page

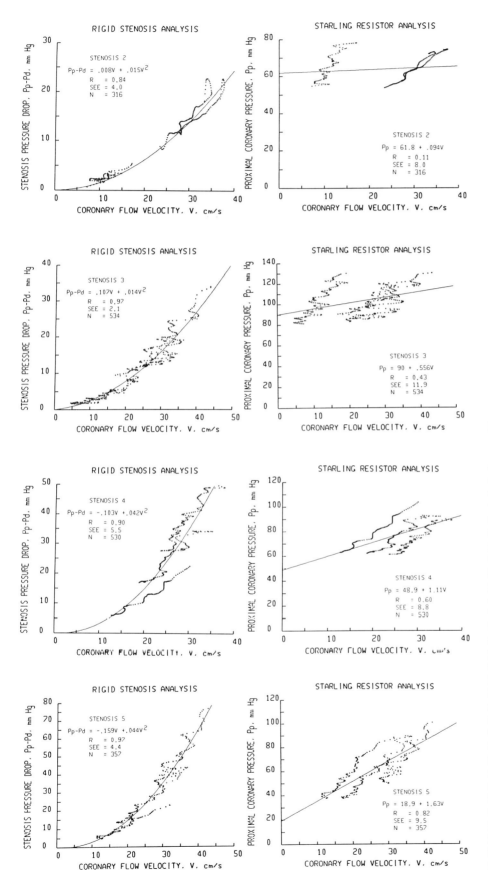

Fig. 6.2 *continued*

high r value (0.986) and a narrow standard error of the estimate (0.53) for 251 data points from 3 diastolic periods over a wide range of coronary flows, thereby indicating very little scatter of measured data about the best-fit quadratic equation. The data from this stenosis did not demonstrate a good fit to the linear equation characterizing a Starling resistor as shown in the right panel. For the second group of stenoses shown, illustrated by stenosis 13, the measured pressure-flow data failed to fit the conventional quadratic equation for a rigid stenosis (left panel). However, the measured pressure flow data did fit the linear relation between proximal coronary pressure, P_1, and coronary flow velocity characteristic of a pressure-gradient decoupled system or a Starling resistor with a high r value of 0.845 and a narrow standard error of the estimate (6.32), indicating little scatter of the measured data around this best-fit equation. All 13 stenoses between these two extremes are plotted. Cardiac cycles with short R-R intervals have fewer data points, owing to a fixed sample rate for digitizing data; for example, for stenosis 1, n = 251, whereas for stenosis 3, n = 534.

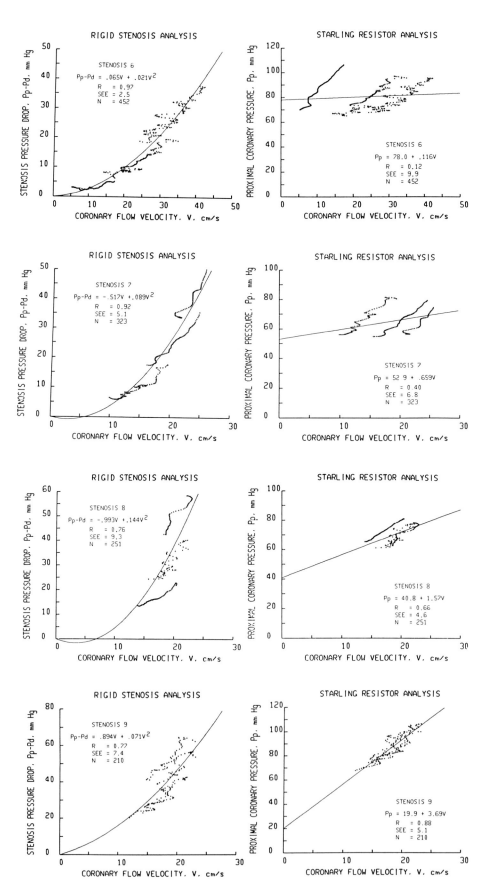

Fig. 6.2 *continued*

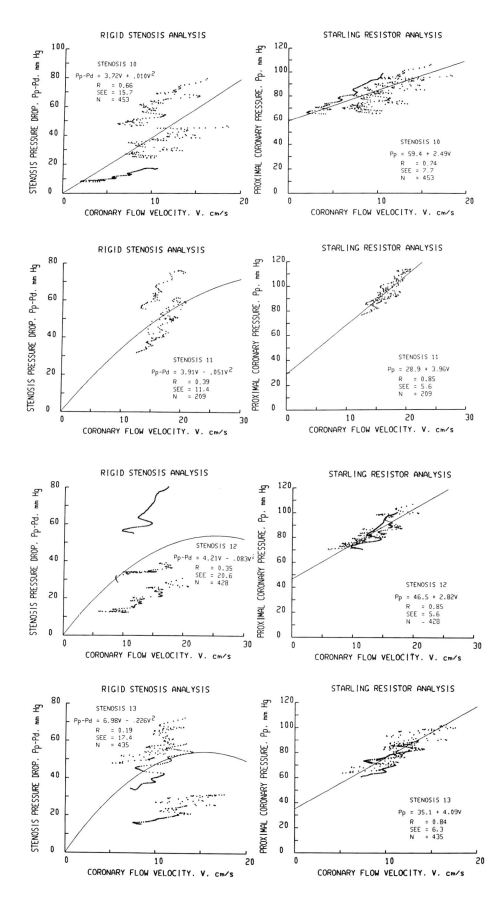

Fig. 6.2 *continued*

Table 6.1 Stenoses Fitting Classic Fluid Dynamics and Starling Resistor Hemodynamics

	Correlation Coefficient, (r) by		Standard Error Estimate, (SEE) by	
Exp. No.	Classic analysis	Starling analysis	Classic analysis	Starling analysis
Stenoses Fitting Classic Fluid Dynamics				
1	.986	.004	0.53	5.08
2	.842	.112	4.03	8.00
3	.965	.426	2.07	11.90
4	.904	.598	5.47	8.81
5	.971	.817	4.42	9.47
6	.969	.120	2.54	9.85
7	.921	.403	5.14	6.82
mean ± S.D.	.937 ± .051	.354 ± .294	3.46 ± 1.80	8.56 ± 2.20
Sig. difference	P = .001		P = .001	
Stenoses Fitting Starling Resistor Hemodynamics				
8	.758	.663	9.29	4.58
9	.767	.878	7.45	5.12
10	.665	.735	15.7	7.72
11	.394	.853	11.4	5.59
12	.347	.851	20.6	5.57
13	.188	.845	17.4	6.32
mean ± S.D.	.520 ± .243	.804 ± .085	13.64 ± 5.08	5.82 ± 1.10
Sig. difference	P = .03		P = 0.01	

sure gradient-flow velocity data did not fit the conventional quadratic equation. No quadratic equation in the form $\Delta P = FV + SV^2$ could be constrained to fit the experimental data points, as evidenced by low correlation coefficients of $r < 0.8$ and a mean r value of .520 ± .243. In addition, visual observation of the scatter in data points around the computer-generated curve reveals that a quadratic equation does not fit these data. Stenoses 8 through 13 thus form a subset of severe stenoses that cannot be adequately described by the conventional quadratic equation for a rigid stenosis.

The alternative analysis, using the linear equation characteristic of a Starling resistor equation, was then applied to all the data of all stenoses, with the results compared between the two subsets. For stenoses 1 through 7, the experimental data that *did* fit the conventional fluid-dynamics quadratic equations for a stenosis *did not* fit the equation $P_1 = P_e + AV$, characteristic of a pressure-gradient decoupled system or Starling resistor, as shown in the right panels of Figure 6.2. Fit of the data to the linear Starling equation was poor, with r values averaging 0.350 ± 0.294. These results demonstrated a unique fit of these stenoses to the standard fluid-dynamic model of stenosis. However, for stenoses 8 through 13, the experimental data that *did not* fit the standard fluid-dynamic quadratic equation for a stenosis *did* fit the linear equation characterizing a pressure-gradient decoupled model or a Starling resistor, as shown in the right panels of Figure 6.2. Correlation coefficients were high, with the average r value being 0.804 ± .085, thereby demonstrating a reasonably unique fit of these stenoses to the pressure-gradient decoupled model describing behavior of a Starling resistor.

Thus, all 13 stenoses were analyzed for uniqueness of fit to the conventional fluid-dynamic quadratic equations for a stenosis and to the linear equation characterizing a pressure-gradient decoupled system consistent with a Starling resistor. The correlation coefficient, r, and standard error of the estimate, SEE, for each method of analysis for each stenosis are listed in Table 6.1. The same stenosis numbering system is used as in the figures. The upper half of Table 6.1 lists the less severe stenoses fitting the conventional quadratic equation. The mean r for fitting the experimental data to the conventional quadratic equation is .937 ± .051, significantly different from the correlation for the same data fit to the linear equation characterizing a pressure-gradient decoupled system or Starling resistor, where the mean r = .350 ± .287, the difference being significant, with P = .001.

The standard error of estimate for the best fit of these stenoses to the conventional quadratic equation is 3.46 ± 1.80, indicating a low degree of data scatter around the best-fit quadratic equation. This standard error of estimate is significantly lower than that for the linear equation characterizing a Starling resistor, 8.56 ± 2.20, with P = .001 for these same stenoses; the larger SEE indicates a significantly larger degree of data scatter and therefore a poorer fit between the data and the equation characteristic of a pressure-gradient decoupled system for stenoses 1 through 7.

The more severe stenoses, 8 through 13, are grouped in the lower half of Table 6.1. The mean r value for fitting the experimental data to the conventional quadratic equation is .520 ± .243, indicating a poor fit as compared to an r of .804 ± .085 for fitting the data to the linear equation character-

Table 6.2 Need Table Title

Stenoses Fitting	Conventional fluid dynamic equations	Equations for Starling resistors
stenosis × sect. area, mm²	0.48 ± .15	0.21 ± .07
	P = .011	
% diameter stenosis, %	61 ± 12	75 ± 3
	P = .038	
measured stenosis *resting* ΔP, mmHg	5 ± 5	19 ± 6
	P = .003	
sets of angiograms	6	4

P value for significance of difference between conventional and Starling equations mean ± 1 standard deviation.

izing a Starling resistor; the difference between these r values is significant at P = .03. The best fit of the data from these stenoses to the conventional quadratic equation results in a larger mean standard error of estimate of 13.64 ± 5.08, indicating great scatter of data as compared to 5.82 ± 1.10, P = .01, for fitting the data to the equation characterizing a Starling resistor. Thus, for stenoses 8 through 13 the coronary flow velocity became uncoupled from and unrelated to the pressure gradient across the stenosis but did correlate with, and depend on, proximal driving pressure alone.

The intraluminal pressure in the stenotic segment cannot be directly measured in vivo. However, the pressure in the coronary artery measured distal to the stenosis demonstrates a profound fall in intraluminal distending pressure during distal coronary vasodilation. For stenoses 1 through 7, the average coronary pressure distal to the stenosis at rest flow was 60 ± 13 mm Hg, falling after coronary arteriolar vasodilation to 42 ± 18 mm Hg. For stenoses 8 through 13, the average coronary pressure distal to the stenosis at rest flow was 55 ± 5 mm Hg, which fell after coronary vasodilation to 22 ± 5 mm Hg. The intraluminal pressure in the stenotic segment itself would probably be less than 22 mm Hg, because of the Bernoulli effect caused by the higher flow velocity in the stenotic segment as compared to that in the larger normal arterial cross-sectional area. The intraluminal pressure in the stenotic segment should not be confused with, and is unrelated to, the distal coronary pressure at which flow ceases or at which the arteriolar or capillary vascular bed "collapses," commonly called the "critical closing pressure."

The dimensions of the stenoses analyzed in this study are presented in Table 6.2. The mean minimum cross-sectional area of the artery at the stenosis was 0.48 ± .15 mm² for those that fit the conventional quadratic equation, as compared to 0.21 ± 0.07 mm² for stenoses that fit the equation characterizing a Starling resistor. This difference was signif-

FIT OF PRESSURE-FLOW DATA TO TESTED MODELS

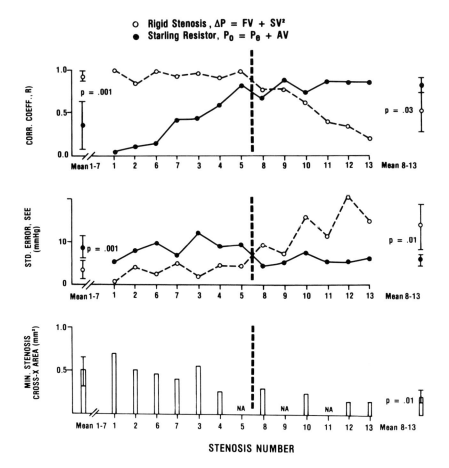

Fig. 6.3 A plot of the correlation coefficient, r, the standard error of estimate, SEE, and the minimum stenosis cross-sectional area for each of the stenoses studied. The bar graphs at the left of the figure indicate the mean values for stenoses 1 through 7, and those at the right indicate the mean values for stenoses 8 through 13. The heavy dashed vertical lines indicate the transition stage at which the standard error of estimate for the best-fit curves of each model cross over each other.

icant, with P = .011. Similarly, the mean percent diameter stenosis at rest flow for the stenoses fitting the conventional equation was 61 ± 12% compared to 75 ± 3% for stenoses demonstrating behavior like a Starling resistor, the difference being significant with P = .038.

It is important to note that the data reflect a continuum of mild to severe stenoses and also variability between different dogs. Thus, there is not a uniform ranking that is applicable to all parameters. Stenoses 8 and 9 are part of a transition zone where it is difficult to determine whether the conventional quadratic equation for rigid stenoses or the linear equation characterizing a pressure-gradient decoupled system is more appropriate. At the opposite ends of the spectrum, stenosis hemodynamics are clearly described by either one equation or the other. This spectrum is illustrated in Figure 6.3, which shows the correlation coefficient, r, standard error of estimate, SEE, and the cross-sectional area of each stenosis.

ANALYSIS OF EXPERIMENTAL OBSERVATIONS

Severe stenoses of coronary arteries of approximately 70%–75% diameter narrowing with segments of flexible walls may not behave according to conventional quadratic equation describing pressure-flow characteristics of most stenoses. Instead, the fluid dynamics of blood flow through these stenoses are best described by a linear equation characteristic of a pressure-gradient decoupled system as seen for a Starling resistor, where flow velocity is linearly related to the coronary driving pressure proximal to the stenosis and is not related to the pressure gradient across the stenosis or to distal coronary pressure.

The following mechanism appears to explain these observations. For a fairly severe stenosis, the total energy content in the proximal coronary artery system consists of a large amount of potential or pressure energy and a low flow velocity or low kinetic energy. In the stenotic segment, however, by Bernoulli's principle, the flow velocity or kinetic energy is high, and potential or pressure energy is low, associated with a fall in intraluminal pressure in the stenotic segment. Thus, in the stenotic segment the pressure energy is converted to kinetic energy, with resulting loss of distending pressure in the lumen of the stenotic segment. At resting conditions this loss of distending pressure may be only modest, insufficient to fall below the collapse pressure of the stenotic segment, P_e. However, with distal coronary vasodilation, the pressure gradient across the stenosis rises dramatically, and distal coronary pressure as well as intraluminal pressure in the stenotic segment correspondingly falls further (1–3). In that case, since intraluminal pressure in the narrowed segment is low even before coronary vasodilation, it may fall below the external pressure, acting to collapse the artery, due to vasomotor tone, arterial elasticity, and/or external compression by a cuff constrictor. When the intraluminal pressure becomes less than the external collapsing pressure, the flexible stenotic segment partially collapses, typically at the distal end for long stenoses (22).

When the arterial segment collapses by this process, flow ceases (or decreases, with incomplete collapse), kinetic energy content of the system falls, and the pressure head or energy content of the system becomes available as intraluminal distending pressure. This restoration of distending pressure opens the flexible segment, flow begins again, and pressure energy is again converted to kinetic energy, with a subsequent fall in intraluminal distending pressure causing collapse again (19–24).

The results of this study demonstrate that, within the range of experimental data, a severely stenotic, flexible-walled coronary artery may, after distal arteriolar vasodilation, behave like a Starling resistor, since flow becomes determined by, and proportional to, aortic pressure. Flow becomes uncoupled from the pressure gradient and therefore independent of the stenosis gradient and distal coronary pressure. The flexible-walled, stenotic coronary artery then meets the criteria of a "vascular waterfall" characteristic of a Starling resistor within the range of measured pressure-flow data.

A GENERAL EQUATION FOR THE FLUID DYNAMICS OF COLLAPSING STENOSES

The observation that collapsing coronary artery stenoses behave like Starling resistors does not provide a complete fluid-dynamic description of the mechanisms involved. A more mechanistic explanation can be provided from a theory of compliant arterial stenoses, whereby both rigid and collapsible stenoses are described in terms of fluid-dynamic behavior, using a more general set of equations than those derived for rigid tubes in vitro. The general equations describing compliant arterial stenoses reduce to conventional fluid-dynamic equations for rigid stenoses if compliance approaches zero.

FLUID-DYNAMIC EQUATIONS FOR COMPLIANT ARTERIAL STENOSES

The following equations and figures for a compliant arterial stenosis were developed in collaboration with Richard L. Kirkeeide.

Pressure drop-velocity relations for severe rigid stenoses have been shown to be of the form

$$\Delta P = C_v V_o + C_i V_o^2 \qquad (1)$$

where C_v and C_i are coefficients calculated from the stenosis geometry and blood properties, V_o is flow velocity proximal to the stenosis, and P is the pressure drop due to the stenosis. This equation describes the proximal-to-distal drop in pressure ($P_o - P_2$) as in the lower panel of Figure 6.4, resulting from (a) frictional losses along the narrowed artery, $C_v V_o^2$, linearly related to velocity and blood viscosity, and (b) inertial losses, $C_i V_o^2$, associated with flow expansion, deceleration, and eddy formation distal to the stenosis. An extensive series of in-vivo experiments using rigid hollowed plugs inserted into various arteries of dogs have validated this relation as well as experiments in vivo by our lab.

The theory assumes that compliant (collapsible) stenoses differ from rigid stenoses only in that their cross-sectional areas (As) vary with pressure. The proximal and distal cross sections of the vessel are also compliant. However, because inclusion of proximal and distal artery compliance into the

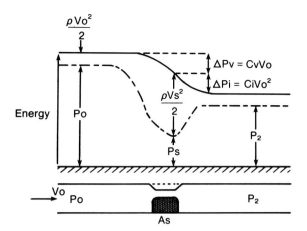

Fig. 6.4 Schematic showing energy on the vertical axis as a function of location along the compliant stenotic artery on the horizontal axis. The various symbols are described in the text of the appendix for the equations used there.

the theory affect only minimally the prediction of pressure drop–velocity relations for numerical simulations of severe coronary stenoses, these effects have been omitted from the following analysis. The pressure drop–velocity relation for compliant stenoses is then similar to the rigid case (Eq. 1) but stenosis area (As) is a variable, i.e.,

$$\Delta P = C_1 (Ao/As)^2 Vo + C_2 (Ao/As - 1)^2 Vo^2 \quad (2)$$

The coefficients C_1 and C_2 are related to the coefficients Cv and Ci in Equation 1 and are calculated from stenosis length (Ls), proximal arterial diameter (Do), blood viscosity (μ), and density (ρ) by the relations:

$$C_1 = 32 (Ls/Do) (\mu/Do) \quad (3)$$

and

$$C_2 = 1.52\rho Do/2 \quad (4)$$

where μ and ρ are the blood viscosity and mass density, respectively.

Compliance of a stenosis is due to a combination of passive and active wall properties associated with the amount of the arterial circumference involved by calcification, the mechanical properties of elastin and collagen, and the amount of vessel smooth muscle tone. The final common effect of all these factors can be expressed by their influence on the stenosis area-pressure relation,

$$As = f(Ps) \quad (5)$$

where f denotes the function relating intra-stenotic pressure to cross-sectional area of the stenosis while that relation exists; its specific form must be either measured experimentally or assumed, as was done in the numerical simulations as follow as a conceptual example. If intra-stenotic pressure (Ps) is measured, then stenotic area is given by Equation 5, and pressure drop across the stenosis for a given velocity is predicted by Equation 2. These equations indicate that although stenosis geometry may depend on pressure, the fluid-dynamic phenomena responsible for viscous shear losses along the stenosis and inertial pressure losses such as turbulence,

flow separation, and flow deceleration, are the same as in rigid stenoses.

Intra-stenotic pressure can also be calculated by considering how flow energy varies between the proximal and stenotic sections of the vessel. The top of Figure 6.4 shows that the total energy proximal to the stenosis is primarily due to pressure (Po) or potential energy. However, at the stenosis the pressure (Ps) decreases from Po by two mechanisms: the increased kinetic energy of stenotic flow (PVs²/2), and the irreversible viscous pressure losses, ΔPv, along the stenosis. In addition, there is conservation of mass-energy principle, expressed as Vs = Vo(Ao/As). Therefore, Ps can be predicted from stenosis geometry and proximal velocity by the relation

$$Ps = Po - \left[\left(\frac{Ao}{As}\right)^2 - 1 \right] P \frac{Vo^2}{2} - Ci \left(\frac{Ao}{As}\right)^2 Vo \quad (6)$$

The behavior of compliant arterial stenoses can now be predicted from the theory, if stenosis geometry and compliance are known. The basic differences between rigid and compliant stenosis behavior can be seen in numerical simulations of coronary stenoses using the following conditions: Proximal pressure (Po) 100 mm Hg, blood viscosity 0.04 poise, density 1 g/mL, proximal arterial diameter (Do) 3 mm, and stenoses length 6mm. Stenosis compliance for the simulations was assumed as shown in Figure 6.5, which relates relative changes in stenosis area, from the fully distended state, As^*, to changes in intra-stenotic pressure relative to proximal pressure (Ps/Po).

The relation of stenosis geometric severity (Ao/As) to proximal flow velocity (Vo) is shown in Figure 6.6 for several different, non-collapsed, but compliant, stenoses. The figure is derived from a combination of Equation 6 and the assumed stenosis compliance shown in Figure 6.5. Each stenosis exhibits quasirigid behavior as flow velocity is initially increased, as indicated by the lower horizontal portion of each curve, for example, segments A–B in Figure 6.6. Further increases in velocity begin to deflate the stenosis, thereby increasing its geometric severity, until at some critical velocity further increases are not permitted by the collapsing stenosis. This critical condition in the compliant stenosis behavior is

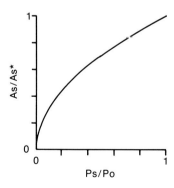

Fig. 6.5 Relation between intra-stenotic distending pressure expressed as a ratio to proximal pressure, Ps/Po, and changing cross-sectional area of the compliant stenosis expressed as a ratio of the cross-sectional area of the partially collapsed stenosis, As, to the fully distended stenosis, As*.

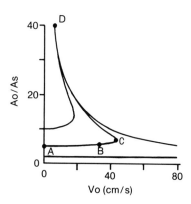

Fig. 6.6 Relation between changing severity of a compliant stenosis expressed as a ratio, Ao/As, and proximal flow velocity, Vo. See text of appendix for discussion of curve and points A, B, and C.

indicated by point C in Figure 6.6 at a velocity of 45 cm/s, which is approximately two times the normal resting velocity. The stenosis is at this point in an unstable state which can lead to a dramatic increase in stenosis severity and fall in arterial flow velocity, shown by the upward left swing of the curve from C to D. The reason for this sudden collapse is that intra-stenotic flow velocity can continue to increase despite the decrease in proximal flow velocity, since stenosis severity increases (worsens) faster than proximal flow velocity decreases. Thus, intra-stenotic pressure continues to fall and the stenosis further narrows. Collapse will continue either until the stenosis assumes a new shape, or until the stenosis and peripheral bed reach a new hydraulic equilibrium in terms of new flows and pressures.

Although all compliant stenoses are theoretically capable of such behavior, vasodilatory capabilities and the characteristics of the stenosis itself will limit the maximal proximal flow velocity attainable. Thus, severe coronary stenoses, with their associated low critical flow velocities, are most likely to exhibit such behavior under physiologic conditions; for example, the fully distended stenosis with a 90% area reduction (Ao/As = 10 at Vo = 0) in Figure 6.7 (solid line) will collapse at a flow velocity of 20 cm/s, which is only slightly greater than resting flow velocity. This pressure drop-velocity relation for the compliant but fully distended stenosis of 90% area reduction is shown in Figure 6.7 along with those predicted if the stenosis were rigid (dashed line). Also shown are the pressure drop–flow relations for more severe, rigid stenoses, AoAs = 15 and 25 (dashed lines). At low velocities, compliant stenoses exhibit the same behavior as rigid stenoses. However, with increasing velocity of flow, the curve swings upward to the critical point where flow is "choked." The curve then swings upward and to the left, signifying the worsening of the hemodynamic severity of the stenosis.

In summary, the developed theory of compliant arterial stenoses shows that the behavior of rigid and collapsible stenosis are fundamentally different in appearance and hemodynamic effect, but can be described from a common set of fluid-dynamic principles if the dependence of geometry on intraluminal pressure is taken into account.

For a severe compliant coronary artery stenosis and distal arteriolar vasodilation, flow velocity increases up to a maximum shown by point C in Figure 6.6 and by the furthest-right point of the solid line in Figure 6.7. At that point, intrastenotic pressure falls sufficiently that the elasticity of the compliant arterial wall of the stenosis causes it to partially collapse. Flow velocity then falls, in association with a higher pressure gradient than for the same velocity in the absence of distal vasodilation. As shown in Figure 6.7 by the solid line, flow velocity is then no longer related to the stenosis pressure gradient according to equations for rigid stenoses. The pressure gradient becomes uncoupled from flow, as shown by Figure 6.7 and observed in experiments reported here. Figure 6.8 illustrates fluttering of the pressure tracing at the unstable point where stenosis collapse begins, in order to further illustrate Starling behavior in these severe flexible stenoses.

Stenosis geometry may also change owing to coronary vasodilation or vasoconstriction of the stenotic segment (4–6), or of the normal coronary artery on either side of the stenotic segment (1–3,26). However, the quantitative effects of vasomotion of the normal artery on either side of a stenotic segment occur primarily with moderate stenoses and are relatively insignificant with severe stenoses, as demonstrated previously by relatively lesser changes in the constants f and s after vasodilation in the presence of a severe stenosis (1–3). In addition, for vasodilation on either side of the stenotic segment, even for moderate stenoses where the effect is greatest, the consequent worsening in percent diameter narrowing accounted for only 16% worsening of the pressure gradient at a given flow (2). In those studies the pressure-flow relations characterizing the stenoses conformed to the conventional quadratic equation, despite different values of f and s accounting for the altered geometry. Therefore, the marked changes in hemodynamic characteristics observed after distal coronary arteriolar vasodilation in severely stenotic, flexible coronary arteries in this study cannot be explained on the basis of large artery vasodilation on either side

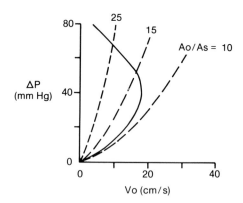

Fig. 6.7 Relation of the pressure drop to flow velocity for a rigid stenosis (dashed line) narrowing the cross-sectional area by 90% (Ao/As = 10) and for a compliant stenosis of the same severity (solid line). Even more severe rigid stenoses (dashed lines, Ao/As = 15 and 25) never demonstrate the "break point" at which the curve bends back toward zero flow velocity, which characterizes a compliant stenosis.

of the stenosis, in that the quadratic form for rigid stenoses could not be fit to the data in these experiments with any values of F and S.

The transition phase from hemodynamic behavior according to the conventional fluid-dynamic quadratic equations for a stenosis to that of a pressure-gradient decoupled system like a Starling resistor is a graded continuum, not a sudden complete change as previously described in the literature. Since our stenoses behaved like Starling resistors, as previously defined (21,23,28,29), but flow did not fall to zero or low fixed levels, there is a relatively stable intermediate, transitional phase where stenoses may behave as Starling resistors without complete collapse of the stenotic segment, as apparent from the equations in the appendix. This fact is fortunate experimentally since, if the transition was sudden and complete from fluid-dynamic behavior characterized by the conventional quadratic equation to complete collapse and cessation of flow, then there would be no range of flow variation over which flow could be demonstrated to uncouple from the pressure gradient. We therefore carefully avoided producing stenoses sufficiently severe that sudden complete collapse occurred but rather studied stenoses where a range of flow could be obtained, in order to demonstrate the altered

pressure-flow relations. With complete collapse of the stenosis, flow would cease and there would be no range of pressure-flow data over which the hemodynamic relations could be studied. For this reason we carried out a limited number of experiments, since it is difficult to obtain data just in the transition phase, as accomplished in these examples. However, statistical analysis that takes into account sample size shows the differences observed to be significant for the number of experiments done.

What is the relevance of our observations to human coronary atherosclerosis in patients with clinical coronary disease? Logan (34) studied the elasticity of human coronary stenoses in 19 patients postmortem by removing the segment of coronary stenosis and perfusing it under controlled conditions while measuring the pressure-flow characteristics. He found that most of the stenoses that he studied demonstrated considerable flexibility and elasticity of the arterial wall of the stenotic segment, with corresponding worsening effects observed on the pressure-flow characteristics of the stenoses. Those stenoses with flexible, eccentric walls had greater pressure losses than predicted from anatomic geometry using conventional fluid-dynamic equations. Brown et al. (4–6) have similarly shown, in patients using quantitative coronary

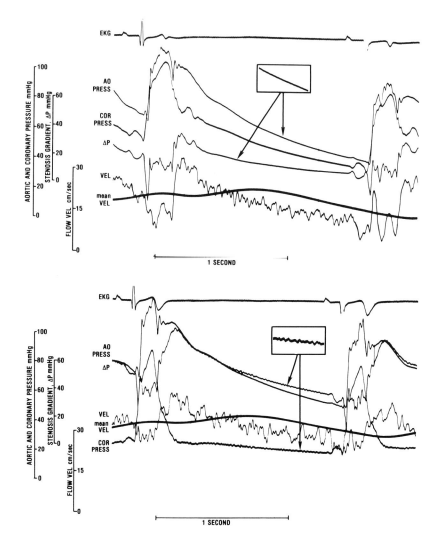

Fig. 6.8 Upper panel shows resting aortic pressure, coronary pressure, pressure gradient, and phasic and mean coronary flow velocity. There is no vibration in the coronary pressure trace. With a small increase in flow after arteriolar vasodilation, the pressure gradient increases markedly, coronary pressure falls, and both demonstrate a characteristic vibration most likely due to "fluttering" of the flexible narrowed coronary artery.

arteriography, that most human coronary stenoses in vivo demonstrate significant changes in dimensions during a variety of manipulations, including coronary vasodilators and handgrip, thereby indicating that stenotic segments of human coronary arteries often have flexible arterial walls.

Since human coronary stenoses may have flexible, vasoactive arterial walls, they may behave like a Starling resistor. These observations represent an additional variation of the constantly expanding theme which we have called "dynamic coronary stenosis" (26), observed in man and in experimental animals.

REFERENCES

1. Gould KL. Pressure-flow characteristics of coronary stenoses in unsedated dogs at rest and during coronary vasodilation. Circ Res 43:242–53, 1978.
2. Gould KL, Kelley KO. Physiologic significance of coronary flow velocity and changing stenosis geometry during coronary vasodilation in awake dogs. Circ Res 50:695–704, 1982.
3. Gould KL, Kelley KO, Bolson E. Experimental validation of quantitative coronary arteriography for determining pressure-flow characteristics of coronary stenoses. Circ 66:930–37, 1982.
4. Brown GB, Josephson MA, Peterson RB, Pierce DC, Wong M, Hecht HS, Bolson E, Dodge HT. Intravenous dipyridamole combined with isometric handgrip for near maximal acute increase in coronary flow in patients with coronary disease. Am J Cardiol 48:1077–85, 1981.
5. Brown BG, Bolson E, Peterson RB, Pierce CD, Dodge HT. The mechanisms of nitroglycerin action: stenosis vasodilation as a major component of the drug response. Circulation 64:1089–100, 1981.
6. Brown BG, Peterson RB, Pierce CD, Bolson EL, Dodge HT. Dynamics of Human Coronary Stenosis: Interactions Among Stenosis Flow, Distending Pressure and Vasomotor Tone in Coronary Artery Disease, ed. Santamore WP and Bove AA. Baltimore: Urban and Schwarzenberg, 1982.
7. Young DF. Fluid mechanics of arterial stenoses. J. Biomechanical Eng 101:157–75, 1979.
8. Mates RF, Gupta RL, Bell AC, Clocke FJ. Fluid dynamics of coronary artery stenosis. Circ Res 42:152–62, 1978.
9. Brown BG, Bolson E, Frimer M, Dodge HT: Quantitative coronary arteriography. Circulation 55:329–37, 1977.
10. Swartz JS, Carlyle PF, Cohn JN: Effect of dilation of the distal coronary bed on flow and resistance in severely stenotic coronary arteries in the dog. Am J Cardiol 43:219–44, 1979.
11. Schwartz JS, Carlyle PF, Cohn JN. Effect of coronary arterial pressure on coronary stenosis resistance. Circulation 61:70–76, 1980.
12. Schwartz JS, Tockman B, Cohn J, Bache RJ. Exercise induced decrease in flow through stenotic coronary arteries in the dog. Am J Cardiol 50:1409–13, 1982.
13. Schwartz JS. Fixed versus non-fixed coronary stenosis: The response to a fall in coronary pressure in a canine model. Cathet Cardiovas Diag 8:383–92, 1982.
14. Walinsky P, Santamore WP, Wiener L, Brest AN. Dynamic changes in the hemodynamic severity of coronary artery stenoses in a canine model. Cardiovas Res 13:113–18, 1979.
15. Santamore WP, Walinsky P. Altered coronary flow responses to vasoactive drugs in the presence of coronary arterial stenosis in the dog. Am J Cardiol 45:276–85, 1980.
16. Santamore WP, Walinsky P, Bove AA, Cox RH, Carey RA, Spann JF. The effects of vasoconstriction on experimental coronary artery stenosis. Am Heart J 100:852–58, 1980.
17. Santamore WP, Kent RL, Carey RA, Bove AA. Synergistic effects of pressure, distal resistance and vasoconstriction on stenosis. Am J Physiol H236–42, 1982.
18. Santamore WP, Bove AA, Carey RA. Tachycardia induced reduction in coronary blood flow distal to a stenosis. Internatl J Cardiol 2:23–37, 1982.
19. Knowlton FP, Starling EH. The influence of variations in temperature and blood pressure on the performance of the isolated mammalian heart. J Physiol 44:206–19, 1912.
20. Holt JP. The collapse factor in the measurement of venous pressure. Am J Physiol 134:292–99, 1941.
21. Holt JP. Flow through collapsible tubes and through in situ veins. IEEE Trans on Biom Eng BME-16 (no. 4):274–83, 1969.
22. Rodbard S, Saiki H. Flow through collapsible tubes. Am Heart J 46:715–25, 1953.
23. Conrad WA. Pressure-flow relationships in collapsible tubes. IEEE Trans on Biom Eng BME-16 (no. 4):284–95, 1969.
24. Shapiro AH. Steady flow in collapsible tubes. Biomech Eng 99:126–47, 1977.
25. Lyon CK, Scott JB, Wang CY. Flow through collapsible tubes at low Reynolds numbers. Circ Res 47:68–73, 1980.
26. Gould KL. Dynamic coronary stenosis. Am J Cardiol 45:286–87, 1980.
27. Riley RL. A postscript to Circulation of Blood: Men and Ideas, The Dickinson Richards Memorial Lecture. Circulation 66:683–88, 1982.
28. Fry DF, Thomas LJ, Greenfield JC. Flow in collapsible tubes (Chart 9) in Basic Hemodynamics, ed. Patel DA and Vaishnav RN. Baltimore: University Park Press, 1980, pp. 407–24.
29. Brower RW, Noordegraaf A. Pressure-flow characteristics of collapsible tubes: a reconciliation of seemingly contradictory results. Ann Biomed Eng 1:333–55, 1973.
30. Downey JM, Kirk ES. Distribution of coronary blood flow across the canine heart wall during systole. Circ Res 34:251–57, 1974.
31. Downey JM, Kirk ES. Inhibition of coronary blood flow by a vascular waterfall mechanism. Circ Res 36:753–60, 1975.
32. Gould KL, Lee D, Lovgren K. Techniques for arteriography and hydraulic analysis of coronary stenoses in unsedated dogs. Am J Physiol 235:H350–56, 1978.
33. Snedecor GW, Cochran WG. Statistical Methods. Ames, Iowa: Iowa State University Press, 1976.
34. Logan SE. On the fluid mechanics of human coronary artery stenosis. IEEE Transactions on Biomed Eng 22:327–34, 1975.

Coronary Flow Reserve

Under resting conditions, coronary blood flow remains normal during progressive coronary artery narrowing until the coronary arterial lumen is severely reduced, to approximately 85% diameter stenosis (1–3), reflecting advanced disease. Consequently, resting coronary flow or myocardial perfusion imaging at rest does not sensitively reflect the presence or severity of coronary artery disease. For this reason the disease is clinically silent until advanced stages when thrombosis, spasm, or minimal further narrowing may cause sudden death, acute myocardial infarction, or angina pectoris.

However, maximum coronary flow, and coronary flow reserve or the capacity to increase flow to high levels in response to exercise stress or pharmacologic coronary arteriolar vasodilators, becomes impaired with mild coronary artery stenosis. This phenomenon of coronary flow reserve in normal and stenotic coronary arteries was first observed experimentally 16 years ago (1), and subsequently related to stenosis geometry and applied clinically by Gould (1–18) as a means of identifying and quantifying the functional or hemodynamic significance of coronary artery stenosis. Coronary flow reserve, illustrated in Figure 7.1, is defined as the ratio of maximum flow or perfusion during stress or pharmacologic vasodilation to resting flow or perfusion (1).

Figure 7.2 relates stenosis severity (horizontal axis) to coronary flow reserve, expressed as the relative increase in flow multiplied by initial baseline resting flow (vertical axis) (1). The dashed line indicates resting flow. The solid line is flow reserve. The grey zone indicates the range for multiple observations. With progressive narrowing, baseline flow remains normal until the coronary artery is narrowed by 80%–85% diameter stenosis. However, coronary flow reserve begins to decrease at 40%–50% diameter stenosis for a vasodilatory stimulus, increasing flow normally to four times baseline. For a stimulus increasing flow to five or six times baseline levels, coronary flow reserve would be reduced by even milder stenoses of 30% diameter.

For the experimental stenoses upon which these figures were based, normal arterial diameter, stenosis length, and physiologic conditions were constant and relatively uniform for each stenosis in a progressive series of experimental coronary artery constrictions. Consequently, percent narrowing related well to flow reserve, with acceptable data scatter (grey area of Figure 7.2). In man absolute dimensions and length are not uniform, with the consequence that percent diameter stenosis is poorly related to coronary flow reserve (11,14,29,33). However, both experimentally and in man we

have shown that directly measured coronary flow reserve is equivalent to, interchangeable with, and predicted by the arteriographic geometry of coronary artery stenoses if all stenosis dimensions are accounted for, including percent stenosis, absolute cross-sectional lumen area, length, and shape (10–18), as reviewed in earlier chapters.

STIMULUS FOR MAXIMAL CORONARY FLOW

The value of coronary flow reserve as a measure of stenosis severity depends on the effectiveness of the vasodilatory stimulus for maximally increasing coronary flow. Therefore, an essential requirement of an imaging method for detecting or assessing severity of coronary artery disease is a potent stimulus for increasing coronary blood flow, in order to maximize regional differences in maximum perfusion caused by flow-limiting stenoses. Since exercise stress is not an optimal stimulus for maximal coronary flow, a potent coronary arteriolar vasodilator is used instead, such as intravenous dipyridamole (5–23), intravenous adenosine (24), or intracoronary papaverine (25). These drugs stimulate an approximately fourfold or higher increase in blood flow through normal human coronary arteries. By measuring coronary flow velocity with a Doppler catheter or by imaging myocardial perfusion at rest in comparison to maximum flow after intravenous dipyridamole, abnormalities in coronary flow reserve and relative distribution of maximum flow are observed that reflect the presence and severity of coronary artery stenoses. Figure 7.1 illustrates this principal as applied clinically by obtaining a radionuclide image of myocardial perfusion at rest and after intravenous dipyridamole.

MECHANISM FOR NORMAL RESTING CORONARY FLOW DESPITE STENOSIS

To explain maintenance of normal resting coronary flow but reduced coronary flow reserve during progressive coronary constriction, consider the stenotic coronary artery as two resistances in series—that is, a narrowed tube and a distal coronary vascular bed, represented schematically in Figure 7.3 (15). Normally, the distal coronary bed resistance at rest is high. The driving pressure for flow is the total pressure gradient across the stenosis and distal vascular bed, which is

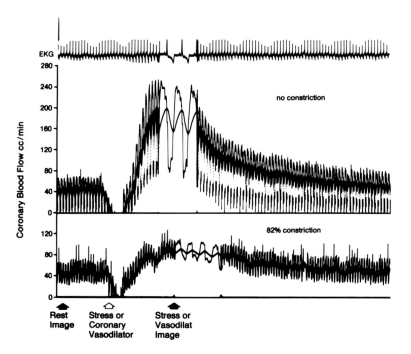

Fig. 7.1 The upper panel records coronary blood flow, measured by electromagnetic flowmeter in a normal artery at rest and following a coronary flow stimulus. Flow normally increases four to five times over baseline levels following pharmacologic exercise stress, thereby indicating a coronary reserve flow of 4 or 5. The lower panel indicates the flow response in the presence of an 82% diameter constriction of the coronary artery. Resting coronary flow is normal, but the increase in flow is blunted by the narrowing, thereby reducing the coronary flow reserve to approximately 2 in this case, as compared to a normal reserve of 4 or 5. Reproduced with permission from Gould KL, Lipscomb K, Hamilton GW, 1974 (1).

approximately central aortic pressure, since venous pressure is relatively small. Flow is therefore determined approximately by aortic pressure divided by the sum of the resistances of the stenosis, R_s, and of the distal vascular bed, R_b, in series. If the distal bed resistance is large compared with the stenosis resistance as normally found at rest, large changes in the stenosis resistance will have little effect on flow, which is determined primarily by distal vascular bed

resistance. Therefore, a progressive stenosis up to a point will have no hemodynamic effect on resting coronary blood flow.

However, as the stenosis becomes sufficiently severe to create a resistance comparable to that of the distal vascular bed, the distal bed vasodilates and loses its ability to autoregulate, and further narrowing will cause a fall in resting coronary blood flow. When the stenosis becomes sufficiently

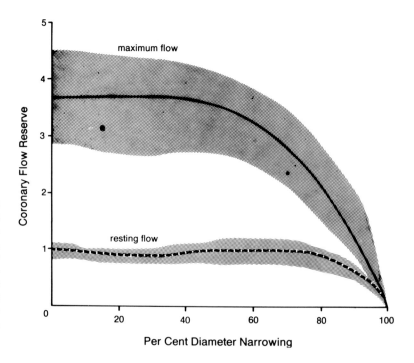

Fig. 7.2 Coronary flow reserve expressed as a ratio of maximum flow to resting flow plotted as a function of percent diameter narrowing. With progressive narrowing, resting flow does not change (dashed lines), whereas the maximum potential increase in flow or coronary flow reserve begins to be impaired at approximately 50% diameter narrowing. The gray areas represent the limits of variability of data about the mean plotted by the solid and dashed lines. Reproduced with permission from Gould KL, Lipscomb K, Hamilton GW, 1974 (1).

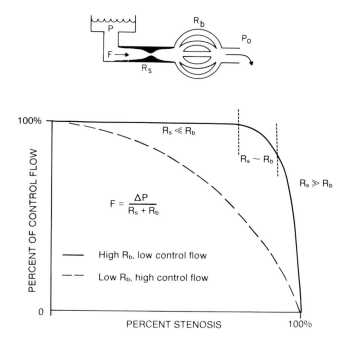

Fig. 7.3 A schematic representing the diseased coronary circulation as two resistances in series. R_s is the resistance of the narrowed artery and R_b is the resistance of the distal vascular bed. The effects of reducing R_b with vasodilators is shown by the dashed line. The equation shows the relation between resistance and flow (F) for various segments of the curves. For a given total pressure gradient across the narrowed tube and distal vascular bed (ΔP), flow is determined primarily by R_b, if R_b is large. Changes in the stenotic resistance, R_s, have little effect until the value of R_s approaches that of R_b. Reproduced with permission from Gould KL, 1985 (15).

severe that its resistance is much greater than that of the distal vascular bed, autoregulation will be lost and flow will be determined predominantly by the stenosis resistance alone. At that point, changes in distal vascular bed resistance will have little effect on blood flow through the stenosis. Thus, as documented experimentally in previous chapters, compensatory vasodilation plays little role in maintaining resting flow in response to progressive stenosis until a 60–70% diameter narrowing.

The coronary vascular system is normally a low-flow, high-resistance circulation at rest. Coronary vasodilators or stress convert this normally low-flow, high-resistance system into a high-flow, low-resistance system, in which coronary stenoses, even mild ones, have greater effects on maximum flow. Such logic explains why imaging regional myocardial perfusion at maximum coronary vasodilation can be used to detect even mild coronary narrowing. This discussion and the schematic in Figure 7.3 have to be qualified by acknowledging that the true venular back pressure to coronary flow may be considerably higher than venous pressure. For example, zero flow pressure of the coronary artery may range from 10–20 mm Hg, which is higher than venous pressure. However, the conceptual explanation of why resting coronary flow remains normal with progressive stenosis is still true.

EFFECT OF SEQUENTIAL STENOSIS IN SERIES ON CORONARY FLOW RESERVE

Figure 7.4 shows the effects on coronary flow reserve of progressive distal constriction in the presence of a fixed proximal constriction in a representative experiment (2). In this dog, coronary flow reserve decreased with a single progressive stenosis, as demonstrated in the results for all stenoses in Figure 7.2. With a fixed proximal stenosis of 75%, coronary flow reserve during progressive distal constriction was shifted downward from flow reserves in the absence of a fixed proximal stenosis. For example, the coronary flow reserve of two 75% constrictions in series was lower than that for a single 75% stenosis. With a critical proximal narrowing of 88% diameter stenosis, coronary flow reserve was eliminated in this experiment, with no capacity for increasing flow in response to vasodilatory stimuli. Adding additional stenoses up to 88% narrowing did not have further effects.

It is a common clinical precept that coronary hemodynamics are determined by the most severe lesion in a coronary artery. Our data indicate that this concept is imprecise. Pressure gradients and resistances of stenoses in series are clearly additive, as demonstrated in previous chapters. However, the effect of stenoses in series on coronary flow and flow reserve is complex. In some circumstances, this concept is accurate. For example, 80% diameter stenosis did not reduce resting

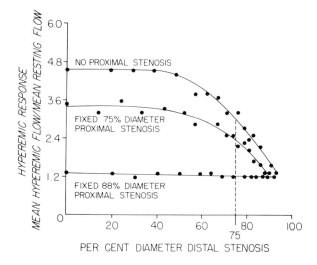

Fig. 7.4 Relation of coronary flow reserve (hyperemic response) after injection of contrast medium to percent diameter constriction of a progressive distal circumflex stenosis with no proximal stenosis, with a fixed proximal stenosis of 75% of arterial diameter, and with a fixed proximal stenosis of 88% of arterial diameter in one dog. The solid lines are the best fit curves to a power series (polynomial). The upper curve is typical for a single stenosis. The middle curve is for an additional fixed proximal 75% diameter stenosis in series with the first 75% diameter stenosis. Coronary flow is reduced more for the two 75% stenoses than for one 75% stenosis alone. For the lower curve, a fixed proximal 88% diameter stenosis was severe enough to prevent significant flow increases over baseline values without added effects of the 75% stenosis. Reproduced with permission from Gould KL, Lipscomb K, 1974 (2).

coronary flow; if in series with 95% stenosis, a degree of constriction that does affect resting flow, the more severe lesion determined the effects on resting flow. Similarly, 30% diameter stenosis alone did not reduce hyperemic response, or coronary flow reserve; if in series with 60% stenosis, a degree of narrowing that does reduce hyperemic response, the more severe lesion also determined entirely the effects on hyperemic flow. However, if both stenoses were moderate and separately severe enough to reduce flow reserve, their effects in series were additive and the more severe lesion did not determine all the effects on flow reserve.

Figure 7.4 illustrates an example. Coronary flow reserve of two 75% stenoses in series is less than that of one 75% stenosis alone. Similarly, two 95% stenoses in series reduce resting flow more than one alone. Thus, the maxim that the more severe lesion determines the hemodynamic effects of stenoses is accurate only when one of the stenoses in series alone has no effect or eliminates flow reserve altogether. Effects of stenosis of intermediate severity that individually reduce resting flow or flow reserve are additive in series.

RELATION OF CORONARY FLOW RESERVE TO PRESSURE GRADIENT ACROSS THE STENOSIS

The relation between coronary flow reserve and the pressure gradient across a stenosis can be derived from a model of the coronary circulation shown in Figure 7.5 (26). Potential collateral connections are represented by a lumped flow path including all flow channels that circumvent the stenosis and anastomose with the myocardial bed. These three vascular elements are linked hemodynamically by the distal coronary pressure, P_c, which is common pressure distal to the stenosis, pressure perfusing the collateral bed, and pressure to the normal myocardial bed. Aortic pressure, P_{Ao}, is the energy source for driving blood through these elements, and the coronary venous pressure, P_v, is the effective back pressure of the system.

Consider conceptually, for simplicity, the model of Figure 7.5 without the systolic changes, vasomotion, or problems of calculating stenosis resistance in vivo. Myocardial blood flow, Q, is determined by the pressure difference across the myocardial bed ($P_c - P_v$) and by the total resistance to flow through the myocardial bed. This resistance, R_b, is due to both intravascular forces (viscous wall shear) and the periodic compression of the vascular bed during systole. It is defined by the relation

$$R_b = (P_c - P_v)/Q \qquad (1)$$

With maximal vasodilation, myocardial resistance falls to about 20% of its resting level. In normal coronary arteries, distal coronary pressure is similar to aortic pressure, and maximal myocardial vasodilation elicits a four- to fivefold increase in coronary flow from its resting level. This response is illustrated by the experimental pressure-flow recordings shown in Figure 3.2A of Chapter 3. The mean resting coronary flow in that figure was about 40 mL/min, increasing to 180 mL/min following a vasodilatory stimulus. Aortic and distal coronary artery pressure showed no significant difference in the absence of a stenosis. The ability of the myocardial bed to produce a four- to fivefold increase in coronary flow is expressed as the artery's normal coronary flow reserve, CFR_n. This important functional characteristic of the coronary circulation is defined as the ratio of the normal maximal coronary flow ($Q_{n,max}$) to its normal resting value ($Q_{n,rest}$):

$$CFR_n = Q_{n,max}/Q_{n,rest} \qquad (2)$$

Under normal conditions, with no significant pressure drop along the artery, coronary collateral flow will be insignificant. Coronary and myocardial flows are therefore equal for normal arteries.

The total flow through the maximally vasodilated normal myocardial bed, $Q_{n,max}$, is described by Equation 1 as

$$Q_{n,max} = (P_{Ao} - P_v)/R_{min} \qquad (3)$$

With a stenosis present, distal coronary pressure is reduced from the aortic pressure by the amount of the pressure drop,

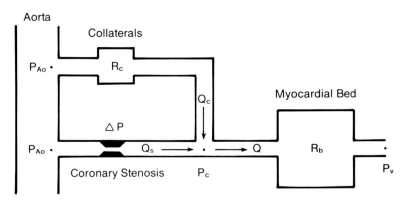

Fig. 7.5 A lumped-parameter model representing the circulation associated with a diseased coronary artery. The myocardial bed distal to the stenotic coronary artery is perfused from both the artery and preformed collateral vessels. The coronary stenosis and collateral vessels influence myocardial flow by changing distal coronary pressure, P_c. P_{Ao} is aortic pressure, P_v is coronary venous pressure, R_c equals collateral resistance, R_b equals resistance of the myocardial bed, Q is myocardial blood flow, Q_s is flow through the stenosis, Q_c is collateral flow, and ΔP equals pressure drop across the stenosis. Reproduced with permission from Wong WH, Kirkeeide RL, Gould KL, 1986 (26).

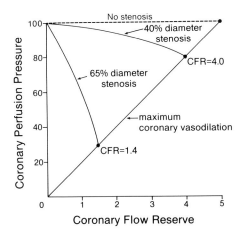

Fig. 7.6 Relation of distal coronary pressure, relative myocardial flow, and stenosis severity. A reduction in coronary flow reserve from 5 to about 4 occurs with a 40% diameter stenosis. Progressive increases in stenosis severity reduce distal coronary pressure and coronary flow reserve. For this simulation, stenoses were assumed to be uniform in cross-section with a length of one normal arterial diameter (3 mm), and normal resting flow rate ($O_{n,rest}$) was 1 mL/s. Reproduced with permission from Gould KL, 1985. (15).

ΔP, across the stenosis and collateral bed combined:

$$P_c = P_{Ao} - \Delta P \qquad (4)$$

Thus, maximal myocardial flow in the presence of a stenosis (Q_{max}) relative to its normal maximum flow rate is written as

$$\frac{Q_{max}}{Q_{n,max}} = 1 - \frac{\Delta P_{max}}{P_{Ao} - P_v} \qquad (5)$$

This equation indicates that the limitation of myocardial flow by the stenosis is directly proportional to the pressure drop across the stenosis, as reviewed in Chapter 3. Mean resting coronary flow was not significantly affected by the stenosis, despite a significant decrease in distal coronary pressure. Following the vasodilatory stimulus, however, coronary flow was increased to only twice its resting level, while distal coronary pressure fell by 60 mm Hg below aortic pressure. This flow limitation represents an approximate 50% decrease in normal coronary flow reserve.

Equation 5 shows that coronary flow reserve is directly related to the maximum pressure drop across the stenosis. As developed in previous chapters, the pressure drop for a given flow is related to the anatomic geometry of the stenosis. Therefore, coronary flow reserve is related to the geometry of the stenosis. This relation between coronary flow reserve, the pressure gradient, and stenosis geometry is the conceptual link between the anatomic and functional characteristics of a coronary artery stenosis.

However, the linear relation between mean pressure gradient and flow described in Chapter 2 and implied in Equation 3 above are due to combined effects of systolic deceleration, diastolic acceleration, and vasomotion occurring in vivo, independent of stenosis severity. Based on phasic and geometric analysis of Chapters 4, 5, and 6, the relation between

flow, distal coronary pressure, and stenosis geometry is a curvilinear relation. When these factors are taken into account, the simple concept expressed by Equation 5 is illustrated correctly by Figure 7.6 (10,26), which graphs Equation 5 based on stenosis geometry and/or diastolic pressure-flow relations. Distal coronary perfusion pressure, P_c, rather than stenosis pressure gradient, is plotted on the vertical axis, with relative myocardial flow ($Q/Q_{n,rest}$) on the horizontal axis (10). Functional effects of a coronary stenosis are most apparent when the distal coronary vascular bed is maximally vasodilated. This condition is indicated in Figure 7.6 by the diagonal straight line, which is the pressure-flow relation (relative flow) of the distal myocardial bed during maximal vasodilation (see Equation 3). Its intercept with the vertical pressure axis is the observed effective 10 mm Hg critical closing pressure of the myocardial bed. For a normal coronary artery with a proximal pressure of 100 mm Hg, a normal coronary flow reserve of 5 is assumed for purposes of illustration. The downward sloping curves show the change in distal coronary pressure associated with increasing flow through the artery when narrowed by stenoses of increasing severity, as expressed by Equation 4. The intersection of the downward curving line characterizing the stenosis with the maximally vasodilated pressure-flow relation of the distal myocardial bed represents the maximal flow possible through the stenosis.

A stenosis with a 40% diameter narrowing, shown in Figure 7.6, reduces the normal flow reserve from 5 to 4 while dropping distal coronary pressure from its normal 100 mm Hg level to 85 mm Hg. As stenosis severity progresses, flow reserve falls until, with a 65% diameter stenosis, flow reserve has fallen to 1.4. Before developing in detail the relations between coronary flow reserve, pressure gradient, and stenosis geometry, the characteristics of flow reserve are reviewed in this chapter, particularly as affected by blood pressure and heart rate.

ABSOLUTE AND RELATIVE CORONARY FLOW RESERVE

The concept of coronary flow reserve, defined as maximum flow divided (normalized) by resting control flow, has evolved into an accepted functional measure of stenosis severity since first proposed (1–4). Its validity has been confirmed and applied clinically by noninvasive imaging (5–22) and by invasive methods such as coronary sinus thermodilution (23), Doppler-tip catheters (27–29), and digital subtraction angiography (25,30). These clinical methods measure pharmacologically induced increases in coronary blood flow, most commonly with intravenous dipyridamole for noninvasive studies and intracoronary papaverine for invasive studies.

Coronary flow reserve has also been theoretically integrated with and experimentally related to the geometric dimensions of stenoses (10–18). The commonly used percent diameter stenosis is poorly related to functional severity of human coronary artery narrowing or coronary flow reserve (10–18,28–33), determined by quantitative coronary arteriography as in Figure 7.7 or by directly measured flow reserve using a Doppler catheter, as in Figure 7.8 (29). Thus, extensive experimental and clinical literature have substantiated the concept of coronary flow reserve.

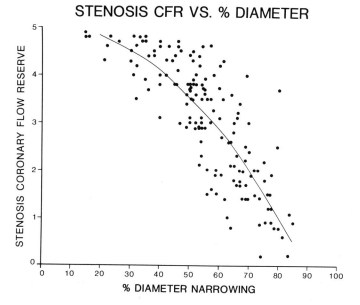

Fig. 7.7 Graph of the relation between stenosis flow reserve and percent diameter narrowing, both determined from automated quantitative arteriographic measurements in 100 patients. Because percent diameter narrowing is only one of several factors used to calculate stenosis flow reserve, the scatter in this relation indicates the importance of those factors other than relative diameter that influence flow impedance of a stenosis. Reproduced with permission from Demer L, Gould KL, Goldstein RA, et al, 1989. (14).

However, changes in aortic pressure and heart rate are known to alter cardiac workload and therefore baseline coronary blood flow, as well as altering maximum coronary flow under conditions of maximal vasodilation (34,35). Consequently, *absolute coronary flow reserve,* as measured by flow-

meter, has also been hypothesized to vary with aortic pressure and heart rate, independent of stenosis geometry due to differential effects of these variables on resting and maximal coronary flow (36,37). Under varying physiologic conditions, or from patient to patient, coronary flow reserve may not

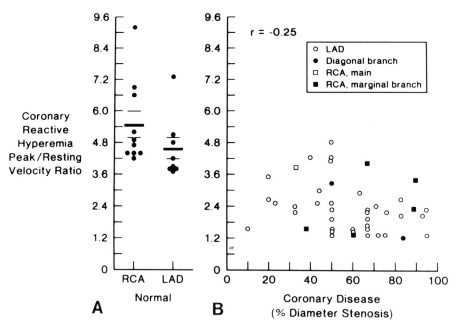

Fig. 7.8 Coronary reactive hyperemic responses obtained in patients with angiographically normal coronary vessels perfusing a normal ventricle (A) and angiographically diseased coronary vessels perfusing a normal ventricle (B). Peak to resting velocity ratio was measured following a 20-s coronary occlusion. The studies were performed at the time of open-heart surgery prior to the pump run. The peak to resting velocity ratio was greater than 3.6 in all normal vessels studied. In patients with coronary obstructive lesions there was a very poor relationship between the percent diameter stenosis and the reactive hyperemic response. RCA is the right coronary artery. These data emphasize the problems in using percent diameter stenosis to predict the physiologic significance of a coronary obstructive lesion. The vast majority of patients included in this study had multivessel coronary artery disease. Reproduced with permission from White CW, Wright CB, Doty DB, et al, 1984 (29).

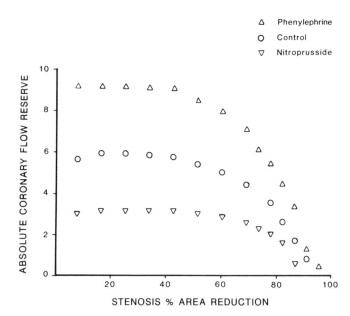

Fig. 7.9 Changes in coronary flow reserve during phenylephrine and nitroprusside infusion during progressive coronary artery stenosis in one experiment. Absolute coronary flow reserve is plotted on the vertical axis, defined as maximum flow divided by resting coronary flow measured by flowmeter. Percent area stenosis is graphed on the horizontal axis measured by the calibrated arterial constrictor confirmed by arteriography, with length and normal diameter remaining constant. Absolute coronary flow reserve showed marked variation for any given fixed stenosis, depending upon aortic pressure. Reproduced with permission from Gould KL, Kirkeeide R, Buchi M, 1990 (12).

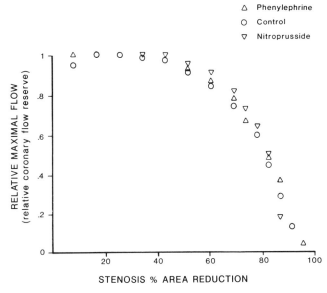

Fig. 7.10 Relative maximum coronary flow or relative flow reserve, defined as maximum flow in the stenotic artery divided (normalized) by normal maximum flow in the absence of the stenosis, showed little variation over a wide range of aortic pressures. Reproduced with permission from Gould KL, Kirkeeide R, Buchi M, 1990. (12).

reliably or specifically reflect severity of coronary artery narrowing, since it may be altered by physiologic factors unrelated to stenosis geometry.

In contrast, relative maximum coronary flow or relative flow reserve, defined as maximum flow in a stenotic artery divided (normalized) by the normal maximum flow in the absence of stenosis, should theoretically be more independent of aortic pressure, heart rate, or varying baseline flow caused by changing cardiac workload. Physiologic variables unrelated to stenosis severity, such as aortic pressure, heart rate, metabolic demand, or vasomotor tone, alter distal coronary bed resistance in series with, and independent of, proximal stenosis resistance. During maximal coronary vasodilation, distal coronary bed resistance is equally minimized for both normal and stenotic arteries. When the maximum flow in the stenotic artery is normalized by normal maximum flow, the term for minimum bed resistance reflecting effects of pressure, heart rate, or vasomotor tone on flow in the numerator and denominator of this ratio cancel out. Therefore, relative differences in regional maximum flow, or relative flow reserve, are determined primarily by proximal stenosis. Relative flow reserve should then measure stenosis severity independent of physiologic variables.

Figure 7.9 shows an example of absolute coronary flow reserve in one experiment at control conditions, during phen-

ylephrine and nitroprusside infusions as the coronary artery was progressively narrowed, with length and normal arterial diameter being constant (12). Absolute coronary flow reserve for a given stenosis ranged from low to high values, depending on aortic pressure and pressure-rate product. For example, for a 65% area narrowing, absolute coronary flow reserve at control conditions was approximately 5.0. For the same stenosis, absolute coronary flow reserve during phenylephrine infusion was approximately 8.0, and during nitroprusside in-

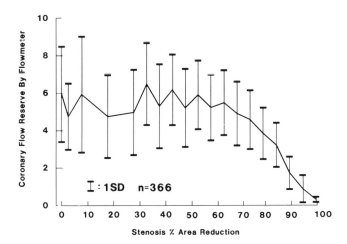

Fig. 7.11 Absolute coronary flow reserve (maximum divided by resting flow) for all experiments over the full range of changes in aortic pressure and stenosis severity. Reproduced with permission from Gould KL, Kirkeeide R, Buchi M, 1990 (12).

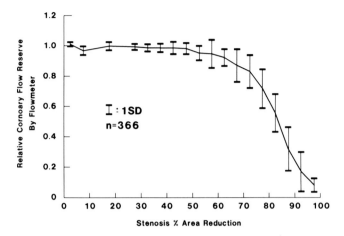

Fig. 7.12 Relative maximum coronary flow or relative flow reserve (maximum flow in stenotic artery divided by normal maximum flow in absence of stenosis) for all experiments over the range of changes in aortic pressure with progressive coronary artery stenosis. Reproduced with permission from Gould KL, Kirkeeide R, Buchi M, 1990 (12).

Table 7.1 Variability of Absolute Coronary Flow Reserve (maximum/resting coronary flow)

% Area stenosis	n	mean CFR	1SD CFR	1SD % of $\overline{CFR}$
0.0	26	5.94	2.54	43%
5.0	5	5.45	2.44	45%
15.0	9	4.62	2.11	45%
25.0	6	4.97	2.27	46%
35.0	41	6.16	2.24	36%
45.0	44	5.89	1.97	33%
55.0	39	5.57	1.80	32%
65.0	43	5.18	1.72	33%
75.0	56	4.17	1.50	36%
85.0	68	2.34	1.24	53%
95.0	29	0.72	0.67	93%
mean	—	—	—	45%

% area stenosis indicates the center of a range of 10% diameter narrowing from 0% to 100%.

n = number of stenoses; CFR = absolute coronary flow reserve; $\overline{CFR}$ = mean values; 1SD = one standard deviation.

Source: Adapted with permission from Gould KL, Kirkeeide R, Buchi M, 1990. Reference 12.

fusion it was 3.0. Thus, for a given fixed stenosis of 65% area narrowing and constant length and absolute dimensions, absolute coronary flow reserve ranged from 3.0 to 8.0, depending upon aortic pressure and heart rate. However, relative maximum flow or relative flow reserve was independent of aortic pressure and heart rate, as seen in Figure 7.10 (12). Relative coronary flow reserve was approximately 0.90 for the 65% stenosis, regardless of physiologic conditions.

For all stenoses with 65% area narrowing, absolute coronary flow reserve averaged 5.2 ± 1.7 (1 SD), a variation of ±33% over the range of aortic pressure and pressure-rate product. By comparison, for the same 65% area stenoses, relative flow reserve averaged 0.90 ± 0.09, a variation of only ±10% over the same range of physiologic variables.

Figure 7.11 shows absolute coronary flow reserve measured by flowmeter for 366 stenoses under a wide range of aortic pressure and heart rate (12). Standard deviations are large, indicating great variability of absolute coronary flow reserve by flowmeter for any given geometrically fixed stenosis. Figure 7.12 shows corresponding values of relative coronary flow reserve, defined as maximum flow in the stenotic artery divided by normal maximum flow in the absence of a stenosis. The standard deviations of relative flow reserve show much less variability during marked changes in aortic pressure and pressure-rate product.

VARIABILITY OF ABSOLUTE VERSUS RELATIVE CORONARY FLOW RESERVE

Table 7.1 shows the systematic variability in absolute coronary flow reserve over the range of aortic pressures and pressure-rate products for all stenoses, from mild to severe narrowing (12). One standard deviation ranged from 2.5 for no coronary narrowing to 0.7 for the more severe narrowings. As a more standardized measure of variability, one standard

deviation was expressed as a percent of the mean absolute coronary flow reserve for each category of stenosis severity. The size of one standard deviation as percent of mean absolute coronary flow reserve for each stenosis severity ranged from ±32% to ±93%, with a mean of ±45% for all stenoses. In other words, a single measurement of coronary flow reserve, on the average, varied by ±45% for fixed stenosis geometry, depending on aortic pressure and pressure-rate product. In contrast, Table 7.2 shows corresponding variability in relative maximum coronary flow or relative flow reserve over the same range of aortic pressures and pressure-rate products for these same stenoses. The standard deviations are mark-

Table 7.2 Variability of Relative Maximum Coronary Flow or Relative Coronary Flow Reserve (maximum flow stenotic artery/normal maximum flow with no stenosis)

% Area stenosis	n	mean RMF	1SD RMF	1SD % of $\overline{RMF}$
0	26	—	—	—
5.0	5	0.99	0.032	3%
15.0	9	1.00	0.025	3%
25.0	6	0.99	0.020	2%
35.0	41	0.99	0.024	2%
45.0	44	0.98	0.039	4%
55.0	39	0.95	0.072	8%
65.0	43	0.90	0.089	10%
75.0	56	0.77	0.132	17%
85.0	68	0.42	0.180	43%
95.0	29	0.14	0.119	83%
mean	—	—	—	17.5%

% area stenosis indicates the center of a range of 10% diameter narrowing for 0 to 100%.

mean = number of; RMF = relative maximum flow; $\overline{RMF}$ = mean values; 1SD = one standard deviation.

Source: Adapted with permission from Gould KL, Kirkeeide R, Buchi M, 1990. Reference 12.

edly lower, averaging ±17.5% of mean relative flow reserve values for each stenosis category of severity, as compared to ±45% for absolute coronary flow reserve (12).

In the intermediate range of severity from 15% to 75% area stenoses, where quantitation of severity is most important clinically, the variability of relative flow reserve ranged from ±2% to ±17%, with a mean of ±6.6%, compared to ±32% to ±46%, with a mean of ±37% for absolute coronary flow reserve. For severe stenoses of 85% area reduction or greater, the variability of absolute and relative coronary flow reserves for fixed stenoses are both fairly large, because maximum flows are so markedly reduced that small variations of flowmeter measurements at resting baseline cause large changes in the denominator of the flow reserve ratio or relative maximum flow ratio. However, these values of flow reserve are so low that this variability does not interfere with the diagnostic identification of severe stenosis.

ABSOLUTE VERSUS RELATIVE CORONARY FLOW RESERVE

Rather than considering absolute coronary flow reserve to be competitive or antithetical to relative flow reserve, our data indicate that these measurements are independent variables providing complementary information. Absolute flow reserve is the flow capacity of the stenotic coronary artery and vascular bed under whatever conditions of pressure, workload, hypertrophy, vasomotor tone, or stenoses are present. It reflects the cumulative summed effects of these various factors without being specific for the mechanism or cause of altered flow reserve. Relative coronary flow reserve reflects more specifically the effects of the stenosis independent of and not affected by the other physiologic variables, if normal maximum flow is high enough. Thus, absolute and relative coronary flow reserve are complementary.

"Balanced" three-vessel coronary artery disease may theoretically cause a false-negative stress perfusion test, depending upon the stress stimulus and the imaging technology, particularly its spatial and contrast resolution. In most hearts affected by coronary artery disease, there is some artery, even a small one, that is unaffected, which serves as a reference area, based on our experience with positron emission tomography (PET). However, small vessel disease, left ventricular hypertrophy, or theoretically "balanced" three-vessel coronary artery disease are potential causes of diffusely impaired flow reserve that must be accounted for in individual patients. For this purpose, some measure of absolute coronary flow reserve is necessary. However, relative flow reserve is also necessary for assessing stenoses, since it is not affected by variability in pressure or heart rate within the same patient or between patients.

RELATION OF RELATIVE AND ABSOLUTE CORONARY FLOW RESERVE TO STENOSIS PRESSURE GRADIENT

Although maximum coronary flow has been related to perfusion pressure (34,35), the effects of varying aortic pressure and cardiac workload on coronary flow reserve in the presence of stenoses has not been previously described, despite controversy about the expected effects (36,37). This study shows that maximum and resting flows may change to different degrees or in different directions, in the same direction, or both, with different alterations in pressure and workload. Consequently, absolute flow reserve may change significantly as a result of physiologic conditions, despite fixed stenosis geometry, whereas relative flow reserve shows much less variability.

The explanation for relative flow reserve being independent of aortic pressure and cardiac workload is theoretically sound, according to readily derived simple equations relating flow reserve to pressure and distal bed resistance (12), as follows:

$$Qr,s = (Pa - \Delta Pr)/Rr = \text{flow in stenotic artery at rest}$$

$$Qm,s = (Pa - \Delta Pm)/Rm = \text{maximum flow in stenotic artery}$$

$$Qm,n = Pa/Rm = \text{maximum flow in normal artery}$$

where Pa is aortic pressure, ΔPr is pressure drop across the stenosis at resting flow, ΔPm is the pressure drop across the stenosis at maximum flow, Rr is distal vascular bed resistance at rest, and Rm is minimum distal vascular bed resistance at maximum flow. By dividing and rearranging:

$$\frac{\text{absolute CFR}}{} = \frac{Qm,s}{Qr,s} = \frac{Pa - \Delta Pm}{Pa - \Delta Pr} \times \frac{Rr}{Rm} \quad (6)$$

$$\frac{\text{relative CFR}}{} = \frac{Qm,s}{Qm,n} = \frac{Pa - \Delta Pm}{Pa} \times \frac{Rm}{Rm} \quad (7)$$

$$= 1 - \frac{\Delta Pm}{Pa}$$

Equation 6 for absolute CFR contains two terms. The first is related to pressure and pressure drop across the stenosis at rest and at maximum flow; the second term is related to distal coronary vascular bed resistance at rest and maximum flow and is therefore dependent on the state of the distal bed. However, Equation 7 for relative CFR has only one term that is related to pressure and pressure drop across the stenosis alone. The resistance terms for the distal coronary vascular bed cancel out. These equations explain why absolute flow reserve is altered by characteristics of the distal coronary vascular bed, independent of and in addition to stenosis severity. Relative coronary flow reserve is altered only by stenosis severity.

LIMITATIONS AND COMPARISON OF ABSOLUTE AND RELATIVE CORONARY FLOW RESERVE IN CLINICAL APPLICATION

Although the experimental methods of this study are well established with unequivocal results, the limitations of the study are related to their clinical applications. There are some qualifications on coronary flow reserve for assessing stenosis severity (13,31–33,36,37), some of which may be related to methodologic differences. However, based on this study, some of the differences may be due in part to determining absolute coronary flow reserve under different conditions or to considering relative versus absolute flow reserve, without specifying which one was measured under what conditions.

The conditions under which absolute and relative coronary flow reserve might fail to reflect stenosis severity would be failure of normal arteries to respond to a vasodilatory stimulus (38) or diffuse global impairment of flow reserve due to small vessel disease (39), and adrenergic coronary vasoconstriction (40), for which absolute flow reserve is necessary.

Absolute coronary flow reserve may also be reduced because of increased resting flow, with no change in maximum flow capacity in left ventricular hypertrophy, both experimentally (41–43) and clinically (44–47). In this instance, relative flow reserve is normal in the absence of stenosis (41,43,47) and is abnormal in the presence of a stenosis, since maximum normal flow is unimpaired. However, in advanced severe hypertrophy due to hypertension or cardiomyopathy, maximum flow may be reduced globally in non-stenotic coronary arteries (42,44,45). Small-vessel disease also reduces maximum flow in the absence of stenosis (39,45,51,53). Consequently, absolute coronary flow reserve in these conditions is impaired, but relative flow reserve is normal. Although theoretically possible, balanced three-vessel disease or diffuse disease would require hemodynamically equal right ostial and left main coronary artery disease that impaired flow reserve to the same extent. Since flow reserve depends on percent narrowing, absolute lumen radius raised to the fourth power, and length and shape, exactly balanced lesions would be unlikely and have not been seen in our experience. In that instance, absolute flow reserve would be reduced, whereas relative flow reserve would be normal.

Finally, awake humans with intact vasomotor reflexes may not show as great changes in flow reserve with altered pressure and heart rate as observed in open-chest anesthetized animals. Nevertheless, for whatever variations there are in aortic pressure and heart rate, relative coronary flow reserve reflects physiologic stenosis severity, despite large variation in absolute flow reserve from whatever cause, provided that normal maximum flow is reached in some part of the heart as a normal reference area. Our experimental observations have been elegantly confirmed in man by R. Watkins (University of Toronto, personal communication, 54), who demonstrated a tight linear relation between coronary flow reserve and heart rate using intracoronary Doppler catheters before and after intracoronary papaverine over a wide range of paced heart rates in patients undergoing clinical coronary arteriography.

CLINICAL IMPLICATIONS

A stress myocardial perfusion image shows relative maximum perfusion (radiotracer uptake) or relative coronary flow reserve. One of the limitations of radionuclide perfusion imaging is considered to be its inability to measure absolute flow and absolute coronary flow reserve. However, despite this purported limitation, perfusion imaging of relative maximal coronary flow or relative flow reserve has been useful for assessing physiologic stenosis severity in the face of greatly changing or widely variant physiologic conditions seen between rest conditions and upright treadmill exercise, bicycle stress, supine exercise, or various pharmacologic

stresses such as dipyridamole and papaverine. The results of our study explain this observation. The stress perfusion image shows relative coronary flow reserve, which is independent of physiologic variables of blood pressure and heart rate. What has long been considered the limitation of stress perfusion techniques is in fact its greatest advantage.

Although direct measures of absolute coronary flow reserve by invasive techniques have provided important research data, they have been of limited diagnostic benefit for assessing stenosis severity in individual patients. The poor correlation between flow reserve and percent narrowing has been ascribed in part to the inadequacy of percent narrowing as a measure of severity (25–29,31–33). However, there is some variability in expected flow reserve even when all other dimensions, such as integrated length and absolute dimensions, as well as percent narrowing, are accounted for (10,12,16). Such variability in directly measured coronary flow reserve for stenoses appears to be out of proportion to their anatomic severity, despite potential limitations in the type of arteriographic analysis of anatomic stenosis severity in some studies (25–29,31–33). As directly examined in a recent clinical study (33), the relatively poor correlation between absolute coronary flow reserve and anatomic severity of stenosis may be due to variability in measurement methodology, poor definition or understanding of what was being measured, and biological variability due to different physiologic conditions.

In order to be optimally effective over the wide range of conditions seen clinically, a method for assessing physiologic stenosis severity should be able to provide measures of both relative and absolute flow reserve. For example, measurement of absolute flow reserve in a coronary artery by a Doppler tip catheter gives the flow response to dipyridamole/papaverine or the effects of diffuse coronary artery disease. However, it may change, owing to varying afterload and baseline pressure-rate product or to physiologic differences between patients that affect flow reserve separate from stenosis geometry. On the other hand, relative coronary flow reserve, as assessed by current standard thallium perfusion imaging, does not adequately reflect the absolute flow response to vasodilatory stimuli or diffuse processes affecting all areas of the heart. Most invasive or noninvasive clinical methods as now used provide measurements of either absolute or relative coronary flow reserve, but not both, with the exception of positron emission tomography, discussed subsequently (12,13,15,18).

Therefore, the optimal noninvasive method would utilize relative coronary flow reserve to assess physiologic stenosis severity *and* absolute flow reserve to assess response to dipyridamole, small-vessel disease, left ventricular hypertrophy, and "balanced" three-vessel disease, as well as coronary artery stenosis.

Although well documented as a functional measure of stenosis severity, the degree of reduction in coronary flow reserve necessary to cause exercise myocardial ischemia by metabolic imaging or ECG changes has not been well described. The relation between reduced flow reserve and exercise-induced ischemia would likely be highly variable, depending on the level of exercise and a large number of unknown biological variables. However, with that qualification, our experience with clinical PET imaging and quantitative

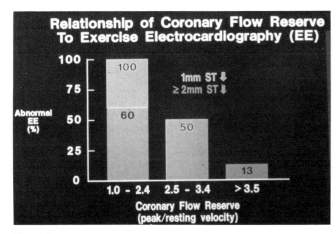

Fig. 7.13 Relation between coronary flow reserve measured by Doppler catheter and ST change on prior exercise ECG (used with permission of R. Wilson, University of Minnesota, pers. comm.).

coronary arteriography suggests that coronary flow reserve must be reduced to around 2.0 before metabolic ischemia by FDG imaging and/or ST change on ECG is observed. Figure 7.13 shows supporting information for this observation (R. Wilson, University of Minnesota, personal communication).

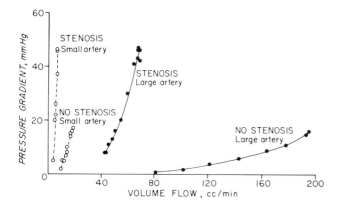

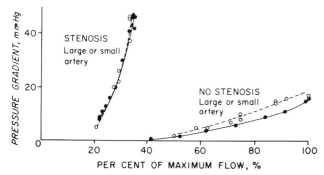

Fig. 7.14 Pressure gradient-volume flow relations of a small and large coronary artery, both with and without a stenosis (upper panel) from direct experimental measurements. In the lower panel, volume flow has been normalized and expressed as percent of normal maximum flow.

Coronary flow reserve was measured by Doppler catheter after intracoronary papaverine at diagnostic arteriography and correlated with the degree of ST change at prior exercise testing. Fairly severe reduction in coronary flow reserve is necessary before definitive ST segment depression appears on stress ECG. However, ischemia with exercise depends on many factors in addition to stenosis severity, thereby making the ischemia–flow reserve relation unpredictable for different patients.

Chapter 5 reviewed the advantages and disadvantages of using pressure gradient–volume flow relations to describe stenosis severity. A significant disadvantage reviewed in Chapter 5 is illustrated in Figure 7.14, upper panel, from experimental measurements. The pressure gradient–volume flow relation appears steeper for small arteries as compared to large arteries, which implies a "worse" stenosis even for a normal artery. Therefore, for comparing stenoses in different-sized arteries, the pressure gradient–volume flow relation is not useful. However, if flow is normalized and expressed as a percent of normal maximum in a given heart, this disadvantage is removed, as shown by the lower panel of Figure 7.14. Therefore, an optimal descriptor of stenosis severity is the pressure gradient–flow relation, where flow is expressed as percent of normal maximum. However, if pressure gradient cannot be measured, the maximum flow per se for each pressure-flow curve reflects stenosis severity. Thus, relative flow reserve and pressure gradient–flow relations normalized to maximum flow are theoretically and experimentally equivalent.

CONCLUSIONS

Absolute and relative coronary flow reserve are independent, complementary variables, which, together, more completely describe physiologic severity of coronary artery narrowing than either one alone. These conclusions have important implications for clinically assessing physiologic stenosis severity noninvasively, by perfusion imaging using positron emission tomography, and by invasive methods, using quantitative coronary arteriography, as discussed in following chapters.

REFERENCES

1. Gould KL, Lipscomb K, Hamilton GW. Physiologic basis for assessing critical coronary stenosis. Am J Cardiol 33:87–94, 1974.
2. Gould KL, Lipscomb K. Effects of coronary stenoses on coronary flow reserve and resistance. Am J Cardiol 34:48–55, 1974.
3. Gould KL, Lipscomb K, Calvert J. Compensatory changes of the distal coronary vascular bed during progressive coronary constriction. Circulation 51:1085–94, 1975.
4. Gould KL, Hamilton GW, Lipscomb K, Kennedy JW. A method for assessing stress induced regional malperfusion during coronary arteriography: experimental validation and clinical application. Am J Cardiol 34:557–64, 1974.
5. Gould KL. Noninvasive assessment of coronary stenosis by myocardial perfusion imaging during pharmacologic coronary vasodilation. I. Am J Cardiol 41:267–78, 1978.
6. Gould KL, Westcott RJ, Albro PC, Hamilton GW. Noninvasive assessment of coronary stenosis by myocardial imaging during pharmacologic vasodilation. II. Clinical methodology and feasibility. Am J Cardiol 41:279–87, 1978.

7. Gould KL. Assessment of coronary stenoses by myocardial perfusion imaging during pharmacologic coronary vasodilation. IV. Limits of stenosis detection by idealized experimental cross-sectional myocardial imaging. Am J Cardiol 42:761–68, 1978.

8. Gould KL, Schelbert HR, Phelps ME, Hoffman EJ. Noninvasive assessment of coronary stenoses with myocardial perfusion imaging during pharmacologic coronary vasodilation. V. Detection of 47% diameter coronary stenosis with intravenous N-13 ammonia and positron emission tomography in intact dogs. Am J Cardiol 43:200–08, 1979.

9. Schelbert HR, Wisenberg G, Phelps ME, Gould KL, Eberhard H, Hoffman EJ, Gomes A, Kuhl DE. Noninvasive assessment of coronary stenosis by myocardial imaging during pharmacologic coronary vasodilation. VI. Detection of coronary artery disease in man with intravenous NH₃ and positron computed tomography. Am J Cardiol 49:1197–207, 1982.

10. Kirkeeide R, Gould KL, Parsel L. Assessment of coronary stenoses by myocardial imaging during coronary vasodilation. VII. Validation of coronary flow reserve as a single integrated measure of stenosis severity accounting for all its geometric dimensions. J Am Coll Cardiol 7:103–13, 1986.

11. Gould KL, Goldstein RA, Mullani NA, Kirkeeide RL, Wong WH, Tewson TJ, Berridge MS, Bolomey LA, Hartz RK, Smalling RW, Fuentes F, Nishikawa A. Noninvasive assessment of coronary stenoses by myocardial perfusion imaging during pharmacologic coronary vasodilation. VIII. Clinical feasibility of positron cardiac imaging without a cyclotron using generator-produced rubidium-82. J Am Coll Cardiol 7:775–89, 1986.

12. Gould KL, Kirkeeide R, Buchi M. Coronary flow reserve as a physiologic measure of stenosis severity. Part I. Relative and absolute coronary flow reserve during changing aortic pressure. Part II. Determination from arteriographic stenosis dimensions under standardized conditions. J Am Coll Cardiol 15:459–74, 1990.

13. Demer L, Gould KL, Kirkeeide RL. Assessing stenosis severity: coronary flow reserve, collateral function, quantitative coronary arteriography, positron imaging, and digital subtraction angiography: a review and analysis. Prog Cardiovas Dis 30:307–22, 1988.

14. Demer LL, Gould KL, Goldstein RA, Kirkeeide RL, Mullani N, Smalling R, Nishikawa A, Merhige M. Diagnosis of coronary artery disease by positron imaging: comparison to quantitative coronary arteriography in 193 patients. Circulation 79:825–35, 1989.

15. Gould KL. Quantification of coronary artery stenosis in vivo. Circ Res 57:341–53, 1985.

16. Gould KL, Kelley KO, Bolson EL. Experimental validation of quantitative coronary arteriography for determining pressure-flow characteristics of coronary stenosis. Circulation 66:930–37, 1982.

17. Gould KL, Kelley KO. Physiologic significance of coronary flow velocity and changing stenosis geometry during coronary vasodilation in dogs. Circ Res 50:695–704, 1982.

18. Gould KL. Identifying and measuring severity of coronary artery stenosis: quantitative coronary arteriography and positron emission tomography. Circulation 78:237–45, 1988.

19. Josephson MA, Brown BG, Hecht HS, Hopkins J, Pierce CD, Petersen R. Noninvasive detection and localization of coronary stenoses in patients: comparison of resting dipyridamole and exercise thallium-201 myocardial perfusion imaging. Am Heart J 103:1008–18, 1982.

20. Leppo J, Boucher CA, Okada RD, Newell JB, Strauss W, Pohost GM. Serial thallium-201 myocardial imaging after dipyridamole infusion. Circulation 66:649–57, 1982.

21. Iskandrian AS, Heo J, Askenase A, Segal BL, Auerbach N. Dipyridamole cardiac imaging. Am Heart J 115:432–43, 1988.

22. Leppo J. Dipyridamole-thallium imaging: The lazy man's stress test. J Nucl Med 30:281–87, 1989.

23. Brown G, Josephson MA, Peterson RB, Pierce CD, Wong W, Hecht HS, Bolson H, Dodge HT. Intravenous dipyridamole combined with isometric handgrip for near maximal acute increase in coronary flow in patients with coronary artery disease. Am J Cardiol 48:1077–85, 1981.

24. Verani MS, Mahmarian JJ, Hixson JB, Boyce TM, Staudacher RA: Diagnosis of coronary artery disease by controlled coronary vasodilation with adenosine and thallium-201 scintigraphy in patients unable to exercise. Circulation 82:80–87, 1990.

25. Vogel RA, LeFree M, Bates E, O'Neill W, Foster R, Kirlin P, Smith D, Pitt B. Application of digital techniques to selective coronary arteriography: use of myocardial contrast appearance time to measure coronary flow reserve. Am Heart J 107:153–64, 1984.

26. Wong WH, Kirkeeide RL, Gould KL. Computer Applications in Angiography in Cardiac Imaging and Image Processing, ed. Collins SM, Skorton DJ. New York: McGraw Hill, 1986.

27. Wilson RF, Laughlin DE, Ackell PH, et al. Transluminal subselective measurement of coronary artery blood flow velocity and vasodilator reserve in man. Circulation 72:82–92, 1985.

28. Harrison DG, White DW, Hiratzka LF, et al. The value of lesion cross-sectional area determined by quantitative coronary angiography in assessing the physiologic significance of proximal left anterior descending coronary arterial stenoses. Circulation 69:1111–19, 1984.

29. White CW, Wright CB, Doty DB, et al. Does visual interpretation of the coronary arteriogram predict the physiologic importance of a coronary stenosis? N Engl J Med 310:819–24, 1984.

30. Nissen SE, Elion JL, Booth DC, Evans J, DeMaria AN. Value and limitations of computer analysis of digital subtraction angiography in the assessment of coronary flow reserve. Circulation 73:562–71, 1986.

31. Marcus ML, Skorton DJ, Johnson MR, Collins SM, Harrison DG, Kerber RE. Visual estimates of percent diameter coronary stenosis: "a battered gold standard." J Am Coll Cardiol 11:882–86, 1988.

32. Gould KL. Percent coronary stenosis: battered gold standard, pernicious relic or clinical practicality? J Am Coll Cardiol 11:886–88, 1988.

33. Zijlstra F, Fioretti P, Reiber JHC, Serruys PW. Which cineangiographically assessed anatomic variable correlates best with functional measurements of stenosis severity?: a comparison of quantitative analysis of the coronary cineangiogram with measured coronary flow reserve and exercise/redistribution thallium-201 scintigraphy. J Am Coll Cardiol 12:686–91, 1988.

34. Dole WP, Montville WJ, Bishop VS. Dependency of myocardial reactive hyperemia on coronary artery pressure in the dog. Am J Physiol 240 (Heart Circ. Physiol) 9:H709–15, 1981.

35. Bache RJ, Schwartz JS. Effect of perfusion pressure distal to a coronary stenosis on transmural myocardial blood flow. Circulation 65:928–35, 1982.

36. Hoffman JIE. Maximal coronary flow and the concept of coronary vascular reserve. Circulation 70:153–59, 1984.

37. Klocke FJ. Coronary blood flow in man. Prog Cardiovas Dis 19:117, 1976.

38. Rossen JD, Simonetti I, Winniford MD, Marcus ML. Coronary dilation with dipyridamole and dipyridamole combined with handgrip (Abstr). Clin Res 35:837A, 1987.

39. Cannon RO, Watson RM, Rosing DR, Epstein SE. Angina caused by reduced vasodilator reserve of the small coronary arteries. J Am Coll Cardiol 1:1359–73, 1983.

40. Schwartz PJ, Stone HL. Tonic influence of the sympathetic nervous system on myocardial reactive hyperemia and on coronary blood flow distribution in dogs. Circ Res 41:51–58, 1977.

41. Marchetti GV, Merlo L, Noseda V, Visiolo O. Myocardial blood flow in experimental cardiac hypertrophy in dogs. Cardiovas Res 7:519–27, 1983.

42. O'Keefe DD, Hoffman JIE, Cheitlin R, O'Neill MJ, Allard JR, Shapkin E. Coronary blood flow in experimental canine left ventricular hypertrophy. Circ Res 43:43–51, 1978.

43. Mueller TM, Marcus ML, Kerber RE, Young JA, Barnes RW, Abboud FM. Effect of renal hypertension and left ventricular hypertrophy on the coronary circulation in dogs. Circulation 42:543–49, 1978.

44. Opherk D, Mall G, Zebe H, Schwarz F, Weihe E, Manthey J, Kubler W. Reduction of coronary reserve: a mechanism for angina pectoris in patients with arterial hypertension and normal coronary arteries. Circulation 69:1–7, 1984.

45. Nitenberg A, Foult JM, Blancet F, Zouioueche S. Multifactorial determinants of reduced coronary flow reserve after dipyridamole in dilated cardiomyopathy. Am J Cardiol 55:748–54, 1985.

46. Goldstein RA, Haynie M, Gould KL. Limited myocardial perfusion reserve in patients with left ventricular hypertrophy (Abstr). Clinical Res 36:279A, 1988.

47. Nitenberg A, Foult JM, Antony I, Blanchet F, Rahali M. Coronary flow and resistance reserve in patients with chronic aortic regurgitation, angina pectoris and normal coronary arteries. J Am Coll Cardiol 11:478–86, 1988.

48. Klocke FJ. Measurements of coronary flow reserve: defining pathophysiology versus making decisions about patient care. Circulation 76:1183–89, 1987.

49. Marcus ML, Wilson RF, White CW. Methods of measurement of myocardial blood flow in patients: a critical review. Circulation 76:245–53, 1987.

50. Marcus ML, Gascho JA, Mueller TM, Eastham CH, Wright CB, Doty DB, Hiratzka LF. The effects of ventricular hypertrophy on the coronary circulation. Basic Res Cardiol 76:575–81, 1981.

51. Strauer BE, Brune I, Schenk H, Knoll D, Perings E. Lupus cardiomyopathy: cardiac mechanics, hemodynamics, and coronary blood flow in uncomplicated systemic lupus erythematosus. Amer Heart J 92:715–22, 1976.

52. Wilson RF, Johnson MR, Marcus ML, Aylward PEG, Skorton DJ, Collins S, White CW. The effect of coronary angioplasty on coronary flow reserve. Circulation 77:873–85, 1988.

53. Marcus ML, Harrison DG, White CW, McPherson DD, Wilson RF, Kerber RE. Assessing the physiologic significance of coronary obstructions in patients: importance of diffuse undetected atherosclerosis. Prog Cardiovas Dis 31:39–56, 1988.

54. Watkins R. Presented at The Scientific Meetings of the AHA Council on Circulation, Durango, Colorado, August 8, 1990.

Quantitative Coronary Arteriography

Quantifying severity of coronary artery stenosis is becoming increasingly important for many reasons, including evaluation of interventions such as cholesterol control, risk factor management, pharmacological agents, percutaneous transluminal coronary angioplasty, thrombolysis, and bypass surgery; clinical decisions on medical versus mechanical treatment of coronary artery stenoses; judgment of adequacy of noninvasive diagnostic techniques; understanding the role of fluid dynamics in localizing atheroma at specific sites of an artery exposed to the same risk factors throughout its length; and in silent coronary artery disease, as the only basis for choosing medical or mechanical intervention to prevent sudden death or acute myocardial infarction.

There are two fundamental ways of describing stenosis severity, based on functional and anatomic approaches (1,2). These anatomic and physiological methods are related but provide independent complementary data; each is essential for judging severity and regression or progression or for making clinical decisions, and each will be briefly reviewed. Coronary flow reserve reflecting functional severity of coronary artery stenoses was reviewed in previous chapters. Quantitative analysis of coronary arteriograms is addressed here.

ANATOMIC-GEOMETRIC ASSESSMENT OF CORONARY STENOSIS SEVERITY

The anatomic-geometric approach uses all of the x-ray-determined geometric dimensions of a stenosis, including percent narrowing, absolute diameter, shape, and length effects (3–13). These dimensions are integrated throughout the length of narrowing to predict with fluid-dynamic equations stenosis resistance (10–13), pressure-flow characteristics of the stenosis (3,4), or coronary flow reserve (1–8). The anatomic approach is an invasive method requiring coronary arteriography, because there is no current way of accurately defining stenosis geometry non-invasively.

Visual interpretations of coronary arteriograms are marked by such great inter-observer and intra-observer variability that a comparison of arteriograms from different patients or at different times from the same patient are of limited value in assessing severity, changes in severity, or functional significance of coronary artery stenosis (14–21). To illustrate this variability of visual estimates of percent diameter stenosis, a graph of individual estimates of percent stenosis compared to a consensus estimate is a scattergram, Figure 8.1

(14). Using size of standard deviation as a measure of variability among different observers, the correlation between individual and consensus readings is approximately midway between random association and complete agreement, and is dependent on which artery is involved, Figure 8.2 (16). The standard deviation as a measure of variability among visual estimates of stenosis severity is greater with more observers and worse in the moderate range of severity, where quantitation is most needed, and is much greater than computerized analysis, Figure 8.3 (11).

For clinical purposes, percent narrowing is commonly used. However, it is an incomplete approximation of the correct anatomic-geometric method for describing severity because it does not account for other important geometric characteristics of stenoses, such as length, absolute cross-sectional luminal area, shape, multiple lesions in series, or eccentric narrowing that may be worse in one view compared with another (1–9). Figures 7.7 and 7.8 of the previous chapter show the poor relation between percent narrowing and functional severity of stenoses in man (22–25).

Absolute cross-sectional lumen area has been proposed as a measure of stenosis severity because it correlated with directly measured coronary flow reserve in the left anterior descending coronary artery (26). However, this association was true only for the left anterior descending artery and did not apply to other coronary arteries for describing stenosis severity. Using minimum absolute diameter or area alone as a measure of severity fails to account for the contributions that percent narrowing, length, and shape make to functional severity. As discussed subsequently, measuring regression or progression of coronary artery disease is not adequate based on any single dimension, because of multidimensional shape changes occurring with regression/progression of disease.

In contrast with single-dimension measures or incomplete approximations of stenosis severity, the validity of quantitative coronary arteriography for predicting the functional pressure-flow characteristics of stenoses has been demonstrated if all the dimensions of the lesion are taken into account, including relative percent narrowing, absolute luminal area, integrated length effects, and shape. Because these multiple dimensions have cumulative hemodynamic effects and interact with each other, they have to be integrated into a single measure of severity for a given stenosis to be practically useful. The most appropriate is flow reserve derived from all geometric dimensions of a stenosis as a standardized, single integrated measure of its severity, reflecting

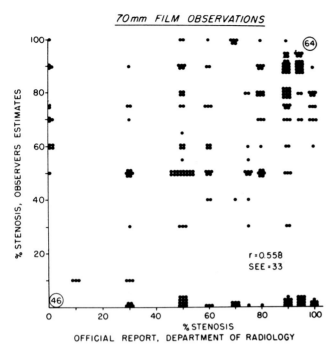

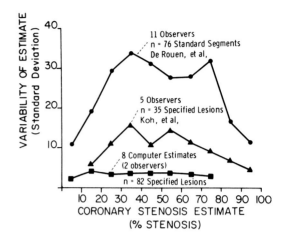

Fig. 8.3 Variability in estimates of percent stenosis in different-sized observer groups for different severity of narrowing. Reproduced with permission from Brown BG, Bolson EL, Dodge HT, 1982. (11).

Fig. 8.1 Relation of individual observer estimates of percent stenosis to the consensus reading. Reproduced with permission from Bjork L, Spindola-Franco H, Van Houten FX, et al., 1975. (14).

the combined effects of percent narrowing, absolute diameter, and length under "standardized" hemodynamic conditions. Determination of stenosis flow reserve by this quantitative analysis of coronary arteriograms correlates well with directly measured flow reserve in animals (5,7) and with maximum regional perfusion defects in patients (6,8). However, in order to derive stenosis flow reserve based on an integrated analysis of stenosis geometry, all of its dimensions need to be extracted from the arteriogram.

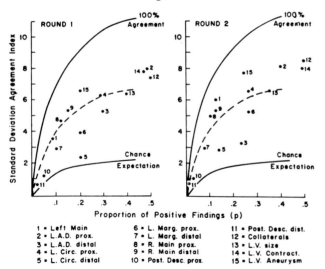

Fig. 8.2 Relation of standard deviation agreement index to proportion of positive findings. Reproduced with permission from Detre KM, Wright E, Murphy ML, et al., 1975. (16).

GEOMETRIC DIMENSIONS FROM CORONARY ARTERIOGRAMS

Quantitative coronary arteriography was originally described by Brown (10–13) and subsequently validated in vivo by Gould et al. (1–9). Our quantitative arteriographic method is similar to that of Brown et al. (10–13) but was developed independently and in parallel, using automated border recognition rather than visual tracing to determine arterial borders and stenosis dimensions on the arteriogram (1–9). Our approach also differs by taking into account length-dependent exit effects not previously accounted for. The Brown method determines stenosis resistance, which, however, is variable, depending on absolute flow as described in Chapter 3. Accordingly, we determine stenosis flow reserve as a single integrated measure of stenosis severity, taking into account all its dimensions independent of physiologic variables, as subsequently reviewed.

Quantitative coronary arteriography (QCA) requires high-quality coronary arteriograms taken in two views, preferably angled at 90° to each other but at any known angle greater than 30° if the isocenter technique is used. The arteriograms may be processed in two different ways. In the first, the images are optically magnified onto a digitizing tablet with the borders of the artery traced visually and thereby digitized for computer processing (1,3,4,10–13). There is some subjectivity in tracing the arterial borders visually.

In the second approach, the entire arteriographic frame is digitized and borders of the artery identified automatically by computer software without visual interpretation other than an operator determined proximal and distal end of the stenosis (5–9,27–33). Our automated computer technique utilizes an edge-detection method, as well as analysis of the absorbance or densitometry (gray scale) diametrically across the artery image (5–9, 31–33). The cross-sectional areas measured by both techniques are automatically compared for each segment of the artery. Disagreements between the two

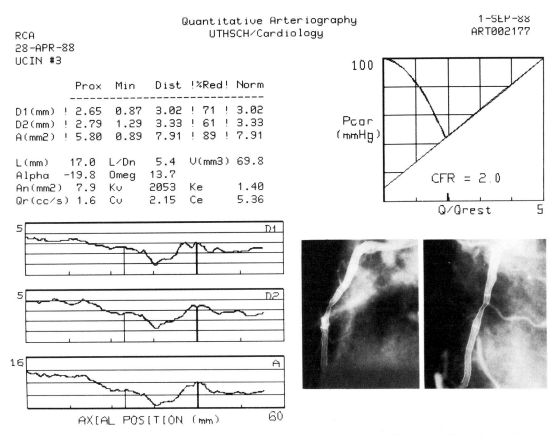

Fig. 8.4 Printout from quantitative coronary arteriography by border recognition analysis of orthogonal arteriographic views. Numbers in upper left show single plane diameters (D_1, D_2) by border recognition and cross-sectional area (A). Dimensions of the proximal (Prox), minimum (Min), distal (Dist), and normal (Norm) segments are shown with percent reduction (% red). Lower left graphs show the diameters in two orthogonal views (D_1, D_2) and cross-sectional area (A) plotted as a function of length along the artery. Although discussed in detail in the next chapter, the arteriographic analysis in the upper right graph shows calculated coronary stenosis flow reserve at standardized conditions of aortic pressure and expected normal flow reserve in the absence of stenosis. In this graph, calculated distal coronary perfusion pressure, P_{COR}, is on the vertical axis. Coronary artery flow (Q) is on the horizontal axis as a ratio to normal flow at rest (Q/Qrest). The straight line indicates the standardized, assumed relation between coronary perfusion pressure and coronary flow under conditions of maximal coronary vasodilation in the absence of a stenosis, as previously described. The downward-curved line is a plot of the relation between P_{cor} and flow defined by stenosis geometry. Coronary flow reserve (CFR) is given by the intersection of the downward-curved line characterizing stenosis severity with the straight upward-slanted line characterizing the CFR-pressure relation in the absence of a stenosis. In this case, coronary stenosis flow reserve is 2.0, as compared with a normal of 5. Reproduced with permission from Demer LL, Gould KL, Goldstein RA, et al., 1989. (8).

methods may occur, especially for eccentric lesions in which the border-recognition technique using orthogonal biplane views is not as accurate as the densitometry technique. However, where other optically dense structures (catheters, other vessels, etc.) are superimposed on the arterial segment of interest, or for foreshortened arteries out of plane, dimensions are best determined by automated border recognition.

An example of automated analysis is illustrated in Figure 8.4 (1), with the arterial borders automatically outlined by the dashed lines. The diameters of the artery are measured at increments along the long axis of the stenosis for purposes of computing the geometric dimensions and integrating lumen area length effects. After the borders of the opacified artery on the arteriogram are identified, the stenosis is analyzed by quantitatively adding the inertial pressure losses to the integrated viscous losses along the length of the stenosis. The final computer printout gives the measured dimensions and predicted pressure drop for a given coronary flow, as well as the pressure gradient–flow relation.

REPRODUCIBILITY AND ACCURACY OF MEASURING PRIMARY DIMENSIONS

Our initial digitizing hardware utilized a Spatial Data Eye Com System, a 512-line video camera and optical magnification, interfaced with a VAX 11/780 computer on which the automated border recognition and densitometric programs operated.

To assess the reproducibility of arteriogram analyses with this system, nine human coronary stenoses were selected, three each from the LCX, LAD, and RCA arteries of differing severities. Each stenosis was then analyzed six times on the basis of six different cine-frames (three consecutive frames at end-diastole for two consecutive cardiac cycles). This sampling method was chosen to include variation in frame selection, arterial image contrast, and user definition of arterial segments of interest. From each set of six analyzed images, the mean value of the parameters in Table 8.1 was calculated and the difference of each measurement from the mean was determined. These differences for all nine stenoses—the parameter mean difference and standard deviation of the differences—were found for all measurements, as shown in Table 8.1. The variability is the same for a similar analysis of experimental arteriograms with a different x-ray system and visually drawn borders, as previously published (3,4).

Accuracy was tested by taking x-rays of a series of progressively smaller tubes having precisely known diameters filled with contrast media and filmed in a tank of scattering media. Figure 8.5 (9) relates automatically measured x-ray diameter on the vertical axis to true known diameter on the horizontal axis in this phantom. The analysis was accurate for measuring absolute diameter to within ± 0.1 mm for phantom sizes down to 0.5 mm. However, in vivo in a beating heart, changing view angles and variable scattering due to differing radiodensity of bone, tissue, and lung may degrade this accuracy.

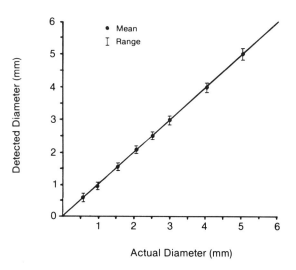

Fig. 8.5 Automated edge detection accuracy. The quantitative analysis system has an accuracy of ± 0.08 mm for x-ray film of phantoms. Correlation of the x-ray-determined diameter and the actual diameter of a phantom constructed from drillings in a plastic block filled with contrast media and submerged in an x-ray scattering medium. The circle stands for the mean; the range bar represents the range. Reproduced with permission from Kirkeeide R, Fung P, Smalling RW, et al., 1982. (9).

A NEW GENERATION SYSTEM FOR QUANTITATIVE ARTERIOGRAPHIC ANALYSIS

The accuracy of diameter measurements from cineangiograms depends on several determinants, such as the intrinsic resolution of the x-ray system (focal spot size, kV, transfer function of the image intensifier, etc.), the contrast medium concentration, the localization of the vessel edge within the edge gradient of the radiographic image, and the film processing and developing. These factors increase the variability of quantitative coronary arteriography, and therefore most investigators have used an automatic edge-detection algorithm to reduce the inherent system variations of diameter measurements from cineangiograms. Several algorithms have been used to locate the vessel edge from coronary angiograms (first or second derivative, base or inflection point of the coronary densogram). Although monoplane projections have been used, biological variations due to eccentric localization of the stenotic lesion and regional differences in coronary vasomotion markedly affect monoplane evaluation of coronary angiograms. Therefore, a new compact system for biplane as well as monoplane analysis of coronary angiograms was developed with new advanced hardware and software for quantitative arteriographic analysis. This system has been developed collaboratively by L. Gould and R. Kirkeeide (physiologic concepts, validation, and stenosis analysis software), the technical group directed by M. Anliker, and the clinical group directed by H. Krayenbuhl of the University of Zurich (hardware and management software) described here, in collaboration with M. Buchi and R. Kirkeeide (34).

The new system has three major components, illustrated in Figure 8.6 (34): (1) A Tagarno 35 CX film projector with 80 frames/s viewing speed and a digital counter interfaced to the workstation, allowing precise frame count and film motion control. A beam splitter directs 50% of the light to the viewing screen and 50% to the CCD (charged coupled device) camera. The bulb current is regulated to prevent line frequency interference with the digitizer. (2) A high resolution (2048 × 3072 pixels) CCD line scanner camera developed at the Institute for Biomedical Engineering in Zurich (35) is used for image digitization with a dynamic range of 12 bits. Since the angiographic technique does not allow resolution below 0.1 mm, the resolution of the CCD camera was limited to 1380 × 1024 pixels to increase computing speed. Inhomogenous

Table 8.1 Reproducibility of Automated QCA

N = 54	Size of One Standard Deviation	
	Units	% of Mean
Diameter, mm	.07	3%
Diameter—dist, mm	.07	4%
Diameter—min, mm	.15	18%
Diameter—% stenosis	5.03	7%
Area—% stenosis	5.10	9%
Area—minimum, mm²	.39	37%
Coronary flow reserve	.36	23%
Calibration factor	.002	2%

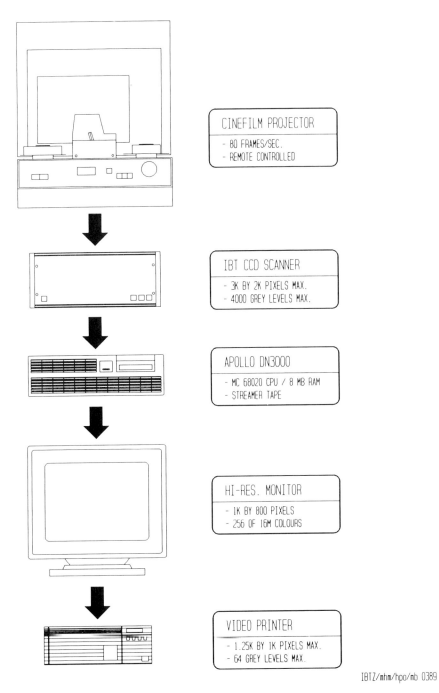

CINEFILM PROJECTOR
- 80 FRAMES/SEC.
- REMOTE CONTROLLED

IBT CCD SCANNER
- 3K BY 2K PIXELS MAX.
- 4000 GREY LEVELS MAX.

APOLLO DN3000
- MC 68020 CPU / 8 MB RAM
- STREAMER TAPE

HI-RES. MONITOR
- 1K BY 800 PIXELS
- 256 OF 16M COLOURS

VIDEO PRINTER
- 1.25K BY 1K PIXELS MAX.
- 64 GREY LEVELS MAX.

IBTZ/mhm/hpo/mb 0389

Fig. 8.6 Diagram of the quantitative coronary arteriography system. Reproduced with permission from Buchi M, Hess OM, Kirkeeide R, et al., in press. (34).

background illumination is corrected by subtraction of a blank image mask before each series of angiograms. (3) The digitized angiograms are stored in an Apollo DN 3000 computer workstation. Pincushion distortion is corrected using an analytic function of radii obtained from a centimeter grid filmed against the input screen of the image intensifier. For further processing, a region of 690 × 512 pixels is chosen by the operator from the digitized full-frame image.

BORDER RECOGNITION SOFTWARE

Arterial lumen borders are determined semi-automatically as follows: The user defines an arterial region-of-interest (ROI) by tracing a mouse-controlled cursor along an approximate centerline of the vessel segment of interest. The ROI is then radially expanded by the user until it exceeds the largest radial dimension of the arterial segment. A dynamic search algorithm then automatically determines the axially directed path of greatest image brightness within the ROI, which then corresponds to a final, computer-generated centerline. This computer-generated centerline and the radial ROI dimension define the ROI in which edge detection and border recognition take place.

Vessel borders are then identified by sequential edge detection and border recognition, each of which is also repeated once. The edge detection process (9) follows the logic outlined in Figure 8.7 (34). At two- to four-pixel intervals along the centerline, image gray levels are scanned transversely to the local centerline using bilinear interpolation. Each scanline is then processed by a subroutine, which computes the first spatial derivative of the scanline. Possible edge points along the scanline are initially approximated as the local maxima and minima of the derivative function whose absolute values exceed 25% of the maximum absolute value of the scanline derivative. Zero to 10 possible edge points may be found for each scanline, depending on the local gray-level terrain. Border recognition follows edge detection, using a dynamic search algorithm derived from the work of Parker et al. (36,37). For this purpose, possible edge-point locations are placed into a two-dimensional matrix, with each row containing one scanline and columns denoting location along the scanline. Points corresponding to derivative maxima are assigned the value 1, minima −1, and 0 for all other matrix elements. The search algorithm then finds the best—that is, most continuous—paths through the possible maxima and minima elements. The second pass through the edge detection-border recognition algorithm follows the same logic, except for the fact that the centerline is automatically defined by computer as the midpoints between the vessel borders found in the first pass.

At this point the user may correct any gross errors made

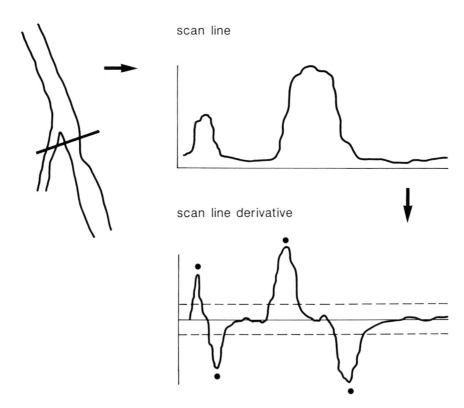

scan line

scan line derivative

Fig. 8.7 Vessel edge detection. Arteriographic views or densograms are taken orthogonal to the centerline of the vessel (scanline). The first derivative of this densogram is automatically determined by the computer, and the local maxima and minima of the derivative whose absolute values exceed 25% of the maximum value (dashed line) are marked as possible edge points (dots). Reproduced with permission from Buchi M, Hess OM, Kirkeeide R, et al., in press. (34).

by the border recognition software. After pointing to a particular suspect edge point on the image display, the user can instruct the system to exclude this point or to make the border connect with or through that point. Only existing edge points, whether they are to be part of the border or not, can be modified by this procedure. The user cannot freely draw any section of vessel border.

DIAMETER MEASUREMENT SOFTWARE

Diameters are automatically derived as the distance between the arterial borders along each diameter perpendicular to the local centerline. Each such diameter is corrected for distortion caused by image blur of the imaging chain, as previously described (9). Each x-ray imaging system blurs the arterial image uniquely, while edge detection based on the first derivative of density introduces a systematic distortion affecting all images presented to the software. Our previous experiments with automated diameter detection have validated corrections for these factors for one particular x-ray system at the University of Texas (9). In the present study, the same correction factors for the systematic distortion of edge detection were applied to the phantom vessel diameter measurements taken at the University Hospital of Zurich and are

denoted as uncorrected measurements in Figure 8.8 (34), that is, uncorrected for the x-ray blur uniquely characteristic of each x-ray system. Based on the differences between these uncorrected and true diameters, a correction look-up table was generated for the imaging chain at the Zurich location. Using this look-up table, "corrected" diameters (second-order correction) were found for each uncorrected diameter measured on the Zurich x-ray system and compared to true diameters of the phantom (Fig. 8.8). We believe that the differences between the uncorrected and corrected diameters are due to differences in image quality that will vary among different laboratories. The arterial lumen area was calculated in monoplane projection assuming a circular geometry, and in biplane projection assuming elliptical geometry.

CALIBRATION OF THE X-RAY AND ANALYSIS SYSTEM

Basically, three methods are available for calibrating the x-ray system or images in order to transform image distances or dimensions in pixels to absolute dimensional equivalents in millimeters. The first two methods use catheter or cardio-marker dimensions, as described by Brown and coworkers

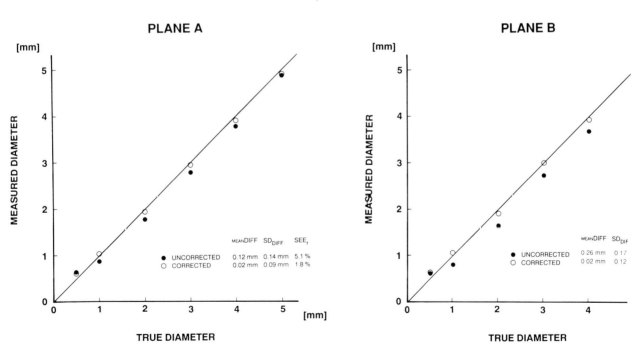

PHANTOM MEASUREMENTS

(100 % CONTRAST)

Fig. 8.8 Correlation between the true and the measured diameters of precision-drilled holes in a plexiglas cube filled with 100% contrast medium. The uncorrected data are represented by the closed symbols and show a slight underestimation for diameters above 1 mm and an overestimation below 1 mm by quantitative coronary arteriography. Data are given for both planes. The corrected data (second-order correction) are represented by the open symbols and show a good correlation with minimal deviations from the line of identity. The standard error of estimate of the mean (SEEr) decreased by this correction from 5% to 1.8% for plane A and from 5.5% to 4.2 for plane B. (mean diff = mean difference; SD diff = standard deviation of the differences.) Reproduced with permission from Buchi M, Hess OM, Kirkeeide R, et al., in press. (34).

(10–13), whereby the calibration factor is derived as the ratio of known object size (mm) in the image field to its apparent size in the image (pixels). For the catheter method, the diameter of the injection catheter is used as the true reference size in mm, and automated edge detection of the catheter x-ray image is used to determine the apparent image size in pixels. The cardiomarker method uses known spacing (20 mm) between thin titanium rings on the catheter. The positions of these rings on the computer screen are marked by the user in each of the orthogonally paired arteriographic views to account for the foreshortening of the catheter with respect to the image intensifier planes. Both of these calibration techniques correct for the differential magnification between the catheter and coronary segment, according to the methods of Brown et al. (10–13).

In our current work, as described here, calibration factors were determined solely by the third available technique, the isocenter method (37). The isocenter is the rotational center of the x-ray system. As shown in Figure 8.9 (34), translating an image distance on the computer screen (Ds, pixels) to its absolute size (D, mm) requires calculation of x-ray beam divergence and size transformations along the imaging chain. Due to the conical divergence of the x-ray beam from the focal spot of the x-ray tube to the input phosphor of image intensifier, the size of the x-ray "shadow" projected onto the input phosphor (Di, mm) is greater than the true object size (D, mm). From the similar triangles in the imaging geometry shown in Figure 8.9, the relative enlargement, Di/D, is equal

to the length ratio Li/L, where Li is the distance between the focal spot of the x-ray tube and the image intensifier, and l is the focal spot to object distance. The ratio of these distances is the correction factor for magnification caused by beam divergence.

Transformation of the input phosphor image along the imaging chain up to the image on the computer screen is corrected by use of an overall size transformation coefficient, the video magnification factor (Mv, mm/pixel). Although Mv depends on each component of the imaging chain for a given x-ray system, only the image intensifier field size and the working image array size are variable, but only within a few fixed options. Therefore, Mv was determined for every combination of array size, image intensifier, and associated various field sizes in the arteriographic systems used in this study. For these options, Mv was determined by analyzing images of a grid field (1-cm squares) filmed with the grid against the protective cover of the image intensifier input phosphor, which is less than 1 cm from the input phosphor itself. As an example of this method, a 7-inch field size (178 mm) digitized on the 1380-pixel-wide matrix gives in an Mv value of about 0.13 mm/pixel. Actual measurements of Mv were 0.105 and 0.104 mm/pixel for the 7-inch field sizes of the AP and lateral imaging chains of the biplane x-ray system, respectively. These lower values for Mv reflect the fact that less than a full 7-inch image intensifier field is digitized by the CCD-camera.

The overall transformation of true object size, D, to digitized image size, Ds, is:

$$D = (D/Di)\ (Di/Ds)\ Ds$$

Since Di/Ds is the video magnification coefficient, Mv, and substituting L/Li for D/Di to correct for beam divergence, this equation becomes:

$$D = (L/Li)\ Mv\ Ds$$

The length ratio, L/Li, is found from the triangulation technique shown in Figure 8.10 (34). From knowledge of the x-ray imaging geometry, the three-dimensional positions of the focal spot of the x-ray tubes (f1 and f2) and the image intensifier impact points (P1 and P2) of the x-rays passing through the studied object (P) are determined with respect to the x-ray system's isocenter point (C).

Wollschlager and coworkers (39) used a spherical coordinate system whose origin is at the x-ray system's isocenter, and small lead spheres on each image intensifier (C1 and C2) to show the projected position of the isocenter in each image. The location of P with respect to C can then theoretically be found from the intersection of the two x-ray vectors, f1-P1 and f2-P2. However, small errors in describing the imaging geometry makes locating an intersection point uncertain (36,39). We have therefore adopted the technique of Parker et al. (36,37), who used the midpoint of the minimum distance vector between the two x-rays instead of the intersection. The relevant length ratio for angiographic view 1, for example, is then given as the ratio of the length of vector f1-P to the length of vector f1-P1.

For the practical application of the isocenter technique, the distances between the x-ray tube and the isocenter (point C in Fig. 8.10), as well as the distance between the isocenter and the image intensifier, must be determined in each patient.

ARTERIOGRAM MAGNIFICATION

CORRECTION

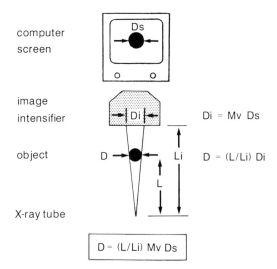

Fig. 8.9 Schematic presentation of the arteriogram magnification correction. The magnification of an object (D) from the input phosphor (Di) along the image chain ending with the magnified object on the computer screen (Ds) can be calculated from the length ratio L/Li and the video magnification factor (Mv). For further explanations see text. Reproduced with permission from Buchi M, Hess OM, Kirkeeide R, et al., in press. (34).

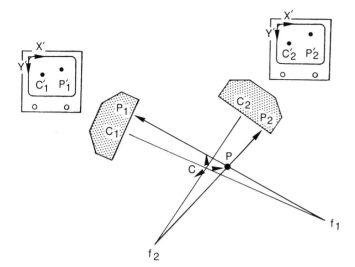

Fig. 8.10 Isocenter method for calibration of the angiogram. With the knowledge of the distance from the focal spot (f1, f2) to the isocenter (C) and from the distance of the focal spot to the projection of the isocenter on the image intensifiers (C1, C2), the calibration factor for any point of interest (P) can be calculated (for further explanations see text). The isocenter is determined once with a phantom, and its projection on the image intensifier (C1, C2) is marked with small lead spheres (2 mm in diameter). Reproduced with permission from Buchi M, Hess OM, Kirkeeide R, et al., in press. (34).

The projection of the isocenter on the image intensifier (C1 and C2) is marked with a small lead sphere on both image intensifiers. With the knowledge of these distances and the projection of the isocenter (C1, C2), the calibration factor for any point of interest (P) can be calculated from the projection of P on the two image intensifiers (P1, P2). In practice, the isocenter points in the RAO and LAO projections C'1 and C'2, as well as the projections of P (P'1 and P'2), are marked on the monitor by a cursor. A computer program based on three-dimensional vectorial geometry, adapted from the work of Wollschlager et al. (39), allows the determination of the magnification factor at the specific point in both projections. This factor corresponds to the ratio D/Ds in Figure 8.9 (34).

The above isocenter calibration method was tested against calibration factors derived from analyses of 1-cm-square grids filmed with varying image geometry. Calibration factors determined by the isocenter method were in the 0.08–0.09 mm/pixel range and were very accurate (within 1% of the grid-based calibration factors), and reproducible (differences between repeated analyses were less than 1%).

ACCURACY AND PRECISION OF PHANTOM MEASUREMENTS

The accuracy of this new system was evaluated using cine-films of a plexiglass phantom with precision-drilled holes which were filled with contrast medium of 50%, 75%, and 100% concentration (iopamidol 755.2 mg/mL, trometamol 1

mg/mL = Iopamiro 370 R). The diameters of the holes ranged from 0.5 to 5.0 mm, with a known accuracy of ±0.01 mm. The plexiglass model was filmed in the center of the image intensifier under 10 cm of water, in both planes.

The accuracy of the quantitative coronary arteriography system was defined as the mean difference between the measured and the true diameters. Precision was defined as the standard deviation of the signed differences (40). Intra- and interobserver variabilities were assessed with a linear regression analysis. Variability is expressed as the standard error of estimate in absolute terms (SEEa) and as the standard error of estimate in percent of the mean vessel area (SEEr).

Quantitative analysis of the filmed plexiglas phantoms showed a good correlation between the true and the measured diameter for both planes (Fig. 8.8). Although the software corrects for distortion in the imaging chain and that associated with the edge detection algorithm, we used a further correction, which is specific for each catheterization laboratory that depends on the individual characteristics of each image intensifier and film processing unit. This so-called second-order correction is based on a look-up table described earlier. After the implementation of this second-order correction, the quantitative analysis of the phantoms showed a clear improvement, with a mean difference of 0.02 mm and SD of the differences of 0.09 mm for plane A, and mean difference of 0.02 mm and SD of the differences of 0.12 mm for plane B, as shown in Figure 8.8 (34). The SEEr was slightly larger for plane B than for plane A. With contrast agent concentrations of 100% and 75%, the accuracy and precision are very good (mean difference < 0.05 mm and SD of the difference < 0.1 mm) but with 50% contrast medium concentration, accuracy and precision are less good (– 0.16 and 0.25 mm, respectively).

The correlation of the data from plane A with the data from plane B showed minimal differences and a small standard deviation of the differences; the standard error of estimate in percent of the mean diameter ranged between 2.5% and 3.1% for the three different contrast medium concentrations (Table 8.2).

This new quantitative analysis system showed excellent accuracy and precision for both planes using 100% and 75% contrast medium concentrations. The results were clearly less good when 50% contrast medium concentration was used, as has also been observed by others (9,29) and suggests that only good-quality angiograms should be used for quantitative evaluation. In the range of the small vessel diameters (<1 mm), overestimation of the true vessel diameter was observed, whereas larger vessel diameters were systematically underestimated by the computer system. These systematic errors have been described by Kirkeeide et al. (9) as due to the relation between vessel size and penumbra, which becomes critical below 1 mm. Since these deviations of the measured vessel diameter from the true vessel diameter are inherent to the system, a second-order correction is used to minimize these over- and underestimations of the true vessel size (Fig. 8.8). Preferably, such a correction should be performed for each individual x-ray system to improve the accuracy of quantitative coronary arteriography. Using this second-order correction, the standard error of estimate in percent of the mean vessel diameter decreased from 5.1% to 1.8% for plane A and from 5.5% to 4.2% for Plane B (Fig. 8.8).

Table 8.2 Phantom Measurements (Diameter Measurements)

	Mean Diff. (mm)	SD Diff. (mm)	r	SEEa (mm)	SEEr (%)
Plane A					
100% contrast	0.020	0.092	0.999	0.046	1.8
75% contrast	−0.037	0.098	0.999	0.079	3.1
50% contrast	−0.158	0.250	0.994	0.184	7.1
Plane B					
100% contrast	0.020	0.124	0.998	0.109	4.2
75% contrast	−0.093	0.301	0.992	0.219	8.2
50% contrast	−0.110	0.374	0.986	0.273	10.1
Plane A vs. Plane B					
100% contrast	−0.002	0.058	0.999	0.064	2.5
75% contrast	−0.147	0.160	0.999	0.083	3.1
50% contrast	−0.060	0.137	0.999	0.082	3.0

Legend: Mean diff = mean difference; SD diff. = standard deviation of the differences; r = correlation coefficient; SEEa = standard error of the estimate in mm; SEEr = standard error of estimate in percent of the mean diameter of the plexiglas holes.

Source: Adapted from Buchi M, Hess OM, Kirkeeide R, et al., in press. Reference 34.

INTRA- AND INTEROBSERVER VARIABILITY OF PATIENTS STUDIES

Intra- and interobserver variability was determined from coronary angiograms of five patients. Two independent observers analyzed the same frame twice. Sixteen normal vessels with a cross-sectional area ranging between 1.0 and 8.7 mm^2 and five stenotic vessel segments with an area ranging between 0.8 and 2.5 mm^2 were analyzed. Intra-observer variability, expressed as the standard error of estimate (SEEa), was 0.072 mm^2 for observer 1 and 0.146 mm^2 for observer 2. The SEE, as percent of the mean vessel area (SEEr), was 2.1% for observer 1 and 4.4% for observer 2. Inter-observer variability was in the same range as the intra-observer variability, with the SEEr being 4.1% for measurement 1 and 3.6% for measurement 2.

SUMMARY OF NEW QUANTITATIVE ANALYSIS SYSTEM

Quantitative coronary arteriography is influenced by multiple biological variables; for example, differences in vasomotor tone, mixing of the contrast medium with blood, errors in calibration as well as variations in the data analysis procedures (quantum noise, electronic noise, errors in analog-to-digital conversion, etc.). These factors influence quantitative evaluation of coronary angiograms as reflected by the intra- and inter-observer variability of quantitative coronary arteriography. For comparison of observers, the effect of coronary vasomotor tone and mixing of the contrast medium were excluded by analyzing the same cineframe by both observers and for both measurements.

Inaccuracies due to calibration were minimized in our study by using the isocenter calibration technique, which proved to be fast, accurate, and reproducible. Thus, varia-

tions in coronary luminal area for the observer comparisons were mainly or exclusively due to variations in the data analysis procedures by different technical staff loading on the film for analysis and choosing stenosis proximal and distal limits, and by hardware-software processing.

Intra-observer variability for biplane measurement was found to be small, namely 2.1% and 4.4% (Table 8.3 and Fig. 8.11) (34). Inter-observer variabilities for biplane measurement were also excellent, being 3.6% and 4.1%, respectively (Table 8.3 and Fig. 8.12) (34). Computer systems based on manual tracings of biplane coronary angiograms showed slightly larger variations for intra- (range 6%–8%) (29) and interobserver (7.9%) (41,42) variabilities.

The new CCD camera system for biplane quantitative coronary arteriography provides an easy, fast determination of absolute coronary dimensions with good accuracy, high reproducibility, and small intra- and interobserver variabilities of less than 5%.

FLUID-DYNAMIC ANALYSIS OF STENOSES FROM AUTOMATED DIMENSIONAL MEASUREMENTS*

The general fluid-dynamic equations for predicting pressure losses across coronary stenoses have been reviewed in previous chapters. However, their application to coronary arteriograms using computer-measured dimensions requires additional discussion here.

The flowfield in the vicinity of a coronary stenosis is shown in Figure 8.13 (43). Immediately upstream from the stenosis, flow is laminar despite being pulsatile, and coronary velocity profiles have a parabolic shape characteristic of fully developed flows in long straight tubes. In the vicinity of branches and highly curved sections of artery, these profiles

* Prepared with R. Kirkeeide, Ph.D.

Table 8.3 Intra- and Interobserver Variability (Cross-sectional Area)

Intraobserver Variability	Mean Diff. (mm²)	SD Diff. (mm²)	r	SEEa (mm²)	SEEr (%)
Observer 1	0.013	0.071	0.999	0.072	2.1
Observer 2	0.016	0.147	0.998	0.146	4.4
Interobserver Variability	Mean Diff. (mm²)	SD Diff. (mm²)	r	SEEa (mm²)	SEEr (%)
Measurement 1	0.053	0.140	0.998	0.137	4.1
Measurement 2	0.058	0.136	0.999	0.123	3.6

Mean diff. = mean difference; SD diff. = standard deviation of the differences; r = correlation coefficient; SEEa = standard error of the estimate in mm²; SEEr = standard error of estimate in percent of the mean vessel area.

Source: Adapted from Buchi M, Hess OM, Kirkeeide RL, et al., in press. Reference 34.

become skewed (44,45). As flow enters the stenosis, it remains laminar while its bulk velocity, V, increases due to the principle of conservation of mass. The blood velocity distribution across the arterial lumen reshapes with this convective acceleration of the flow. The basis for this reshaping of flow profile upon entering the stenosis is the increased wall friction acting to retard the flow and to shear off the endothelial cells from their foundations. This wall friction, combined with convective acceleration, "stretches" the velocity profiles along the vessel axis.

From the proximal end of the stenosis to the section of minimal lumen area of the artery, pressure falls by two mechanisms: viscous wall shear (wall friction) and an exchange of potential energy (pressure) for kinetic energy of flow asso-

ciated with flow acceleration. Since viscous losses are irreversible, the progressive fall in the total flow energy along this section of the stenosis is due to viscous losses, ΔP_v (bottom panel of Fig. 8.13). Viscous losses are directly proportional to the flow velocity proximal to the stenosis (V_s) and are given by

$$\Delta P_v = C_v V_s \qquad (1)$$

where C_v is the viscous pressure loss coefficient, dependent on the viscosity of blood and the geometric characteristics of the stenosis. An analytic expression for C_v will subsequently be presented.

The flowfield from the minimal area of the stenosis into the distal, enlarged vessel segment undergoes further major

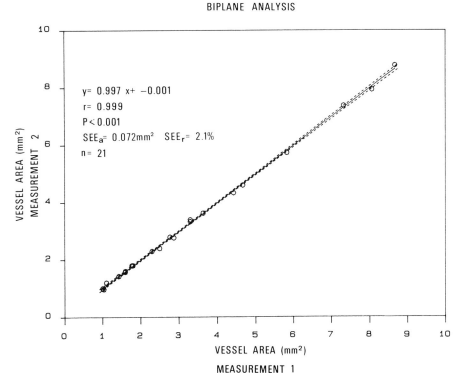

INTRAOBSERVER VARIABILITY   (OBSERVER 1)
BIPLANE ANALYSIS

y= 0.997 x+ −0.001
r= 0.999
P< 0.001
SEEa= 0.072mm²   SEEr= 2.1%
n= 21

VESSEL AREA (mm²)
MEASUREMENT 2

VESSEL AREA (mm²)
MEASUREMENT 1

Fig. 8.11 Intraobserver variability for repeated measurements of the luminal vessel area of the same angiographic frame. Twenty-one vessel segments were analyzed twice by the same observer. There was excellent correlation with a standard error of estimate (SEEa) of 0.072 mm². The standard error of estimate in percent of the mean vessel area (SEEr) amounted to 2.1% (observer 1). (P = probability; r = correlation coefficient.) Reproduced with permission from Buchi M, Hess OM, Kirkeeide R, et al., in press. (34).

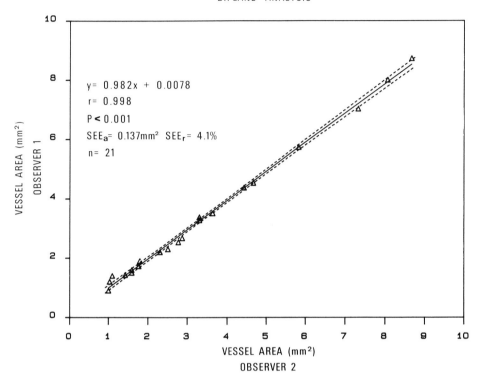

INTEROBSERVER VARIABILITY (MEASUREMENT 1)

BIPLANE ANALYSIS

$y = 0.982x + 0.0078$
$r = 0.998$
$P < 0.001$
$SEE_a = 0.137 mm^2$ $SEE_r = 4.1\%$
$n = 21$

Fig. 8.12 Interobserver variability for luminal vessel area determined by two independent observers. There was an excellent correlation between the two observers, with a standard error of estimate (SEEa) of 0.137 mm². The standard error of estimate in percent of the mean vessel area (SEEr) amounted to 4.1% (measurement 1). Other abbreviations as in Figure 8.7. Reproduced with permission from Buchi M, Hess OM, Kirkeeide R, et al., in press. (34).

change, causing kinetic energy loss and therefore pressure loss or a pressure gradient across the stenosis. As the flow moves along the stenosis, its axially directed momentum increases in proportion to the proximal-to-minimal vessel area ratio (Ao/As). When the flow emerges from the narrowing, its momentum keeps it moving along the vessel axis, not permitting it to expand radially as the lumen enlarges. Therefore, the bulk of flow separates from endothelium to form a high-velocity jet that is surrounded by low-velocity, recirculating eddies. The jet expands distally as it interacts with its surrounding eddies and thereby decelerates, producing turbulence.

Such turbulence is frequently "heard" as murmurs or bruits in peripheral and cerebrovascular disease (46), but is difficult to appreciate with coronary disease, owing to the masking sounds of the heart and the acoustic properties of the chest. Pressure losses associated with the expansion of the stenotic lumen accumulate with the diffusion of the jet and its accompanying disordered flow. At or distal to the point of reattachment of the flow profile, the ordered flow is reestablished, comparable to the arterial segment upstream to the stenosis. The net expansion associated pressure loss is ΔP_e (Fig. 8.13). Pressure losses accompanying an abrupt expansion reflect the change in flow momentum and kinetic energy between the flow separation point (where the jet first forms) and the site where ordered flow is reestablished. These losses are dependent on the square of the flow velocity as follows:

$$\Delta P_e = C_e V_s^2 \qquad (2)$$

where C_e is the coefficient of expansion pressure loss and is related to the blood mass, density, and stenosis geometry; V_s is the flow velocity distal to the stenosis, which for the case shown in Figure 8.13 equals the flow velocity proximal to the stenosis.

Pulsatility of coronary blood flow is of minor importance in determining pressure losses across moderately-to-severely stenotic coronary arteries, for several reasons. Rapid changes in coronary flow are confined to the brief periods of isovolumetric contraction and relaxation of the ventricle. During the remainder of the cardiac cycle, time-dependent changes in flow are much smaller, and instantaneous pressure losses across the stenosis are dominated by the viscous and abrupt expansion mechanisms. Progressively severe coronary stenoses damp the coronary flow waveform, thereby reducing its pulsatile nature, as shown in Chapters 4, 5, and 6, particularly at elevated flow conditions. Thus, at least for the purposes of analyzing the mean or instantaneous diastolic pressure drops across a clinically significant coronary stenosis, blood flow can be considered as varying but quasi-steady (47,48) with regard to inertial losses associated with pulsatility, as opposed to inertial losses due to stenosis expansion.

FLOWFIELD

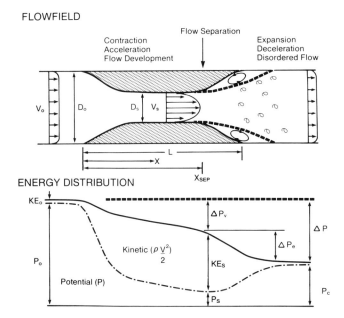

Fig. 8.13 Flowfield (top panel) and energy distribution (bottom panel) along an idealized coronary stenosis. The stenosis flowfield is dominated by the constricted arterial lumen, which accelerates the flow and alters the velocity distribution (profiles) across the lumen, and by the abrupt lumen expansion at the distal end of the stenosis, which causes the flow to separate and the distal flowfield to become disordered. The flow's total energy (bottom panel, solid heavy line) falls along and distal to the stenosis, owing to viscous losses (ΔP_v) and expansion losses (ΔP_e). Pressure falls within the stenosis owing to the high kinetic energy of the intrastenotic flow; however, part of this energy may be recovered when the flow decelerates beyond the stenosis. The total, irreversible pressure loss across the stenosis, ΔP, is the sum of viscous and expansion losses. V_s = flow velocity; D_o = diameter of artery before stenosis; D_s = diameter at the stenosis; L = length of stenosis; KE_o = original (prestenosis) kinetic energy; P_{Ao} = aortic pressure; and P_c = distal coronary pressure. Reproduced with permission from Wong WH, Kirkeeide R, Gould KL, 1986. (43).

CALCULATING THE PRESSURE DROP-FLOW CHARACTERISTICS OF CORONARY STENOSES

From the preceding discussion, the total mean pressure drop (ΔP) across a stenosis is described as the sum of the viscous and expansion losses. Combining Equations 1 and 2, ΔP is given by

$$\Delta P = C_v V_s + C_e V_s^2 \qquad (3)$$

An alternative but equivalent relation for expressing the pressure drop across stenoses uses the volume flow rate through the stenosis, Q_s, instead of V_s (these two flow descriptors being related by the lumen area in the normal vessel segment, $Q_s = V_s A_o$). In this case,

$$\Delta P = C'_v Q_s + C'_e Q_s^2 \qquad (4)$$

where $C'_v = C_v/A_o$ and $C'_e = C_e/A_o^2$. Equations 3 and 4 yield the same results in fluid-dynamic terms for rigid tubes but are not equivalent for vasoactive arteries in vivo, as reviewed in previous chapters. The choice of using velocity or flow equation for characterizing a stenosis can be made on the basis of whether one measures flow velocity, V_s, or the volume flow rate, Q_s. Implications associated with this choice were discussed at length in previous chapters. Based on the traditional fluid-dynamic approach, the velocity equation will be developed, but in later discussion will be adapted for volume flow.

Hydraulic and in vitro experiments have shown that the viscous loss coefficient C_v can be computed from the geometry of a stenosis by an equation in the form

$$C_v = \frac{4\mu}{1333 D_o} \int K \frac{A_o D_o^2}{A D_h^2} \frac{dx}{D_o} \qquad (5)$$

where A_o and D_o are the normal arterial lumen area and diameter, respectively. A and D_h are the local lumen area and hydraulic equivalent diameter (defined below), which vary along the length of the stenosis, and μ is the absolute viscosity of blood. The integration is performed from the proximal end of the stenosis to the assumed point of flow separation, which is the minimal cross-sectional area section of the stenosis. In applying this formula to the data obtained from computer analysis of biplane arteriograms, the integral sign is replaced by a summation sign and the differential distance dx is replaced by the finite distance along the reconstructed three-dimensional vessel centerline at which orthogonal diameters have been determined.

The numeric constant 1,333 expresses the equivalence, 1 mm Hg = 1,333 dyne/cm². It is therefore necessary that all variables be expressed in the centimeter-gram-second system of units [i.e., flow velocity (cm/s), area (cm²), diameter (cm), incremental length (cm), and viscosity (dyne-s/cm²)]. The hydraulic diameter is defined as the ratio of four times the lumen area to the wetted circumference (4A/C). For the case in which only two orthogonal diameters are available to describe the lumen shape, the hydraulic diameter is expressed as

$$D_h = \left(\frac{2a^2 b^2}{a^2 + b^2} \right)^{1/2} \qquad (6)$$

where a and b are the orthogonal diameters at a specific position along the vessel's centerline as determined, for example, by quantitative arteriography.

The coefficient K in Equation 5 is a dimensionless variable that depends on the shapes of the velocity profiles along the stenosis. If the velocity profiles were everywhere parabolic in shape, K would be a constant equal to 8 and could be brought outside of the integral. Extensive hydraulic and in-vitro experiments with a wide variety of modeled coronary stenoses generally support this assumption (3,4,47–51), despite more precise and complex formulas for C_v that don't contribute much to final accuracy. For purposes of discussion here, we shall use Equation 5 with a K value of 8.

The expansion pressure loss coefficient C_e in Equation 2 is computed by the equation

$$C_e = \frac{P}{2} \frac{K_e}{1333} \left(\frac{A_d}{A_{s,min}} - 1 \right)^2 \qquad (7)$$

where A_d is the normal vessel area distal to the stenosis, $A_{s,min}$ is the minimal cross-sectional area along the stenosis, and P is the mass density of blood (taken as 1.06 g/mL). The constant K_e, like the variable K in Equation 5, depends on velocity profile shape. The relevant velocity profiles for K_e are those at the minimal area and distal normal sections. Brown and colleagues (10–13) originally assumed K_e to be equal to 1.0, implying the velocity profiles to be everywhere flat along the expansion segment. Experimental findings, however, point to a larger value of K_e for arterial flow conditions. Seeley and Young (49) recommended a K_e value of 1.5, based on results from hydraulic tests of various stenosis models, a value that was also found applicable to stenoses of canine femoral and carotid arteries (48).

However, our hydraulic studies (50,51) indicate the new observation that K_e is directly related to the length of the stenosis, L_s, proximal to its minimal area section. The observation implies that longer stenosis entrance sections permit the velocity profiles to develop more fully, which then augment exit losses. This entrance effect can be accounted for by expressing K_e as a linear function of L_s (50,51), for example, by the relation

$$K_e = 1.21 + 0.08(L_s/D_o) \qquad (8)$$

where D_o is the absolute vessel diameter proximal to the stenosis. The constant 1.21 in this expression reflects the expansion losses found with very short stenoses, approaching the configuration of a sharp orifice, a condition that Mates et al. (47) accounted for by the use of an entrance loss coefficient.

After the diameter and area functions along a coronary stenosis have been determined by quantitative analysis of the coronary arteriogram, the hydraulic diameters along the stenosis are computed using Equation 6. From these data, the viscous pressure loss coefficient is determined with Equation 5, and the expansion pressure loss coefficient is computed from Equations 7 and 8. The resulting numeric values for C_v and C_e are substituted into Equation 3 to yield the pressure drop-flow characteristic of the stenosis in terms of flow velocity. Dividing C_v and C_e by the normal lumen area yields the coefficients C_v' and C_e', respectively, which can be substituted into Equation 4 to define the hemodynamic characteristics of the stenosis in terms of the volume flow rate.

From these equations the functionally significant geometric characteristics of coronary stenoses are the proximal normal-to-stenotic area ratio (or absolute lumen area alone in the flow equation), the normal diameter-to-stenotic hydraulic diameter ratio (or the absolute hydraulic diameter for the flow equation), stenosis length up to the minimal area section (in relative or absolute terms), the distal normal-to-minimal stenotic area ratio, and the absolute diameter of the normal vessel in which the stenosis developed. Among these parameters, stenosis area and hydraulic diameter (in relative or absolute terms) and the flow through the stenosis (V_s or Q_s) are major determinants of the hemodynamic severity of the stenosis, since they are raised to the second power.

The graphs shown in Figures 5.3 through 5.5 demonstrate the pressure drop–flow relations for stenoses of progressive geometric severity (3). With increasing flow through the stenoses, the pressure drop–flow relations curve nonlinearly up-

ward, owing to the nonlinear dependence of the expansion pressure losses on flow. The directly measured pressure gradient–flow relations for stenoses are graphed with the pressure drop-flow relations predicted by quantitative analysis of the biplane arteriograms for the same stenoses, using the above hemodynamic equations for C_v and C_e. The close correspondence between the in-vivo measured and angiographically predicted pressure drop–flow relations illustrated in Figure 5.5 have validated quantitative coronary arteriography for whatever vasoactive state of the artery is present at the time of arteriography (3). Additional in-vivo studies with femoral and carotid arterial stenoses, using equations similar to those above, also show good correlation between the geometry-predicted and experimentally measured pressure drop–flow relations (48).

However, expressing stenosis severity in terms of pressure gradient–flow equations or graph is too technical and fluid-dynamically oriented for routine physiologic or clinical applications. Accordingly, the next chapter develops the concept of stenosis flow reserve as a simply expressed, single number derived from all stenosis geometry that defines stenosis severity suitably for physiologic and clinical use.

REFERENCES

1. Gould KL. Quantification of coronary artery stenosis in vivo. Circ Res 57:341–53, 1985.
2. Gould KL. Identifying and measuring severity of coronary artery stenosis: quantitative coronary arteriography and positron emission tomography. Circulation 78:237–45, 1988.
3. Gould KL, Kelley KO, Bolson EL. Experimental validation of quantitative coronary arteriography for determining pressure-flow characteristics of coronary stenosis. Circulation 66:930–37, 1982.
4. Gould KL, Kelley KO. Physiologic significance of coronary flow velocity and changing stenosis geometry during coronary vasodilation in dogs. Circ Research 50:695–704, 1982.
5. Kirkeeide R, Gould KL, Parsel L. Assessment of coronary stenoses by myocardial imaging during coronary vasodilation. VII. Validation of coronary flow reserve as a single integrated measure of stenosis severity accounting for all its geometric dimensions. J Am Coll Cardiol 7:103–13, 1986.
6. Gould KL, Goldstein RA, Mullani NA, Kirkeeide RL, Wong WH, Tewson TJ, Berridge MS, Bolomey LA, Hartz RK, Smalling RW, Fuentes F, Nishikawa A. Noninvasive assessment of coronary stenoses by myocardial perfusion imaging during pharmacologic coronary vasodilation. VIII. Clinical feasibility of positron cardiac imaging without a cyclotron using generator-produced rubidium-82. J Am Coll Cardiol 7:775–89, 1986.
7. Gould KL, Kirkeeide R, Buchi M. Coronary flow reserve as a physiologic measure of stenosis severity. Part I. Relative and absolute coronary flow reserve during changing aortic pressure. Part II. Determination from arteriographic stenosis dimensions under standardized conditions. J Am Coll Cardiol 15:459–74, 1990.
8. Demer LL, Gould KL, Goldstein RA, Kirkeeide RL, Mullani N, Smalling R, Nishikawa A, Merhige M. Diagnosis of coronary artery disease by positron imaging: comparison to quantitative coronary arteriography in 193 patients. Circulation 79:825–35, 1989.
9. Kirkeeide RL, Fung P, Smalling RW, Gould KL. Automated evaluation of vessel diameter from arteriograms. Computers in Cardiology, Proc IEEE Computer Soc 215–18, 1982.
10. Brown BG, Bolson EL, Frimer M, Dodge HT. Quantitative coronary arteriography. Circulation 55:329–37, 1977.
11. Brown BG, Bolson EL, Dodge HT. Arteriographic assessment of coronary atherosclerosis. Review of current methods, their limitations, and clinical applications. Arteriosclerosis 2:2–15, 1982.
12. Brown BG, Lee AB, Bolson EL, Dodge HT. Reflex constriction of

significant coronary stenosis as a mechanism contributing to ischemic left ventricular dysfunction during isometric exercise. Circulation 70:18–24, 1984.

13. Brown BG, Bolson E, Peterson RB, Pierce CD, Dodge HT. The mechanism of nitroglycerine action: stenosis vasodilation as a major component of the drug response. Circulation 64:1089–100, 1981.

14. Bjork L, Spindola-Franco H, Van Houten FX, Cohn PF, Adams DF. Comparison of observer performance with 16 mm cinefluorography and 70 mm camera fluorography in coronary arteriography. Am J Cardiol 36:474–78, 1975.

15. DeRouen TA, Murray JA, Owen W. Variability in the analysis of coronary arteriograms. Circulation 55:324–28, 1977.

16. Detre KM, Wright E, Murphy ML, Takaro T. Observer agreement in evaluating coronary angiograms. Circulation 52:979–86, 1975.

17. Myers MG, Shulman HS, Saibil EA, Naqvi SZ. Variation in measurement of coronary lesions on 35 and 70 mm angiograms. Am J Roentgenol 130:913–15, 1978.

18. Zir LM, Miller SW, Dinsmore RE, Gilbert JP, Harthorne JW. Interobserver variability in coronary angiography. Circulation 53:627–32, 1976.

19. Vlodav Z, Frech R, Van Tassel RA, Edwards JE. Correlation of the antemortem coronary arteriogram and the postmortem specimen. Circulation 47:162–69, 1973.

20. Grondin CM, Dyrda I, Pasternac A, Campeau L, Bourassa MG, Lesperance J. Discrepancies between cineangiographic and postmortem finding in patients with coronary disease and recent myocardial revascularization. Circulation 49:703–08, 1974.

21. Hutchins GM, Bulkley BH, Ridolfi RL, Griffith LSC, Lohr FT, Piasio MA. Correlation of coronary arteriograms and left ventriculograms with postmortem studies. Circulation 56:32–37, 1977.

22. White CW, Wright CB, Doty DB, et al. Does visual interpretation of the coronary arteriogram predict the physiologic importance of a coronary stenosis? N Engl J Med 310:819–24, 1984.

23. Marcus ML, Skorton DJ, Johnson MR, Collins SM, Harrison DG, Kerber RE. Visual estimates of percent diameter coronary stenosis: "a battered gold standard." J Am Coll Cardiol 11:882–86, 1988.

24. Gould KL. Percent coronary stenosis: battered gold standard, pernicious relic or clinical practicality? J Am Coll Cardiol 11:886–88, 1988.

25. Marcus ML, Harrison DG, White CW, McPherson DD, Wilson RF, Kerber RE. Assessing the physiologic significance of coronary obstructions in patients: importance of diffuse undetected atherosclerosis. Prog CV Dis 31:39–56, 1988.

26. Harrison DG, White DW, Hiratzka LF, et al. The value of lesion cross-sectional area determined by quantitative coronary angiography in assessing the physiologic significance of proximal left anterior descending coronary arterial stenoses. Circulation 69:1111–19, 1984.

27. Sanders WJ, Alderman EL, Harrison DC. Coronary artery quantification using digital imaging processing techniques. Computers in Cardiology, Proc IEEE Computer Soc, 15–19, 1979.

28. Selzer RH, Blankenhorn DH. The identification of the variation of atherosclerosis plaques by invasive and noninvasive methods. In Atherosclerosis Clinical Evaluation and Therapy, ed. Lenzis and GC Descovich. Boston, MTP Press Lt, 453–465, 1982.

29. Spears JR, Sandor T, Baim DS, Paulin S. The minimum error in estimating coronary luminal cross-sectional area from cineangiographic diameter measurements. Cathet Cardiovas Diag 9:119–128, 1983.

30. Spears JR, Sandor T, Als AV, Malagold M, Markis JE, Grossman W, Serur JR, Paulin S. Computerized image analysis for quantitative measurement of vessel diameter from cineangiograms. Circulation 68:453–461, 1983.

31. Kirkeeide RL, Wustin B, Gottwik M. Computer-assisted evaluation of angiographic findings. In Thrombose und Atherogenese, Pathophysiologie und Therapie der arteriellen Verschlusskrankheit,

ed. K Breddin. Baden-Baden: Gerhard Witzstrock Verlag, 1981, pp. 414–17.

32. Kirkeeide RL, Smalling RW, Gould KL. Automated measurement of artery diameter from arteriograms. Circulation 66 (suppl. II):325, 1982.

33. Kirkeeide RL, Fung P, Smalling RW, Gould KL. Automated evaluation of vessel diameter from arteriograms. Computers in Cardiology, Proc IEEE Computer Soc, 215–18, 1982.

34. Buchi M, Hess OM, Kirkeeide RL, Suter T, Muser M, Osenberg HP, Niederer P, Anliker M, Gould KL, Krayenbuhl HP. Validation of a new automatic system for biplane quantitative coronary arteriography. Internatl J CV Imaging (in press).

35. Muser M, Leemann TH. A high resolution digital image scanner for use in photogrammetry. Proc ISPRS Intercomm Conf on fast processing of photogrammetric data, Zurich, 1987.

36. Parker DL, Wu J, Pope DL, Van Bree R, Caputo GR, Marshall HW. Three-dimensional reconstruction and flow measurement of coronary arteries using multi-view digital angiography. In New Developments in Quantitative Coronary Arteriography, ed. JHC Reiber, PW Serruys. Kluwer Academic Publishers, Dordrecht, Netherlands, 1988, pp. 225–47.

37. Pope PL, Parker DL, Clayton PD, Gustafson DE. Left ventricular border recognition using a dynamic search algorithm. Radiology 155:513–17, 1985.

38. Wollschlager H, Lee P, Zeiher AM, Solzbach U, Bonzel T, Just H. Improvement of quantitative coronary angiography by calculation of exact magnification factors. Comput Cardiol:483–86, 1985.

39. Wollschlager H, Lee P, Zeiher A, Solzbach U, Bonzel T, Just H. Mathematical tools for spatial computations with biplane isocentric X-ray equipment. Biomed Technik 31:101–06, 1986.

40. Reiber JHC, Serruys PW, Kooijman CJ, Wijns W, Slager CJ, Gerbrands JJ, Schuurbiers JCH, Den Boer A, Hugenholtz PG. Assessment of short-, medium-, and long-term variations in arterial dimensions from computer-assisted quantitation of coronary cineangiograms. Circulation 71:280–88, 1985.

41. Gaglione A, Hess OM, Corin WJ, Ritter M, Grimm J, Krayenbuehl HP. Is there coronary vasoconstriction after intracoronary beta-adrenergic blockade in patients with coronary disease? J Am Coll Cardiol 10:299–310, 1987.

42. Gage JE, Hess OM, Murakami T, Ritter M, Grimm J, Krayenbuehl HP. Vasoconstriction of stenotic coronary arteries during exercise in patients with classic angina pectoris: reversibility by nitroglycerine. Circulation 73:865–76, 1986.

43. Wong WH, Kirkeeide RL, Gould KL. Computer applications in angiography. In Cardiac Imaging and Image Processing, ed. S.M. Collins and D.J. Skorton. New York: McGraw Hill, 1986.

44. Nerem RM, Rumberger JA, Gross DR, Muir WW, Geiger GL. Hot film coronary artery velocity measurements in horses. Cardiovas Res 10:301–13, 1976.

45. Wells MK, Winter DC, Nelson AW, McCarthy TC. Blood velocity patterns in coronary arteries. J Biomech Eng 99:26–32, 1977.

46. Kirkeeide RL, Young DF. Wall vibrations induced by flow through simulated stenoses in models and arteries. J Biomech 10:431–41, 1977.

47. Mates RE, Gupta RL, Bell AC, Klocke FJ. Fluid dynamics of coronary artery stenosis. Circ Res 42:151–62, 1976.

48. Young DF, Cholvin NR, Kirkeeide RL, Roth AC. Hemodynamics of arterial stenoses at elevated flow rates. Circ Res 41:99–107, 1977.

49. Seeley BD, Young DF. Effect of geometry on pressure losses across models of arterial stenoses. J Biomech 9:439–48, 1976.

50. Lipscomb K, Hooten S. Effect of stenotic dimensions and blood flow on the hemodynamic significance of model coronary arterial stenoses. Am J Cardiol 42:781–92, 1978.

51. Siebes M, Gottwik M, Schlepper M. Qualitative and quantitative experimental studies on the evaluation of model coronary arteries from angiograms. Computers in Cardiology, Proc IEEE Computer Soc 211–14, 1982.

Stenosis Flow Reserve by Quantitative Arteriography

Previous chapters have described the pressure gradient–flow relation for defining functional or hemodynamic severity of coronary artery stenoses and related it to anatomic geometry from arteriograms. Coronary flow reserve has also been observed to be a functional measure of severity and related to pressure gradient or gradient flow equations. The final step toward integrating functional-hemodynamic and anatomic-geometric characteristics of coronary stenoses is to relate coronary flow reserve to stenosis geometry.

In practical application, the stenosis pressure-flow relation is too awkward for clinical or physiologic use. Stenosis resistance cannot be interpreted quantitatively without knowing absolute coronary flow. Therefore, despite sophisticated automated arteriographic analysis and experimental validation, quantitative coronary arteriography is not widely used, probably for two reasons. The first is lack of a readily accessible film workstation with appropriate analysis software, and the second is that there has been no simple way of expressing the results that is both well founded scientifically and intuitively relevant clinically.

Consequently, we developed the concept of stenosis flow reserve (1–7) as a single measure of severity derived from all integrated stenosis geometry. It is conceptually clinically and physiologically oriented, is related to coronary flow reserve, as directly measured in the experimental laboratory by flowmeter or radiolabeled microspheres, is related to stenosis geometry by fluid-dynamic equations, is independent of other physiologic variables (heart rate, blood pressure), and has been validated in two separate experimental studies (1,3). Finally, the clinical value of stenosis flow reserve has been demonstrated in man by its good relation to quantitative perfusion defects using dipyridamole PET perfusion imaging (2,5). Reversal of coronary artery stenoses has also been documented by stenosis flow reserve, despite multidimensional shape changes of coronary stenoses during cholesterol-lowering therapy, as reviewed in a subsequent chapter.

A major conceptual difficulty in assessing the effect of a coronary stenosis on blood flow is that myocardial perfusion is an integrated response of an anatomic-hemodynamic system in which the coronary stenosis is but one component. Current measures of stenosis severity, such as coronary flow reserve, are affected not only by anatomic severity but also by the characteristics of the distal vascular bed. Therefore, the approach we took was that of component testing, whereby the stenosis was quantified from geometry as an isolated part of the total system by imposing standardized physiologic conditions. Our approach is conceptually similar to testing an isolated component of an electronic circuit. The information so gained describes the stenosis as an isolated part and as an integrated unit of the whole system.

Accordingly, the approach to this problem requires consideration of two different basic concepts about how stenosis severity is quantified. The first considers the stenotic coronary vascular system as an entire integrated system, in which coronary flow reserve depends not only on stenosis configuration but also on aortic pressure, coronary vascular tone, collateral flow, the effectiveness of the coronary vasodilator stimulus, and normal coronary flow reserve in the absence of a stenosis. The second approach considers the anatomic stenosis as a component separate from the overall coronary vascular system, such that its effects can be quantified independently of all these other variables in the system. For coronary flow reserve, a total system response, to correlate with the component characteristic of stenosis configuration, other physiologic variables affecting coronary flow reserve must be accounted for or standardized. The relation between stenosis configuration and functional effects of other variables can be understood only by separately analyzing responses of the components of the system as well as the total system. The purpose of this chapter is to provide the theoretical basis and experimental validation for using coronary flow reserve as a single measure of stenosis severity accounting for all its geometric characteristics. It therefore establishes the relation between functional or physiologic and anatomic descriptors of stenosis severity that are both clinically applicable.

THEORETICAL BASIS FOR STENOSIS FLOW RESERVE

Consider the schematic at the top of Figure 9.1 (1), illustrating a stenosis in the coronary system with a pressure source, aortic pressure (P_a), a stenotic artery with flow (Q) through

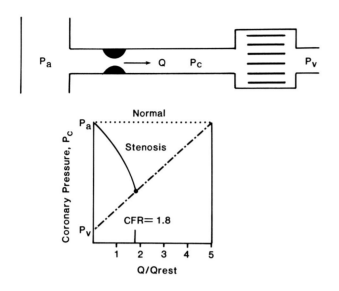

$$P_c = P_a - [A(Q/Q_{rest}) + B(Q/Q_{rest})^2]$$

Stenosis Pressure Drop

Fig. 9.1 Top: Schematic of a stenotic coronary artery and distal bed. P_a = aortic pressure, Q = coronary flow, P_c = distal coronary perfusion pressure, and P_v = effective coronary back pressure. Middle: In this graph, P_c is plotted on the vertical axis and coronary artery flow (Q) is plotted on the horizontal axis as a ratio to normal flow at rest (Q/Q_{rest}). The dash-and-dot line plots the relation between coronary perfusion pressure and coronary flow under conditions of maximal coronary vasodilation in the absence of a stenosis, as previously documented experimentally (10). The solid line is a plot of the relation between P_c (coronary pressure distal to the stenosis) and flow in the presence of a stenosis. This solid line is the graphic plot of the equation at the bottom of the figure derived in the text. A and B are terms related to stenosis geometry. CFR = coronary stenosis flow reserve. Reproduced with permission from Kirkeeide R, Gould KL, Parsel L, 1986. (1).

it, a pressure distal to the stenosis, coronary perfusion pressure (P_c), a distal bed with a resistance (R), and an effective coronary back pressure (P_v), which is the critical closing pressure of the vascular bed or coronary venous pressure, whichever is higher. The resistance (R) is a lumped value for the combined total resistances of all blood vessels distal to the stenosis (distal coronary artery, arterioles, capillaries, venules, and veins), as caused by both intravascular flow phenomenon (viscous shear) by extravascular compression and by vascular smooth muscle tone.

Flow through the coronary vascular bed can be described by the following conventional equation:

$$Q = \frac{P_c - P_v}{R} \tag{1}$$

Under conditions of maximal coronary dilation in the absence

of a stenosis, this equation becomes:

$$Q_{n,m} = \frac{P_a - P_v}{R_m} \tag{2}$$

where $Q_{n,m}$ is normal maximal coronary flow and R_m is minimal coronary vascular resistance during maximal coronary vasodilation.

Coronary flow reserve (CFR) is defined as the ratio of maximal to resting flow (Q_m/Q_r), where Q_r is coronary flow at rest, as follows: CFR = Q_m/Q_r. In the absence of a stenosis, normal coronary flow reserve is defined as follows: CFR_n = $Q_{n,m}/Q_{n,r}$, where CFR_n is the normal coronary flow reserve at a given aortic pressure in the absence of a stenosis.

Equation 2 can then be rewritten as:

$$Q_{n,r} = \frac{P_a - P_v}{R_m} \frac{1}{CFR_n} \tag{3}$$

where $Q_{n,r}$ is normal coronary flow at rest in the absence of a stenosis. With a stenosis present, flow expressed in relative terms as a ratio to flow at rest $Q/Q_{n,r}$ is obtained by dividing Equation 3 into Equation 1, yielding:

$$\frac{Q}{Q_{n,r}} = CFR_n \frac{P_c - P_v}{P_a - P_v} \frac{R_m}{R}$$

which can be arranged to give the following:

$$P_c = \frac{P_a - P_v}{CFR_n} \frac{R}{R_m} \frac{Q}{Q_{n,r}} + P_v \tag{4}$$

This equation has the form as follows: y = mx + b, where y is the distal coronary pressure (P_c), x is coronary flow expressed as a ratio to the normal flow at rest ($Q/Q_{n,r}$), m is the slope of the pressure-flow relation characteristic of the myocardial bed, and P_v is the pressure at which flow ceases. The behavior of Equation 4 is depicted in Figure 9.2A (1) as a family of lines representing different degrees of coronary vasodilation, that is, for various values of R/R_m. The heavy solid line indicates the condition of maximal vasodilation such that in Equation 4, R/R_m = 1. The slope of the pressure-flow relation for the myocardial vascular bed is then (P_a − P_v)/CFR_n. Myocardial vasoconstriction relative to maximal vasodilation would then be represented by lines of increasing slope where R/R_m > 1.

The effect of a coronary stenosis is to decrease coronary pressure (P_c) below its normal aortic pressure value by the amount of the stenosis pressure drop (ΔP), that is,

$$P_c = P_a - \Delta P \tag{5}$$

Extensive studies (4,12,22) have shown that the pressure drop across a coronary stenosis is described by an equation having the general form:

$$\Delta P = fQ + sQ^2 \tag{6}$$

where fQ represents pressure losses due to viscous wall shear along the stenotic lumen, which are linearly related to the flow rate through the stenosis (Q); sQ^2 reflects pressure losses associated with the abrupt expansion and deceleration of the flow as it exits the stenosis as related to the square of the blood flow. The coefficients f and s are determined by the detailed configuration of a coronary stenosis (that is, its length, axial and cross-sectional shapes, the diameter of the

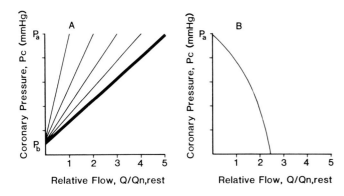

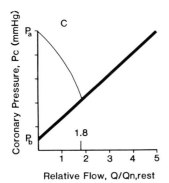

Fig. 9.2 Panel A: Relation between coronary flow and coronary perfusion pressure (P_c) under conditions of maximal coronary vasodilation is indicated by the heavy solid line (10). P_a = normal aortic pressure; P_b = back pressure in an occluded coronary artery. Panel B: Relation between distal coronary perfusion pressure (P_c) and coronary flow is expressed as a ratio to normal flow at rest for a coronary artery stenosis ($Q/Q_{n, rest}$). This line represents the distal coronary perfusion pressure resulting from the pressure gradient across the stenosis, which in turn is determined by stenosis configuration. Panel C is a superimposition of the graphs in A and B. The intersection of the two graphs gives the coronary flow reserve (1.8) for that particular stenosis of known dimensions and that coronary vascular bed under conditions of maximal coronary vasodilation. Reproduced with permission from Kirkeeide R, Gould KL, Parsel L, 1986. (1).

normal artery, the minimal cross-sectional area of the stenosis); f and s are also related to the viscosity and density of blood, but these are relatively constant in most circumstances. We have previously shown that the coefficients f and s in Equation 6 can be accurately predicted by quantitative coronary arteriography (1–9).

Combining Equations 5 and 6 produces an equation for the coronary pressure that can be maintained for a given pressure and coronary stenosis, that is:

$$P_c = P_a - fQ - sQ^2 \qquad (7)$$

To express flow relative to control at rest, these pressure-loss terms can be multiplied and divided by $Q_{n,r}$ to make the

terms in Equation 7 comparable with those in Equation 4:

$$P_c = P_a - fQ_{n,r}\left(\frac{Q}{Q_{n,r}}\right) - sQ_{n,r}^2\left(\frac{Q}{Q_{n,r}}\right)^2 \qquad (8)$$

The graphic form of this equation is plotted in Figure 9.2B. As (relative) coronary flow increases, the distal coronary pressure decreases nonlinearly, owing to the pressure losses across the stenosis until maximal coronary vasodilation is reached. As shown in Figure 9.2C, which graphs Equations 4 and 8 simultaneously, this flow-limiting condition occurs when the pressure-flow curve for the stenosis (Eq. 8, Fig. 9.2B) intersects the pressure-flow relation for the maximal vasodilated distal bed without a stenosis (Eq. 4 with $R/R_m = 1$ and heavy line in Fig. 9.2A). That intersection point gives the coronary flow reserve for that stenosis and that distal coronary vascular bed under conditions of maximal coronary vasodilation.

For the final composite graph in Figure 9.1, the coronary pressure distal to a stenosis (P_c) is plotted on the vertical axis. Coronary artery flow is plotted on the horizontal axis as a ratio to normal flow at rest ($Q/Q_{n,r}$). The dash-and-dot line graphs the relation between coronary perfusion pressure and coronary flow under conditions of maximal coronary vasodilation, as documented experimentally by Bache and Schwartz (10). It describes the pressure-flow relation of the coronary vascular bed at maximal vasodilation, that is, it gives the maximal flow possible after maximal coronary vasodilation for a given perfusion pressure (P_c). P_v is the coronary pressure at zero flow, or the back pressure of the completely occluded coronary artery; P_a is aortic pressure. For a normal, nonstenotic coronary artery, the perfusion pressure is aortic pressure, and the normal maximal increase in coronary flow is assumed to be five times flow at rest at a mean aortic pressure of 100 mm Hg, as shown by the dotted line.

The solid line in Figure 9.1 is a plot of the relation between distal coronary pressure (P_c) and flow (expressed as a ratio to control flow at rest) after coronary vasodilators in the presence of a stenosis. The solid line is the graphic plot of the equation at the bottom of the diagram derived in the Appendix. The terms A and B are related to stenosis geometry as follows: A = (f)($Q_{n,r}$) and B = (s)($Q_{n,r}^2$). The coefficients f and s, described earlier, are derived from arteriographic stenosis geometry. Thus, for a given stenosis the relation between P_c and flow ($Q/Q_{n,r}$) is determined by measuring mean aortic pressure (P_a), the coefficients f and s from arteriographic geometry and normal flow at rest ($Q_{n,r}$) (or flow velocity if the diameter of the artery is known from the arteriogram). With known values of P_a, f, s, and $Q_{n,r}$, the solid line can be graphed for any stenosis.

The point at which the solid curved line (characteristic of the stenosis) intersects the linear dash-and-dot line (the maximal flow possible for a given coronary perfusion pressure under conditions of maximal coronary vasodilation) gives the coronary flow reserve for that particular stenosis at that particular pressure. For the example shown, the solid line intersects the dash-and-dot line at a coronary flow reserve of 1.8. Therefore, the maximal flow achievable for that stenosis at that aortic pressure is 1.8 times flow at rest, or coronary flow reserve of 1.8. The distal coronary perfusion pressure (P_c) is about one-third the aortic pressure at that point.

PHYSIOLOGIC VARIABLES

The relative importance of physiologic variables on coronary flow reserve depends on what question one wishes to ask about stenosis severity, which in turn depends on a total systems analysis or a component analysis. For example, consider two patients with geometrically identical coronary stenoses under identical physiologic conditions, except that aortic pressure is lower in one than the other. That patient with lower aortic pressure will have a lower coronary flow reserve due to a lower perfusion pressure (Fig. 9.1) (1). At one extreme, if he were dead, his coronary flow reserve would be zero despite identical stenoses. Therefore, to compare stenoses in these two patients, one would need to calculate the expected coronary flow reserve under assumed standardized conditions of aortic pressure, such as 100 mm Hg, even if one of the patients did not actually have a measured mean aortic pressure of 100 mm Hg.

Similarly, one of those two patients might not be responsive to coronary vasodilators, such that his normal maximal coronary flow in the absence of stenosis would be only three times resting control levels at normal aortic pressure rather than five times. A stenosis that limited coronary flow to four times levels at rest would cause no limitation to flow in that case, because distal vascular bed resistance would be higher than the resistance caused by the stenosis. The distal bed resistance rather than the stenosis would therefore limit the increase in flow, and there would be no perfusion defect caused by the stenosis in that patient. However, if a normal coronary flow reserve in the absence of a stenosis were assumed to be five as a standardized condition, then the severity of a stenosis could be described in terms of limited coronary flow reserve for comparison with other stenoses, independent of that patient's state of vasomotor tone. A similar argument can be made for each of the other physiologic variables affecting coronary flow reserve, such as coronary flow at rest and the extent of collateralization.

STANDARDIZED CONDITIONS

To compare severity of stenosis in different individuals or of the same stenosis at different times, flow reserve should be determined under assumed standardized conditions even if those conditions are not actually present in a given patient. A set of useful or representative standardized conditions for humans would be a mean aortic pressure of 100 mm Hg, a normal maximal coronary flow of five times the levels at rest, a coronary flow velocity at rest of 15 cm/s, and the assumption of no collateral flow. By assuming these standardized conditions for our analysis, we can define stenosis severity in various patients regardless of a wide variety of physiologic conditions, ranging from hypertension to no blood pressure (death) or from no collateral flow to collateral equal to normal arterial flow. We refer to this approach as component analysis; that is, one component of the coronary vascular system, the stenosis, is analyzed as if separate from the rest of the system under standardized conditions.

On the other hand, stenosis severity can be evaluated by directly measuring the actual coronary flow reserve in a given patient. However, it may be different from the measurement at a different time or for a different patient with the same anatomy due to different physiologic variables. In principle, it would be necessary to measure directly the physiologic conditions affecting coronary flow reserve, such as aortic pressure, normal maximal coronary flow, flow velocity at rest, and the amount of collateral flow in order to compare stenosis severity at different times or in different patients. Therefore, the poor correlation between individual stenosis dimensions and measured coronary flow reserve reported for large numbers of subjects (13–16) might be expected not only because of the use of one geometric dimension (percent stenosis or absolute lumen area) but also because physiologic conditions other than stenosis configuration affecting coronary flow reserve may not have been standardized or accounted for. The use of standardized physiologic conditions in determining coronary flow reserve is a way of compartmentally analyzing the stenosis separately from the rest of the cardiovascular system in intact subjects.

COLLATERAL FLOW

The physiologic variable of collateral flow, in particular, requires further mention here although analyzed in detail in a subsequent chapter. For purposes of discussion, let us assume that the vascular bed supplied by a stenotic coronary artery had such large collaterals from another artery that myocardial perfusion reserve measured by radiolabeled microspheres was normal, whereas coronary flow reserve measured in the stenotic artery directly by flowmeter was reduced. Under the assumed standardized conditions excluding collateral flow, the arteriographically determined stenosis flow reserve would be reduced and would not equal the directly measured myocardial perfusion reserve in that subject. However, stenosis flow reserve would be correct if the intent were to analyze the stenosis itself separately from the rest of the cardiovascular system, as if in the absence of collateral circulation. Regardless of how the heart adapted with collaterals to bypass the stenosis, the flow reserve in the stenosis per se would be reduced, as would be intuitively necessary for collaterals to develop.

Only by such compartmental analysis of a stenosis—independent of the collateral supply—could its severity be established, as if in comparison with other stenoses in other subjects under standardized conditions of no collateral flow. Stenoses of equal geometric severity may have different functional effects, depending on the physiologic condition of collateral channels, independent of configuration. Comparison of the functional effects of stenoses then requires standardized physiologic conditions if the functional effects are to reflect differences in geometric severity only.

DYNAMIC STENOSES

Another physiologic variable potentially affecting the relation between measured and arteriographically determined flow reserve is dynamic change in stenosis severity (8,9,12,17,18). Coronary artery spasm, collapsing stenoses, or worsening percent narrowing due to vasodilation of normal segments may cause changes in stenosis configuration and therefore in coronary flow reserve. Such changes in configuration would have to be measured by arteriograms taken during the state of altered configuration to determine the corresponding altered coronary flow reserve. However, the basic relation between configuration and flow reserve should remain as previously shown.

VASCULAR BED SIZE

The final difficulty in interpreting quantitative arteriography in functional terms relates to the size of the distal vascular bed and the absolute arterial diameter. Even if all the dimensions of a stenosis are known, including absolute diameter, one does not know what the absolute diameter of the artery normally should be (or was, in the absence of atherosclerosis) to supply that distal vascular bed with adequate flow. In other words, even if quantitative arteriography could precisely predict what coronary flow and distal coronary pressure were at a given aortic pressure, one would not know whether that blood flow was appropriate for the vascular bed size. This problem also relates to where absolute dimensions are measured. A given absolute dimension may be normal for a distal segment of coronary artery but would indicate severe narrowing if present more proximally in that artery. However, directly measured coronary flow reserve accounts for diffuse disease of an artery. It would be decreased in a diffusely narrowed artery relative to the size of its distal vascular bed. By comparison, a normal artery of equal size relative to its smaller distal bed would have a normal coronary flow reserve. Quantitative coronary arteriography, to date, is applied to segmental stenoses and does not account for diffuse atherosclerosis without segmental narrowing. However, we are developing an extension of quantitative arteriography to the entire coronary vascular tree that does account for diffuse and segmental coronary atherosclerosis.

EXPERIMENTAL VALIDATION OF STENOSIS FLOW RESERVE

Absolute coronary flow reserve reflects physiologic stenosis severity but is altered by several physiologic factors unrelated to stenosis severity, such as aortic pressure, heart rate, vasomotor tone, hypertrophy, and so on. Since coronary flow reserve is defined as maximum flow divided (normalized) by resting baseline flow, any conditions which alter either maximum or resting flow may also change flow reserve, unrelated to stenosis severity. Accordingly, a change in flow reserve could reflect a change or difference in aortic pressure or workload rather than a change or difference in stenosis severity.

The problem of changing physiologic variables was obviated by assuming "standardized" theoretical values for aortic pressure and normal maximum flow in the absence of coronary artery stenosis, in the equations for determining coronary stenosis flow reserve from geometric dimensions alone. Accordingly, there can be no variability in stenosis flow reserve due to extraneous physiologic variables unrelated to stenosis severity.

However, stenosis flow reserve determined by quantitative analysis of stenosis dimensions might not equal directly measured coronary artery flow reserve in a given patient at a specific time, because the physiologic variables for the patient might not be the same as those arbitrarily assumed for the "standardized" geometric analysis. On the other hand, stenosis flow reserve based on anatomic geometry using standardized values of aortic pressure and normal flow reserve reflect anatomic severity with sufficient precision to permit interventional decisions or the comparing of stenosis severity between patients or in the same patient at different times, since it should theoretically be independent of varying or different physiologic conditions.

Therefore, assessing physiologic stenosis severity by *invasive methods* requires asking: 1) Is accurate, direct measurement of absolute coronary flow reserve, as by flowmeter, Doppler catheter, or microspheres, the optimal, accurate measure of physiologic stenosis severity? Should we therefore focus on better invasive methods to measure directly absolute coronary flow or absolute flow reserve? or 2) Is stenosis flow reserve derived from all stenosis dimensions on arteriograms with assumed "standardized" aortic pressure and normal maximum flow reserve the optimal, accurate, and consistent measure of physiologic stenosis severity needed for invasive clinical procedures?

MEASURED AND ASSUMED STANDARDIZED VARIABLES

For each stenosis in our validation study (3), P_a was chosen to be 110 mm Hg which was mean aortic pressure for all experiments; f and s were determined by quantitative analysis of coronary arteriograms, as described in previous chapters. Flow velocity at rest for medium-sized arteries 3 to 5 mm in diameter in a number of species have been observed to be 10 to 20 cm/s (mean 15) (11), confirmed in our own laboratory (8,9,12). Because coronary flow velocity at rest cannot be measured clinically by noninvasive means, we chose a flow velocity at rest of 15 cm/s; the validity of this assumption is justified by published data (8,9,11,12) and confirmed by the accuracy of the arteriographically predicted flow reserve compared with directly measured coronary flow reserve (1,3), as described subsequently. Normal coronary flow reserve in the open-chest dog studies subsequently described averaged six times baseline in the absence of stenoses. Accordingly, normal flow reserve was chosen as 6. With values of P_a, f, s, and $Q_{n,r}$, a diagram giving arteriographically predicted coronary flow reserve like that in Figure 9.2 was plotted for each stenosis on the computer analysis printout. For every stenosis, coronary flow reserve was also measured directly by flowmeter and compared with that predicted from arteriographic film dimensions.

EXPERIMENTAL VALIDATION OF STENOSIS FLOW RESERVE BY QUANTITATIVE CORONARY ARTERIOGRAPHY

Figure 9.3 illustrates from an experimental arteriogram the automatic, quantitative coronary arteriographic analysis (3). Dimensions and cross-sectional lumen area of the proximal, minimum, distal, and normal segments and percent diameter and area reduction were measured and plotted as a function

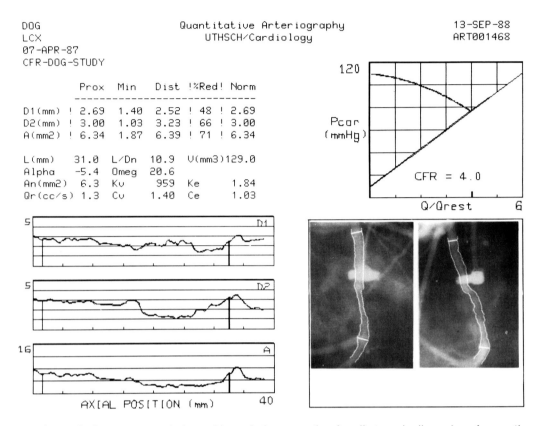

Fig. 9.3 Automated quantitative coronary arteriographic analysis accounting for all stenosis dimensions from orthogonal arteriographic views. Numbers in upper left show single plane diameters (D₁, D₂) by border recognition and cross-sectional lumen area (A). Dimensions of the proximal (Prox), minimum (Min), distal (Dist), and normal (Norm) segments are shown with percent reduction (% red). Lower left graphs show the diameters in two orthogonal views (D₁, D₂) and cross-sectional area (A) plotted as a function of length along the artery. Upper right graph shows calculated coronary stenosis flow reserve at standardized conditions of aortic pressure (110 mm Hg) and expected normal flow reserve of 6 in the absence of stenosis. In this graph, calculated distal coronary perfusion pressure, Pcor, is plotted on the vertical axis. Coronary artery flow (Q) is plotted on the horizontal axis as a ratio to normal flow at rest (Q/Qrest). The straight line graphs the standardized, assumed relation between coronary perfusion pressure and coronary flow under conditions of maximal coronary vasodilation in the absence of a stenosis, as previously described. The downward-curved line is a plot of the relation between Pcor and flow defined by stenosis geometry. Coronary stenosis flow reserve (CFR) is given by the intersection of the downward-curved line characterizing stenosis severity with the straight upward-slanted line characterizing the CFR-pressure relation in the absence of a stenosis. In this case, coronary stenosis flow reserve is 4.0, as compared with a normal of 6. Reproduced with permission from Gould KL, Kirkeeide R, Buchi M, 1990. (3).

of length along the artery in the lower left side of Figure 9.3. Stenosis flow reserve was calculated for standardized conditions of aortic pressure at 110 mm Hg and expected normal flow reserve of 6 in the absence of the stenosis. Distal coronary perfusion pressure, calculated from stenosis dimensions, is graphed in the upper right side of Figure 9.3 against coronary artery flow, expressed as a ratio to normal resting flow. The straight line in this graph shows the observed, experimental relation between coronary perfusion pressure and coronary flow under conditions of maximum coronary vasodilation in the absence of a stenosis, as previously described (1–10). The downward-curved line is a graph of the relation between coronary perfusion pressure and flow derived by stenosis geometry. Arteriographic stenosis coronary flow reserve is given by the intersection of the downward-curving line characterizing stenosis severity with the straight upward slanted line characterizing the flow reserve–coronary pressure relation in the absence of a stenosis. In this case,

arteriographic stenosis coronary flow reserve was 4, as compared to the standard chosen normal of 6 for these open chest experimental studies. For chronically instrumented intact experimental preparations, the normal flow reserve is 5. The higher normal coronary flow in open chest-preparations is probably due to anesthesia and inhibition of vasoconstriction and is normally present in awake intact preparations.

ARTERIOGRAPHIC STENOSIS FLOW RESERVE VERSUS DIRECTLY MEASURED CORONARY FLOW RESERVE BY FLOWMETER

To illustrate principles, Figure 9.4 shows directly measured coronary flow reserve by flowmeter in one experiment at 148 mm Hg and 93 mm Hg as the coronary artery was progressively narrowed (3). Flowmeter-measured coronary flow re-

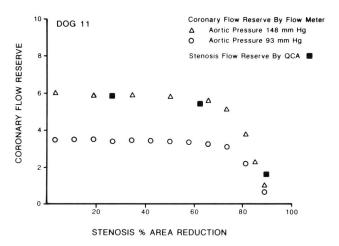

Fig. 9.4 Changes in coronary flow reserve at high and low aortic pressure, graphed as a function of percent area narrowing. The closed triangles are directly measured coronary flow reserve by flowmeter at aortic pressure of 148 mm Hg, and the open circles are measurements at 93 mm Hg, during progressively severe coronary stenosis. The solid squares indicate arteriographically determined stenosis flow reserve by quantitative coronary arteriography (QCA) based on geometric dimensions. Reproduced with permission from Gould KL, Kirkeeide R, Buchi M, 1990. (3).

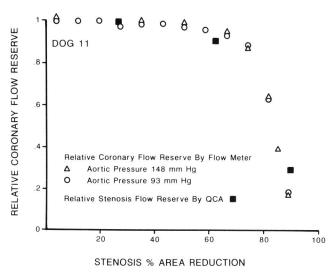

Fig. 9.5 Directly measured relative maximum flow or relative coronary flow reserve by flowmeter at the two different aortic pressures shown in the previous figure. The vertical axis shows relative flow reserve in the stenotic artery as a fraction of normal maximum flow, as measured by flowmeter, with progressive coronary stenosis. The solid squares indicate arteriographically determined relative stenosis flow reserve (QCA). Reproduced with permission from Gould KL, Kirkeeide R, Buchi M, 1990. (3).

serve for any given stenosis ranged from low to high values, depending on aortic pressure and pressure-rate product. For example, for a 68% area narrowing, directly measured coronary flow reserve by flowmeter at 148 mm Hg was 5.8, whereas at 93 mm Hg it was approximately 3.8. Thus, for a given fixed stenosis of 68% area narrowing, constant length, and normal proximal and distal diameter, directly measured coronary flow reserve by flowmeter ranged from 3.8 to 5.8, depending on afterload. Therefore, directly measured flow reserve did not specifically define functional stenosis severity.

Figure 9.4 also shows arteriographic stenosis flow reserve using a fixed standardized aortic pressure of 110 mm Hg and a fixed maximum normal flow reserve of 6, regardless of the actual aortic pressure or normal maximum flow reserve under different conditions of aortic pressure and heart rate. Arteriographic stenosis flow reserve corresponded closely to directly measured flow reserve by flowmeter at the higher pressure. This equivalency of arteriographic stenosis flow reserve and directly measured coronary flow reserve by flowmeter illustrates the accuracy of the arteriographic method in an example where the physiologic and "standardized" conditions were comparable.

ARTERIOGRAPHIC RELATIVE STENOSES FLOW RESERVE VERSUS DIRECTLY MEASURED RELATIVE CORONARY FLOW RESERVE

For this same experimental example, Figure 9.5 (3) illustrates that for the 68% area stenosis, relative maximum flow or relative flow reserve by flowmeter is 0.90 (90%) of normal max-

imum regardless of afterload conditions as described in Chapter 7. Relative stenosis flow reserve can also be derived from the arteriographic dimensions and expressed as a fraction of the normal "standardized" value by dividing arteriographic stenosis flow reserve by the standardized normal value of six times baseline for these experiments. Figure 9.4 (3) graphs arteriographically determined relative stenosis flow reserve against relative flow reserve by flowmeter for progressively severe stenosis; there is close correspondence of the values measured by both methods.

For 52 coronary artery stenoses, arteriographic stenosis flow reserve was compared to coronary flow reserve measured directly by flowmeter, while aortic pressure was increased by approximately 40% by phenylephrine and decreased by approximately 40% by nitroprusside (3). Figures 9.6 and 9.7 show for these experiments the mean changes in pressure, heart rate, pressure-rate product, normal resting, maximum, and flow reserve in nonstenotic coronary arteries before stenoses were applied (3).

Figure 9.8 shows arteriographic stenosis flow reserve for all stenoses over the range of pressures and heart rate observed for progressively severe stenoses with standard deviation bars of ± 1 (3). The 1-SD limits of absolute coronary flow reserve by flowmeter for the same 52 stenoses are reproduced from Figure 7.11 as the shaded area for comparison to stenosis flow reserve by quantitative arteriography. The standard deviations for arteriographic stenosis flow reserve are much smaller than for direct flowmeter measurements over the range of pressure and pressure rate products observed. Therefore, arteriographic measurements using standardized conditions are more specific measures of stenosis

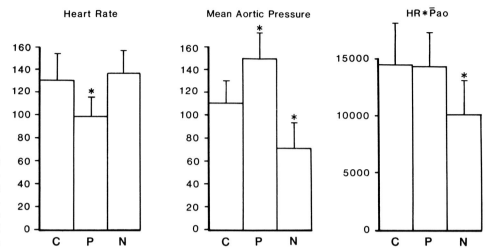

Fig. 9.6 Effects of nitroprusside (N) and phenylephrine (P) on aortic pressure, heart rate, and the product of aortic pressure and heart rate (HR) (Pao). C = control; *p < 0.01. Values are mean ± 2 SD. Reproduced with permission from Gould KL, Kirkeeide R, Buchi M, 1988. (3).

severity than directly measured flow reserve by flowmeter under changing physiologic conditions.

Figure 9.9 shows arteriographic- and flowmeter-measured relative flow reserve for the same 52 experimental stenoses over the range of pressures and heart rates observed (3). The gray area represents the limits of relative flow reserve by flowmeter for the same 52 stenoses from Figure 7.12. Arteriographic relative stenosis flow reserve correlates closely with relative flow reserve by flowmeter; both show comparable, relatively little scatter, thereby indicating (a) the accuracy of arteriographic analysis for assessing physiologic severity of stenoses over a wide range of physiologic conditions; and (b) the validity and importance of "normalizing" for different physiologic conditions either by relative flow reserve measured with flowmeters or by standardized conditions using quantitative arteriography.

COMPARISON OF VARIABILITY IN FLOW RESERVE MEASUREMENTS OVER A RANGE OF STENOSIS SEVERITY UNDER DIFFERENT PHYSIOLOGIC CONDITIONS

Figure 9.10 shows the relative size of one standard deviation expressed as percent of the mean coronary flow reserve at each category of stenosis severity, for absolute and relative coronary flow reserve measured by flowmeter and for stenosis flow reserve determined by quantitative arteriography over the range of changing aortic pressure/pressure-rate products (3). This figure demonstrates that the variability in apparent stenosis severity based on flowmeter-measured coronary flow reserve at different aortic pressures is eliminated by arteriographic stenosis flow reserve using "standardized"

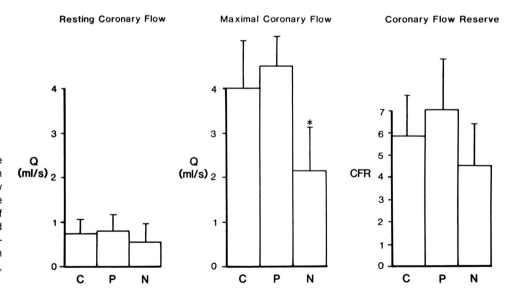

Fig. 9.7 Effects of nitroprusside (N) and phenylephrine (P) on rest and maximal coronary flow (Q) and coronary flow reserve (CFR), defined as the ratio of maximal to rest flow, measured by flowmeter. C = control. Reproduced with permission from Gould KL, Kirkeeide R, Buchi M, 1988. (3).

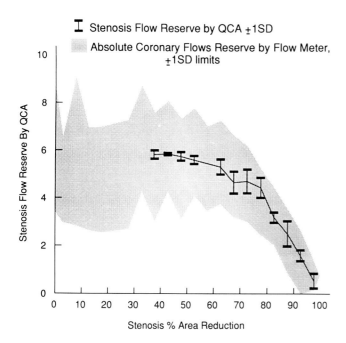

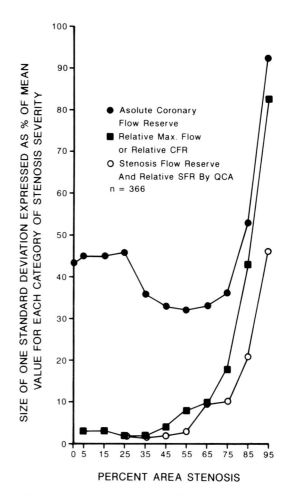

Fig. 9.8 Arteriographic stenosis flow reserve (max/resting) by quantitative coronary arteriography (QCA) derived from all geometric dimensions of percent narrowing, absolute cross-sectional lumen area, and integrated length effects for those categories of progressively severe coronary stenoses shown in previous figures. The error bars indicate ± 1 standard deviation for 52 arteriograms. The shaded area indicates limits of 1 standard deviation for flowmeter-measured absolute coronary flow reserve from Figure 7.11. Reproduced with permission from Gould KL, Kirkeeide R, Buchi M, 1990. (3).

Fig. 9.10 Size of one standard deviation expressed as percent of the mean value of each category of stenosis severity for directly measured coronary flow reserve (CFR) by flowmeter, for relative flow reserve by flowmeter, and for arteriographic stenosis flow reserve (SFR) and relative stenosis flow reserve by quantitative coronary arteriography (QCA). Reproduced with permission from Gould KL, Kirkeeide R, Buchi M, 1990. (3).

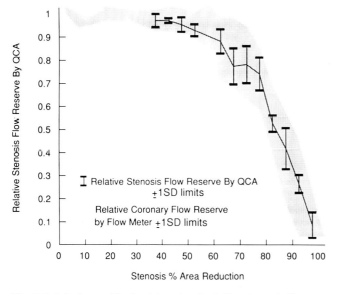

Fig. 9.9 Arteriographically determined relative stenosis flow reserve by quantitative coronary arteriography (QCA), graphed as a function of progressive stenosis severity. The shaded area indicates the limits of 1 standard deviation for flowmeter-measured relative flow reserve from Figure 7.12. Reproduced with permission from Gould KL, Kirkeeide R, Buchi M, 1990. (3).

physiologic conditions or by flowmeter-determined relative flow reserve. At very severe stenoses, the percent errors for all measurements of flow reserve are large, owing to measured values so small that the noise inherent in the measurements causes a large percent error. However, for such severe stenoses, flow reserve measurements are so low that these percent errors are of no clinical consequence, since they indicate very severe narrowing.

Due to the large variation in directly measured coronary flow reserve by flowmeter at different aortic pressure/pressure-rate products, it is not possible to correlate directly measured coronary flow reserve to arteriographic stenosis flow reserve, since the gold standard using flowmeters changes so greatly under changing physiologic conditions. However, in Figure 9.11 it is evident that arteriographic stenosis flow reserve (QCA) derived from all geometric dimensions of percent narrowing, absolute cross-sectional lumen area, and integrated length correlate with directly measured coronary flow

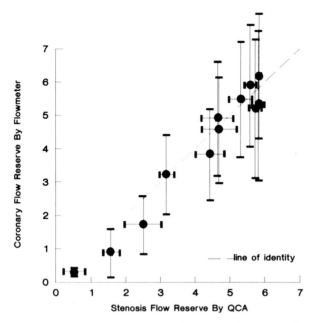

Fig. 9.11 Correlation between directly measured coronary flow reserve by flowmeter and arteriographic stenosis flow reserve by quantitative coronary arteriography (QCA). The error bars indicate mean ± 1 standard deviation. The variability for directly measured coronary flow reserve by flowmeter is considerably larger than that for arteriographic stenosis flow reserve for the same stenoses, from mild to severe coronary narrowing. Reproduced with permission from Gould KL, Kirkeeide R, Buchi M, 1990. (3).

reserve by flowmeter (3). The standard deviations for the arteriographic measurements are much smaller than for directly measured absolute flow reserve by flowmeter over the range of aortic pressures.

Figure 9.12 shows the comparable correlation between relative flow reserve by flowmeter and arteriographic relative stenosis flow reserve (3). The correlation is also good, and the size of one standard deviation is more comparable for the flowmeter and arteriographic measurements, because the effects of changing aortic pressure/pressure-rate product have been normalized out of both.

Our studies demonstrate that stenosis flow reserve determined by coronary arteriographic analysis of all stenosis dimensions provides an accurate invasive measure of physiologic stenosis severity, independent of widely varying aortic pressure and cardiac workload. Arteriographic stenosis flow reserve is more a consistent, specific functional (invasive) measure of stenosis severity than direct measurement of absolute coronary flow reserve by flowmeter, because the effect of physiologic variables other than stenosis severity are eliminated. These findings may also explain in part why direct measurements of coronary flow reserve by invasive techniques have been of limited diagnostic benefit for assessing stenosis severity in individual patients (13–16,19–21). The variability between directly measured flow reserve and anatomic severity could perhaps be explained in part by differences in physiologic conditions not accounted for in those studies.

CLINICAL RELEVANCE

Direct invasive measurements of absolute coronary artery flow and absolute flow reserve may be of limited value in some circumstances for assessing physiologic stenosis severity, since they are altered by physiologic variables unrelated to stenosis severity, particularly left ventricular hypertrophy (22–28), small-vessel disease (29–31), cardiomyopathy (30), sympathetic tone (32), or failure to respond to vasodilatory stimuli such as dipyridamole (33), and in the immediate post-angioplasty period (34). Therefore, stenosis flow reserve determined from arteriographic analysis of all stenosis dimensions may be the best available invasive approach for assessing integrated functional severity in such patients.

Rather than considering the arteriographic approach as competitive to direct flow measurements, we would like to emphasize that these two approaches provide independent, complementary data. *Invasive directly measured coronary flow reserve by flowmeter or Doppler catheter* reflects the flow capacity of the coronary vascular system for whatever conditions of pressure, vasomotor tone, hypertrophy, or narrowed coronary arteries are present. Although indicating the cumulative summed effect of these various factors, it is not specific for cause or mechanism of reduced flow reserve and is therefore not specific for stenosis severity. *Stenosis flow reserve derived from arteriographic analysis of stenosis dimensions, using standardized values of pressure and normal maximum flow, is a specific invasive descriptor of functional stenosis severity independent of all the physiologic conditions that may affect flow reserve. Relative coronary flow re-*

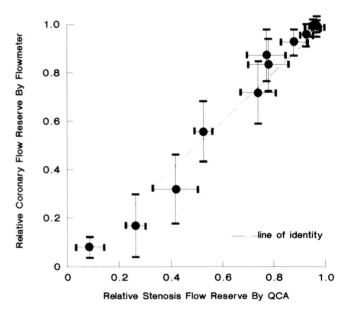

Fig. 9.12 Correlation between directly measured relative coronary flow reserve by flowmeter and arteriographically determined relative stenosis flow reserve by quantitative coronary arteriography (QCA). The error bars indicate mean ± 1 standard deviation. Reproduced with permission from Gould KL, Kirkeeide R, Buchi M, 1990. (3).

serve by noninvasive perfusion imaging is the most specific noninvasive measure of stenosis severity, with little variability due to changing pressure/workload; however, its interpretation as a measure of stenosis severity must be conditional upon some area of myocardium demonstrating normal absolute flow reserve. *Absolute coronary flow reserve by noninvasive perfusion imaging* is necessary for assessing responsiveness to dipyridamole, small-vessel disease, or left ventricular hypertrophy, as described earlier. Relative stenosis flow reserve by quantitative coronary arteriography has no advantage over stenosis flow reserve, since the effects of varying physiologic conditions are eliminated by our arteriographic method.

Arteriographic stenosis flow reserve may not equal the directly measured coronary flow reserve by flowmeter or Doppler catheter in a given subject at a given time, because the pressure and normal maximum flow for the patient at the time of direct-flow measurements might not be the same as those assumed for the "standardized" arteriographic analysis. However, from another point of view this apparent disadvantage of the arteriographic approach is also its major benefit, because arteriographic stenosis flow reserve allows comparison of complex lesions of different shapes in different patients without misleading effects on flow reserve due to differences in physiologic conditions among the patients, as distinct from stenosis geometry.

LIMITATIONS OF QUANTITATIVE CORONARY ARTERIOGRAPHY AS CURRENTLY APPLIED

There are some conceptual and practical problems with quantitative coronary arteriography for determining stenosis flow reserve. High-quality arteriograms are required, as is careful attention to film quality and overlapping structures. Densitometry is highly dependent on angulation and therefore requires orthogonal views and angulation correction, even though the densitometry is carried out in one plane. High-quality arteriographic workstations for multiview, high-resolution, three-dimensional analysis of stenoses will be required for routine clinical applications of these concepts.

As currently applied, all quantitative coronary arteriography addresses the severity of discrete segments of an artery. As currently used, it does not account for diffuse coronary artery disease, since it is applied to discrete segments of the artery. In addition, in diffuse disease of a coronary artery there may be no discreet stenosis or normal segment of that artery that serves as a normal size reference for determining percent narrowing (35). In this instance, directly measured absolute coronary flow reserve by flowmeter or Doppler catheter contributes important, independent information not obtainable by quantitative coronary arteriographic analysis *as currently applied* to discrete segments of the involved artery. However, directly measured coronary flow reserve by flowmeter or Doppler tip catheter as a reflection of diffuse coronary artery disease will still depend on extraneous physiologic variables unrelated to the anatomic severity of the disease, such as hypertrophy, hypertension, and small-vessel disease. Thus, there are limitations for each approach to stenosis quantitation, which must be applied

with knowledge of what it means and where it is applicable (36).

The optimal solution for the above limitations to quantitative coronary arteriography as currently applied is to extend the angiographic methodology for analyzing discrete segments of the coronary artery to its entire epicardial length by integrating the geometric dimensions from origin to distal segments. However, this approach requires knowing what the arterial size should be or has been for the size of its distal vascular bed in the absence of diffuse disease. Several approaches to accomplish this end currently look promising but require further investigation.

Finally, quantitative coronary arteriography has been validated in three previous separate, independent experimental studies (1,3,8), but all utilized cine x-ray film. With the diagnostic utility of quantitative coronary arteriography for routine clinical applications demonstrated (2,5), the next major technological advance needed is online applications to digital subtraction arteriography. Currently, major interventional decisions are made on the basis of visual severity estimates that are limited for objectively discriminating small changes in stenosis dimensions having major hemodynamic consequences. With growing use of PTCA in patients with symptoms controllable by medical therapy, some objective measure of severity is needed as a guide to intervention and for following its results.

REFERENCES

1. Kirkeeide R, Gould KL, Parsel L. Assessment of coronary stenoses by myocardial imaging during coronary vasodilation. VII. Validation of coronary flow reserve as a single integrated measure of stenosis severity accounting for all its geometric dimensions. J Am Coll Cardiol 7:103–13, 1986.
2. Gould KL, Goldstein RA, Mullani NA, Kirkeeide RL, Wong WH, Tewson TJ, Berridge MS, Bolomey LA, Hartz RK, Smalling RW, Fuentes F, Nishikawa A. Noninvasive assessment of coronary stenoses by myocardial perfusion imaging during pharmacologic coronary vasodilation. VIII. Clinical feasibility of positron cardiac imaging without a cyclotron using generator-produced rubidium-82. J Am Coll Cardiol 7:775–89, 1986.
3. Gould KL, Kirkeeide R, Buchi M. Coronary flow reserve as a physiologic measure of stenosis severity. Part I. Relative and absolute coronary flow reserve during changing aortic pressure. Part II. Determination from arteriographic stenosis dimensions under standardized conditions. J Am Coll Cardiol 15:459–74, 1990.
4. Demer L, Gould KL, Kirkeeide RL. Assessing stenosis severity: coronary flow reserve, collateral function, quantitative coronary arteriography, positron imaging, and digital subtraction angiography: a review and analysis. Prog CV Dis 30:307–22, 1988.
5. Demer LL, Gould KL, Goldstein RA, Kirkeeide RL, Mullani N, Smalling R, Nishikawa A, Merhige M. Diagnosis of coronary artery disease by positron imaging: comparison to quantitative coronary arteriography in 193 patients. Circulation 79:825–35, 1989.
6. Gould KL. Quantification of coronary artery stenosis in vivo. Circ Res 57:341–53, 1985.
7. Gould KL. Identifying and measuring severity of coronary artery stenosis: quantitative coronary arteriography and positron emission tomography. Circulation 78:237–45, 1988.
8. Gould KL, Kelley KO, Bolson EL. Experimental validation of quantitative coronary arteriography for determining pressure-flow characteristics of coronary stenosis. Circulation 66:930–37, 1982.
9. Gould KL, Kelley KO. Physiologic significance of coronary flow velocity and changing stenosis geometry during coronary vasodilation in dogs. Circ Res 50:695–704, 1982.

10. Bache RJ, Schwartz JS. Effect of perfusion pressure distal to a coronary stenosis on transmural myocardial blood flow. Circulation 65:928–35, 1982.
11. Caro CG, Pedley TJ, Seed WA. Mechanics of the circulation. In Cardiovascular Physiology, ed. AC Guyton. London: Med Tech Publ, 1978.
12. Gould KL. Pressure-flow characteristics of coronary stenoses in unsedated dogs at rest and during coronary vasodilation. Circ Res 43:242–53, 1978.
13. White CW, Wright CB, Doty DB, et al. Does visual interpretation of the coronary arteriogram predict the physiologic importance of a coronary stenosis? N Engl J Med 310:819–24, 1984.
14. Marcus ML, Skorton DJ, Johnson MR, Collins SM, Harrison DG, Kerber RE. Visual estimates of percent diameter coronary stenosis: "a battered gold standard." J Am Coll Cardiol 11:882–86, 1988.
15. Gould KL. Percent coronary stenosis: battered gold standard, pernicious relic or clinical practicality? J Am Coll Cardiol 11:886–88, 1988.
16. Zijlstra F, Fioretti P, Reiber JHC, Serruys PW. Which cineangiographically assessed anatomic variable correlates best with functional measurements of stenosis severity?: a comparison of quantitative analysis of the coronary cineangiogram with measured coronary flow reserve and exercise/redistribution thallium-201 scintigraphy. J Am Coll Cardiol 12:686–91, 1988.
17. Gould KL. Dynamic coronary stenosis. Am J Cardiol 45:286–92, 1980.
18. Gould KL. Collapsing coronary stenosis—a Starling resistor. Internatl J Cardiol 2:39–42, 1982.
19. Vogel RA, LeFree M, Bates E, O'Neill W, Foster R, Kirlin P, Smith D, Pitt B. Application of digital techniques to selective coronary arteriography: use of myocardial contrast appearance time to measure coronary flow reserve. Am Heart J 107:153–64, 1984.
20. Vogel RA. The radiographic assessment of coronary blood flow parameters. Circulation 72:460–65, 1985.
21. Nissen SE, Elion JL, Booth DC, Evans J, DeMaria AN. Value and limitations of computer analysis of digital subtraction angiography in the assessment of coronary flow reserve. Circulation 73:562–71, 1986.
22. Opherk D, Mall G, Zebe H, Schwarz F, Weihe E, Manthey J, Kubler W. Reduction of coronary reserve: a mechanism for angina pectoris in patients with arterial hypertension and normal coronary arteries. Circulation 69:1–7, 1984.
23. Goldstein RA, Haynie M, Gould KL. Limited myocardial perfusion reserve in patients with left ventricular hypertrophy. Clinical Res 36:279A, 1988 (abstract).
24. Marcus ML, Gascho JA, Mueller TM, Eastham CH, Wright CB, Doty DB, Hiratzka LF. The effects of ventricular hypertrophy on the coronary circulation. Basic Res Cardiol 76:575–81, 1981.
25. Marchetti GV, Merlo L, Noseda V, Visiolo O. Myocardial blood flow in experimental cardiac hypertrophy in dogs. Cardiovas Res 7:519–27, 1983.
26. O'Keefe DD, Hoffman JIE, Cheitlin R, O'Neill MJ, Allard JR, Shapkin E. Coronary blood flow in experimental canine left ventricular hypertrophy. Circ Res 43:43–51, 1978.
27. Mueller TM, Marcus ML, Kerber RE, Young JA, Barnes RW, Abboud FM. Effect of renal hypertension and left ventricular hypertrophy on the coronary circulation in dogs. Circulation 42:543–49, 1978.
28. Nitenberg A, Foult JM, Antony I, Blanchet F, Rahali M. Coronary flow and resistance reserve in patients with chronic aortic regurgitation, angina pectoris and normal coronary arteries. J Am Coll Cardiol 11:478–86, 1988.
29. Cannon RO, Watson RM, Rosing DR, Epstein SE. Angina caused by reduced vasodilator reserve of the small coronary arteries. J Am Coll Cardiol 1:1359–73, 1983.
30. Nitenberg A, Foult JM, Blancet F, Zouioueche S. Multifactorial determinants of reduced coronary flow reserve after dipyridamole in dilated cardiomyopathy. Am J Cardiol 55:748–54, 1985.
31. Strauer BE, Brune I, Schenk H, Knoll D, Perings E. Lupus cardiomyopathy: cardiac mechanics, hemodynamics, and coronary blood flow in uncomplicated systemic lupus erythematosus. Am Heart J 92:715–22, 1976.
32. Schwartz PJ, Stone HL. Tonic influence of the sympathetic nervous system on myocardial reactive hyperemia and on coronary blood flow distribution in dogs. Circ Res 41:51–58, 1977.
33. Rossen JD, Simonetti I, Winniford MD, Marcus ML. Coronary dilation with dipyridamole and dipyridamole combined with handgrip (Abstr). Clin Res 35:837A, 1987.
34. Wilson RF, Johnson MR, Marcus ML, Aylward PEG, Skorton DJ, Collins S, White CW. The effect of coronary angioplasty on coronary flow reserve. Circulation 77:873–85, 1988.
35. Marcus ML, Harrison DG, White CW, McPherson DD, Wilson RF, Kerber RE. Assessing the physiologic significance of coronary obstructions in patients: importance of diffuse undetected atherosclerosis. Prog CV Dis 31:39–56, 1988.
36. Klocke FJ. Measurements of coronary flow reserve: defining pathophysiology versus making decisions about patient care. Circulation 76:1183–89, 1987.

10

Reversal by Risk Factor Modification

SUMMARY OF MAJOR TRIALS FOR MODIFYING CORONARY HEART DISEASE

Most major trials to modify coronary risk factors, particularly cholesterol, have utilized as endpoints either cardiac events, death, myocardial infarction, and/or angina pectoris. These studies were based either on primary prevention in large numbers of subjects without known heart disease at entry, or on secondary prevention in patients with clinical coronary artery disease manifest by prior myocardial infarction, sudden death, or angina pectoris. Another type of secondary intervention trial utilizes coronary arteriography to follow regression or progression of coronary artery stenoses. As background, the outcomes of cholesterol lowering and/or risk factor change in 16 major trials are briefly reviewed here.

RELATION BETWEEN CHOLESTEROL AND ISCHEMIC HEART DISEASE

Extensive epidemiologic data links four major risk factors to ischemic heart disease: smoking, hypercholesterolemia, family history, and hypertension. Of the modifiable risk factors, cessation of smoking and control of hypertension are accepted as beneficial. Since some controversy exists about the relative risk of moderately elevated serum cholesterol, this risk factor will be reviewed briefly. The association between cholesterol level and mortality due to ischemic heart disease is summarized by Figure 10.1 from the National Cholesterol Education Program (1). Similar data from Framingham support a relation between serum cholesterol and cardiovascular mortality for 31–39 year old men, Figure 10.2 (2). However, for women and older men, 56–65 years old, there is little association between cholesterol and cardiovascular mortality in the 30-year follow-up of the Framingham study, Figure 10.3 (2).

PRIMARY PREVENTION TRIALS

Each of the following tables summarizes the sample size, entry criteria, duration of follow-up, type of intervention, and outcome. The Helsinki Heart Study (3) reported a 37% re-

duction in nonfatal myocardial infarction over 5 years associated with an 8.5% reduction in total cholesterol (TC) by treatment with gemfibrozil (Table 10.1). There was no difference in total mortality between the control and treated groups. The LRC-CPPT trial (4) reported 19% lower coronary events, 9.8% versus 8.1%, associated with an 8% reduction in total cholesterol by treatment with cholestyramine (Table 10.2). There was no difference in total mortality between treated and control groups. The World Health Organization Study (5), with follow-up at 5 and 13 years, reported no difference in cardiac events between controls and those treated with clofibrate (Table 10.3). However, there was a 25% reduction in nonfatal myocardial infarction in the treated group, but also an 11% excess total mortality in the treated group. The WHO European Collaborative Group (6) reported no benefit on cardiac events or total mortality between controls and

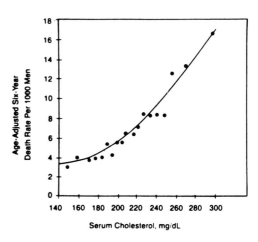

Fig. 10.1 Relation of serum cholesterol to coronary heart disease death in 361,662 men 35 to 57 years of age during an average follow-up of 6 years in MRFIT study. Each point represents the median value for 5% of the population. Key points are as follows: 1) risk increases steadily, particularly above levels of 200 mg/dl; and 2) the magnitude of the increased risk is large, four-fold in the top 10% as compared with the bottom 10%. Reprinted with permission from Arch Intern Med, 1988. (1).

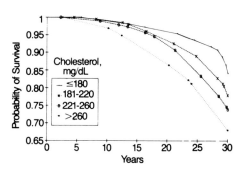

Fig. 10.2 Risk of dying in 30 years, according to total cholesterol, based on Framingham Heart Study men aged 31 to 39 at entry to study. Thirty-year mortality by serum cholesterol level at examination 2 for men aged 31 to 39 years. Reprinted with permission from Anderson KM, Castelli WP, Levy D, 1987. (2).

multiple risk factor modification without cholesterol-lowering drugs (Table 10.4). However, in the Belgian subset of this study, with 17% lowering of total cholesterol, cardiac deaths declined 24%. MRFIT (7) reported no benefit of multiple risk factor modification with decreases in total cholesterol of only 5%–7% (Table 10.5).

The Oslo Study (8) of diet and smoking cessation found a 47% reduction in cardiac events from 2.2% to 1.0% and a decrease in total mortality from 3.8% to 2.6% (Table 10.6). In the Finnish Mental Hospital Study (9), a 41% decrease in cholesterol was associated with a fall in cardiac mortality from 14.1% to 6.6% without differences in total mortality (Table 10.7).

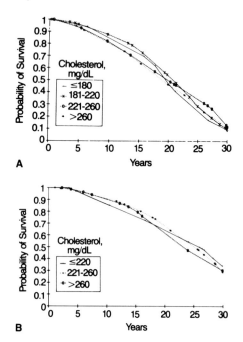

Fig. 10.3 (A) Thirty-year mortality by serum cholesterol level at examination 2 for men aged 56 through 65. **(B)** Thirty-year mortality by serum cholesterol level at examination 2 for women aged 56 through 65 years. There is no risk of higher mortality related to cholesterol levels in these groups. Reproduced with permission from Anderson KM, Castelli WP, Levy D, 1987. (2).

Table 10.1 Helsinki Heart Study (4,081 men, TC 289 mg/dL, 5 yrs)*

	Control	Gemfibrozil
TC reduction	8.5%	
Cardiac events	4.1%	2.7%
Total mortality	2.1%	2.2%

*No benefit on total mortality; 37% reduction in nonfatal MI

Source: Adapted with permission from Frick MH, Elo O, Haapa V, et al., 1987. Reference 3.

Table 10.2 LRC–CPPT (3,806 men, TC 265 mg/dL, 7 yrs)*

	Control	Cholestyramine
TC reduction	8%	
Cardiac events	9.8%	8.1%
Total mortality	3.7%	3.6%

*CHD 19% lower in treatment group; no beneficial effect on total mortality

Source: Summarized from JAMA, 1984. Reference 4.

Table 10.3 World Health Organization Study (15,745 men, TC 249 mg/dL, 5 & 13 yrs)*

	Control	Clofibrate
TC reduction	9%	
Cardiac events	3.5%	3.6%
Total mortality	7.9%	8.6%

25% reduction of nonfatal MI in Rx group; 11% excess mortality with clofibrate Rx

*Age-standardized death rate per 1,000 per annum

Source: Summarized from Oliver MF, Heady JA, Morris JN, et al., 1984. Reference 5.

Table 10.4 WHO European Collaborative Group (49,781 men, TC 217 mg/dL, 6yrs)*

	Control	Rx
TC reduction	1.2%	
Cardiac events	3.3%	4.2%
Total mortality	3.2%	4.0%

*In Belgian subset, 17% reduction of TC associated with 24% decline in CHD

Source: Summarized from European Heart J, 1983. Reference 6.

Table 10.5 MRFIT Study (12,866 men, high cholesterol, HTN, smoking, 7 yrs)*

	Control	Rx
TC reduction	5.5%	7.0%
Cardiac events	1.9%	1.8%
Total mortality	4.1%	4.0%

*No difference between Rx and controls

Source: Summarized from JAMA, 1982. Reference 7.

Table 10.6 Oslo Study (1,232 men, TC 329 mg/dL, 5 yrs)*

	Control	Rx
TC reduction	13%	
Cardiac events	2.2%	1.0%
Total mortality	3.8%	2.6%

*47% reduction of CHD in Rx group

Source: Summarized from Hjermann I, Holme I, Byre KV, et al., 1981. Reference 8.

Table 10.7 Finnish Mental Hospital Study (4,000 men, control crossover 12-yr trial, TC 268 mg %)*

	Control	Diet
Cardiac mortality	14.1%	6.6%
All mortality	36.0%	32.0%
Cholesterol change		−41.0%

*Polyunsaturated fat substitute decreased CV mortality

Source: Summarized from Turpeinen O, 1979. Reference 9.

SECONDARY INTERVENTION TRIALS

The Wadsworth Veterans Administration Hospital Study (10) reported a decrease in cardiac events from 14% to 9.6% associated with a 13% lowering of total cholesterol by diet (Table 10.8). There was no benefit on total mortality. The Coronary Drug Project (11) reported little benefit of clofibrate but a 12% reduction in cardiac events and 11% reduction on total mortality in the niacin-treated group (Table 10.9). The Stockholm Ischemic Heart Disease Secondary Prevention Study (12) reported a 26% reduction in total mortality in the group treated with clofibrate and niacin as compared to controls (Table 10.10). For patients over 60 years old, the comparative reduction in mortality was 28%.

Although suggestive, these intervention trials did not consistently demonstrate the benefit on cardiac events or mortality that might be expected from the correlation between cholesterol and mortality suggested in Figure 10.1.

Taylor et al. (13) have estimated the months added to life expectancy as a function of a lifelong reduction in serum cholesterol, based on published data, Figure 10.4 and Table 10.11. In high-risk groups, cessation of smoking and blood pressure control clearly extended life expectancy by 2 to 6 years. In comparison, reduction of serum cholesterol up to 6%–7% extended life expectancy by only a few months. Reduction of serum cholesterol by 20% extended life expectancy

Table 10.8 Wadsworth Veterans Administration Hospital Study (846 men, TC 233 mg/dL, 8 yrs)

	Control	Diet
TC reduction		13%
Cardiac events	14.0%	9.6%
Total mortality	42.0%	41.0%

Source: Adapted from Datyon S, Pearce ML, Hashimoto S, et al., 1969. Reference 10.

Table 10.9 Coronary Drug Project (8,341 men, S/P MI, TC 235 mg/dL, 5 and 15 yrs)*

	Control	Clofibrate	Niacin
TC reduction	26.0%	6.4%	10.0%
Cardiac events	26.0%	23.0%	23.0%
Total mortality			
at 5 years	21.0%	20.0%	22.0%
at 15 years	57.0%	56.0%	51.0%

*12% reduction of cardiac events in Rx; total mortality in nicotinic acid group 11% lower than controls at 15 years

Source: Summarized from JAMA, 1975. Reference 11.

Table 10.10 Stockholm IHD Secondary Prevention Study (555 men, S/P MI, TC 252 mg/dL, 5 yrs)*

	Control	Clofibrate and Nicotinic Acid
TC reduction		13%
Cardiac events	26.4%	16.8%
Total mortality	29.7%	21.9%

*26% reduction of total mortality in Rx group; 28% reduction of mortality in Rx group for patients above 60 years

Source: Summarized from Carlson LA, Rosenhawer G, 1988. Reference 12.

Table 10.11 Risk Factor Changes and Life Expectancy in Patients at Hgh Risk*

	Cholesterol Reduction			Smoking Reduction		Blood Pressure Reduction
Age (yrs)	3%	6.7%	20%	Program	Quit	
			months			
Women						
20	2	4	12	17	37	19
40	4	9	24	17	37	26
60	5	11	29	11	23	22
Men						
20	2	4	11	32	70	24
40	3	7	18	29	63	34
60	1	2	5	15	32	24

*High risk is defined as systolic blood pressure, cigarette smoking habit, and total serum cholesterol level each at the 90th percentile of the age- and sex-specific population distribution and high-density-lipoprotein cholesterol level at the 10th percentile of the age- and sex-specific population distribution

Source: Summarized from Taylor WC, Pars TM, Shepard DS, et al., 1987. Reference 13.

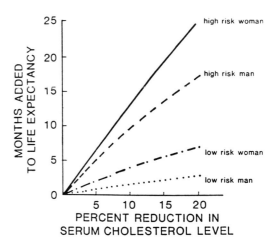

Fig. 10.4 Calculated change in life expectancy from a lifelong program to lower cholesterol level, as a function of the amount of cholesterol reduction for persons aged 40 with an initial cholesterol level at the 90th percentile of the age- and sex-stratified population distribution. Discount rate = 0%; lag period = 3 years. Reproduced with permission from Taylor WC, Pars TM, Shepard DS, et al., 1987. (13).

by 6 months to 2 years. His model suggests a linear relation between extended life expectancy and percent reduction in serum cholesterol. However, it also suggests that greater reductions in cholesterol than achieved in most previous large scale trials would be needed for beneficial effects.

Finally, Stamler and Shekelle (14,15) have reported evidence that reduction in dietary cholesterol independent of serum cholesterol may be beneficial. Based on long-term follow-up of the Chicago Western Elective Study, they estimated a 37% reduction in risk of death, equivalent to an extension of life expectancy by 3.4 years, associated with low dietary cholesterol intake in part, independent of serum cholesterol.

ARTERIOGRAPHIC TRIALS

Seven previous coronary arteriographic trials of cholesterol lowering by diet and/or drugs have been reported (16–23). The study by Kuo et al. (Table 10.12) (16), and the Leiden Intervention Trial (Table 10.13) (17), suggested that progression of stenoses was prevented by cholesterol lowering, but these studies had no untreated control group for comparison to those treated with diet and drugs. Studies by Nash et al. (Table 10.14) (18) and Nikkila et al. (Table 10.15) (19) showed prevention of progression of stenoses by cholesterol-lowering drugs in comparison to untreated controls which, however, were not randomized, and therefore were subject to potential selection bias. In a randomized controlled trial of clofibrate, Cohn et al. (Table 10.16) (20) showed equal progression of disease in 63% and 69% of treated and control groups, respectively, without regression observed. The NHLBI Type II Coronary Intervention Study (Table 10.17) (21) was a randomized, controlled trial of diet and cholestyramine with less arteriographic progression, 32%, in the treated group as compared to progression of 49% in the control group, a significant difference. However, these differences are not large with 32% of the treated group still showing progression of disease, and no regression occurred. The CLAS Trial (Table 10.18) (22) was the first randomized controlled arteriographic trial of diet, colestipol, and niacin, showing 16% regression in treated patients based on visual estimates by blinded arteriogram readers, as compared to 2% regression in control groups. Appearance of new lesions was prevented in the treatment group, and global severity scores were significantly less in the treated group as compared to controls. However, in the treated group, 39% still showed progression of disease, indicating a high failure rate from the viewpoint of individual patient therapy.

None of the above studies utilized automated quantitative coronary arteriography or measured all stenosis dimensions in order to define the geometric changes in toto oc-

Table 10.12 Kuo et al.—Angiographic Study (25 patients, familial type II HLP, TC 437 mg/dL, 7 yrs)

	Diet and Colestipol
TC reduction	38%
No change	67%
No regression observed	

HLP = hyperlipoproteinemia

Source: Summarized from Kuo PT, Hayase K, Kostis JB, et al., 1979. Reference 16.

Table 10.13 Leiden Intervention Study (Arteriography) (39 patients with documented CAD,* TC 267 mg/dL, 2yrs)**

	Diet (< 100 mg cholesterol/day)
TC reduction	10%
No change	46%
Progression	54%

*At least 1 vessel with 50% stenosis

**Correlation with TC/HDL ratio; no progression observed with TC/HDL ratio < 6.9

Source: Summarized from Arntzenius AC, Kromhout D, Barth JD, et al., 1985. Reference 17.

Table 10.14 Nash et al.—Angiographic Study (42 patients with CHD,* TC 280 mg/dL, 2 yrs)**

	Control	Colestipol
TC reduction	1.7%	20.0%
No change	53.0%	88.0%
Progression	47.0%	12.0%

*> 50% stenosis of nongraft vessels

**Less progression in treatment group (only 1 case of progression with TC <220 mg/dL)

Source: Summarized from Nash DT, Gensini G, Esente P, 1982. Reference 18.

Table 10.15 University of Helsinki Prospective Angiographic Study (48 patients, TC 298 mg/dL, 7 yrs)*

	Control	Diet and Drugs*
TC reduction		18%
Cardiac mortality	35%	13%
No change	8%	32%
Progression	38%	17%

*No progression correlated with HDL/TC ratio

**Clofibrate or nicotinic acid or both

Source: Summarized from Nikkila EA, Viikinkoski P, Valle M, et al., 1984. Reference 19.

Table 10.16 Cohn et al.—Angiographic Study (40 men, S/P CABG, TC 260 mg/dL, 1 yr)*

	Control	Clofibrate
TC reduction	+3.0%	3.3%
Progression	63%	69%

*No regression observed; no diffeence between groups

Source: Summarized from Cohn K, Sakai FJ, Langston MF, 1975. Reference 20.

Table 10.17 NHLBI Type II Coronary Intervention Study (Arteriography) (116 men with Type II HLP, TC 331 mg/dL, 5 yrs)*

	Control	Diet and Cholestyramine
TC reduction		17%
Progression	49%	32%

*Little regression noted; less progression in treatment group

Source: Summarized from Brensike JF, Levy RI, Kelsey SF, et al., 1984. Reference 21.

Table 10.18 CLAS (Arteriography) (188 men with CAD, S/P CABG, TC 246 mg/dL, 2 yrs)*

	Control	Colestipol and Niacin
TC reduction	4.0%	26.0%
Global scores	0.8	0.3
Regression	2.4%	16.2%

*Significant regression observed in treatment group; new lesions formation reduced in both coronary arteries and bypass grafts

Source: Adapted with permission from Blankenhorn DH, Nessim SA, Johnson RL, et al., 1987. Reference 22.

curring with regression or progression. Finally, the post-treatment cholesterol levels remained fairly high in these studies, averaging 252, 222, 270, 256, 244, and 240, and decreasing below 200 (to 180) only in the CLAS study, which also reported the best results up to that time. The percent decreases of cholesterol in these studies averaged -3%, -20%, -38%, -17%, -18%, -10%, and -26%. Despite these ranges of change, significant progression occurred in substantial numbers of treated patients, thereby making individual responses to therapy unpredictable from the viewpoint of individual patient management. Accordingly, a collaborative trial between the University of California at San Francisco and the University of Texas at Houston was undertaken to make intense, comprehensive change of alterable risk factors in order to determine whether regression or cessation of progression could be achieved more predictably as therapy for individual patients.

This reversal trial (23,24) was a randomized, controlled, blinded, arteriographic study to determine whether change of risk factors stops progression or causes regression of coronary artery stenosis and whether stenosis shape changes or remolds with progression or regression of coronary atherosclerosis in man, such that no single dimension reflects the essential changes observed. The rationale for the study was that lifestyle change had not been previously shown to reverse coronary narrowing, and no prior arteriographic study utilized automated quantitative analysis, or measured all stenosis dimensions to determine the overall shape change in stenosis geometry and related fluid-dynamic characteristics during progression or regression of coronary atherosclerosis in patients.

The initial report of the Lifestyle Heart Trial (23,24) describes in detail the experimental design, patient demographics, randomization, the lifestyle intervention, and overall results based on the traditional measure of coronary artery disease severity, percent diameter stenosis, measured by automated quantitative arteriographic analysis. However, as reviewed in earlier chapters, percent stenosis is an incomplete measure that does not account for changes in length, absolute diameters, or shape. In the literature, the meaning and significance of percent narrowing is open to question (33–38). There are also complex changes in different primary stenosis dimensions in different directions. The interactions between these primary dimensional changes may profoundly affect the fluid-dynamic characteristics of stenoses that simply are not accounted for or described by percent narrowing.

Automated quantitative, arteriographic analysis was used for several reasons. Most prior studies have not shown any changes or only mild changes by visual inspection. Visual interpretations of arteriograms are marked by such great inter-observer and intra-observer variation that comparisons of arteriograms from different subjects or the same subject at different times have very limited quantitative accuracy for assessing severity or changes in severity of stenoses (25–29); variations of 36% to 100% have been reported in visual estimates of percent diameter stenosis. Furthermore, percent diameter narrowing has been shown to reflect poorly the physiologic significance of coronary artery stenoses (30–38) and, as shown subsequently, percent diameter stenosis may improve despite progression of disease when all integrated dimensional changes are accounted for. Finally, the reproducibility of automated quantitative coronary arteriographic analysis of primary dimensions has been shown to be $\pm$ 3% to $\pm$ 5% in absolute dimensions (not percent stenosis), with a precision in phantoms of $\pm$ 0.1 mm (32–35,39–43), so that small changes in stenosis geometry could be reliably measured in control and treated groups.

STUDY PATIENTS

Patients were male or female, 35 to 70 years old, had documented coronary artery disease by arteriography, had no recent myocardial infarction or lipid-lowering drugs, and had left ventricular ejection fraction >25%.

Risk factor modification consisted of a vegetarian, low-cholesterol (less than 5 mg per day), low-fat (less than 10% of calories) diet with 15% protein and 75% complex carbohydrates augmented with vitamin B-12. Patients stopped smoking, practiced stress management, and participated in moderate aerobic exercise on a daily basis. Group reinforcement for adherence to the lifestyle change program was developed by an initial week-long retreat and twice-weekly group sessions during the treatment.

QUANTITATIVE CORONARY ARTERIOGRAPHY

The cardiac catheterization laboratories were calibrated for quantitative arteriographic analysis with meticulous records of the view angles, x-ray exposures, image intensifier, x-ray tube, and patient distances, and reference catheter dimensions were maintained. Follow-up arteriograms utilized these same characteristics in order to reproduce views and exposures as closely as possible on follow-up studies.

The arteriograms were analyzed in pairs (initial and follow-up studies) side by side by a technician blinded to clinical data or group assignment, using automated border recognition and stenosis analysis techniques in order to avoid the potential bias, imprecision, and uncertainties of visual interpretation.

Cine-arteriographic frames of orthogonal views were digitized for each stenosis involving a major artery. Absolute and relative stenosis dimensions were measured with a computer program providing automatic detection of vessel borders, previously illustrated in the chapter on quantitative coronary arteriography. The primary stenosis dimensions measured by the automated arteriographic program include proximal diameter and cross-sectional area, minimal diameter and area, distal diameter and area, exit angle, and calculated measures of severity including percent diameter stenosis, percent area narrowing, integrated length-area effects, and stenosis flow reserve, as described in previous chapters (33–35,38–44).

Figure 10.5A illustrates an example of the automated arteriographic analysis for a clinical study. The standardized conditions for a clinical analysis were a mean pressure of 100 mm Hg and a normal maximum flow reserve of 5 (24). The pressure-flow relation, shown as the downward-curved line, was derived from arteriographic dimensions. Stenosis flow reserve was determined as the intersection of the downward-curved line, characterizing stenosis severity based on all stenosis dimensions, with the upward straight line characterizing maximum flow for given pressure. Flow is expressed as a relative multiple of rest flow, Q/Qrest, under standardized hemodynamic conditions of aortic pressure and normal standardized maximum flow reserve of five times baseline. In this example, coronary stenosis flow reserve (CFR) was 2.0, indicating a maximum increase of two times baseline through a stenosis of the geometry shown at 100 mm Hg and a normal flow reserve of 5 in the absence of disease.

Figure 10.5B illustrates three sequential studies on the same patient, each separated by approximately 1½ years (24). For this patient the first study showed moderate severity of 39% diameter narrowing, with a stenosis flow reserve of 4.3 at baseline. The patient did not wish to change his diet or lifestyle and 1½ years later developed worsening angina pectoris. Repeat coronary arteriography at that time showed progression of disease, with 77% diameter narrowing and a stenosis flow reserve of 1.0. Motivated by worsening symptoms and fairly marked anatomic progression of disease, he began a stringent vegetarian diet and lifestyle change with relief of symptoms, and approximately 1½ years later showed regression, with improvement to 59% diameter narrowing and a stenosis flow reserve of 2.4.

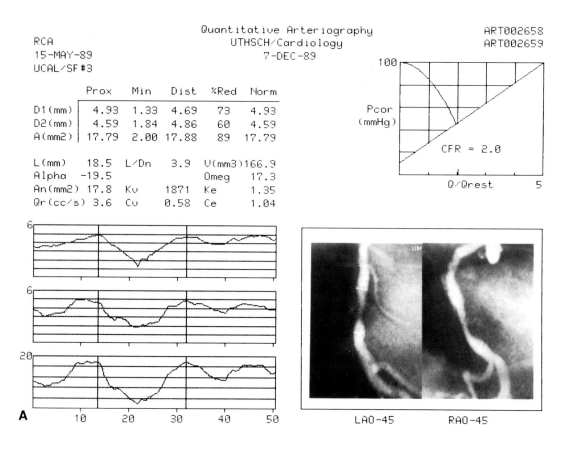

Fig. 10.5A Quantitative coronary arteriographic analysis of a coronary artery stenosis, taking into account relative percent narrowing, absolute cross-sectional luminal area, and integrated length effects to derive coronary stenosis flow reserve (CFR), for standard physiologic conditions of 100 mm Hg aortic pressure and a normal maximal flow reserve of 5 for clinical studies. In the upper left are orthogonal single plane diameters (D1, D2) and cross-sectional luminal area (A) by both biplane border recognition and densitometry for proximal (Prox), minimal (Min), distal (Dist), and normal (Norm) coronary segments with percent reduction (% Red). An is normal cross-sectional area; Qr is rest flow; Kv and Cv are coefficients related to viscous losses dependent on geometry of the stenosis; Ke and Ce are coefficients of momentum losses dependent on entrance and exit geometry of the stenosis; V is intraluminal volume in the stenotic segment; L is length; L/Dn is length/diameter ratio. In the lower left are diameters in two orthogonal views (D1, D2) and cross-sectional luminal area (A) plotted as a function of lesion length (L) along the artery (axial position). The upper right shows distal coronary perfusion pressure (Pcor) on the vertical axis and coronary flow (Q) as a ratio to normal flow at rest (Qrest) on the horizontal axis. Calculated coronary flow reserve (CFR) was 2, as compared with a normal value of 5. Reproduced with permission from Gould KL, Ornish D, Kirkeeide R, 1990. (24).

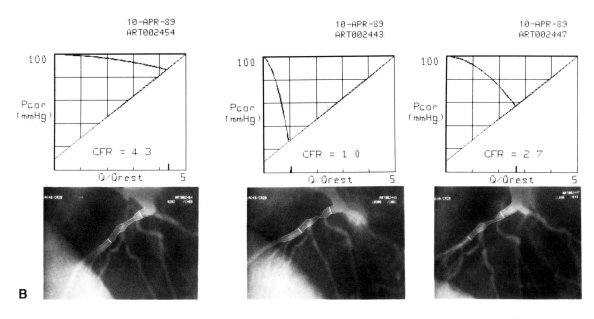

Fig. 10.5B Three sequential arteriographic studies in the same patient, each approximately 18 months apart. There was progression of stenosis severity between the first and the second study before the patient was willing to undertake diet and lifestyle change of risk factors. After undertaking risk factor modification, regression occurred between the second and the third study. Reproduced with permission from Gould KL, Ornish D, Kirkeeide R, 1990. (24).

Since different stenosis dimensions often change in opposite directions, definitions of progression, regression, and molding of stenoses are necessary. Figure 10.6 illustrates what we have termed simple regression, in which all primary dimensions of proximal, minimum, and distal diameters improve, the exit angle becomes smaller or more streamlined, percent diameter narrowing decreases, and stenosis flow reserve increases. In simple progression, all of these measurements become worse.

Figure 10.7 shows more complex changes, in which (top panel) proximal and distal diameters worsen (progression) and the narrowest segment remains unchanged (stabilization or no progression), while percent diameter lessens and stenosis flow reserve increases, reflecting overall improvement or diminution in severity (regression). The middle panel of Figure 10.7 shows worsening of distal and proximal diameters, enlargement or regression of the narrowest segment, and lessening of percent diameter stenosis, with more improvement in stenosis flow reserve. We term this pattern remolding, or a shape change of the stenosis that leaves a diffusely narrower artery than normal but with less segmental narrowing and improved flow capacity. Since the overall flow capacity

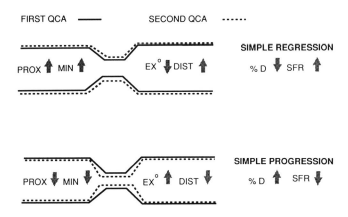

Fig. 10.6 Patterns of changing coronary artery stenoses. QCA = quantitative coronary arteriography, showing simple progression and simple regression. PROX = proximal, MIN = minimum, and DIST = distal diameters. EX° = exit angle, % D = percent diameter stenosis, and SFR = stenosis flow reserve accounting for all stenosis dimensions.

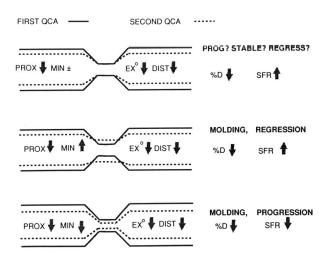

Fig. 10.7 Patterns of changing coronary artery stenoses; complex changes of stenosis dimensions in opposite directions with shape change or remolding during progression or regression.

or stenosis flow reserve is improved, this pattern of remolding is more clearly characteristic of regression. The lowest panel of Figure 10.7 shows narrowing of proximal and distal segments to a greater extent than the narrowest segment, thereby causing percent diameter stenosis to improve but stenosis flow reserve to become worse, indicating worsening flow capacity, a pattern that is one form of remolding with progression of disease. Several other combinations of opposite changes in different dimensions can be envisioned, the net effects of which are measured in toto only by stenosis flow reserve accounting for or integrating all these changes together.

The changes in stenosis geometry reported here are mean values. Stenoses are irregular, eccentric, of varying shapes and lengths, and behave individually, unrelated to the changes in other stenoses of the same patient. The schematics of stenoses shown here therefore indicate average changes and may not reflect actual appearance of all stenoses.

Since this data focuses on changes in stenosis geometry, stenoses that progressed to occlusion or occluded arteries that opened during the trial in both control and treatment groups (a total of six) were excluded from analysis in this report, because potentially large incremental changes due possibly to thrombosis or thrombolysis could bias mean values of shape change, owing to atheromatous alterations in other stenoses. Analysis of all data, including stenoses progressing to occlusion or occluded arteries opening during the trial, showed greater, more significant differences between control and treated groups but was not different from the more conservative results excluding those instances, as reported here. Of 48 patients enrolled, 7 did not have follow-up angiographic data as described in the initial report (23,24), and for this analysis one additional patient was excluded because his only endpoint was a total occlusion that became patent. Therefore the data base for this material is 40 patients (24). All exclusions were made before the data was analyzed.

Eighteen patients with 87 coronary artery stenoses were suitable for analysis in the control group, and 22 patients with 105 stenoses were suitable in the treated group, a total of 40 patients having 192 stenoses, or 4.8 stenoses per patient. The mean interval between the first and second arteriogram was 15 ± 3 months as either a control or treatment subject.

Table 10.19 lists the dimension changes in control and treated groups, with the statistical significance of each change (24). Figure 10.8 schematically illustrates these changes and the statistical significance of the difference in each dimensional change between the control and the treated subjects. In both groups, proximal and distal diameters both significantly decreased. The minimum diameter decreased further or progressed in controls but did not progress in the treated group. Percent diameter stenosis and stenosis flow reserve worsened in the controls and improved in the treated group, and the changes from the first to the second study between the control and treated groups were statistically significant.

Table 10.20, Table 10.21, and Figure 10.9 show the changes in stenosis dimensions for lesions that were initially mild (stenosis flow reserve ≥ 3) or initially severe (stenosis flow reserve <3) at the baseline entry study. For baseline mild

Table 10.19 Stenosis Dimension Changes

Controls	Prox	Min	EX°	Dist	% DS	SFR
n = 87	mm	mm	deg	mm	%	
QCA 1	3.07	1.75	12.7	2.84	42.7	3.90
QCA 2	2.98	1.64	14.0	2.71	44.4	3.79
Δ QCA 2 − 1	− 0.10	− 0.12	+ 1.14	− 0.14	+ 1.75	− 0.11
P for Δ	0.01	0.001	NS	0.000	NS	NS
Treated						
n = 105						
QCA 1	2.86	1.67	16.0	2.67	40.1	3.94
QCA 2	2.78	1.67	16.1	2.55	38.0	4.07
Δ QCA 2 − 1	− 0.08	+ 0.007	− 0.91	− 0.11	− 2.1	+ 0.13
P for Δ	0.02	NS	NS	0.001	0.03	0.03
P for ΔT vs ΔC	NS	0.008	NS	NS	0.006	0.01

% DS = prcent diameter stenosis; SFR = stenosis flow reserve; QCA = quantitative coronary arteriography; C = control; T = treated; NS = not significant and n = number of stenoses

Source: Adapted with permission from Gould KL, Ornish D, Kirkeeide R, et al., 1990. (24).

lesions (Table 10.20) of the control group, proximal, minimum, distal diameters, percent diameter stenosis, and stenosis flow reserve all worsened significantly, reflecting simple progression of all dimensions. Baseline mild lesions in the treatment group remained stable, with proximal and minimum diameters, percent diameter stenosis, and stenosis flow reserve all remaining stable, indicating that progression was prevented; distal diameter decreased slightly (but significantly) but had no effect on flow reserve (24).

Baseline severe lesions of the control group showed no significant change during the study (Table 10.21). Baseline severe lesions of the treated group showed statistically significant more narrowing of proximal and distal diameters, enlargement of the minimum diameter, a decrease of 9.3% di-

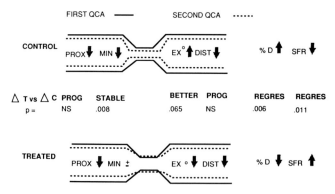

Fig. 10.8 Comparison of stenosis dimensional changes from initial (QCA 1) to follow-up arteriograms (QCA 2) between control and treated (Rx) groups. T = change in treated group, ± = no change, C = change in the control group.

Table 10.20 Baseline Severity and Stenosis Dimension Changes*

Mild, Control	Prox	Min	EX⁰	Dist	% DS	SFR
n = 74	mm	mm	mm	mm	%	
QCA 1	3.15	1.91	12.2	2.94	38.2	4.26
QCA 2	3.04	1.78	13.7	2.82	40.8	4.07
ΔQCA 2 − 1	−0.11	−0.14	+1.47	−0.12	+2.6	−0.19
P for Δ	0.015	0.001	NS	0.004	0.015	0.011
Mild, Treated						
n = 88						
QCA 1	2.83	1.81	10.7	2.65	35.0	4.33
QCA 2	2.76	1.78	10.2	2.55	34.3	4.32
ΔQCA 2 − 1	−0.06	−0.03	−0.54	−0.09	−0.7	−0.01
P for Δ	NS	NS	NS	0.006	NS	NS

* Mild = baseline stenosis flow reserve (SFR) ≥3; % DS = percent diameter stenosis; SFR = stenosis flow reserve; QCA = quantitative coronary arteriography; C = control; T = treated; NS = not significant; n = number of stenoses

Table 10.21 Baseline Severity and Stenosis Dimension Changes*

Severe, Control	Prox	Min	EX⁰	Dist	% DS	SFR
n = 13	mm	mm	deg	mm	%	
QCA 1	2.59	0.82	15.7	2.30	68.4	1.82
QCA 2	2.60	0.89	15.7	2.12	65.1	2.17
ΔQCA 2 − 1	+0.00	+0.06	−0.05	−0.17	−3.3	+0.35
P for Δ	NS	NS	NS	NS	NS	NS
Severe, Treated						
n = 17						
QCA 1	3.06	0.96	16.3	2.79	66.5	1.94
QCA 2	2.87	1.14	12.7	2.55	57.2	2.79
ΔQCA 2 − 1	−0.19	+0.17	−3.6	−0.24	−9.3	+0.85
P for Δ	0.014	0.002	NS	0.048	0.001	0.000

* Severe = baseline stenosis flow reserve (SFR) <3; % DS = percent diameter stenosis; SFR = stenosis flow reserve; QCA = quantitative coronary arteriography; C = control; T = treated; NS = not significant; n = number of stenoses

ameter stenosis units, and an improvement of stenosis flow reserve of 0.85, all statistically significant improvement. These changes reflect remolding of the stenosis, with regression toward a diffusely smaller artery than normal having less segmental narrowing and improved flow capacity. Figure 10.9 summarizes these changes where the dashed lines indicate statistically significant changes on the second arteriogram compared to the entry study.

Figure 10.10 summarizes the dimensional changes in relation to adherence to the risk modification program as described in detail previously for the combined control and treated groups. For this analysis, the combined groups were divided into subgroups of poor adherence (adherence score of ≤ 0.75), good adherence (adherence score of > 0.75 but ≤ 1.15) and those who excelled in risk factor management (adherence score of >1.15). Poor adherence was associated with statistically significant progression of disease, good adherence with stabilization or cessation of progression, and the highest adherence scores were associated with stabilization of minimum diameter (no progression), significant decrease in percent diameter narrowing, and improved stenosis flow reserve, indicating regression.

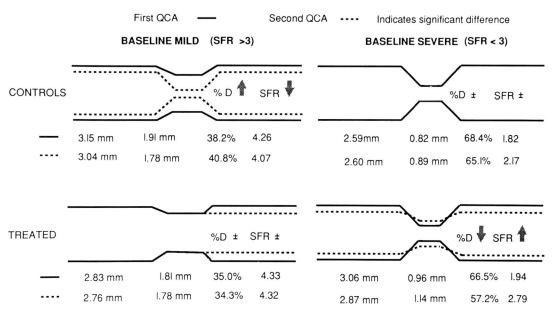

Fig. 10.9 Stenosis change related to baseline severity in treated and control groups. Reproduced with permission from Gould KL, Ornish D, Kirkeeide R, et al., 1990. (24).

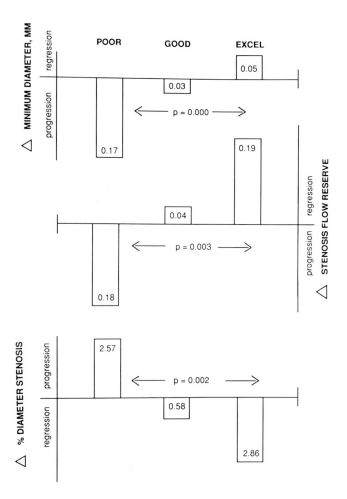

Fig. 10.10 Stenosis change related to adherence to the risk modification program. Numbers in the bars indicate mean absolute changes between the initial and follow-up arteriograms.

Figure 10.11 shows the dimensional changes in relation to adherence to the risk modification program for all patients in the combined control and treated groups together, categorized by baseline stenosis severity at the initial entry study (24).

Baseline mild lesions (stenosis flow reserve ≥3, Figure 10.11A) in the poor adherence group showed statistically significant progression of all dimensions, whereas groups with good and excellent adherence showed no progression. Baseline severe lesions (stenosis flow reserve < 3, Figure 10.11B) in the poor and good adherence groups remained stable without further progression. Baseline severe stenoses in the group that excelled in adherence to the program showed statistically significant regression of minimum diameter, percent diameter stenosis, and stenosis flow reserve. Therefore, good adherence to the lifestyle program prevented progression of milder stenoses, but more vigorous adherence was required for regression of severe coronary artery stenoses.

These data demonstrate that intense lifestyle modification of risk factors stops progression of mild to moderate coronary artery stenoses and causes regression of severe stenoses, leaving residual milder diffuse narrowing of the artery but less severe segmental stenoses and improved flow reserve. Complex shape changes or remolding of coronary stenoses occur with progression or regression, such that no single anatomic dimension alone describes the changes seen.

SIGNIFICANCE OF CHANGES IN STENOSIS SHAPE

Mean absolute changes of stenosis dimensions were small but statistically significant and were internally consistent from several points of view. Progression was associated with poor adherence to the program, stabilization of stenoses with good adherence, and regression with those having the highest adherence scores, changes consistent with a dose response of risk factor modification. This dose effect of risk factor modification is maintained for preventing progression of mild stenoses and causing regression of severe ones. Finally, severe stenoses showed greater regression than milder ones, reflecting a reasonable theoretical expectation that removal of a small amount of cholesterol from a severe stenosis having a small circumference would cause more improvement and a larger increase in minimum diameter than the same amount of cholesterol removed from a mild stenosis having a large circumference.

The results of this study are also consistent with pathologic changes reported in the literature, indicating the persistence of a fibrosed, diffusely but less severely, narrowed coronary artery having less segmental narrowing in the treatment group as compared to controls (45–48). Several reports have described different rates of progression/regression of different parts of atherosclerotic arteries, depending on their histologic maturity and the duration/degree of serum/dietary cholesterol changes (46,48,49). In primates with dietary coronary atherosclerosis, early atheroma may progress in severity in the six months after decrease in serum cholesterol levels, whereas more mature lesions regress, owing to differential content of cholesterol, cholesterol esters, and foam cells in different layers of early versus mature lesions (49). Therefore, different arterial segments evolve through phases of maturation from different starting points and at different rates, as is consistent with our observations of opposite changes in some dimensions, particularly depending on initial severity.

Finally, if the absolute dimension changes reported here are expressed as a percent change from baseline, the regression becomes even more apparent. For example, in Figure 10.9, for severe baseline stenoses (stenosis flow reserve < 3), the minimum diameter increased by 0.17 mm as compared to a mean minimum diameter of 0.96 mm at baseline, an approximately 18% improvement. In this same group, the percent diameter stenosis change was −9.3% stenosis diameter units from a mean baseline severity of 67% diameter narrowing, or a 14% improvement. More importantly in this group, stenosis flow reserve improved by 0.85 over a baseline stenosis flow reserve at entry of 1.9, *or a 45% improvement*

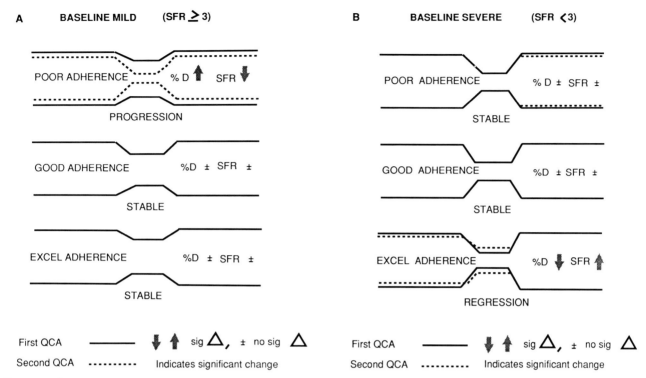

Fig. 10.11 Stenosis change related to both baseline severity and adherence to the program of risk modification (**A**) for mild baseline stenoses with stenosis flow reserve ≥ 3 and (**B**) for severe baseline stenoses with stenosis flow reserve <3. Reproduced with permission from Gould KL, Ornish D, Kirkeeide R, et al., 1990. (24).

in stenosis flow reserve, all statistically significant changes with P values of 0.002 or less. The physiologic importance of these changes are best indicated by stenosis flow reserve, accounting for the integrated, total effects of all dimensional changes. Since the flow effects are a function of arterial radius raised to the fourth power, small changes in diameter or radius have proportionately much larger effects on the flow capacity.

CLINICAL IMPLICATIONS

Our analysis of stenosis shape indicates that intense lifestyle modification of risk factors can stop progression of mild coronary artery stenoses and cause molding with regression of more severe narrowing. However, many individuals may not be willing or able to make such intense lifestyle changes. The question then is whether there is a trade-off between duration and intensity of lifestyle modification that would have intermediate effects on shape or change some dimensions more than others, since different dimensions clearly change in different directions and to differing degrees, all affecting severity. Since the time course of changes in different dimensions varies, would less intense lifestyle change over a long period of time be as effective or alter shape differently, compared to these intense modifications over a shorter period? Or, phrased differently, is there a threshold level of risk factor modification necessary for a given therapeutic benefit on severity, and is that threshold the same for all stenosis dimen-

sions? Our results are consistent with some form of approximate threshold dose effect of risk factor modification for a given endpoint; that is, poor adherence was associated with progression, good adherence with stopping progression, and those excelling in risk modification had regression. However, different stenosis dimensions responded differently. Whether further molding and regression develops in future years in the good adherence group, rather than just the halt of progression, will be determined by subsequent follow-up now under way.

IMPORTANCE OF SEPARATE RISK FACTORS ON STENOSIS SHAPE CHANGE

The problem of intensity and duration of risk factor modification is also related to the question of the relative contribution made by each separate risk factor modification toward the beneficial effects observed. Since the cause of coronary atherosclerosis and its progression appears to be multifactorial, the causes or mechanisms of stopping progression or of regression are also probably multifactorial. One might anticipate that it would be experimentally difficult to separate the relative contributions of lowering dietary cholesterol and fat independently of serum cholesterol, stress management, exercise, and/or stopping smoking. Consequently, it is unclear whether dietary change will be effective without stress management, or without the modest levels of exercise used.

Thus, there is no indication to what extent compromises or trade-offs can be made in the comprehensive intensive lifestyle alterations used here and still achieve a beneficial effect.

Regression and shape changes observed here did not correlate well with serum total cholesterol, HDL, or LDL levels. However, the average cholesterol in this study was not as high as in previous studies, and the range of cholesterol values were fairly narrow. Different risk factors may be of relatively greater or lesser importance, depending on the severity of other risk factors. In addition, a reasonable explanation may be hypothesized from experimental studies indicating that 75% of the variability in serum cholesterol response to dietary cholesterol is due to genetic differences in cholesterol absorption and metabolism. Thus, there appears to be genetically determined susceptibility to coronary atherosclerosis, independent of exposure to known risk factors (50). Consistent with these observations, dietary fat content has recently been shown to be a risk factor independent of serum cholesterol (14,15). Stress has also been demonstrated to play an important role in experimental atherosclerosis, in association with cortisol levels (51,52). Therefore, the fact that regression/progression correlated better with overall adherence scores than with serum cholesterol alone is reasonable, since more of the multifactorial causes associated with progression/regression are accounted for in the adherence scores as opposed to the single risk factor of serum cholesterol.

Finally, our results imply that measurements of a single anatomic stenosis dimension fails to describe the extensive remolding that characterizes regression in man. Future studies will have to take the multiple dimensions of coronary artery stenoses into account, since shape change or remolding of coronary artery lesions appears to be an important characteristic of regression/progression in man as well as experimental animals.

This study demonstrates the feasibility of risk factor modification in man for improving the geometry of coronary artery stenosis consistent with regression in severity, if all dimensions and overall shape of stenoses are accounted for. Further follow-up and confirmatory studies will be necessary to determine the general applicability of intense risk factor modification, with or without cholesterol-lowering drugs, for treatment of patients with coronary atherosclerosis and their effects on the severity and morphology of coronary artery stenoses. The concurrent study by Brown et al. (53) in abstract also showed reversal of coronary artery stenoses by a combination of diet and drugs based on percent stenosis.

FOLLOWING CHANGES IN STENOSIS SEVERITY BY PET

Positron emission tomography (PET) of cardiac perfusion and metabolism is described in subsequent chapters. However, it is important here to correlate the arteriographic changes in this reversal trial with changes in myocardial perfusion by PET. Standard rest-dipyridamole PET scans were obtained using the perfusion tracers ^{82}Rb or ^{13}N ammonia before and after the control or treatment period. PET images were displayed in quantitative polar map displays, as described in later chapters, and visually interpreted by readers blinded to clinical results or arteriographic findings. Figure 10.12 illustrates three sequential PET tomographs at rest (upper row) and after dipyridamole (lower row) taken one year apart while the patient was on a vegetarian diet, with marked cholesterol lowering. The severity of the inferior defect on the dipyridamole scan progressively decreases with improved maximum perfusion, associated with arteriographic regression. Preliminary data (54) is shown in Figure 10.13 and Table 10.22. As a group, patients who showed worsening PET scans during

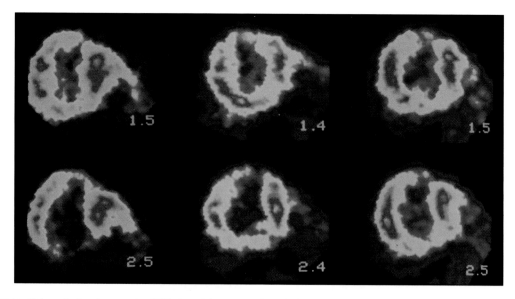

Fig. 10.12 Myocardial perfusion images by PET at rest (upper row) and after dipyridamole (lower row), taken at 12-month intervals on a low-fat vegetarian diet. The initial inferior perfusion defect after dipyridamole becomes progressively better on each subsequent study, correlating with regression by coronary arteriography.

CAD PROGRESSION/REGRESSION BY PET AND QCA

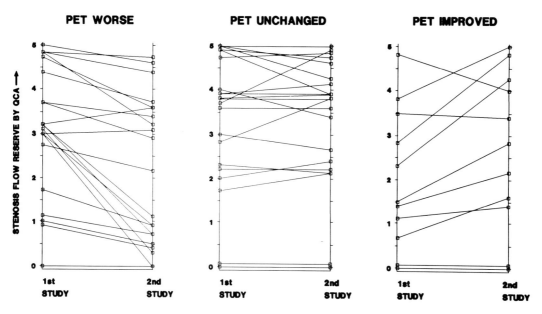

Fig. 10.13 Changes in stenosis flow reserve by quantitative coronary arteriography for patients whose second PET scan as compared to the entry study was worse, unchanged, or better after one year, on intense risk modification program or as a control.

the study on the average had progression of arteriographic disease, with a fall in arteriographic stenosis flow reserve, as shown in Table 10.22. Patients with progression by PET had, on the average, progression in arteriographic flow reserve; patients with no change on PET scans show, on the average, no arteriographic progression, and those with improved PET scans had arteriographic regression.

Figure 10.13 shows individual correlation of visually interpreted PET with quantitative arteriography. Although there was some disagreement between changes in PET and changes in arteriography, in general, PET perfusion imaging paralleled arteriographic changes. Quantitative analysis of the PET data and larger numbers are currently being analyzed to determine the accuracy of PET for following regression or progression of coronary artery stenosis. Preliminary data available indicate that arteriographic anatomic regression or progression of coronary artery stenosis of the degree described here is associated with corresponding functional changes in the stenosis, that is, improvement or worsening of dipyridamole perfusion defects by cardiac PET. Improved flow capacity by PET in these patients may not only be due to regression of the stenosis but also to changes in endothelial function, known

to occur with cholesterol lowering, that favor coronary vasodilation and less platelet activation.

CLINICAL REGIMEN FOR REVERSAL OF CORONARY ARTERY STENOSES

Since both lifestyle risk factor modification and cholesterol lowering by drugs cause regression of coronary artery stenoses, the author uses a combined approach at the University of Texas. This risk factor modification program is outlined in Table 10.23. The criteria for various intensity levels of risk factor modification and/or drugs for lowering cholesterol are outlined in Table 10.24. These criteria for patients without known coronary artery stenoses are similar to the recommendations of the National Cholesterol Education Program (1) or other consensus recommendations (55–57). However, for patients identified as having coronary artery stenosis by arteriography or by PET, we attempt more vigorous risk factor modification than recommended by the National Cholesterol Education Program, by lifestyle change as well as cholesterol lowering by drugs, as outlined in Table 10.25 and Table 10.26.

Table 10.22 CAD Progression/Regression by PET and QCA

PET	Mean QCA	P*
Worse	$3.1 \pm 1.4 \rightarrow 2.1 \pm 1.7$	< 0.01
Unchanged	$3.3 \pm 1.6 \rightarrow 3.4 \pm 1.6$	> 0.10
Improved	$2.0 \pm 1.6 \rightarrow 2.7 \pm 1.8$	< 0.05

* paired t-test

Table 10.23 Modifying Risk Factors

Stop smoking
Control hypertension
Control cholesterol
    Optimize weight
    Exercise in moderation

Table 10.24 University of Texas Modified Rx of Hypercholesterolemia with No CAD

TC (mg/dL)	LDL	Risk Factors	Rx
< 200	< 130	no	none
200–260	130–160	no	diet
		yes	diet
> 260	> 160	no	diet
		yes	diet, drugs
HDL < 35		no	diet, exercise
		yes	diet, exercise, drugs

For the many patients with coronary artery disease who cannot or will not maintain a diet of less than 10% fat, we accept a diet of less than 15%–20% fat that is "near"-vegetarian, augmented by occasional fish, chicken, or turkey, and drug therapy with a goal of total cholesterols below 150 mg/dL. Further studies are now under way to test the relative effectiveness of a strict vegetarian lifestyle program as compared to somewhat less strict lifestyle modification augmented by cholesterol-lowering drugs.

Table 10.25 University of Texas Modified Rx of Hypercholesterolemia with CAD

	Strict diet, 10% fat Resin, Lovastatin, ASA		
Goal:	TC	LDL	HDL
	< 160	< 120	> 45

Table 10.26 Strict Diet

Total fat	10% of total calories*
Carbohydrates	75%
Protein	15%
Cholesterol	5 mg/day

* Total calories for lean body weight

REFERENCES

1. Report of the National Cholesterol Education Program Expert Panel on Detection, Evaluation, and Treatment of High Blood Cholesterol in Adults. Arch Intern Med 148:36–69, 1988; NIH pub no. 88-2926, 1987.
2. Anderson KM, Castelli WP, Levy D. Cholesterol and mortality: 30 Years of Follow-up from the Framingham Study. JAMA 257:2176–80, 1987.
3. Frick MH, Elo O, Haapa V, et al. Helsinki heart study: primary prevention trial with gemfibrozil in middle-aged men with dyslipidemia. N Engl J Med 317:1237–45, 1987.
4. The Lipid Research Clinics Coronary Primary Prevention Trial. I. Reduction in incidence of coronary heart disease. II. The relationship of reduction in incidence of coronary heart disease to cholesterol lowering. JAMA 251:351–74, 1984.
5. Oliver MF, Heady JA, Morris JN, Cooper J. WHO cooperative trial on primary prevention of ischemic heart disease with clofibrate to lower serum cholesterol: final mortality follow-up: report of the committee of principal investigators. Lancet 2:600–04, 1984.
6. World Health Organization European Collaborative Group. Multifactorial trial in the prevention of coronary heart disease: 3. Incidence and mortality results. European Heart J 4:141–47, 1983.
7. Multiple Risk Factor Intervention Trial Research Group. Multiple Risk Factor Intervention Trial: risk factor changes and mortality results. JAMA 248:1465–77, 1982.
8. Hjermann I, Holme I, Byre KV, Leren P. Effect of diet and smoking intervention on incidence of coronary heart disease. Report from the Oslo Study Group of a randomized trial in healthy males. Lancet 2: p 1303–10, 1981.
9. Turpeinen O. Effect of cholesterol lowering diet on mortality from coronary heart disease and other causes (The Finnish Mental Hospital Study). Circulation 59:1–7, 1979.
10. Datyon S, Pearce ML, Hashimoto S, Dixon WJ, Tomiyasu U. A controlled clinical trial of a diet high in unsaturated fat in preventing complications of atherosclerosis. Circulation 39 (suppl II):1–62, 1969.
11. The Coronary Drug Project. Clofibrate and niacin in coronary heart disease. JAMA 231:360–81, 1975.
12. Carlson LA, Rosenhawer G. Reduction of mortality in the Stockholm Ischemic Heart Disease Secondary Prevention Study by combined treatment with clofibrate and nicotinic acid. Acta Med Scand 223:405–18, 1988.
13. Taylor WC, Pars TM, Shepard DS, Romaroff AL. Cholesterol reduction and life expectancy: a model incorporating multiple risk factors. Ann Intern Med 106:605–14, 1987.
14. Stamler J, Shekelle R. Dietary cholesterol and human coronary heart disease. Arch Pathol Lab Med 112:1032–40, 1988.
15. Shekelle RB, Stamler J. Dietary cholesterol and ischemic heart disease. Lancet 1:1177–79, 1989.
16. Kuo PT, Hayase K, Kostis JB, Moreyra AE. Use of combined diet and colestipol in long-term (7–7½ years) treatment of patients with type II hyperlipoproteinemia. Circulation 59:199–214, 1979.
17. Arntzenius AC, Kromhout D, Barth JD, Reiber JHC, Bruschke AVG, Buis B, VanGent CM, Kempen-Voogd N, Strkwerda S, Van der Velde EA. Diet, lipoproteins, and the progression of coronary atherosclerosis. The Leiden Intervention Trial. N Engl J Med 312:805–11, 1985.
18. Nash DT, Gensini G, Esente P. Effect of lipid-lowering therapy on the progression of coronary atherosclerosis assessed by scheduled repetitive coronary arteriography. Internat J Cardiol 2:43–55, 1982.
19. Nikkila EA, Viikinkoski P, Valle M, Frick MH. Prevention of progression of coronary atherosclerosis by treatment of hyperlipidemia: a seven year prospective angiographic study. Brit Med J 289:220–23, 1984.
20. Cohn K, Sakai FJ, Langston MF. Effect of clofibrate on progression of coronary disease: a prospective angiographic study in man. Am Heart J 89:591–98, 1975.
21. Brensike JF, Levy RI, Kelsey SF, Passamani ER, Richardson JM, Loh IK, Stone NJ, Aldrich RF, Battaglini JW, Moriarty DJ, Fisher MR, Friedman L, Friedewald W, Detre KM, Epstein SE. Effects of therapy with cholestyramine on progression of coronary arteriosclerosis: results of the NHLBI Type II coronary intervention study. Circulation 69:313–24, 1984.
22. Blankenhorn DH, Nessim SA, Johnson RL, Sanmarco ME, Azen SP, Cashin-Hemphill L. Beneficial effects of combined colestipolniacin therapy on coronary arteriosclerosis and coronary venous bypass grafts. JAMA 257:3233–40, 1987.

23. Ornish D, Brown SB, Scherwitz LW, Brown SB, Billings JH, Armstrong WT, Ports TA, McLanahan SM, Kirkeeide RL, Brand RJ, Gould KL. Can lifestyle changes reverse coronary heart disease? Lancet 336:129–133, 1990.

24. Gould KL, Ornish D, Kirkeeide RL, Brown S, Stuart Y, Jones D, Billings J, Armstrong W, Ports T, Scherwitz L. Improved stenosis geometry by quantitative coronary arteriography after risk factor change in man. (in press).

25. Bjork L, Spindola-Franco H, Van Houten FX, Cohn PF, Adams DF. Comparison of observer performance with 16 mm cinefluorography and 70 mm camera fluorography in coronary arteriography. Am J Cardiol 36:474–78, 1975.

26. DeRouen TA, Murray JA, Owen W. Variability in the analysis of coronary arteriograms. Circulation 55:324–28, 1977.

27. Detre KM, Wright E, Murphy ML, Takaro T. Observer agreement in evaluating coronary angiograms. Circulation 52:979–86, 1975.

28. Zir LM, Miller SW, Dinsmore RE, Gilbert JP, Harthorne JW. Interobserver variability in coronary angiography. Circulation 53:627–32, 1976.

29. Myers MG, Shulman HS, Saibil EA, Naqvi SZ. Variation in measurement of coronary lesions on 35 and 70 mm angiograms. Am J Roentgenol 130:913–15, 1978.

30. Gould KL, Lipscomb K, Hamilton GW. Physiologic basis for assessing critical coronary stenosis. Am J Cardiol 33:87–94, 1974.

31. Gould KL. Dynamic coronary stenosis. Am J Cardiol 45:286–92, 1980.

32. Gould KL, Kelley KO, Bolson EL. Experimental validation of quantitative coronary arteriography for determining pressure-flow characteristics of coronary stenosis. Circulation 66:930–937, 1982.

33. Gould KL. Quantitation of coronary artery stenosis in vivo. Circ Res 57:341–53, 1985.

34. Gould KL. Identifying and measuring severity of coronary artery stenosis. Quantitative coronary arteriography and positron emission tomography. Circulation 78:237–45, 1988.

35. Kirkeeide RL, Gould KL, Parsel L. Assessment of coronary stenoses by myocardial perfusion imaging during pharmacologic coronary vasodilation. VII. Validation of coronary flow reserve as a single integrated functional measure of stenosis severity reflecting all its geometric dimensions. J Am Coll Cardiol 7:775–85, 1986.

36. White CW, Wright CB, Doty DB, Hiratza LF, Eastham CL, Harrison DG, Marcus ML. Does the visual interpretation of the coronary arteriogram predict the physiological significance of a coronary stenosis? N Engl J Med 310:819–24, 1984.

37. Marcus ML, Skorton DJ, Johnson MR, Collins SM, Harrison DG, Kerber RE. Visual estimates of percent diameter coronary stenosis: "a battered gold standard." J Am Coll Cardiol 11:882–85, 1988.

38. Gould KL. Percent coronary stenosis: battered gold standard, pernicious relic or clinical practicality? J Am Coll Cardiol 11:886–88, 1988.

39. Gould KL, Goldstein RA, Mullani NA, Kirkeeide R, Wong G, Smalling R, Fuentes F, Nishikawa A, Matthews W. Noninvasive assessment of coronary stenoses by myocardial perfusion imaging during pharmacologic coronary vasodilation. VIII. Clinical feasibility of positron cardiac imaging without a cyclotron using generator-produced rubidium-82. J Am Coll Cardiol 7:775–89, 1986.

40. Demer LL, Gould KL, Goldstein RA, Kirkeeide RL, Mullani NA, Smalling RW, Nishikawa A, Merhige ME. Assessment of coronary artery disease severity by positron emission tomography: comparison to quantitative arteriography in 193 patients. Circulation 79:825–35, 1989.

41. Kirkeeide RL, Fung P, Smalling RW, Gould KL. Automated evaluation of vessel diameter from arteriograms. Computers in Cardiology, Proc IEEE Computer Soc 215–18, 1982.

42. Kirkeeide RL, Smalling RW, Gould KL. Automated measurement of artery diameter from arteriograms. Circulation 66 (suppl. II):325, 1982.

43. Kirkeeide RL, Buchi M, Demer LL, Gould KL. Afterload affects flow reserve of stenotic coronary arteries. Circulation 76 (suppl. IV):386, 1987.

44. Gould KL, Kirkeeide RL, Buchi M. Coronary flow reserve as a physiologic measure of stenosis severity. Part I. Relative and absolute coronary flow reserve during changing aortic pressure and cardiac workload. Part II. Determination from arteriographic stenosis dimensions under standardized conditions. J Am Coll Cardiol 15:459–74, 1990.

45. Armstrong ML, Heistad DD, Marcus ML, Piegors DJ, Abboud FM. Hemodynamic sequelae of regression of experimental atherosclerosis. J Clin Invest 71:104–13, 1983.

46. Malinow MR. Atherosclerosis: Progression, regression and resolution. Am Heart J 108:1523–37, 1984.

47. Wissler RW, Vesselinovitch D. Regression of atherosclerosis in experimental animals and man. Mod Concepts CV Disease 46:27–32, 1977.

48. Roberts WC. Coronary arteries in fatal acute myocardial infarction. Circulation 45:215–30, 1972.

49. Small DM, Bond MG, Waugh D, Prack M, Sawyer JK. Physiochemical and histological changes in the arterial wall of nonhuman primates during progression and regression of atherosclerosis. J Clin Invest 73:1590–605, 1984.

50. Clarkson TB, Weingand KW, Kaplan JR, Adams MR. Mechanisms of atherogenesis. Circulation 76 (suppl I):20–28, 1987.

51. Schneiderman N. Psychophysiologic factors in atherogenesis and coronary artery disease. Circulation 76 (suppl. I):41–47, 1987.

52. Clarkson RB, Kaplan JR, Adams MR, Manuck SB. Psychosocial influences on the pathogenesis of atherosclerosis among nonhuman primates. Circulation 76 (suppl I):29–40, 1987.

53. Brown GB, Lin JT, Schaefer SM, Kaplan CA, Dodge HT, Albers JJ. Niacin or Lovastatin, combined with colestipol regresses coronary atherosclerosis and prevent clinical events in men with elevated apolipoprotein. Circulation 80:II–266, 1989.

54. Gould KL, Buchi M, Kirkeeide RL, Ornish D, Stein E, Brand R. Reversal of coronary artery stenosis with cholesterol lowering in man followed by arteriography and positron emission tomography. J Nucl Med 30:845, 1989 (abstract).

55. Guide to Clinical Preventive Services Report of the US Preventive Services Task Force, ed. M. Fisher. Baltimore: Williams and Wilkins, 1989.

56. American Heart Association Conference Report on Cholesterol. Circulation 80:715–48, 1989.

57. Consensus Development Conference. Lowering blood cholesterol to prevent heart disease. JAMA 253:2080–83, 1985.

Positron Emission
Tomography of the Heart

11

Principles of Cardiac Positron Emission Tomography

The purpose of cardiac PET is to determine accurately, non-invasively, in either symptomatic or asymptomatic man, the presence or severity of coronary artery stenosis and myocardial viability for choosing and following effects of interventions such as cholesterol control, risk factor management, pharmacological agents, percutaneous transluminal coronary angioplasty, and bypass surgery. An objective basis for clinical decisions on dietary, medical, or mechanical treatment of coronary artery disease becomes particularly important if it is clinically silent, as is increasingly recognized. Non-invasive cardiac imaging should provide sufficiently accurate functional information to indicate catheterization for arteriography, with mechanical intervention based on the non-invasive test. Therefore, it should not only be a reliable guide to managing symptomatic coronary artery disease in traditional or interventional cardiology but should also provide the basis for vigorous medical management of asymptomatic coronary atherosclerosis to achieve stenosis regression and prevent sudden death or myocardial infarction.

As reviewed here, positron imaging of the heart with either generator-produced rubidium-82, cyclotron-produced nitrogen 13-ammonia, or fluoro-18-deoxyglucose (FDG) is optimal for accurate non-invasive diagnosis of coronary artery disease in symptomatic or asymptomatic patients (1–8), including "balanced" three vessel disease (9,10), for assessing physiological stenosis severity (1 4,9 14), for imaging myo cardial infarction (15–27), for determining myocardial viability and/or ischemia (13–18,20–27), for assessing effects of interventions such as thrombolysis on metabolism (24), PTCA on coronary flow reserve (28), bypass surgery on coronary flow and metabolism (16,17), for following progression or regression of coronary artery disease during risk factor treatment (29), and for evaluating collateral function non-invasively (30–32). Positron imaging, therefore, provides a physiological or functional basis for specific therapeutic approaches in the management of heart disease, whether silent or symptomatic, that is not possible with any other technology.

In traditional medical practice, the patient and physician wait until symptoms bring the patient to medical attention designed to salvage or preserve myocardium late in the pathophysiologic course of coronary atherosclerosis. Although re-active treatment triggered by symptoms appropriately remains central to cardiovascular medicine, advanced diagnostic and therapeutic technology provide opportunity for an alternative approach. Positron emission tomography has sufficient accuracy for the diagnosis of coronary artery disease in symptomatic or asymptomatic individuals that it permits economical noninvasive identification and dietary/medical therapy for reversal of coronary atherosclerosis, shown to be feasible with sufficiently vigorous risk factor management (33,34). Such therapy may not be appropriate for the general population or for individuals without known coronary artery stenosis. It is therefore individual, specific preventive intervention. For severe silent disease, mechanical intervention may also be indicated to prevent myocardial infarction or sudden death.

BASIC PRINCIPLES

A positron is a positively charged electron emitted by unstable atoms in the process of radioactive decay, such as generator-produced rubidium-82 or cyclotron-produced carbon-11, oxygen-15, nitrogen-13, and fluorine-18. This positron travels several millimeters in tissue and annihilates with a negative electron, giving off two 511-keV photons in opposite directions. The annihilation photon pair can be detected with a pair of radiation detectors connected through a coincidence counting circuit, so that one decay is recorded if both detectors are activated simultaneously by the photon pair, shown in Figure 11.1.

Radioactive decays occurring outside the sample volume between the detectors are excluded from the count data, since an unpaired photon striking only one of the detectors is not counted. Collimation, or exclusion of stray radiation, is therefore accomplished electronically with coincidence counting rather than solely with lead collimators, as in single-photon imaging. Coincidence counting has several attributes that make PET uniquely quantitative and accurate for clinical imaging, including accurate attenuation correction of emission data and electronic collimation that provides higher efficiency, more counts, and better statistics, all of which are the basis for better spatial and contrast resolution than with single photon systems.

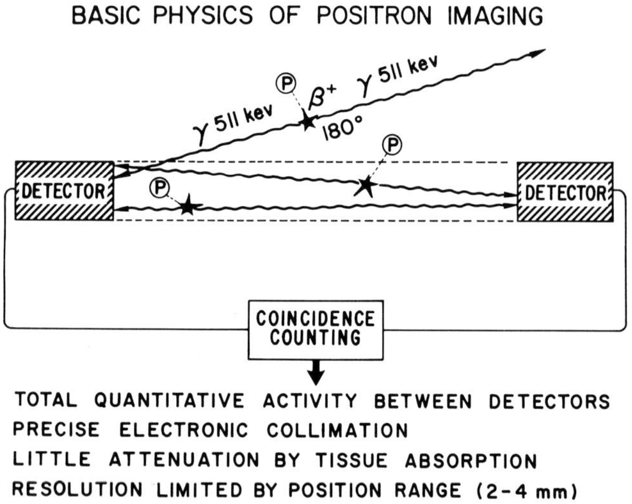

BASIC PHYSICS OF POSITRON IMAGING

TOTAL QUANTITATIVE ACTIVITY BETWEEN DETECTORS
PRECISE ELECTRONIC COLLIMATION
LITTLE ATTENUATION BY TISSUE ABSORPTION
RESOLUTION LIMITED BY POSITION RANGE (2-4 mm)

Fig. 11.1 Positron radionuclides decay by emitting a positive electron or positron, e+, which travels several mm in tissue before annihilating in interaction with a negative electron, e−, giving off two 511-keV photons 180° apart. These paired photons are detected by coincidence counting in such a way that positron decay outside of the volume subtended by the coincidence detectors is excluded. The activity in the volume subtended by the detectors can therefore be quantified.

A positron camera has four components: the scintillation detector-photomultiplier tube (PMT) modules, the gantry housing these detectors with its patient pallet, the electronics, and the computer systems. The design of each of these components and their interrelation is crucial for diagnostic accuracy, for patient volume throughput, and for using ultrashort half-life, generator-produced Rb-82 for routine clinical studies without the expense of a cyclotron. The relation between essential design features of a PET scanner and its clinical performance are described in a later chapter, but the basic principles are outlined here.

Generically, PET cameras contain 1,000 to 1,500 detectors in three to eight banks of rings, attached to photomultiplier tubes (PMT) in ratios ranging from one to eight detectors for each PMT. Scintillations from the coincidence detectors cause electronic signals from the PMTs, which are converted to digital information and processed in a computer to reconstruct a tomographic image, as shown in Figure 11.2, like a CT scanner. However, the source of radiation is a positron tracer, not an external x-ray tube. In order to optimize spatial sampling, the banks of detectors are wobbled in an eccentric path around the subject, with each coincidence decay assigned a spatial location in the wobble path. A transmission image for attenuation correction is obtained by placing a ring of activity around the patient for imaging the target organ before injection of the radiotracer. The positron radiotracer is then injected intravenously and an emission image obtained by back projection techniques. The emission image is corrected for attenuation loss, random coincidences, scattered radiation, deadtime losses, wobble, and variation in detector sensitivity. If done correctly, a quantitative three-

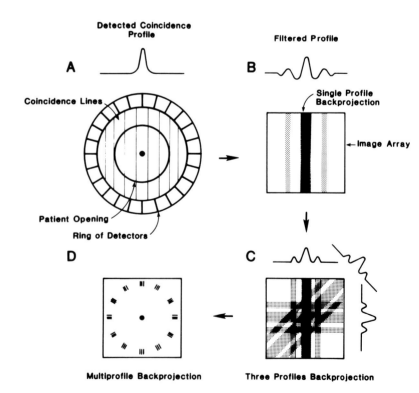

Fig. 11.2 A tomographic image is reconstructed by back projection with appropriate filters and corrections.

dimensional image of the radiotracer activity can be obtained for the organ imaged. A PET scanner is shown in Figure 11.3.

In comparison to the standard single photon radionuclides used in clinical nuclear medicine, positron radiotracers have two additional unique characteristics. The first is that their half-life is short, ranging from 75 s to 110 min. Consequently, several sequential studies may be repeated at one sitting, before and after an intervention. However, the chemistry for labeling radiotracers must be efficient, with high yields. For the ultrashort half-life tracers, like ^{82}Rb (half-life = 75 s) or ^{15}O (half-life = 121 s), the PET scanner must be able to accept very high count rates of up to 0.3 to 1.0 × 10^6 counts/s in order to obtain adequate count statistics for a good image in the brief period of usable radioactivity. The second characteristic is that positron tracers are analogues of elements normally present in metabolism and therefore a wide range of biological compounds can be labeled for in-vivo studies. The most important positron radiotracers currently used for clinical cardiac applications are generator-produced ^{82}Rb (1,4,12,19,26,35–39) and cyclotron-produced ^{13}N ammonia (40–42), ^{15}O water (43,44), and fluoro-18-deoxyglucose (FDG) (15), as discussed subsequently, although many others are used for research.

Quantitative PET imaging refers to reconstruction of tomographic images that quantitatively reflect or recover the actual or true distribution of activity in the target organ or field of view, undistorted by tissue attenuation, which is corrected by the transmission scan. This type of quantitative data recovery also depends on the technical characteristics of the camera and the duration of imaging permitted by the half-life of the positron tracer, as discussed in a later section.

In addition, quantitation involves measurement of biological processes such as myocardial perfusion in cc/min/g or glucose uptake in grams of glucose per gram of myocardium per minute. These biological quantitative measurements require both quantitative imaging of activity distribution and a model of radiotracer behavior in vivo that relates the imaged activity to biological units being measured, as discussed subsequently.

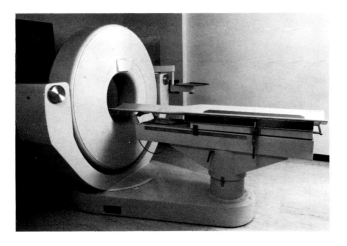

Fig. 11.3 A multi-slice clinical PET scanner (Positron Corp, Houston).

CLINICAL SUMMARY OF CARDIAC PET

Clinical and experimental studies currently support the clinical applications for cardiac PET listed below. The major applications are discussed in detail in subsequent chapters.

Noninvasive Diagnosis of Coronary Artery Disease in Either Symptomatic or Asymptomatic Patients

The sensitivity and specificity of diagnosing coronary artery disease by positron emission tomography (1–8), as compared with automated quantitative coronary arteriography, are both 95% to 98% in symptomatic or asymptomatic individuals, including balanced three-vessel disease (9,10). False negative studies are usually associated with distal coronary stenoses or disease of smaller arteries; false positives are usually associated with nonatheromatous coronary artery abnormalities such as spasm or thrombi (4). This application is discussed in several later chapters.

Assessment of the Physiologic Severity of Coronary Artery Stenosis or Changes in Stenosis Severity

As previously reviewed, percent diameter narrowing is not an adequate standard for quantifying stenosis severity of coronary artery narrowing (1–4,9–14,45–50); this observation has been confirmed by others (51–54). It does not account for the effects of diffuse disease, eccentricity, stenosis length, absolute cross-sectional area, entrance and exit shape, or absolute dimensions on flow or flow capacity. It is also limited by substantial inter- and intraobserver variability. Alternative invasive approaches providing fluid-dynamically correct measurements of graded stenosis severity utilize quantitative arteriographic methods to calculate stenosis resistance (51), pressure-flow curves (49,50), or coronary flow reserve (1–12,31), as reviewed in previous chapters and developed more subsequently.

The quantitative severity of PET perfusion defects after dipyridamole reflects the anatomic severity of the coronary artery stenosis as determined by automated, quantitative coronary arteriography, taking into account length, absolute dimensions, shape, and percent narrowing of the stenosis (1–4,9–13,28,29). Therefore, noninvasive positron emission tomography provides assessment of the physiologic severity of coronary stenoses, as well as changes in severity after an intervention such as thrombolysis (24), bypass surgery (16,17), PTCA (28), or cholesterol lowering (29). With accurate quantitation of stenosis severity, binary analysis based on sensitivity and specificity become inadequate or even misleading for validating or describing diagnostic value. Consequently, this capacity of PET is one of its unique strengths, demonstrable by comparison to an appropriate arteriographic gold standard that takes into account all stenosis dimensions. Comparison of two non-invasive methods—for example, PET versus single proton emission computed tomography (SPECT)—using arteriographic percent diameter stenosis as the standard may be misleading or may inappropriately favor one or the other non-invasive method, since percent stenosis has little relation to coronary flow reserve

serve (1–4,9–12) except in cases of very severe narrowing. Several later chapters expand on these issues.

Imaging Myocardial Ischemia, Infarction, and Viability

The location and extent of myocardial infarction (15–27) and myocardial ischemia or viability (13–19,20–27) may be imaged by positron emission tomography with or without reperfusion, using generator-produced [82]Rb or cyclotron-produced ^{13}N ammonia and FDG, in order to determine if bypass surgery or PTCA is indicated. Documentation of this application is reviewed in a subsequent chapter.

Identification and Assessment of Significant Collateral Function in Man by Imaging Coronary Steal During Dipyridamole-Handgrip Stress

Coronary steal occurs under conditions of near-maximum coronary vasodilation if collaterals provide a significant proportion of resting myocardial perfusion. A fall in absolute myocardial uptake of activity, after injection of a perfusion tracer, during dipyridamole vasodilation as compared to rest then indicates coronary steal and the presence of significant collaterals (30–32). Because it is physiologically complex and uniquely assessed by PET, myocardial steal is addressed in more detail in a chapter on this topic.

Dilated Cardiomyopathy

Dilated cardiomyopathy unrelated to coronary artery disease may also be diagnosed by positron imaging as an enlarged, poorly functioning heart with no resting or stress perfusion defects typical of ischemic cardiomyopathy due to coronary artery disease.

Left Ventricular Function and Wall Thickening

By gating the positron emission tomographs with the ECG, left ventricular pumping function and wall thickening may be assessed regionally in three dimensions (1,55). Since there are many other less expensive, simpler measures of left ventricular function, gated PET has not been developed clinically. However, as PET comes to be recognized as a noninvasive substitute for diagnostic catheterization, recording first-pass gated blood pool for LV function as a part of routine perfusion studies will likely become common in order to obtain complete cardiac evaluation as at cardiac catheterization for the basic questions of arterial patency, myocardial viability, stress underperfusion, and left ventricular function.

12

PET Perfusion Imaging

The physiologic principles of PET perfusion imaging for identifying and assessing severity of coronary artery stenosis are derived directly from the concepts of relative and absolute flow reserve discussed in previous chapters. Flow through moderately severe coronary artery stenosis is generally normal at rest unless unstable angina is present. Exercise or coronary vasodilators increase flow through the stenosis, but only to submaximal levels, thereby producing a disparity in regional perfusion relative to areas supplied by a normal coronary artery. This disparity in regional perfusion at high coronary blood flow is imaged as a means of identifying coronary artery disease non-invasively with perfusion tracers. The quantitative severity of defect on an image of absolute coronary flow reserve is proportional to the severity of the stenosis.

With marked increases in coronary flow, functionally mild, early coronary artery stenoses can be identified before symptoms or myocardial infarction occur, thereby allowing medical therapy aimed at reversal of coronary atherosclerosis. However, with only modest increases in coronary flow, as during exercise stress, only severe coronary stenoses can be identified. An inadequate stimulus for increasing coronary flow or an inadequate perfusion imaging agent or technique will limit the ability to detect or quantify coronary stenoses by perfusion imaging. Based on animal studies (9,45–50,56), and as confirmed in man (1,4), there are three essential principles of an imaging method for detecting and assessing severity of coronary artery disease: (a) cross-sectional positron tomography in order to avoid overlapping structures and to obtain depth-independent resolution for accurate quantitative measurements of coronary blood flow; (b) a myocardial perfusion imaging agent, which is taken up or deposited in myocardium in proportion to flow at high coronary blood flows up to five times resting control levels; and (c) a potent stimulus for increasing coronary flow in order to image the regional disparities in maximum perfusion caused by stenosis. Figure 12.1 demonstrates these principles (57). In the top panel, resting coronary flow and distribution are normal despite a severe stenosis. After intravenous dipyridamole, flow increases to four times baseline (middle panel) in the normal area but is restricted to a two-times increase in the diseased area. An average ratio of 2.4 to 1 or 150% difference between the normal and affected areas is the minimum that is visible as a relative perfusion defect on planar thallium image in experimental animals, as illustrated in Figure 12.2

(45). With PET, a difference of only 15% can be detected—that is, an abnormal area that is 85% of normal maximum.

Figure 12.3 (57) shows the problem of an inadequate stimulus for increasing flow or inadequate uptake of radionuclide perfusion tracer at high flows. No perfusion defect is seen because flow in the abnormal area is similar to flow in the normal area, which fails to increase flow anywhere in the heart over the limit of maximum flow imposed by the stenosis.

The ratio of radionuclide activity after dipyridamole (or stress) to the activity at rest is an index of absolute flow reserve. It is only an *index* of absolute flow reserve, because flow-dependent extraction and arterial input function of the radionuclide are not usually accounted for in clinical images. The ratio of activity in a perfusion defect to the normal maximum activity in the distribution of normal coronary arteries on the dipyridamole (or stress) image is an index of relative coronary flow reserve. It is also only an index, unless flow-dependent extraction is accounted for. With quantitation of PET perfusion imaging to account for arterial input function and flow-dependent radionuclide extraction, absolute and relative coronary flow reserve are both quantitatively measured by PET. In Figure 12.1, an additional observation needs emphasis. An abnormality or defect on an image of absolute coronary flow reserve will appear visually more severe or intense than the corresponding defect on the relative flow reserve image, because the range of absolute flow reserve values is greater (1 to 5) than for relative flow reserve (0.0 to 1.0). For the same color-display scale, this greater range of values heightens contrast of the perfusion defect on an image of absolute coronary flow reserve. Quantitative PET is addressed in a subsequent chapter.

CLINICAL PROCEDURE

All of the examples and data on cardiac perfusion imaging by PET in this book utilized the following protocol. Patients were fasted and caffeine, theophylline, and cigarettes were withheld for 8 h prior to study. Twelve-lead ECG and Dynamap blood pressure cuff were attached to monitor the patient. Fluoroscopy was used to mark the cardiac borders for patient positioning. PET scans for this book were obtained as previously described (1,4,12,19,28,29), with the first-prototype University of Texas multi-slice tomograph utilizing cesium fluoride detectors and a narrow coincidence window of 6 nsec that reduces randoms and increases count rate capacity, as

143

REST NO IMAGE DEFECT

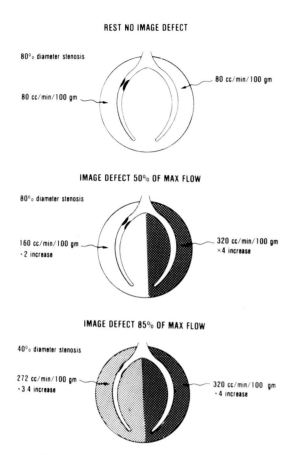

IMAGE DEFECT 50% OF MAX FLOW

IMAGE DEFECT 85% OF MAX FLOW

Fig. 12.1 Schema demonstrating the principle for detection of coronary artery disease by perfusion imaging under conditions of maximum coronary vasodilation. With an 80% diameter narrowing, coronary flow reserve is limited to approximately a two-times increase over resting levels, as compared to a four-times increase in non-stenotic arteries. The abnormal area, therefore, has 50% less activity, reflecting a 50% decrease in flow as compared to normal maximum. A milder stenosis of approximately 40% diameter narrowing will produce a relative defect of approximately 15% below maximum flow, indicating a mild lesion. Reproduced with permission from Gould, 1986. (57).

is essential for obtaining adequate counts with ultra short half-life tracers. Reconstructed resolution was 12 to 14 mm FWHM, consistent with the range of cardiac motion on ungated images.

Using a plexiglass ring containing 3 mCi of Gallium 68, transmission images to correct for photon attenuation were obtained over 20–30 min to contain 200 million counts. Emission images of 15 to 25 million counts were obtained over 6 min following intravenous injection of 40–50 mCi of generator-produced rubidium-82 (^{82}Rb), or over 15–20 minutes following 15–20 mCi of cyclotron-produced ^{13}N ammonia. To allow for blood pool clearance, image acquisition was begun 80 s after starting the infusion of ^{82}Rb. There was a 3-min delay after ammonia administration.

At 10 min after administration of the first dose of ^{82}Rb or 40 min after ^{13}N ammonia, dipyridamole (0.142 mg/kg/min) was infused for 4 min. Two minutes after the infusion was

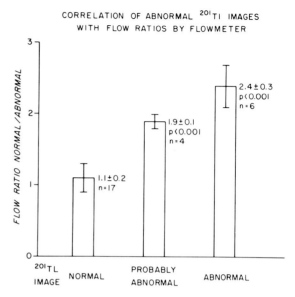

Fig. 12.2 Ratio of maximal flow in the normal coronary artery to maximal flow in the stenotic coronary artery during coronary vasodilation, related to abnormalities in myocardial images of thallium-201 injected after intravenous administration of dipyridamole. Values expressed as mean ± 1 SD. Reproduced with permission from Gould KL, 1978. (46).

completed, 25% of the pre-determined maximal handgrip was held with one hand for 4 min. Two minutes after starting the handgrip, a second dose of the same amount of the same tracer was injected, and imaging was repeated. For those patients developing significant angina, aminophylline (125 mg) was given intravenously.

For patients undergoing exercise treadmill testing, ^{13}N ammonia was used at rest. Forty minutes later, the patient was moved from the PET camera to the treadmill for a standard Bruce symptom limited exercise test. At peak symptom limited exercise, a second dose of ^{13}N ammonia was injected intravenously, and the patient continued exercising for 45–60 s. On termination of exercise, the patient was repositioned in the PET scanner and image acquisition was begun immediately, collecting 15 to 20 million counts over 15–20 min. ECG and blood pressure were monitored throughout exercise stress. Both dipyridamole infusion and exercise testing were supervised by a physician.

THREE-DIMENSIONAL RESTRUCTURING ALGORITHM AND POLAR MAP DISPLAY FOR PET IMAGES

The set of transaxial cardiac images obtained from PET is oriented in a transverse plane perpendicular to the axis of the body. Since the heart is positioned with its long axis to the left and downward relative to the body axis, the transverse slices are not oriented for the most advantageous analysis. For effective quantification, the transaxial or acquisition data is restructured into slices perpendicular to the long axis of the heart, called short-axis views, as previously described (10). The three-dimensional restructuring algorithm for gen-

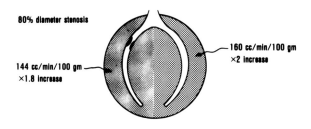

IMAGE DEFECT 90% OF SUBMAX FLOW

80% diameter stenosis

144 cc/min/100 gm
×1.8 increase

160 cc/min/100 gm
×2 increase

NO IMAGE DEFECT

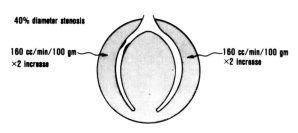

40% diameter stenosis

160 cc/min/100 gm
×2 increase

160 cc/min/100 gm
×2 increase

Fig. 12.3 The limitations of this approach are apparent if the vasodilatory stimulus is inadequate. In the top panel, flow increased only two times in the normal artery, which is not sufficient to cause a difference in comparison with the abnormal area. Under these conditions, a milder stenosis is not identified because maximum coronary vasodilation is not achieved. Reproduced with permission from Gould KL, 1986. (57).

erating true short and long axis views from PET transaxial cardiac images has been validated by testing with computer-generated and phantom data sets (10). Restructured short-axis views serve as input data to a routine that computes polar coordinator maps for rest and stress images, as previously described.

COMPARATIVE ANALYSIS OF REST AND STRESS PET STUDIES

A set of four specialized polar coordinate maps reflecting relative regional activity distribution at *rest* and *stress,* the *change in absolute activity,* and *change in relative activity distribution* from rest to stress is created, utilizing rest and stress polar coordinate maps as input. The *rest and stress* polar maps are scaled from zero to maximum radioactivity, 100%, in order to reflect relative regional distribution of activity throughout the myocardium during rest and stress on the same scale. These two "scaled" polar maps are produced by an algorithm that searches the original rest and stress polar coordinates for maximum activity and determines the average of the top 5% of the activity values (10). The routine assigns a value of 100% to the regions where activity is equal to or greater than the average maximum value, and computes values for all other regions of the scaled polar maps using the equation:

$$\text{Scaled Activity Value} = \frac{\text{Activity Value}}{\text{Maximum Activity Value}} \times 100$$

These scaled polar maps are displayed by grouping the scaled activity values into ranges of 5%, with a discrete color scale that uses one color to represent each 5% of activity. The

stress polar map represents relative flow reserve throughout the left ventricle.

An *absolute ratio polar map* is computed by an algorithm using original rest and stress polar coordinate maps as input data, normalizes the two maps to compensate for differences in injected dose, and produces a ratio map by dividing the values of the dose-corrected stress polar map by those of the dose-corrected rest polar map. The resulting absolute ratio polar map provides an index of absolute coronary flow reserve (1–4,9,10), as contrasted with the relative flow reserve map indicated above. The importance and value of assessing both relative and absolute coronary flow reserve were discussed in previous chapters.

The *relative ratio polar map* shows the relative regional change in activity from the scaled rest to stress images. It is generated by an algorithm that divides the values of the stress scaled polar map (0 to 100%) by the values of the rest scaled polar map (0 to 100%), producing relative ratio values on a scale of 0.0 to 2.0, with the same restriction on widely deviant relative ratio values (9,10).

QUANTITATIVE ANALYSIS OF REGIONAL ACTIVITY

In order to quantitate relative regional activity, all polar maps are divided into fixed sections representing the lateral, anterior, septal, inferior, and apical quadrant of the polar display. A minimum algorithm for each quadrant of each polar map determines the lowest average 5% of the data as the regional minimum activity value. The mean algorithm determines, for each of the polar maps, the mean activity level in each of the five regions (9,10).

A fractionation routine provides the percent of the cardiac image with given relative activity levels for each of the specialized polar maps. The algorithm scans the rest and stress scaled circumferential profile values, counting the number of profile values in the ranges of 0 to 20%, 21% to 40%, 41% to 60%, 61% to 80%, and 81% to 100% of normal (maximum) activity. The number of profile values within each range is divided by the total number of profile values to produce five fractions describing the frequency of specific activity levels in each scaled polar map.

STATISTICAL ANALYSIS FOR SIGNIFICANCE OF ABNORMALITIES

The standard deviation blackout routine automatically identifies regions for each polar map that have values that deviate significantly from standard normal values, based on studies of 30 disease-free individuals. The blackout algorithm creates standard deviation blackout polar maps by performing sector-by-sector comparisons of polar map images from an individual study with sets of normal standard deviation images of 1.5, 2.0, and 2.5 standard deviations. The blackout routine then computes the percent of circumferential profile units that are blacked out in the lateral, anterior, septal, inferior, and apical regions of each of the standard deviation polar maps. Thus, the percent of the cardiac image that falls beyond 1.5, 2.0, or 2.5 standard deviations from normal is automatically determined regionally and for the whole heart for each of the four specialized polar maps (10).

DISPLAY AND USER INTERACTION

A user-friendly, menu-driven program displays essential visual and quantitative information by a single command key. Rest and stress transverse, long, and short axis, and polar coordinate map-image sets are displayed with a selectable format for a complete study presentation or slice-by-slice comparison on three video planes of the monitor. The intensities of rest and stress–paired tomographic sets for a whole heart can be independently altered without affecting the automated quantitative routines. The scaled absolute ratio and relative ratio polar maps are displayed along with related quantitative information on the same video screen as the long-axis views and original polar coordinate maps. With button functions, the user can select any of the quantitative information, minima, means, and fractional breakdowns, for display on the screen next to the appropriate polar map. The display routine allows the user to overwrite the four specialized polar maps with a chosen set of standard deviation (1.5, 2.0, or 2.5) blackout polar maps. The percent of blacked-out profile units in a region for the selected standard deviation is written on the screen next to the appropriate blackout polar maps (10).

The display program has a routine for entering into the display a visual interpretation of the study for the scaled absolute ratio and relative ratio polar maps. After visual interpretation is completed, the display routine prompts the user by a simple screen menu to enter codes describing visual intensity and size of abnormalities in each region and over the entire map, for each of the four polar maps. After visual interpretation is completed, the display routine prompts the user to enter clinical information, which, with visual interpretations, is written in a record file that can be accessed by statistical and database routines. The comprehensive rest-stress display and restructuring routines form a highly integrated software package for generating, analyzing, storing, and recalling short- and long-axis views, polar coordinate maps, and quantitative data with a minimum amount of user interaction. The entire analysis, including display of all quantitative data and visual interpretation, can be carried out in two to five minutes, depending on the speed of visual interpretation. The paired display is also used for stress-stress comparison before and after the control or treatment period (10,29), in order to evaluate progression or regression.

ERROR ANALYSIS OF ROI STATISTICS FOR THE 3D RESTRUCTURING ALGORITHM

Errors introduced into a data set by interpolation procedures were 2.36% on the average, computed from all ROI data after three-dimensional rotation (10). For ROIs with less than 10 pixels, the average error was 4.29%, while the average error for ROIs containing 10 or more pixels was 2.10%. Thus, the average error increased by a factor of two when the ROI size was less than 10 pixels.

Accordingly, data in a region of interest taken from a myocardial image that has been rotated and interpolated once in three dimensions will have a value that is, on average, within 2.36% of the value in the comparable region of interest from the original cardiac image. For quantitative analysis, no region of interest containing less than 20 pixels was utilized, and edge regions were excluded from the quantitative analysis of polar coordinate maps carried out after rotation. Consequently, the actual error is considerably less than 2.36%. Partial volume errors are minimized by quantifying midwall peak (average top 2%) activity profiles for relative distribution, relative ratios, or changes in activity.

RADIONUCLIDES FOR CLINICAL PET PERFUSION IMAGING

The most commonly used PET perfusion radionuclides for clinical cardiac studies are nitrogen-13 ammonia and rubidium-82. ^{13}N ammonia for studies in this book was produced using a 35 meV Scanditronix, positive-ion, variable energy cyclotron (1). Our method utilizes the (p,α) reaction on oxygen-16 in water [^{16}O(p,α)^{13}N]. The water target was bombarded for 2 min with a proton beam of up to 40 μA at 17.2 meV. Production is typically 250–300 mCi of ^{13}N at the end of bombardment, for a yield of 3 mCi/μA per min. The yield of ^{13}N is obtained largely in the form of nitrate. Then, 30 cc of bombarded water is transferred to a 50-cc flask equipped with a short-path distillation head containing sodium hydroxide. Titanium trichloride is added to produce titanium (OH$_3$), a strong reducing agent that converts the ^{13}N nitrate to ^{13}NH$_3$, which is then recovered as approximately 40 mCi in 2–4 cc of distillate within 5 min. Fluorine-18 formed from the p,n reaction on ^{18}O, comprising 2% of total activity, and other contaminants knocked out of the foil by the proton beam are removed by the distillation, thereby providing a final product free of chemical and radionuclide contaminants. Ten to 20 mCi of ^{13}NH$_3$ was injected intravenously for clinical studies, and positron imaging was carried out as described in the following section on imaging protocol.

Rubidium-82 for studies in this book was eluted from an ^{82}Sr-^{82}Rb generator (Squibb) using a 50-cc syringe driven by a microprocessor-controlled motor connected to an on-line radiation monitor that provided preset volume, dose, and dose rate of ^{82}Rb to the patient (1,35–39). Typically, with a fresh generator, 30–50 mCi were injected in a 10-cc volume over 20–25 s. Toward the end of the useful life of the generator (5 weeks), volumes of 30–40 cc were required to deliver 30–50 mCi of ^{82}Rb. With a half-life of only 75 s, approximately one-half to two-thirds of this activity reaches the arterial circulation, with the balance decaying in transit through the infusion tubing, the venous system, and the lungs.

Rubidium is an alkali metal analogue of potassium and is similar in its chemical and biologic properties. It is rapidly concentrated by the myocardium with a first-pass extraction of 50%–60% at resting flow levels, which falls to 25%–30% at high flows (37–39). By comparison, first-pass myocardial extraction of ^{13}NH$_3$ is somewhat higher, 70% falling to approximately 35% at high flows (40–42). With appropriately larger doses of Rb (50 mCi), images are comparable to those of ^{13}NH$_3$ (18 mCi) (1,4).

Rubidium-82, because of its short half-life (75 s), is the agent of choice for repeated or sequential myocardial imaging. It is particularly useful in acute clinical situations in which the patient's condition is changing rapidly, or for studies before and after an intervention, such as dipyridamole stress and PTCA.

For clinical cardiac PET studies without a cyclotron, the source of ^{82}Rb is its parent strontium-82, by a generator that uses hydrous SnO_2 as the inorganic absorbent. This generator has the lowest ^{82}Sr breakthrough level of all systems tested thus far, can be efficiently eluted with isotonic saline of physiologic pH, and delivers ^{82}Rb in a small eluate volume.

The use of short-lived, positron-emitting ^{82}Rb in cardiovascular nuclear medicine requires a system for a rapid elution of a ^{82}Rb generator and on-line injection of the generator eluate. The ^{82}Rb Infusion System (Squibb, New Brunswick, NJ) incorporates features for efficient elution and precisely controlled delivery of a sterile solution of ^{82}Rb in saline. It has been designed to deliver a uniform, non-pulsating flow of eluent. The system has preformed sterile, disposable plastic tubing, one-way valves, and a syringe that are electromechanically actuated to provide the eluent flow by positive flow pump action. The syringe plunger is bidirectionally actuated by a low-friction, recirculating ball screw jack that is coupled to a stepper motor through a reduction gear. The speed of the motor driving the syringe plunger, and hence the infusion rate, is regulated automatically by a radiation monitor in line with the infusion tubing to deliver a predetermined dose and dose rate.

The components of the system—pump, fluid tubing, filters, one-way valves, electronic control modules, shielded vault for the ^{82}Rb generator, shield for the waste container, and dosimeter—are self-contained on a stainless steel mobile cart. The elution and injection procedure is fully defined by the settings of the controls on the electronics modules for the infusion and dosimetry systems. Settings include eluted volume to be delivered, flow rate, dose to be delivered, dose rate, and patient volume to be delivered.

COMPARISON OF ^{82}Rb AND ^{13}N AMMONIA

There are significant advantages and disadvantages of using either ^{13}N ammonia or ^{82}Rb. The advantages of ^{13}N are as follows: (a) The first-pass extraction fraction of ^{13}N ammonia is approximately 60% to 70% (40–42), as compared with 50% to 60% for ^{82}Rb (37–39). The slightly better extraction of ^{13}N ammonia indicates that it may give slightly better contrast between areas of high and low flow reserve in the images. (b) The longer half-life of ^{13}N ammonia (9.9 min) as compared with that of ^{82}Rb (75 s) allows longer counting times, for better accumulated counting statistics by a slow camera not designed to accept high count rates. The long half-life also permits injection of the perfusion tracer during vigorous exercise, with subsequent imaging of the ^{13}N ammonia trapped in the myocardium under conditions of stress and imaged later at rest. Diagnostic accuracy is the same for ^{13}N ammonia and ^{82}Rb (1,4), as shown by the two identical images in Figure 12.4.

However, the disadvantage of ^{13}N ammonia for perfusion imaging is that it requires an on-site cyclotron, whereas ^{82}Rb is generator-produced and therefore more economical. The shorter half-life of ^{82}Rb does not call for the 40-min decay time between rest and stress images required by ^{13}N am-

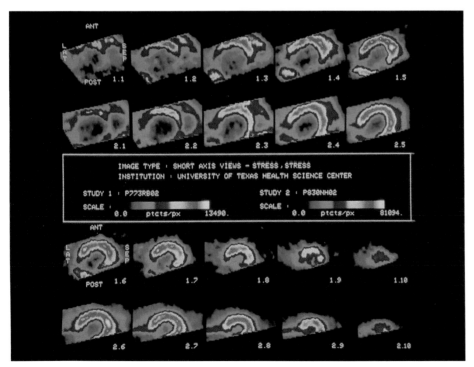

Fig. 12.4 (A) Comparison of short-axis PET of ^{13}N ammonia (upper of each paired row of images) compared to ^{82}Rb (lower of each paired row of images), showing an identical inferior defect at rest. (*continued*)

A

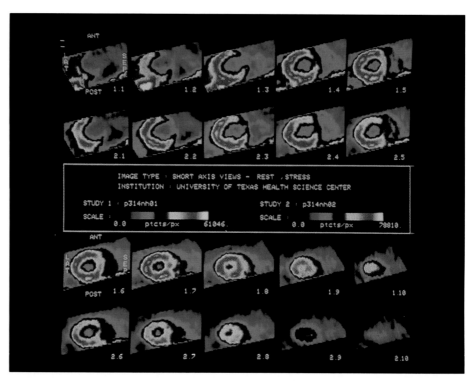

B

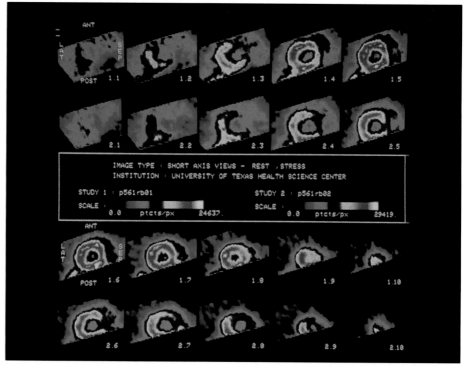

Fig. 12.4 (*cont.*)(**B**) Short-axis views with ¹³N ammonia at rest (upper of each paired row of images) and after dipyridamole (lower of each paired row of images) with an anterior septal defect. (**C**) Short-axis rest dipyridamole images with ⁸²Rb in another patient with similar anterior septal defect but with more severe apical involvement in addition to anterior and septal defects.

C

monia. Acquisition time for a cardiac study with [82]Rb is 6 min, as compared with 15–20 min for ^{13}N ammonia. Therefore, a rest-dipyridamole study with [82]Rb requires approximately 1 h, whereas with ^{13}N ammonia it requires 2½ hours, thereby decreasing patient throughput volume, which is essential for economical operation. With the fixed cost of a [82]Rb generator, the cost per study goes down as patient volume rises, whereas with ^{13}N ammonia the unit cost of radionuclide does not fall. Perfusion imaging with [82]Rb is therefore more economically feasible, with the additional advantage that repeated studies may be done more rapidly because of its shorter half-life.

Although less expensive than a cyclotron, the cost of [82]Rb has been set fairly high by its manufacturer, such that a less expensive perfusion imaging agent, generator-produced copper-62 PTSM is becoming an important alternative (58,59).

CLINICAL EXAMPLES AND EXPLANATION OF PET IMAGES

Figure 12.5 shows the orientation of cardiac tomographic image planes viewed as if looking down from above on one's own sectioned heart (10). Tomographs of vertical hearts tend to be doughnut-shaped, whereas in horizontal hearts they are horseshoe-shaped. Figure 12.6 shows the distribution of the coronary arteries as viewed from above, with the vascular bed of the left anterior descending coronary artery at the top of each image, the left circumflex artery on the left, and the right coronary artery on the right side and in inferior sections (10). Figure 12.7 illustrates in the top panel that the tomo-

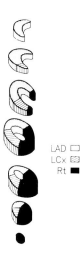

Fig. 12.6 Distribution of coronary arteries on tomographic myocardial perfusion images, oriented as if looking down on the heart from above. Reproduced with permission from Hicks K, Ganti G, Mullani N, et al., 1989. (10).

graphic image planes are acquired perpendicular to the long axis of the body and therefore cut the heart at an oblique semi-long axis angle; this is called the acquisition view (10). These data are then rotated into true short- and long-axis views for a complete three-dimensional analysis and interpretation.

Figure 12.8 shows rest-stress PET of generator-produced [82]Rb in a patient with severe three-vessel coronary artery dis-

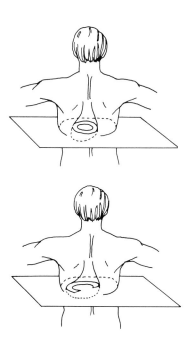

Fig. 12.5 Orientation of cardiac cross-sectional tomograms as if looking down on the heart from above. The tomographic sections in patients with vertical hearts tend to be doughnut-shaped images, whereas those from patients with horizontal hearts appear as horseshoe-shaped images. Reproduced with permission from Hicks K, Ganti G, Mullani N, et al., 1989. (10).

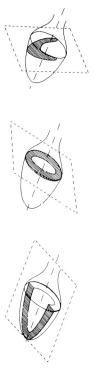

Fig. 12.7 Orientation of tomographic image planes as acquired in the top panel, in true short-axis view in the middle panel and in true long-axis views in the lower panel. Reproduced with permission from Hicks K, Ganti G, Mullani N, et al., 1989. (10).

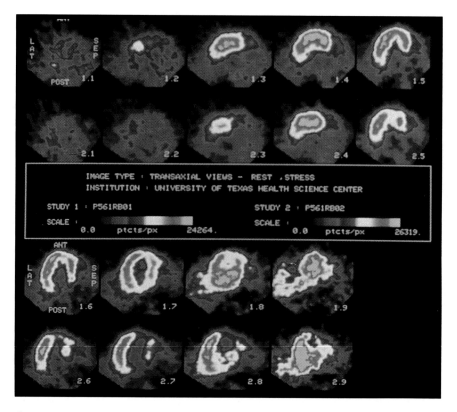

A

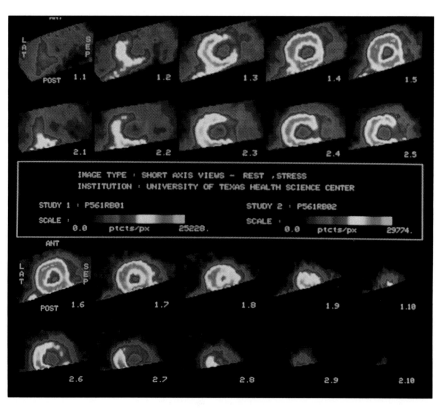

B

Fig. 12.8 Rest-stress ⁸²Rb images of a patient with three-vessel coronary artery disease. For details of the display, see text. (**A**) Acquisition view looking down from above. (**B**) True short-axis views. (**C**) True horizontal and vertical long-axis views, with polar map displays of minimum activity in each quadrant and whole heart. (**D**) Mean activity in each quadrant (upper four polar maps) and fraction of each quadrant and whole-heart image outside of 2.5 SD from normals (lower four polar maps). Reproduced with permission from Hicks K, Ganti G, Mullani N, et al., 1989. (10).

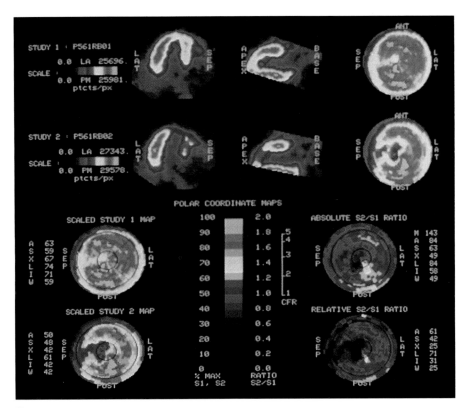

C

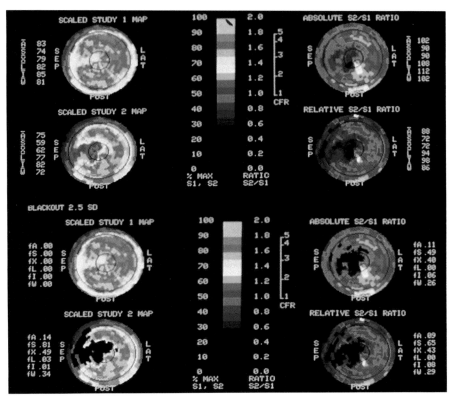

D

ease as imaged in the acquisition view (panel A), in true short-axis views (B), and in horizontal and vertical long-axis views (panel C) (10). Rest images are shown in the upper row of each pair of images (study 1); the dipyridamole stress images are in the lower row (study 2). The number after the decimal is the image plane for both study 1 and study 2. In the system of color coding, white indicates the highest flow, red next-highest, yellow intermediate, and green and blue indicate the lowest relative flows. The tomographs in the horizontal long-axis views (top images of panel C) are oriented as if looking down from above with the anterior or apex at the top of each image, the left lateral free wall on the left, and the muscular septum on the right, with the AV ring and/or inferior myocardium at the bottom. In the true short-axis views of panel B, the image planes are arranged from the AV ring at the upper left to the apex at the lower right, with the anterior wall being up, the free LV wall on the left, and the septum on the right of each tomograph. The open "C" shape in the basal short-axis views in the upper left images of panel B is due to the membranous septum of the left ventricular cavity, which is avascular and therefore appears as a defect although actually it reflects normal anatomy.

The resting tomographs of Figure 12.8 show a small apical defect, indicating a small myocardial scar. With dipyridamole stress, the anterior, septal, and apical myocardium show a defect in both short- and long-axis views. The inferior and lateral myocardium do not show a definite stress perfusion defect on tomographic views that can be identified, however, when the entire set of data is analyzed together on the polar coordinate maps.

Panel C shows horizontal (left) and vertical (right) long-axis views of the heart. Rest images are shown in the top row, with dipyridamole stress images in the second row of the top half of the figure. The horizontal long-axis views are oriented as if looking down from above. The vertical long-axis tomographs are oriented as if looking at the left side of the body cut head to toe. Anterior myocardium is at the top, inferior at the bottom, apex at the left, and the AV ring on the right.

Tomographic data is summarized in a polar display as if looking at the patient from the outside toward the apex of the left ventricle located in the center of the bull's-eye, with the outer rim of the bull's-eye corresponding to the AV ring. Polar displays on the left (lower half of figure) show the relative activity on a scale of 0 to 100%, with rest being the upper (S1) and stress being the lower (S2) of the polar maps on the left side of the panel. The upper right polar map (in the lower half of the figure), labeled absolute S2/S1 ratio (ABS S2/S1), shows the absolute counts of the stress image divided by the rest image, displayed on a scale from 0 to 2.

Increase in activity is shown by warm colors (yellow, orange, red, white) indicating ratios greater than one (blue), which reflect increased radiotracer uptake and perfusion due to dipyridamole. Beside the scale for absolute S2/S1 radiotracer uptake ratio (stress/rest) is a scale of coronary flow reserve values, derived by a two-compartment model accounting for extraction-dependent flow derived from animal studies. The lower right polar display, labeled relative S2/S1 ratio (REL S2/S1) shows the relative distribution of flow at rest divided by the relative distribution of activity on the stress image (relative instead of absolute values), also on a

scale of 0 to 2. It therefore maps the relative change in activity from rest to stress, or the change in relative coronary flow reserve.

Letters and numbers beside each polar map show quantitative results. For regions of the heart, A = anterior, S = septal, X = apex, L = lateral, I = inferior. The numbers beside each region indicate the minimum activity as a percent of normal areas (100%). For letters with a bar, such as Ā, the numbers indicate mean activity of all pixels (rather than minimum) for that quadrant of the polar map as percent of normal areas shown in D, the upper set of four polar maps. The blacked-out polar maps in D, the lower set, show those areas that are greater than 2.5 standard deviations away from normals. For black-out figures, the numbers beside the area, such as fA, give the fraction of the quadrant or whole heart, fW, that is 2.5 SD beyond the normal range (or 2.0 or 1.5 SD, electively). By using a single push-button command, the minimum, the average, or other analytical data can be instantaneously displayed beside the appropriate polar coordinate map. The fractions, f, beyond 2.5 SD limits therefore provide the size of the area involved. The percent of each quadrant in short-axis views falling in 20% ranges of activity from 0–20% to 80–100% at rest and stress may also be displayed beside polar map coordinates (not shown).

For the example in Figure 12.8, the visual inspection of the polar map display (panel C) and the quantitative analysis shows considerably more information than could be obtained from visual inspection of the tomographic views alone. The polar map S2 shows not only a severe decrease in relative activity of the anterior, septal, and apical areas but also a mild decrease in the inferior septal area not apparent on tomographic views but confirmed by the minimum activity decreasing on S2 (stress) compared to S1 (rest). The lateral wall also shows a visual and quantitative decrease in activity, reflecting a mild relative decrease throughout the lateral quadrant with stress, that is not apparent on the tomographic views. In the polar map on the upper right (C), the absolute S2/S1 ratio shows that at least one part of the heart located inferior-laterally responded with a flow reserve of 2.8 (times baseline). Flow reserve in the rest of the heart was severely depressed, indicating three-vessel disease that was worse for the LAD proximal to the first septal perforator, with "balanced" disease of the left circumflex and right coronary arteries. The relative flow reserve defect on S2 is not as apparent as the marked defect of absolute flow reserve on S2/S1, as is consistent with the discussion of the previous chapter.

In addition, parts of the anterior septum and the apex show a decrease in absolute counts, with an absolute ratio of less than one on the absolute S2/S1 ratio polar map. A fall in absolute activity after dipyridamole as compared to rest indicates myocardial steal, and hence the presence of collaterals to viable myocardium. The 2.5-SD black-out display (panel D, lower four polar maps) indicates that after dipyridamole (S2), 14% of the anterior wall quadrant is beyond 2.5 SD of normals, as is 81% of the septum, 49% of the apex, and 34% of the whole heart. On the S2/S1 absolute ratio polar map, approximately 26% of the whole myocardium shows myocardial steal and is therefore viable, collateralized myocardium, mostly in the anterior, septal, and apical regions.

Thus, the location, intensity, size, statistical significance of, and presence of collateralized viable myocardium can be automatically quantitated.

In order to illustrate further the application of assessing both absolute and relative coronary flow reserve clinically, Figure 12.9 illustrates an example of a PET study at rest and after dipyridamole stress, using generator-produced [82]Rb that shows mild "balanced" three-vessel disease (9). The rest study (S1, upper left polar map) is normal. Since it was obtained after dipyridamole, the stress study (S2, lower left polar map) reflects regional relative coronary flow reserve on the same scale of 0 to 100% and is abnormal. Every quadrant in the stress study shows a fall in relative minimum intensity from 82% to 73% of normal in the anterior (A) quadrant, from 73% to 65% of normal intensity in the septal (S) quadrant, from 68% to 50% of normal intensity in the apex (X), and from 74% to 67% of normal intensity in the inferior quadrant, with the high lateral quadrant showing no relative defects, 67% to 66%. However, S2 doesn't show a localized regional or sharply circumscribed relative flow reserve defect.

The upper right polar map, labeled ABS S2/S1, shows the absolute activity in the stress study (S2) divided by the absolute activity in the rest study (S1) expressed as absolute coronary flow reserve, using a model accounting for radionuclide extraction, dose, and cardiac output changes. In this instance, the maximum regional coronary flow reserve located in the anterior-lateral area of the heart in response to

dipyridamole was 4.0 (times resting levels), indicating that this patient responded well to dipyridamole in a small artery to the high anterior lateral myocardium. Since flow reserve was reduced to every quadrant of the heart except to this high anterior lateral area, the PET scan was interpreted without knowledge of clinical data or arteriograms as showing mild to moderate "balanced" three-vessel disease. Thus, despite "balanced" three-vessel disease affecting all major arteries of the heart, at least some part of the myocardium responded well to this vasodilatory stimulus as a normal reference area. By using measures of both relative and absolute coronary flow reserve, balanced three-vessel disease was identified. Coronary arteriography confirmed 50% to 60% diameter narrowing of the three major coronary arteries, thereby allowing medical management and cholesterol lowering therapy.

The entire quantitative analysis requires 26 s to complete on reconstructed, rotated images, with each set of parameters displayed instantaneously on coded push-button command. A simple menu-driven visual interpretation can be coded in quickly while viewing the images and quantitative data beside them. Table 12.1 shows the printed report of all quantitative analysis for Figure 12.8, done automatically in addition to the visual interpretation for each quadrant in the whole heart (10).

The two-study display format can also be used for assessing changes in two sequential stress studies for purposes

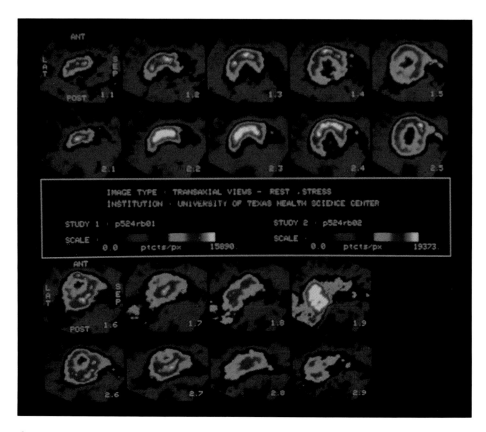

Fig. 12.9 PET images of generator-produced [82]Rb in acquisition (A), (*continued*)

A

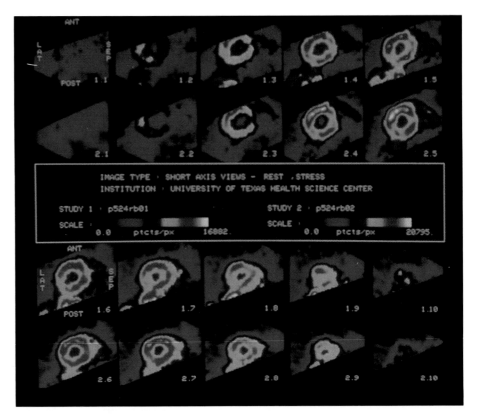

B

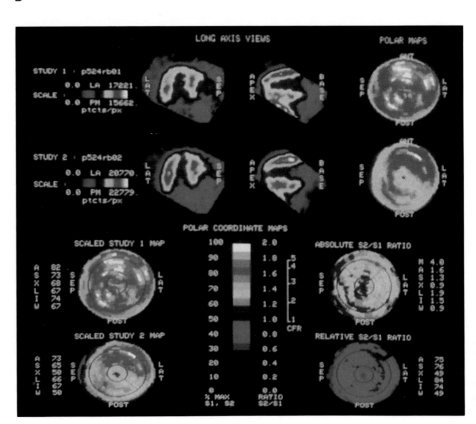

Fig. 12.9 (continued)

short-axis **(B)**, and horizontal (upper left) and vertical (upper right) long-axis views **(C)** of the heart of a patient with mild, "balanced" three-vessel coronary artery disease presented in the same format. See text for details. Reproduced with permission from Gould KL, Kirkeeide R, Buchi M, 1990. (9).

C

Table 12.1 Quantitative PET Analysis UTHSC Tofpet V1.1

PET no: 561	PET ID: p561	Study 1: P561REST	Study 2: P561DIPY
ST date: 3/4/87	RD date: 8/24/88	Tracer S1: Rb	Tracer S2: Rb
Reader: Gould	Quality: Excellent		
Angina: Y	ST: Y	Bkgd S1(%): 22.02	Bkgd S2(%): 19.89
T: Y	Aminophyllin: Y	Bkgd S1(px): 7216.	Bkgd S2(px): 6517

Polar Map	RGN	RGN % Min	RGN % Mean	Regional Fractions 1.5 SD	Regional Fractions 2.0 SD	Regional Fractions 2.5 SD	Whole PCM Fractions		Diagnosis Visual RGN	Inten	Size
S1	A	63	83	0.00	0.00	0.00	All regions		dA	normal	normal
	S	59	74	0.01	0.00	0.00	>0.8	0.45	dS	normal	normal
	X	67	79	0.00	0.00	0.00	>0.6	0.55	dX	normal	normal
	L	74	82	0.00	0.00	0.00	>0.4	0.00	dL	normal	normal
	I	71	85	0.00	0.00	0.00	>>0.2	0.00	dI	normal	normal
	W	59	81	0.00	0.00	0.00	>0.0	0.00	dW	normal	normal
S2	A	50	75	0.31	0.16	0.14	All regions		dA	mild	large
	S	48	59	1.00	0.96	0.81	>0.8	0.19	dS	severe	large
	X	42	62	0.57	0.52	0.49	>0.6	0.51	dX	severe	large
	L	61	77	0.19	0.10	0.03	>0.4	0.30	dL	mild	large
	I	42	82	0.11	0.08	0.01	>0.2	0.00	dI	modrt	medium
	W	42	72	0.48	0.40	0.34	>0.0	0.00	dW	severe	large
S2/ S1 ABS CFR	A	0.8	1.1	0.32	0.24	0.11	MX 5%	2.83	dA	mild	large
	S	0.6	0.9	1.00	0.90	0.49	>1.4	0.01	dS	severe	large
	X	0.5	0.9	0.89	0.56	0.40	>1.25	0.03	dX	severe	large
	L	0.8	1.4	0.24	0.08	0.00	>1.1	0.17	dL	mild	large
	I	0.6	1.6	0.22	0.14	0.06	>0.9	0.48	dI	modrt	medium
	W	0.5	1.1	0.63	0.42	0.26	<0.9	0.31	dW	severe	large
S2/ S1 REL CHG	A	61	88	0.29	0.17	0.09	All regions		dA	mild	large
	S	42	72	1.00	0.76	0.65	>1.0	0.12	dS	severe	large
	X	25	72	0.55	0.48	0.43	>.66	0.63	dX	severe	large
	L	71	94	0.11	0.01	0.00	>.33	0.24	dL	mild	large
	I	31	98	0.17	0.11	0.08	<.33	0.00	dI	modrt	medium
	W	25	86	0.45	0.35	0.29			dW	severe	large

Source: Adapted from Hicks K, Ganti G, Mullani N, et al., 1989. Reference 10.

of evaluating regression/progression of coronary artery disease. Figure 12.10A shows long-axis views and quantitative polar displays of ^{13}N ammonia and treadmill exercise *stress image* before (S1) and the *stress* image (S2) after a six-month period of anti-arrhythmic therapy with no symptoms or clinical event in a patient with prior painless sudden death due to coronary artery disease (10). However, there is obvious progression of the stress perfusion defect antero-apically and laterally, confirmed by quantitative analysis, in addition to a severe inferior defect also present at rest (not shown), indicating a scar. This patient therefore had three-vessel coronary artery disease involving an occluded right coronary artery, moderate and only moderately progressive mid-LAD disease, and markedly progressive severe LCX disease.

Figure 12.10B (upper four polar maps) shows that on the initial stress image (S1) 13% of the heart was beyond 2.5 SD from normals, progressing on the second stress image (S2) six months later to 43% of the heart outside 2.5 SD. Figure 12.10B (lower four polar maps) also shows the stress perfusion image (S1) and the fasting metabolic image using FDG (S2) during stress, showing marked uptake laterally in the

area of worsening stress defect, indicating metabolic ischemia. Inferiorly there is no perfusion or metabolic activity, thereby indicating myocardial scar. In the anterior apical region there is a moderately worsening perfusion defect but no glucose uptake, thereby indicating that the moderate impairment of relative coronary flow reserve in the mid-anterior wall did not cause metabolic ischemia.

Although this patient had ventricular tachycardia controlled on anti-arrhythmics, and no symptoms, on the basis of this much progression of silent coronary artery disease over a six-month period by PET, repeat catheterization was done. It showed that the LAD had progressed from 50% to 70% diameter stenosis and the left circumflex had progressed from no stenosis to near-occlusion. Despite no symptoms and a controlled arrythmia, bypass surgery was carried out because of the progression of disease. This example therefore demonstrates visual and quantitative progression of perfusion defects and metabolic ischemia surrounding a fixed scar, with sufficient accuracy to indicate a major intervention despite no change in symptomatic status.

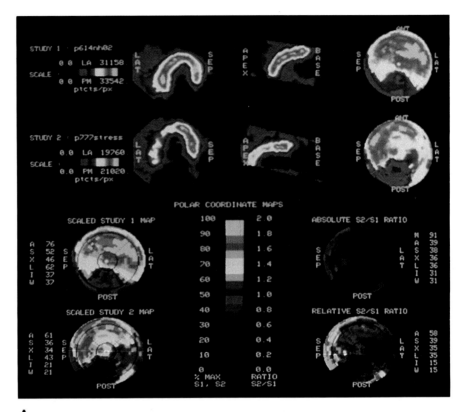

A

Fig. 12.10 Horizontal and vertical long-axis views with quantitative polar map displays of a patient showing progression of silent coronary artery disease, with worsening of anterior and lateral stress perfusion defects over a six-month period. Treadmill exercise stress and ^{13}N ammonia was used in this example. **A** shows the comparison of stress images before (scaled study 1) and stress images after (scaled study 2) the six-month period, with relative defect intensity displayed. The upper four polar maps of **B** show that on the initial stress image (scaled study 1), 13% of the heart was beyond 2.5 SD from normals, progressing to 43% of the heart six months later. The lower four polar maps in **B** compare the final stress perfusion image (scaled study 1) to the fasting FDG at stress (scaled study 2). There is a fixed inferior scar with no perfusion or FDG uptake, a severe reversible stress perfusion defect laterally that takes up FDG on a fasting ischemia protocol, indicating viable, ischemic myocardium, and a less severe anterior apical perfusion defect that does not cause ischemia because there is no glucose uptake in that area. Reproduced with permission from Hicks K, Ganti G, Mullani N, et al., 1989. (10).

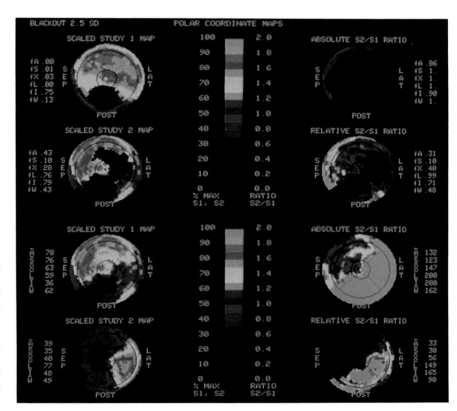

B

SENSITIVITY AND SPECIFICITY OF PET PERFUSION IMAGING

The sensitivity and specificity of diagnosing coronary artery disease by PET in comparison to automated quantitative coronary arteriography are both 95%–98% in symptomatic or asymptomatic individuals (1–8), including balanced three-vessel disease (9,10). False-negative studies are usually associated with distal coronary stenoses of moderate severity or disease of smaller arteries, in which arterial bed size is small, minimizing the defect intensity or the contrast between normal and abnormal areas. False positives are usually associated with nonatheromatous coronary artery abnormalities such as spasm, thrombi, myocardial muscle bridge, or readily identifiable technical artifacts that allow correct interpretation. Although this diagnostic accuracy is better than for other non-invasive technologies for evaluating coronary artery disease, measuring diagnostic accuracy by the endpoints of sensitivity and specificity fails to account for the quantitative capacity of PET to assess severity and size of involved areas rather than just presence or absence of disease.

Most reports on the diagnostic accuracy of myocardial perfusion imaging have used sensitivity/specificity to describe the relation between perfusion image defects and arteriographically documented disease. This method requires binary (positive or negative) classification of both imaging and arteriographic results. Perfusion images have been classified as normal/abnormal, and arteriographic stenosis severity has usually been described in terms of a threshold percent diameter narrowing, such as 50% stenosis, as the criterion for presence of coronary artery disease.

There are three limitations to this use of sensitivity/specificity analysis for assessing accuracy of non-invasive tests for coronary disease. First, coronary atherosclerosis is not an all-or-none condition. Binary classification requires arbitrary threshold criteria and creates artificial classifications for a disease that has a continuous spectrum of severity by both arteriography and perfusion imaging. Thresholds that yield optimal sensitivity and specificity values for one test may yield falsely lower values for a different but more accurate test if its detection threshold is different. For example, an imaging test capable of detecting 40% stenoses may have low specificity according to a 60% stenosis criterion but high specificity according to a 40% stenosis criterion. Second, sensitivity and specificity are markedly affected by disease severity and distribution in the study population (60–62). A sample population with a high frequency of mild disease will be distributed centrally near the threshold values, where scatter is more likely to lower sensitivity and specificity. A sample population with a high prevalence of severe disease causing good contrast between normal and abnormal areas of an image will produce good sensitivity/specificity. Thus, the sensitivity and specificity found in one population may not apply to a different population. The most severe test for a non-invasive method is a low-prevalence, asymptomatic population.

To overcome the limitations of sensitivity/specificity as endpoints of effectiveness, analysis of test results as continuous variables has been proposed; however, this requires quantitative analysis of PET scans and quantitative arteriography (1–4,9,12,45–50,63).

In addition to these limitations, we have also shown that percent diameter narrowing is not an adequate standard for quantifying stenosis severity of coronary artery narrowing (1–4,9–12,45–50), as also confirmed by others (51–54). Percent stenosis does not account for the effects of diffuse disease, eccentricity, stenosis length, absolute cross-sectional area, entrance and exit shape, and absolute dimensions on flow or flow capacity. It is limited by substantial inter- and intraobserver variability.

Alternative approaches providing fluid dynamically correct measurements of graded stenosis severity utilize quantitative arteriographic methods to calculate stenosis resistance (51), pressure-flow curves (49,50), or stenosis flow reserve (1–12,50), as described in previous chapters.

Quantitative coronary arteriography predicts the functional pressure-flow characteristics of stenoses directly measured by flowmeter if all the dimensions of the lesion are taken into account, including relative percent narrowing, absolute luminal area, shape, and integrated length effects (1–12,49,50). Because these multiple dimensions have cumulative hemodynamic effects and interact with each other, they are combined by fluid-dynamic equations into a single measure of stenosis severity that is applicable clinically, stenosis flow reserve. Stenosis flow reserve is the same as coronary flow reserve, but instead of being measured directly by flowmeter, stenosis flow reserve is derived from all geometric dimensions of the narrowing (1–4) as a standardized, single, integrated measure of its severity for standardized conditions of pressure and normal reference vasodilator reserve, as described in previous chapters. Thus, we use the term "stenosis flow reserve" in reference to calculated coronary flow reserve derived from anatomic stenosis dimensions by quantitative analysis of coronary arteriograms. We use the term coronary

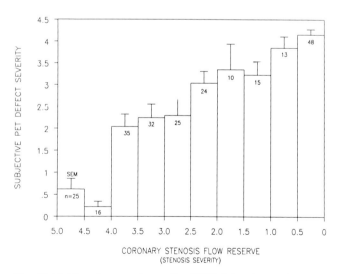

Fig. 12.11 Visually scored severity of PET defect from 0 (normal) to 5 (severe defect), related to stenosis flow reserve by automated quantitative coronary arteriography.

flow reserve for flow reserve directly measured by a flow-meter, Doppler catheter, or perfusion imaging. The concept of arteriographic stenosis flow reserve has been well developed theoretically, validated by comparison with directly measured flow reserve experimentally (2,9), and proven clinically valuable by comparison with regional PET perfusion defects in patients (1,4). Therefore, stenosis flow reserve provides the best arteriographic definition of stenosis severity, suitable as a gold standard for comparison to noninvasive imaging. Using stenosis flow reserve as the gold standard, PET has a diagnostic accuracy of 95%–98%, even in asymptomatic patients (1,4).

The quantitative severity of coronary artery stenoses correlates with severity of the corresponding PET perfusion defect on rest-dipyridamole studies. Severity of PET perfusion defects read by two readers blinded to clinical or arteriographic data and graded visually a severity scale from 0 (normal) to 5 (most severe) correlate well with arteriographic severity of disease. This relation between defect severity by PET and stenosis flow reserve by quantitative coronary arteriography is shown in Figure 12.11. Further analysis to compare automated measure of PET severity, independent of visual interpretation, to automated quantitative coronary arteriography is currently underway.

13

Quantitation of PET Perfusion Images

PET is regarded as a quantitative imaging modality. However, there are two forms of quantitation which are commonly confused. Most importantly, the term quantitative imaging refers to reconstruction of tomographic images that quantitatively reflect or recover the actual or true distribution of activity in the target organ or field of view. This type of quantitative data recovery depends on the technical characteristics of the camera and the duration of imaging permitted by the half-life of the positron tracer, as discussed in a later chapter.

The second type of quantitation involves measurement of biological processes, such as myocardial perfusion in cc/min/g or glucose uptake in grams of glucose per gram of myocardium per minute. Biological quantitative measurements require both quantitative imaging of activity distribution and a model of radiotracer behavior in vivo that relates the imaged activity to biological units being measured, for example, blood flow. Historically, biological measurements were considered to be the greatest potential advantage of PET. However, recent data suggests that the value of absolute biological measurements may be less useful than relative quantitative distribution of activity.

There are two basic problems with biological quantitation. The first is whether the assumptions inherent in every model apply in vivo under conditions seen clinically, and therefore whether absolute measurements can be made accurately. The second limitation is whether absolute biological measurements are valuable per se, even if they could be made accurately with the model chosen. For example, measurement of absolute myocardial perfusion in cc/min/g has been made with a variety of models using [82]Rb (10,37–39), ^{13}N ammonia (40–43), or [15]O water (43–44) in order to determine absolute coronary flow reserve, reflecting stenosis severity, and absolute coronary flow, reflecting myocardial ischemia.

However, idealized exact measures of absolute coronary flow and flow reserve by calibrated flowmeter in animals is highly variable and may be an unsatisfactory measure of stenosis severity under changing physiologic conditions and workload (9), as described in previous chapters. Relative maximum flow distribution or relative flow reserve, without determining absolute flow, is a more reliable measure of stenosis severity (9). Similarly, absolute flow measurements have not been particularly useful for determining when myocardial ischemia or necrosis occurs, since demand is not taken into account; however, relative flow distribution expressed in relative terms as percent of normal areas corre-lates well with arteriographic severity (1,4,9,12,28,29), exercise or pacing ischemia (6,13,14), or necrosis (16,64–66), as well or better than absolute flow measurements. Uptake of positron-labeled glucose analogues relative to uptake of a perfusion tracer, without the calculation of absolute glucose uptake, has also proven very useful clinically (15,17,18,21–23). Similar conclusions have been reached about absolute measurements of glucose metabolism in the brain, where visual interpretation of images has proven to be clinically more useful than absolute quantitative measurements (67). Thus, the value of cardiac PET resides in its accurate quantitation of regional radiotracer distribution.

Although measuring absolute myocardial perfusion in cc/min/g may not be very useful clinically, the measurement of both relative and absolute coronary flow reserve is important for assessing stenoses. To the extent that a flow model can improve these functional measures of stenosis severity, it may serve a practical role. In this context, basic tracer kinetic principles for the most clinically used PET perfusion tracers, ^{13}N ammonia and [82]Rb, are discussed.

PRINCIPLES OF QUANTITATIVE MODELS

Quantitative analysis of PET data will depend on the tracer used, the organ being studied, the behavior of the tracer in that organ, the way in which the tracer is injected, and, finally, the function being analyzed. Once this information is defined, a "model" is formulated to describe mathematically the kinetics of that tracer in that organ. Therefore, a model is simply the equation that describes the behavior of the tracer. This model forms the link between the physiological or metabolic characteristics of the tracer and the quantitative data obtained from a positron camera. Count data obtained with the camera over time are then inserted into the mathematical expression of the model in order to obtain the final desired physiologic measurement, such as blood flow, blood volume, or metabolic rates in the organ.

THE SIMPLEST ONE-COMPARTMENT MODEL

In the simplest model, a sample volume of an organ image is treated as a volume of myocardium that has a characteristic arterial input and venous output of the radiotracer. We call this example a one-compartment model because the analysis of the delivery and exit of the isotope to and from that region is based on the single volume of tissue being imaged.

From the basic physical principle of conservation of mass, we can then reason that the amount of tracer in the sample volume of tissue at any one time is equal to the activity delivered to it minus the activity that has egressed from it. Thus, if we are observing the passage of the tracer through the sample volume of tissue with an external detector, such as a positron camera, the image that we see is the difference between the total cumulative activity delivered to the tissue minus the total activity leaving that tissue. The activity left in the tissue at any instant in time is called the residual tracer deposited in the sample volume.

A mathematical expression for the residual is shown below, where $R(T)$ is the residual amount of tracer in the tissue at any one time, T.

$$R(T) = \int_0^T FC_a(t)\,dt - \int_0^T FC_v(t)\,dt \qquad (1)$$

where F is flow in milliliters per minute per gram (mL/min/g) of tissue, $C_a(t)$ is the arterial tracer concentration, and $C_v(t)$ is the venous concentration of the tracer. The integration sign represents a summation of the total amount delivered to or leaving the sample volume between the time $t = 0$ and $t = T$. The product of total flow and arterial concentration FC_a is the instantaneous total amount of radiotracer delivered at any one time and has units of

$$\frac{cc}{min} \times \frac{cts}{cc} \quad or \quad \frac{cts}{min}$$

This simple equation then forms the basis for most mathematical analyses of tracer kinetics for a single-compartment model.

THE CONCEPT OF EXTRACTION

The analysis of PET data using the single-compartment model will depend on the metabolic characteristics of the tracer in the sample volume of tissue. The behavior of a tracer in the tissue characteristically falls into one of three categories: (1) the tracer is not extracted, taken up, or trapped in the tissue; (2) the tracer is totally extracted, taken up, or trapped in the tissue; or (3) the tracer is partially extracted in the tissue. A variation on (2) and (3) is that the tracer is partially or completely extracted but is partially or completely metabolized into other compartments within the myocardial cells, or is washed out of the field as a metabolic product. The concept of extraction of the tracer by the organ being imaged is therefore a fundamental one, which describes the function of the organ (i.e., how it handles that tracer) and is central to all quantitative imaging. The residual tracer retained in the tissue is what we see on heart images: that is, a picture of thallium or rubidium retained in the heart muscle.

NON-EXTRACTED TRACERS

Let us consider as an example the case of a non-extracted tracer, such as ^{11}C-labeled carbon monoxide, used to produce ^{11}C-labeled carboxyhemoglobin. Since carboxyhemoglobin is bound to red cells, the tracer will be confined to the capillary

vascular space and will not cross capillary membranes. If the initial injection of a tracer is in the form of a sharp bolus of activity, then the concentration of the tracer as it is delivered to the region of interest will be fairly sharply defined in time, as shown in the upper panel of Figure 13.1 (68). Since there is no extraction of that tracer in the tissue, the total amount delivered by the arterial blood has to equal the amount that egresses from the tissue through the venous drainage. Thus, the venous concentration, as shown in the middle panel of Figure 13.1, will be slightly delayed, owing to the time required for the tracer to pass through the capillaries. The venous concentration curve will also have a broader shape, due to the various lengths of capillaries and therefore different capillary transit times.

An external detector records the passage of the bolus of activity through the capillaries in the region of interest and thereby records the residual tracer, as shown in the lower panel of Figure 13.1. Since the tracer is not extracted or trapped in the myocardium in this example, the residual function, after the time for the bolus to pass through the region, must be zero, since the input and the output are equal.

The importance of how the tracer is injected can be analyzed by assuming that the tracer is injected as a slow infusion producing a constant blood concentration in time. For a constant infusion or slow injection, the concentration of the tracer at the arterial and the venous side will be equal and constant during the infusion period, and the residual activity will also be constant. A PET image obtained under these circumstances will show the tracer in the blood pool, and if the concentration of the tracer is also measured, an estimate of the organ blood volume can be obtained from this data. Therefore, non-extracted tracers are typically used to measure the blood volume of an organ.

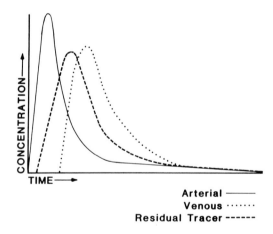

Fig. 13.1 Schematic time-activity curves for a non-extracted tracer, such as ^{11}C-labeled carboxyhemoglobin, will have the form of a sharply defined bolus that passes through a region of myocardial tissue. Since the tracer does not cross capillary membranes, the total amount delivered in arterial blood will be matched by the amount present in venous drainage (slightly delayed because of the time required for tracer to pass through the capillaries), leaving no residual activity. Reproduced with permission from Gould KL, Mullani N, Wong WH, et al., 1986. (68).

TOTALLY EXTRACTED TRACERS

The second type of tracer is totally extracted, taken up, or trapped in its first pass through tissue. If the tracer is totally extracted, none of it leaves through venous drainage, and therefore the concentration of the tracer in the venous side is zero, as shown in the upper panel of Figure 13.2 (68). Recall from Equation 1 that the residual tracer in the tissue is the difference between the total arterial activity delivered and the activity drained through veins from the sample volume. Since the venous concentration is zero, then the total activity leaving the region of interest is zero, and therefore the second term on the right-hand side of Equation 1 is zero. A simpler equation then remains, which describes the amount of residual tracer as a function of flow multiplied by the arterial concentration of the tracer:

$$R(T) = \int_0^T FCa(t)\, dt \qquad (2)$$

Since the total amount of activity delivered to the tissue region of interest is the product of the flow multiplied by the arterial concentration of the tracer, Equation 2 can be rearranged such that flow is equal to the amount of residual tracer divided by the total arterial concentration accumulated over time (A) (i.e., integrated arterial concentration-time curve). Thus,

$$F = \frac{R}{A} = \frac{R(T)}{\int_0^T C_a(t)\, dt} \qquad (3)$$

The amount of residual tracer R can be measured noninvasively by PET as well as the arterial concentration of tracer accumulated over time, or arterial input function, which is the denominator term. Regional blood flow can then

be computed for any organ. Labeled microspheres are totally extracted tracers for which this equation applies. However, for clinical applications there are no current perfusion radiotracers that are 100% extracted.

PARTIALLY EXTRACTED TRACERS

The third type of tracer is one that is partially extracted in the tissue and is characteristic of most metabolic or perfusion radiotracers in clinical use. Images of partially extracted radiotracers are harder to interpret than for the totally extracted or non-extracted tracers, owing to the variation in extraction of the tracer at higher blood flows. As shown in Figure 13.3 (68), a certain fraction, E, of these tracers will be

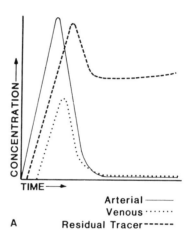

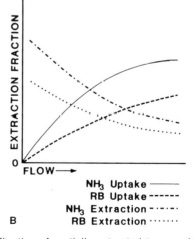

Fig. 13.3 Kinetics of partially extracted tracers. **(A)** Schematic time-activity curves demonstrate partial tissue uptake of tracer, with the remainder appearing in the venous drainage. **(B)** Uptake and extraction fraction of two partially extracted tracers, ^{13}N ammonia and ^{82}Rb, are shown as a function of flow. Extraction of these and similar tracers falls off at higher flows because shortened residence time in the capillary bed reduces uptake across capillary membranes. Reproduced with permission from Gould KL, Mullani N, Wong WH, et al., 1986. (68).

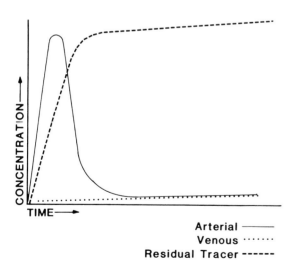

Fig. 13.2 Schematic time-activity curves for a tracer that is totally extracted, taken up, or trapped in its first pass through tissue will show no venous drainage. Residual concentration reaches a maximum plateau value, which can be measured noninvasively by positron emission tomography. Reproduced with permission from Gould KL, Mullani N, Wong WH, et al., 1986. (68).

extracted or taken up by the tissue as the tracer passes through the organ, and the remainder will egress through the venous drainage. Equation 1 can therefore be rewritten by expressing the venous concentration of the tracer as what is left over after extraction from arterial blood. The term for the venous drainage would then be written as $(1-E)$ times the arterial concentration, as in Equation 4.

$$R(T) = \int_0^T FC_a(t)\, dt - (1 - E) \int_0^T FC_a(t)\, dt \qquad (4)$$

This equation can then be simplified to represent the amount of residual tracer R, as in Equation 5.

$$R(T) = E \int_0^T FC_a(t)\, dt \qquad (5)$$

The relation between the arterial concentration, the venous concentration, and the residual tracer for a partially extracted tracer is illustrated in Figure 13.3. Flow can be computed as the amount of residual tracer divided by the product of extraction multiplied by the accumulated arterial input, as in Equation 6:

$$F = \frac{R(T)}{E \int_0^T C_a(t)\, dt} \qquad (6)$$

where F is blood flow or perfusion in the tissue volume imaged, R is the amount of residual tracer activity or uptake in that volume of tissue, the integral term is the accumulated arterial concentration (integrated time-activity curve), and E is the fraction or percent of tracer extracted and taken up into the tissue on the first passage of the tracer through the vascular bed of the sample volume. In practice, R, E, and integrated arterial input are measured with the PET camera or assumed, and F is calculated from these measured values.

THE TWO-COMPARTMENT MODEL—AN EXAMPLE WITH CLINICAL APPLICATION USING ⁸²RB IN THE HEART

Data obtained with partially extracted tracers, such as ^{82}Rb, are a good example of a kinetic model with clinical application. However, a tracer such as ^{82}Rb, which is partially extracted in the heart, is not extracted at all in the brain, since the rubidium ion does not cross the blood/brain barrier. Thus, analysis of a partially extracted tracer in different organs requires an understanding of the kinetics of that tracer in each specific organ being studied.

Myocardial extraction of rubidium requires analysis with a slightly more complex model that has two compartments instead of the one-compartment model discussed above. Rubidium is an analogue of potassium and is taken up rapidly by the myocardial cell, where it is retained for a long time within the cell. The amount of ^{82}Rb extracted by the cell will be a fraction E of the total rubidium in the blood on its first pass through the myocardium. Therefore, the amount of radioactivity detected by PET from a small region of the myocardium will consist of that activity trapped in the cell plus the free circulating activity passing through the sample volume without being taken up into the cells. Analysis of the activity data collected by PET allows the separation of these

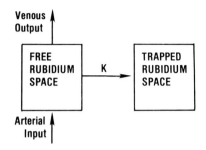

Fig. 13.4 The two-compartment model, showing the relationship between free (circulating) and trapped radiotracer, using ^{82}Rb as an example. The radioactivity measured by an external detector from a small region of myocardium will consist of that activity trapped or extracted by the cells, plus the free activity in the vascular or interstitial space (radioactivity not taken up into cells). Normally, ^{82}Rb does not return to the free space once trapped in the cell. Reproduced with permission from Mullani N, Goldstein RA, Gould KL, et al., 1983. (38).

two components by using a two-compartment model shown in Figure 13.4 (37–39,68). The two compartments are the free rubidium space, consisting of the vascular plus interstitial spaces, and the trapped rubidium or intracellular space. An average or lumped rate constant, K, is used to represent mathematically the net transfer rate of rubidium from the free space to the trapped space, since backward leak of ^{82}Rb back out of the cell does not occur for viable cells.

Therefore, the total tracer activity in the myocardial sample volume detected by PET, P(t), can be mathematically described as the sum of the free activity F(t) and the activity trapped in the myocardial cells M(t), as follows:

$$P(t) = F(t) + M(t) \qquad (7)$$

The free activity F(t) can in turn be mathematically characterized by a suitable experimentally validated exponential function such as

$$F(t) = bte^{-at} \qquad (8)$$

where b and a are constants. The trapped activity M(t) can then be obtained by subtracting the free activity from the total activity P(t) measured by PET at each instant in time after an intravenous injection of rubidium. This procedure for separating the two components of the observed PET data is shown in Figure 13.5 (37–39,68). This illustration demonstrates the rubidium activity detected over the myocardium by an external detector and the best computer-generated "fit" of the two-compartment model to the actual recorded activity from the heart. The first-pass extraction is determined as the activity trapped in the myocardium divided by the total activity measured by PET at the time of peak counts. It is expressed as the fraction of total delivered tracer extracted into the myocardium on first pass through the tissues. Flow can then be determined by using this extraction fraction in Equation 6 and by measuring final myocardial uptake as well as the arterial concentration of tracer by PET.

Thus, we have theoretically shown with a single practical example using rubidium how the data collected by PET can be analyzed to determine two important biological processes,

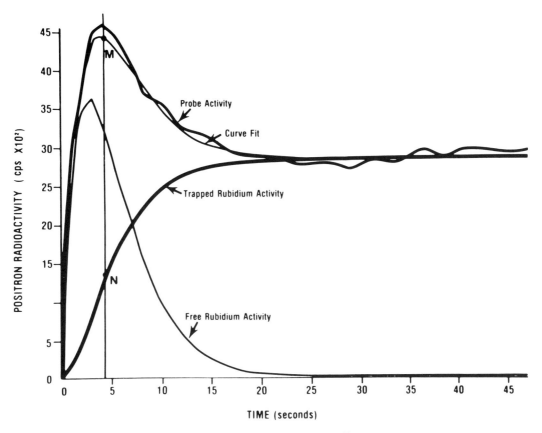

Fig. 13.5 Separation of the two components of observed myocardial uptake of [82]Rb into free activity (in the vascular and interstitial space) and trapped activity (in the intracellular space) can be accomplished by analysis using a two-compartment model. Extraction fraction is computed by dividing the trapped rubidium activity (N) by total activity delivered to myocardium (M) at the time of peak counts. Reproduced with permission from Goldstein RA, Mullani N, Fisher D, et al., 1983. (39).

extraction fraction and flow. The extraction fraction of a given compound by an organ is an important descriptor of its metabolic behavior and/or the function of the cell membrane, quantified as the rate and extent to which the tracer is taken up or released from the cell. Normal myocardial cells retain rubidium, while necrotic cells release rubidium, as detailed in a later chapter. Thus, information about the extent of cellular injury as well as the mechanism (i.e., a measured reduction in flow) can be obtained by quantitative analysis of PET images.

MODELS FOR METABOLIZED SUBSTRATES—THREE OR MORE COMPARTMENTS

The multicompartmental approach to modeling the tissue described above can also be expanded to three anatomic subcompartments, which are the capillary bed, the interstitial space, and the cellular space. The boundaries between the spaces, that is, the capillary wall and the cellular membrane, determine the rate of transport of a tracer, and intracellular trapping or metabolism determines its subsequent fate. The rates at which a tracer is transported from one compartment to the other can be represented by a series of rate constants describing the rate of transport across each boundary in both directions, into as well as out of the cell. With a more complex multicompartmental model, estimates may be obtained of the individual rate constants for each membrane and the amount of tracer in each compartment. This information in turn provides greater insights into the behavior or fate of the tracer or its products in each of the compartments and transport of each tracer by each of the different membranes.

For example, the extraction of [82]Rb in the normal myocardium indicates that rubidium behaves as an analogue for potassium and is trapped in the cellular space. The cell membrane offers great resistance to the egress of rubidium from the cell under normal circumstances. However, in necrotic myocardial tissue the cell membrane is damaged, thereby allowing leakage of rubidium or potassium out of the cell. Therefore, measuring the rate at which rubidium leaves myocardial tissue can provide valuable information about the integrity of the cell membranes after injury. Similarly, the rate at which rubidium is transported across the blood/brain barrier can be used to measure the integrity of the blood/brain barrier after a stroke. Normal brain tissues do not allow the passage of rubidium across the cerebral capillary wall until the blood/brain barrier is damaged through some injury.

Modeling the metabolic processes in tissues requires even more complex models with more compartments. The added compartments are needed in order to describe the different paths of the metabolic cycle within the cell. We will not elaborate on these models, which are mathematically complex and predominantly for research purposes. The principles of quantitative imaging are better illustrated by the simpler models described above, which also have clinical relevance.

Having reviewed some fundamentals of tracer kinetics and of the quantitative analysis of PET data, we may now consider some of their clinical applications.

FLOW MODEL FOR DETERMINING ABSOLUTE AND RELATIVE CORONARY FLOW RESERVE NONINVASIVELY BY PET

Based on the above discussion, myocardial flow (F) can be determined with a diffusible extracted tracer such as ^{13}N ammonia or ^{82}Rb after intravenous injection based on the generic expression

$$Flow = \frac{myocardial\ uptake}{(extraction)\ (total\ delivered\ dose)}$$

Extraction is the percent of radionuclide extracted by the organ in the first pass of radiotracer through that organ. Total delivered dose is the integrated time-arterial concentration of radionuclide during the time of myocardial uptake. Mathematically this expression is written as follows:

$$F = \frac{U_T}{E \int_0^T C_a\ dt}$$

where F is flow in mL/min/g, U_T is uptake in counts/s/g at time T after injection of tracer, E is the first-pass extraction fraction of radioactivity taken up in myocardium, and $\int_0^T C_a dt$ is the integrated time-arterial concentration C_a during uptake U_T.

In order to interpret and apply clinical quantitative imaging techniques, it is useful to understand the basic concepts of how metabolic or flow tracers behave in the body. The clearest way of explaining these concepts is to begin with a simple animal model and then extend that idea to the more imperfect, realistic approaches for humans.

For measuring blood flow using labeled microspheres in experimental animals, the above equation is used with the extraction equal to one, or 100%, since the microspheres are completely trapped in the capillaries of the tissue after left atrial injection. At the time of injection, an arterial reference sample is withdrawn at a known rate and volume in order to determine the arterial-time dose delivered to all arterial beds. The animal is then sacrificed or the tissue biopsied for invitro counting in order to determine myocardial tissue uptake; flow is calculated using a form of this equation with extraction equal to one. This microsphere technique requires left atrial injection distal to lung capillaries, which would trap the microspheres if injected intravenously. Left atrial injection also ensures proper mixing of the tracer at ostia of the coronary arteries. It also requires tissue samples, for the

counting of myocardial uptake of activity. It is, therefore, not suitable for patient or noninvasive studies.

In contrast, diffusible tracers are only partially extracted with extraction fractions less than one, or less than 100%. The percent of tracer extracted depends on flow and falls as flow increases. Since extraction is variable and dependent on flow, accurate flow determinations require measuring extraction of the radiotracer in its first pass through the organ after intravenous injection. Figure 13.6 (57) illustrates these concepts.

How are these ideas related to a clinician looking at the radionuclide image of a patient's heart or other organ? The picture the clinician looks at with current imaging techniques, such as positron tomography or the standard gamma camera, shows the distribution of tracer uptake in the organ. As shown above, uptake is the product of flow and extraction and is therefore only an indirect index of perfusion, as follows:

$$F \times E = \frac{U_T}{\int_0^T C_a\ dt}$$ or

$$visual\ image = F \times E = \frac{myocardial\ uptake}{delivered\ dose}$$

Since the dose delivered to the heart or arterial input is the same for the various regions of an organ for a given single injection, relative regional uptake in an abnormal region (R) compared to normal (R_n) of an organ is given by a simplified equation:

$$\frac{F \times E}{F_n \times E_n} = \frac{R}{R_n}$$

where $F \times E$ equals relative regional myocardial uptake in the distribution of the stenotic artery and the normal (n) artery.

Thus, the image the clinician sees is a picture of the regional values of extraction of the tracer multiplied by flow, or regional $E \times F$.

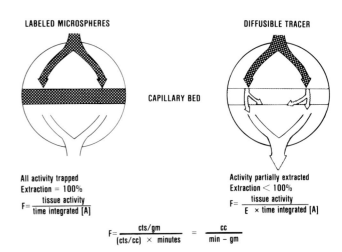

Fig. 13.6 Simplified conceptual equations illustrating the method for determining blood flow with either microspheres or a diffusible tracer. Reproduced with permission from Gould KL, 1986. (57).

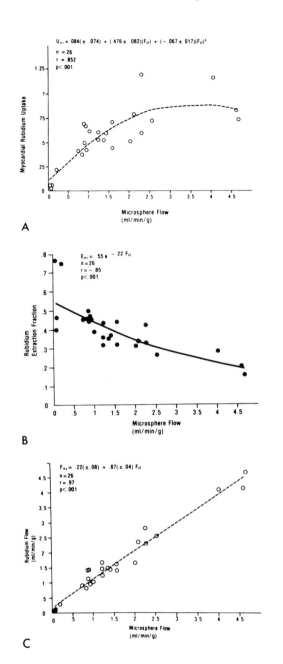

Fig. 13.7 (A) Relation between myocardial uptake (normalized for arterial input) of rubidium and microsphere-determined flow (Fμ) under control conditions. Radiotracer uptake, which is the product of flow and extraction, is linearly related to flow up to 2.5 times normal, but overestimates low flow rates and underestimates the high flows.

(B) Relation between extraction of rubidium (E_Rb) and microsphere-determined flow (Fμ) under controlled flow conditions. Extraction decreases at high flow because of decreased residence time; hence, product of flow and extraction (i.e., uptake) underestimates high flow.

(C) Relation between rubidium-determined flow (F_Rb) and microsphere-determined flow (Fμ) under controlled conditions. Rubidium values were obtained by dividing uptake by extraction as determined by the model. All panels reproduced with permission from Goldstein RA, Mullani N, Fisher D, et al., 1983. (39).

This relative uptake of activity is linearly related to flow at normal control levels of myocardial flow for ^{13}N ammonia and [82]Rb. However, at high flow it underestimates true flow, since extraction decreases at high flow because of decreased residence time of the tracer in capillaries, with less time for extraction or exchange across the capillary membrane, as illustrated in Figure 13.3B. Very low flow is somewhat overestimated because extraction is increased, owing to long residence time.

Therefore, the final, most important concept is that the image seen by the clinician shows the regional distribution in the organ of the net uptake of radionuclide tracer as affected by flow-dependent extraction fraction and volume of flow delivering tracer to the myocardial bed.

According to the equations above, the image of a perfusion scan shows relative distribution of radionuclide uptake, which is not the same as relative flow distribution, because flow-dependent extraction has not been accounted for at resting conditions. Radiotracer extraction fraction is approximately uniform for resting myocardial flow, since the relative range of resting flows are relatively narrow, that is, 0 to 1. Accordingly, a perfusion image at rest reasonably reflects relative distribution of perfusion. However, after intravenous dipyridamole, coronary flows may range from resting levels up to 5 times baseline. In this case, the image does not reflect flow distribution as well as at rest, owing to decreasing extraction fraction at high flows in some areas of the heart. A stress perfusion image would accurately show relative flow reserve, as discussed in earlier chapters, if regional variation in extraction fraction associated with regional differences in maximum flow were accounted for.

Absolute flow reserve can be qualitatively assessed as the ratio of the stress perfusion image to the rest perfusion image. However, this image ratio is the stress/rest radionuclide uptake ratio. It is not a flow ratio, because of lower extraction at high flows during which the stress image was obtained. In addition, the total dose of perfusion radiotracer delivered to the heart decreases if cardiac output increases after dipyridamole or stress conditions. The upper panel of Figure 13.7 shows the proportionate decrease in radionuclide uptake as flow increases, owing to falling extraction at higher flows (38,39).

Therefore, for measuring absolute flow reserve, radiotracer extraction as well as the effect of altered cardiac output on the radiotracer dose injected or arterial input function must be accounted for. Consequently, the relation between coronary flow reserve, radiotracer extraction, and arterial input function are described below as a simple practical model applicable to clinical studies that improves diagnostic information and relates the PET perfusion image to the concepts of coronary flow reserve developed in prior chapters.

RELATION OF CORONARY FLOW AND FLOW RESERVE TO EXTRACTION FRACTION, CARDIAC OUTPUT, AND ARTERIAL INPUT FUNCTION

As flow increases, the fraction of radiotracer extracted on first pass through the coronary vascular bed falls from 50% to 25% in open-chest dogs, as shown in the middle panel of Figure

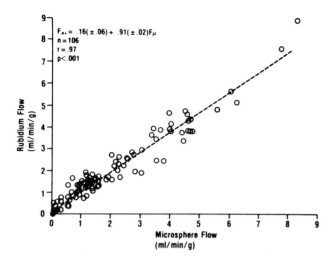

Fig. 13.8 Composite results for flow by rubidium (F_{Rb}) compared with flow by microspheres ($F\mu$). Data represent all injections done under control conditions and after interventions. Reproduced with permission from Goldstein RA, Mullani N, Fisher D, 1983. (39).

13.7 (38,39). The equation relating extraction fraction to flow from Figure 13.7 is $E = .55e^{-.22F}$. If extraction fraction and arterial input function are measured experimentally, flow measured by ^{82}Rb and detector probes over the heart equals that by microspheres shown in the lowest panel of Figure 13.7 and in Figure 13.8 (39). The relation between coronary flow reserve, extraction fraction, and arterial input, based on the above experimental observations for a two-compartment model, can be derived as follows:

$$\frac{U_s}{U_r} = \frac{F_s}{F_r} \times \frac{E_s}{E_r} \times \frac{A_s}{A_r}$$

where U is uptake, F is flow, E is extraction, A is integrated arterial input, and the subscript r is rest and s is dipyridamole stress. Using our empirically derived relation between extraction and flow by microspheres, $E = 0.55e^{-.22F}$ (37–39), this equation can be written as:

$$\frac{U_s}{U_r} = \left(\frac{A_s}{A_r}\right) \frac{F_s}{F_r} e^{.22(Fr - Fs)}$$

U_s/U_r and arterial input function ratios A_s/A_r are determined from the PET scan and flow reserve F_s/F_r determined from a look-up table. If the same dose of radionuclide is injected at rest and stress, this equation reduces to:

$$\frac{U_s}{U_r} = \frac{CO_r}{CO_s} \left(\frac{F_s}{F_r}\right) e^{.22(Fr - Fs)}$$

where CO is cardiac output at rest and stress. As an example, cardiac output increases by approximately 25% to 50% after dipyridamole (69–74) where:

$$\frac{CO_r}{CO_s} = \frac{1}{(\%\Delta CO + 1}$$

or, conservatively, for a maximum of 50% increase in cardiac output

$$CO_r/CO_s = 0.67$$

This equation then becomes:

$$\frac{U_s}{U_r} = .67 \left(\frac{F_s}{F_r}\right) e^{.22(Fr - Fs)}$$

Based on this equation, a look-up table gives values of F_s/F_r or coronary flow reserve for observed values of U_s/U_r by PET in order to show feasibility. Myocardial extraction and uptake of ^{13}N ammonia also decreases at elevated flow. With a similar empirical equation relating extraction or uptake to flow, flow values can then be determined by a similar model (75). Figures 12.8 and 12.9 in the preceding chapter show a clinical PET study incorporating this model to give absolute coronary flow reserve on the CFR scale beside the upper right polar map labeled absolute S2/S1 ratio.

Figure 13.9 summarizes the relation between true coronary flow reserve, as measured by flowmeter (horizontal axis), and the expected or theoretical flow reserve that would be observed by PET for various changes in extraction and cardiac output based on the above equation. The straight line shows the ideal relation if extraction or cardiac output did not change from rest to stress or was accounted for. The uppermost curved line of Figure 13.9 shows the expected

Rb UPTAKE RATIO vs CORONARY FLOW RESERVE

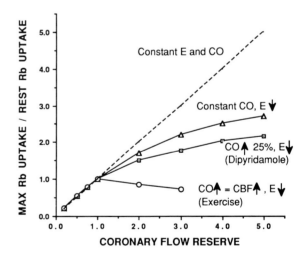

Fig. 13.9 Relation between coronary flow reserve by flowmeter (horizontal axis) and myocardial uptake reserve (vertical axis) for a radionuclide perfusion tracer with (a) constant extraction fraction, cardiac output (CO), and dose at all flows from rest to a maximum of four times baseline (dashed line); (b) a falling extraction fraction as flow increases, according to the equation given in the text, but with constant cardiac output ($\triangle$—$\triangle$); (c) a falling extraction fraction, according to the equation in the text, and 25% increase in cardiac output as occurs with dipyridamole (▣—▣); (d) a falling extraction fraction and an increase in cardiac output comparable to that which may occur with exercise stress ($\bigcirc$—$\bigcirc$).

measured flow reserve by the radionuclide method if at a four-times increase in flow, extraction of radiotracer fell to half of its value at resting flow with no change in cardiac output. If extraction fraction were constant and cardiac output increased by 100%, coronary flow reserve by the radionuclide technique would also be erroneously low, corresponding to this same line. In reality, both occur as in the middle curved line of Figure 13.9, that is, extraction fraction falls at higher flows and cardiac output rises. The best approximation to reality is a fall in extraction by the above equation and an average increase of 25% in cardiac output after dipyridamole, in a total of 106 patients from five studies in which cardiac output was measured before and after intravenous dipyridamole (69–74). Consequently, the radiotracer uptake ratio of the stress to rest images is only 2 to 1 for a flow ratio of 4 to 1. This analysis explains why the range of the uptake ratios on the stress/rest ratio image is only 1.0 to 2.0 in Figures 12.8 and 12.9, corresponding to flow ratios of 1 to 4.

This analysis also explains the reported fall in myocardial thallium uptake during exercise stress, whereas with dipyridamole stress, myocardial uptake of thallium increases in the same patients (47,48). With exercise, cardiac output usually increases as much or more than coronary blood flow. Extraction fraction also falls as coronary flow increases during stress. The cumulative effect of a fall in extraction and increase in cardiac output comparable to the increase in coronary blood flow makes myocardial radionuclide uptake and activity in the heart during stress lower than at rest, as shown by the lowest curve in Figure 13.9. This apparent paradox of lower cardiac radionuclide activity despite increasing coronary flow is due to the falling extraction fraction at high coronary flows, combined with a rise in cardiac output to the same extent as coronary flow. With dipyridamole, coronary flow increases proportionately much more than cardiac output. Therefore, myocardial radionuclide activity after dipyridamole is greater than at rest, whereas myocardial activity with exercise stress is less than at rest (47,48).

ROLE OF HANDGRIP IN DIPYRIDAMOLE PERFUSION IMAGING

Originally, handgrip during dipyridamole was reported to increase coronary flow more than dipyridamole alone, based on coronary sinus thermodilution measurements (74). However, direct arterial flow velocity measurements with a Doppler catheter do not confirm this augmentation of coronary artery flow by handgrip (76). However, handgrip with dipyridamole reflexly increases aortic pressure (47,48) and aortic impedance, thereby limiting the increased cardiac output compared to that after dipyridamole without handgrip. Therefore the potential benefit of adding handgrip to dipyridamole for perfusion imaging may be to reduce the increase in cardiac output after dipyridamole, thereby minimizing differences in arterial input function at rest and stress. Minimizing or accounting for these differences make the measurement of absolute coronary flow reserve more accurate.

The coronary flow reserve scale in Figures 12.8 and 12.9 uses a constant ratio of resting to stress cardiac output of 0.67 (reflecting a CO of 50% with dipyridamole in man) which may not hold true for all individual patients. Accordingly,

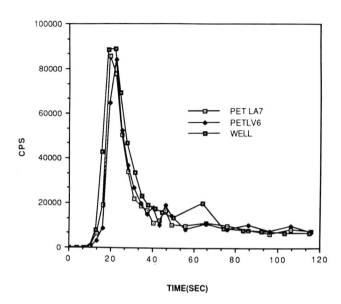

Fig. 13.10 Arterial input function by serial blood sampling and by serial 3-s PET images.

flow reserve would be more accurately measured if arterial input formation were determined for each patient. Figure 13.10 shows an experimental arterial input function obtained by serial PET images every three seconds as activity passes through the left ventricular blood pool. The first activity curve is that obtained by direct arterial blood sampling at the aortic root in order to illustrate that the arterial input function determined by noninvasive PET is comparable to direct blood sampling. The second curve is from PET images displaced by the transit time through the same catheter, which is known and readily shifted to the left.

Although feasible, measuring arterial input function by PET is now a research procedure, because it is time-consuming and virtually all PET cameras saturate at the high count levels present with passage of the full-dose bolus of radionuclide through the left ventricle. Consequently, we are now developing a very fast camera capable of accepting these very high count rates and a simple method for determining arterial input corrections for measuring absolute coronary flow reserve automatically on a routine basis.

APPLICABILITY TO HUMANS OF THE FLOW MODEL DERIVED FROM EXPERIMENTAL DATA

The relation between myocardial flow determined by radiolabelled microspheres and ^{82}Rb first-pass myocardial extraction is described experimentally by the empirical equation $E = 0.55e^{-0.22F}$, where F is flow in cc/min/g and E is first-pass extraction as analyzed in the previous section. Based on this relation, coronary flow reserve is related to myocardial uptake of ^{82}Rb by the equation derived previously:

$$\frac{U_s}{U_r} = \frac{CO_r}{CO_s} \frac{F_s}{F_r} e^{0.22(Fr - Fs)}$$

where, as defined previously, U_s is myocardial [82]Rb uptake after dipyridamole, U_r is uptake at rest, CO is cardiac output after dipyridamole, CO_r is cardiac output at rest, F_s is flow after dipyridamole, and F_r is flow at rest. The essential term that determines the relation between maximum to rest uptake ratio, U_s/U_r, and coronary flow reserve, F/F_r, is the constant 0.22 of the exponential expression.

The question then is whether this constant, 0.22, in the exponential term determined for dogs experimentally is approximately the same in humans. This constant can be estimated in humans by substituting known observed values for maximum flow reserve and rubidium maximum/rest uptake ratio after dipyridamole into the equation and solving for the value of x.

$$\frac{U_s}{U_r} = \frac{CO_r}{CO_s} \frac{F_s}{F_r} e^{x(Fr - Fs)}$$

Using Doppler catheters, F_s/F_r after dipyridamole in man averages approximately 4.0 (71). The ratio of maximum myocardial [82]Rb uptake to resting uptake, U_s/U_r, averages approximately 2.0 in over 200 dipyridamole clinical PET studies. Since the average increase in cardiac output after dipyridamole is 25% over resting cardiac output (69–74), the ratio $CO_r/CO = 0.8$. Substituting these values into the above equation and solving for x gives a value of 0.22 for humans, the same as that determined independently in animal experiments. Therefore, this equation appears appropriate for determining coronary flow reserve, F_s/F_r, based on PET measurements of U_s/U_r and measured arterial input function at rest and after dipyridamole in individual patients.

Figure 13.10 graphs myocardial [82]Rb uptake ratio for dipyridamole/rest, U_s/U_r, to coronary flow reserve, F/F_r, using the above equations. The dashed line shows the linear relation between rubidium uptake ratio and coronary flow reserve if extraction, E, and cardiac output, CO (or arterial input function) during dipyridamole were constant and the same as at rest. It is equivalent to or corresponds to coronary flow reserve measured by PET from U_s/U_r, using our flow model giving true coronary flow reserve. The upper curve shows U_s/U_r by PET if cardiac output, CO (or arterial input function), were constant or accounted for without correction for falling myocardial extraction, E, of [82]Rb at higher flows. The middle curve shows U_s/U_r by PET for increasing flow reserve observed experimentally and in humans with falling extraction and a 25% increase in cardiac output after dipyridamole. By using our flow model, this line is corrected to the dashed line. This analysis also explains why the range of radionuclide uptake ratios of stress/rest images is only 1.0 to 2.0 in Figures 12.8 and 12.9, corresponding to flow reserves of 1.0 to 4.0.

After dipyridamole, coronary blood flow increases by approximately 4.0 times baseline flow, or a 300% increase, associated with a 25% increase in cardiac output. With treadmill exercise stress, the cardiac output increases approximately as much as coronary flow, owing to peripheral mode work demands. Coronary flow increases at most by approximately 100%, to 2 times baseline. As apparent from the above equations, if cardiac output increases to the same extent as coronary flow during exercise, the rubidium uptake ratio on a perfusion scan, U_s/U_r, falls, owing to falling extraction as coronary flow increases. Therefore, myocardial radiotracer uptake during exercise stress is lower than at rest, as reported for thallium-201 in humans (47,48). The lower curve shows

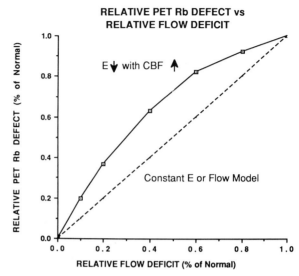

RELATIVE PET Rb DEFECT vs RELATIVE FLOW DEFICIT

E↓ with CBF↑

Constant E or Flow Model

RELATIVE PET Rb DEFECT (% of Normal)

RELATIVE FLOW DEFICIT (% of Normal)

Fig. 13.11 Severity relative perfusion defect by flowmeter (horizontal axis) and by PET (vertical axis), uncorrected for (solid line) and corrected for (dashed line) falling extraction at high flows.

this relation for exercise that explains the apparent paradox of decreased radionuclide uptake by myocardium during exercise as compared to rest. For this reason, dipyridamole is a better stress for evaluating coronary flow reserve than is exercise. In addition, flow increases more after dipyridamole than after exercise stress, thereby creating greater relative disparities in regional maximal radiotracer uptake that are more readily imaged.

Perfusion images after dipyridamole show relative distribution of maximum radionuclide uptake, reflecting relative distribution of maximum flow. The intensity of relative perfusion defects after dipyridamole can then be expressed as a percent of normal maximum of adjacent normal areas of myocardium. The severity of the PET defect is then described by a similar equation, as follows:

$$\frac{U_s}{U_n} = \frac{F_s}{F_n} \times e^{0.22(Fn - Fs)}$$

where U_s and F_s are, as before, radionuclide uptake and flow after dipyridamole in the area of the stenotic artery, but U_n and F_n are maximum uptake and flow in normal areas of myocardium without a stenotic arterial supply on the stress image. Relative maximum radionuclide uptake and relative maximum flow distribution are measured after dipyridamole only, unrelated to resting values. Accordingly, changes in cardiac output or arterial input function from rest to stress are not relevant, and the cardiac output term drops out of the above equation. Consequently, the quantitative defect in relative radionuclide uptake on a perfusion image differs from the true perfusion deficit only by the effects of falling extraction at high flows. Consequently, the relative uptake defect on a PET scan more nearly approximates the relative perfusion defect, as in Figure 13.11. The straight line shows the linear relation between relative perfusion defect by PET using our model, as compared to the true perfusion defect after dipyridamole. We are currently developing automated software for correcting PET data to provide true relative flow reserve for routine clinical studies.

Coronary Collateral Function
Assessed by PET

Coronary steal is conventionally defined as a fall in absolute coronary perfusion (cc/min/g) of collateralized myocardium after coronary arteriolar vasodilation, usually after intravenous dipyridamole. It has been studied experimentally (30–32,77–79), modeled theoretically (31), and demonstrated by PET imaging in humans (30,79), and occurs in 10% to 30% of patients with coronary artery disease undergoing dipyridamole perfusion imaging, as evidenced by chest pain, ECG changes, and abnormal perfusion scans (4,32,79–81). The mechanism is a fall in perfusion pressure at the origin of collateral vessels, due to proximal stenoses of coronary arteries supplying the collaterals or to proximal viscous friction developing at high flow rates even in normal arteries from which the collaterals arise. Expressed in terms of circuit models, decreased collateral flow (steal) is due to proportionately greater increase in conductance of the normal vascular bed in parallel with the relatively low, fixed conductance of the collateral bed, which cannot compensate further for the fall in pressure at their origin (31) associated with high flow in the artery supplying the collaterals.

In view of these mechanisms, the term "steal" is a misnomer, since blood is not "stolen" from the collateralized bed by backward flow through collateral channels to the normal vascular bed. It merely reflects a fall in collateral flow during arteriolar vasodilation below resting control levels, thereby producing ischemia. While developing only in the presence of severe coronary artery stenosis, collaterals in humans protect the myocardium from necrosis and deteriorating contractile function, if sufficiently developed over prolonged time periods before occlusion occurs (80,82). Severity of stenosis and the length of time it is present prior to occlusion are recognized factors in collateral development.

Coronary subendocardial steal is defined as a fall in absolute subendocardial perfusion, with a rise or no change in subepicardial perfusion, after coronary arteriolar vasodilation following intravenous dipyridamole. As recently demonstrated (83), subendocardial steal may occur with severe coronary artery stenosis in the absence of collaterals. The mechanisms are similar to those outlined above. At normal resting conditions with severe stenosis, resting flow and/or distal coronary pressure are reduced enough to stimulate compensatory subendocardial vasodilation, thereby using up its limited flow reserve. Subendocardial conductance is therefore relatively fixed. In these circumstances, intravenous di-

pyridamole then causes subepicardial arterioles to vasodilate proportionately more than subendocardial arterioles. Consequently, absolute perfusion falls in the subendocardium, owing to greater increase in conductance of subepicardial vessels that are in parallel with relatively fixed conductance vessels of the subendocardium, which cannot compensate for the fall in distal pressure. As discussed in Chapter 3, with this fall in coronary perfusion pressure, subendocardial filling may be delayed, thereby causing subendocardial ischemia, particularly with tachycardia occurring after intravenous dipyridamole. The necessary conditions for subendocardial steal without collaterals are a severe stenosis which produces maximally vasodilated, fixed conductance, subendocardial arterioles, and a fall in distal pressure after dipyridamole, which causes lower subendocardial perfusion and causes tachycardia. Thus, the mechanisms for coronary collateral steal and subendocardial steal are similar but the anatomy producing them is different.

Clinically, coronary steal, as manifested by chest pain and ST depression after intravenous dipyridamole, is usually a sign of severe coronary artery disease with viable myocardium. Steal in the absence of collaterals, that is, subendocardial steal, is not commonly seen clinically, since these patients often have severe or unstable angina at rest and are therefore likely to be excluded from dipyridamole stress. Uncommonly, a severe stenosis will demonstrate collapse (84) after dipyridamole, as described in Chapter 6, with a fall in coronary flow below resting control levels that mimics steal without collaterals. However, in the majority of patients undergoing appropriate dipyridamole perfusion imaging by PET, coronary steal is a sign of collaterals providing significant resting flow rather than subendocardial steal without collaterals.

Figure 14.1 illustrates clinical coronary steal demonstrated by positron emission tomography (PET) as a fall in stress activity below resting levels. PET also provides the percent of the heart outside 2.5 SD from normal which, for the polar map of absolute stress/rest ratio of Figure 14.1, indicates the percent of the heart that is collateralized.

Clinically, myocardial steal is therefore an important, useful diagnostic sign seen during dipyridamole perfusion imaging; it is associated with severe defects and indicates severe coronary artery disease and viable myocardium, most commonly associated with significant collateral supply but oc-

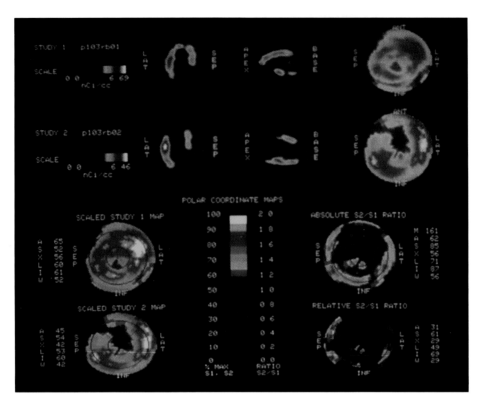

Fig. 14.1A PET image of generator-produced [82]Rb in horizontal (left upper tomographs) and vertical (right upper tomographs) long-axis views. Rest images are shown in the upper row, and dipyridamole stress images in the lower row. In the system of color coding, white is the highest, red next-highest, yellow intermediate, and green and blue lowest relative flows. Tomographs are oriented as if looking down from above with the anterior or apex at the top of each image (ANT), the left lateral free wall on the left (LAT), and the muscular septum (SEP) on the right with the atrioventricular ring and/or inferior myocardium at the bottom (INF). Resting tomographs show a small inferior apical defect, indicating a small myocardial scar. With dipyridamole stress, myocardial activity increases appropriately in inferolateral areas. The anterior and apical myocardium shows a severe stress defect extending laterally. Tomographic data can be summarized in a polar display as if looking from outside the body at the apex of the left ventricle located at the center of a bullseye, where the outer rim of the bullseye corresponds to the atrioventricular ring. Polar displays (lower left) show the relative defect on a scale from 0% to 100%, with rest being the upper (Study 1) and the stress the lower (Study 2) of the left polar maps. The numbers beside the polar maps indicate mean activity of each quadrant; A = anterior, S = septal, X = apex, L = lateral, I = inferior. The right polar map labeled S2/S1 absolute ratio (upper right) shows the absolute counts of the stress image, divided by the rest image displayed on a scale from 0 to 2. Increase in activity is shown by warm colors, indicating ratios >1 or an increase in absolute activity reflecting increased perfusion on the dipyridamole image. Blue areas indicate an absolute fall in activity, with a corresponding fall in perfusion during dipyridamole stress consistent with myocardial steal in a large area supplied by collaterals. The lower right polar display labeled S2/S1 percent ratio illustrates the change in the relative distribution of flow at stress normalized to rest (instead of the absolute values). Reproduced with permission from Gould KL, 1989. (32).

casionally without collaterals. Out of 1,100 cardiac PET studies, including approximately 75 with steal visible by PET, two patients had such well-developed collaterals that they showed no steal and no perfusion defect on dipyridamole PET imaging. In both of these patients the occluded artery filled by collaterals during arteriography at the same rate and visual flow velocity as the other normal non-stenotic coronary arteries.

THE BASIS FOR CORONARY STEAL BY PET: COLLATERAL NETWORK MODEL

The relation of steal to coronary flow reserve is best described by a hydraulic model shown in Figure 14.2 (31). Flow through the supply artery, the left circumflex (LCx) in this example,

divides at the origin of the collaterals, represented by the crossing channel between left anterior descending (LAD) and LCx. When flow increases in the supply artery in response to distal arteriolar vasodilation, the distal pressure in the supply artery falls, owing to a finite viscous resistance along its length, shown by subsequent experimental and theoretic evidence. This fall in distal supply artery pressure, which may be marked in the presence of a proximal stenosis, results in lower perfusion pressure to the collateral channels, with a corresponding fall in collateral flow.

At rest, the two vascular beds may receive equal flow despite the added resistance of the collateral vessels, because the collateral-dependent arteriolar bed dilates in order to maintain adequate flow. This compensatory vasodilation causes a loss of vasodilatory reserve in the collateral-dependent bed. With administration of a potent coronary arteriolar

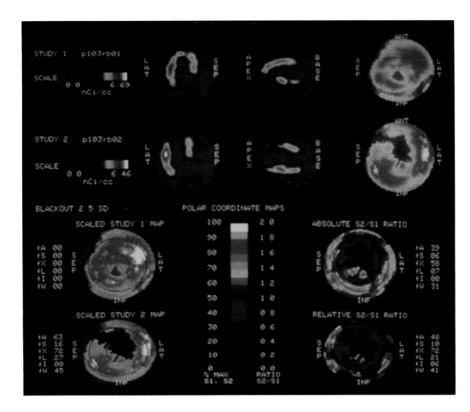

Fig. 14.1B Activity outside 2.5 SD compared with normal subjects appears as blacked-out areas. The numbers beside the polar map indicate the percent of the heart outside 2.5 SD. Thus, polar maps demonstrate a small inferior apical resting defect (Study 1) and a severe large stress defect of anterior, apical, and apical lateral myocardium (Study 2), involving 45% of the heart. Of this large area of viable myocardium, 31% shows collateralized myocardium associated with myocardial steal, as seen in the polar display of S2/S1 absolute ratios (upper right). PET imaging therefore has correctly demonstrated the extent and severity of coronary artery disease with collaterals, confirmed by arteriography. Reproduced with permission from Gould KL, 1989. (32).

vasodilator, such as dipyridamole, the collateral-dependent bed undergoes less net change in resistance than the supply artery bed. The greater decrease in vascular bed resistance of the supply artery, as compared to the higher resistance collaterals, causes more of the supply artery flow to go to its own capillary bed with a fall in flow through the collateral bed. In Figure 14.2 (31), consider that at rest, 50 mL/min flows antegrade through a severely stenotic LAD and 50 mL/min flows through the collateral channel from the LCx to produce 100 mL/min to the distal LAD bed. With arteriolar vasodilation, forward flow through the LAD increases to 60 mL/min, but collateral flow falls to 25 mL/min, owing to decreased coronary perfusion pressure (P), associated with the normal four- to five-times increase in LCx flow. The total flow to the LAD bed then is 85 mL/min, an absolute decrease in flow to the LAD bed, or myocardial steal. There is no reversal of collateral flow, only a decrease in absolute flow.

Three reasonable assumptions are involved in this explanation of coronary steal:

1. Collateral resistance is not negligible.
2. Pressure of the supply artery at the origin of collaterals falls with distal vasodilation, either with or without a stenosis of the supply artery.
3. The collateral-dependent bed lacks adequate vasodilatory reserve to prevent steal, since it is already vasodilated to some extent in compensation for the increased resistance of the collaterals. These assumptions are justified in the following sections.

COLLATERAL RESISTANCE

Schaper et al (85–89) studied chronically occluded, collateralized coronary arteries of dogs, using implanted arterial pressure catheters. They found that pressure distal to the occlusion (P_2 in Fig. 14.2) decreased markedly with administration of coronary arteriolar vasodilators; this pressure drop indicates significant flow-limiting resistance in the collateral vessels. They also measured the pressure-flow relation of collaterals by using radioactive microspheres. Their results indicated that the combined resistance of the collaterals and the distal vascular bed supplied by the collaterals was about

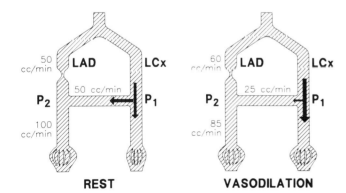

Fig. 14.2 Hydraulic model illustrating coronary steal. For this example, the LCx is the supply artery, with the vascular distribution of the LAD being supplied by collaterals from the LCx coronary artery. P_1 is the perfusion pressure at the origin of the collaterals from distal circumflex branches. P_2 is the perfusion pressure of the vascular distribution of the LAD coronary artery, which is severely stenotic. Reproduced with permission from Demer L, Gould KL, Kirkeeide R, 1988. (31).

10 times the minimal normal vascular bed resistance. With chronic occlusion, more extensive collaterals developed with time and collateral resistance fell. However, collateral resistance following 4 to 18 weeks of occlusion still measured approximately four times the normal minimal vascular bed resistance.

Using open-chest, instrumented dogs, Wusten et al (85) reported collateral perfusion values averaging 31% of normal resting values following acute LAD occlusion in beagles. Mongrel dogs, known to have less well-developed collaterals by anatomic criteria, had collateral perfusion of only 8.6% of normal after LCx coronary artery occlusion. Thus, the resistance of collaterals is not negligible even when they are well developed.

COLLATERAL SUPPLY PRESSURE WITH ARTERIOLAR VASODILATION

Becker (90,91) studied coronary steal by measuring flow with radiolabeled microspheres before and after intravenous administration of dipyridamole in dogs with only native collaterals and acute LAD occlusion. In the first set of experiments (90), coronary steal was not demonstrated. Following LAD occlusion, perfusion of the distal LAD bed was low and did not significantly decrease with dipyridamole-induced vasodilation. In a later, separate set of experiments (91), noncritical stenoses were added to the supply artery proximal to the takeoff of collaterals. In this preparation, steal was demonstrated. Accordingly, Becker concluded that steal occurs only when there is a stenosis in the collateral supply artery.

The stenosis of the supply artery in Becker's second preparation for inducing steal generated a mean pressure gradient of 30 mm Hg under high flow conditions, sufficient to halve the peak reactive hyperemic response from 400% to 200%. The corresponding resistance, 2×10^4 dynes/cm^5, can be calculated from the general equation for pressure loss across a stenosis using Becker's data. However, Becker's all-or-none conclusion that a proximal narrowing of the supply artery is necessary for steal is not entirely correct; his data are also consistent with two different interpretations. The first is that there were no collaterals or poorly developed collaterals and steal could not occur in the first set of experiments. The second is that steal requires only measurable resistance in the proximal supply artery, but not necessarily a stenosis, particularly at high flows. After a potent vasodilator stimulus and rise in flow, the proximal resistance in a normal artery up to the origin of the collaterals may be sufficient to cause a significant fall in pressure, where greater pressure drop along the artery is associated with greater steal after arteriolar vasodilators. Even in the absence of stenosis, substantial resistance develops, owing to viscous friction along the length of a normal coronary artery proximal to the collateral takeoff. For example, Wyatt et al. (92) found a 20% decrease in pressure from the aorta to the origin of collaterals by cannulation of the recipient bed artery at resting flow. Patterson and Kirk (93) found that 12% of total vascular resistance in a normal supply artery occurred proximal to the origin of collaterals. They demonstrated significant coronary steal in dogs with acute LAD occlusion and normal collateral supply arteries, using both retrograde flow and microsphere techniques.

The amount of inherent resistance expected along a normal coronary artery would depend on its length, diameter, and flow. It can be calculated from the following relation:

$$P = f'Q \quad \text{where} \quad f' = \frac{8\pi\mu l}{A^2}$$

where P is the difference in pressure between aorta and origin of collaterals at the arteriolar bed, f' is the coefficient of pressure loss due to viscous friction along this length of artery, μ is viscosity of blood, l is the length of the artery, and A is the mean cross-sectional area of the arterial lumen. For this equation, non-Newtonian characteristics of blood and viscoelasticity of the vessel wall are excluded for simplicity, and the approximate or expected resistance of the proximal portion of a normal artery with diameter uniformly tapering from 3 mm to 1 mm over a 6-cm distance can be calculated. At resting flow, supply pressure to collaterals originating beyond the 6-cm point would be 6 mm Hg less than aortic pressure at resting flows. However, at maximal flows, the pressure gradient would increase to 30 mm Hg, resulting in a 30–mm Hg drop in the distal pressure of the supply artery, sufficient to cause steal in this model. Therefore, proximal resistance of the supply artery may be caused not only by a proximal stenosis but also by the viscous friction along the length of a normal artery proximal to the origin of collaterals.

This viscous pressure loss along a normal artery may be magnified by larger than normal flow in the supply artery to well-developed collaterals, because viscous resistance is flow-dependent, as shown by the above equation. Even at rest, flow through the proximal supply artery may increase to two times its normal resting flow in the presence of collaterals feeding a large collateralized bed. Proximal resistance may then increase five to ten times with vasodilation and higher flow in the supply artery. Thus, conditions for steal may occur following a strong vasodilator stimulus owing to any proximal resistance from either a normal or stenotic supply artery. These directional changes in arteriolar pressure after administration of coronary arteriolar vasodilators have been confirmed by direct experimental measurements (94).

VASODILATORY RESERVE OF THE COLLATERAL-DEPENDENT BED

Relating the effects of antegrade coronary flow with vasodilatory reserve of the collateral-dependent vascular bed requires more detailed analysis, because the interactions are too complex to predict intuitively. For example, coronary arteriolar vasodilation may cause more, or less, net perfusion of the collateralized bed as antegrade flow rises through the normal or stenosed native artery. Whether flow increases or decreases to the collateral-dependent bed depends on the exact values of resistance, pressure drop, and degree of increase in flow through the supply artery.

These hemodynamic changes may be systematically analyzed using a general network model, which is an electrical analogue of the collateralized coronary circulation with five resistance elements, known as the Wheatstone bridge, shown in Figure 14.3 (31). Its first element represents the left main coronary artery with two branches, the LCx and LAD coronary arteries. The cross-element represents collateral vessels. Two

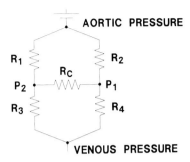

Fig. 14.3 The model network analyzed as an electrical analogue. R_1 represents the resistance of the LAD coronary artery and branches; R_2, the resistance of the LCx coronary artery and branches; R_3, the resistance of the distal vascular bed of the LAD artery; R_4, the resistance of the distal vascular bed of the LCx coronary artery; R_c, the resistance of the collateral connections; P_1, the perfusion pressure to the collateral bed and distal circumflex bed; P_2, the perfusion pressure to the distal LAD bed. This electrical circuit is called a Wheatstone bridge. For details of the computer simulation, see the text. Reproduced with permission from Demer L, Gould KL, Kirkeeide R, 1988. (31).

parallel lower branches represent resistance of the vascular coronary beds. Flow rejoins in the venous circulation. The supply voltage is equivalent to aortic pressure.

ASSUMPTIONS FOR NETWORK ANALYSIS

For this network analysis, several simplifying assumptions are made in the computer simulations:

1. Steady state is assumed—that is, the phasic changes in coronary flow are not incorporated into this model.

2. Coronary vascular capacitance is considered negligible.

3. Multiple collateral channels are lumped into a single resistance element.

4. Collateral resistance is fixed with respect to time, because collaterals do not demonstrate normal vasodilation and autoregulation.

5. All parameters are normalized with respect to well-defined values for purposes of generalization; for example, stenosis length is expressed as relative to normal vessel diameter, and resistance values are normalized with respect to minimal distal resistance after vasodilators, as reported in the literature. Similarly, relative conductance is normalized with respect to minimal distal resistance. The ratio of distal resistance at rest to minimum distal resistance during vasodilation is set at five, reflecting the approximate five-times increase in flow after a potent coronary arteriolar vasodilator.

6. Autoregulation is incorporated by allowing independent internal adjustment of resistance in the distal bed of the collateral-dependent artery (R_3) and resistance of the distal bed of the supply artery (R_4) by means of a feedback loop. The program simulates physiologic autoregulation by having the resistance vessels "dilate" in response to decreased flow, thus augmenting flow to a level such that either demand flow or minimal resistance is reached.

Aortic and venous pressures are chosen to be 100 and 10 mm Hg, respectively. Resting flow is set at 1 ml/min/g. LAD and LCx bed sizes are set at 100 g each. Input variables include (1) percent area reduction and length of proximal arterial stenoses, (2) flow demand for each distal bed (either resting demand or maximum vasodilation), and (3) collateral resistance. Since myocardial steal occurs at the levels of the perfused capillary bed, we use the term myocardial perfusion reserve as the ratio of myocardial perfusion after dipyridamole to myocardial perfusion at rest. The term myocardial perfusion reserve is equivalent to coronary flow reserve except that myocardial perfusion is measured by radiolabeled microspheres or by PET rather than by periarterial flowmeter.

RESULTS OF NETWORK ANALYSIS

This network model predicts a curvilinear relation between myocardial perfusion reserve (MPR) and collateral conductance, shown in Figure 14.4. Since resting collateral flow accounts for a progressively greater proportion of resting flow, that is, with increasing collateral conductance, myocardial perfusion in the collateral-dependent bed falls below resting values after administration of potent coronary arteriolar vasodilators. MPR therefore falls progressively below one. This decrease in MPR as the collateral conductance increases indicates coronary steal, which in turn identifies collaterals. With poorly developed collaterals or decreasing collateral conductance, MPR approaches a value of one, reaching one in the absence of significant resting collateral flow and rising above one with antegrade flow. For purposes of comparison to the conductance values of Figure 14.4, the conductance of a normal coronary vascular bed may be estimated using approximate values of the aortic-venous pressure gradient and maximum flow. For normal patients with a resting myocardial perfusion of 1 mL/min/g, maximum perfusion would be about

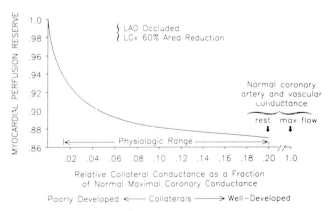

Fig. 14.4 Effect of collaterals on myocardial perfusion reserve of the LAD bed. The network model predicts an inverse curvilinear relation between myocardial perfusion reserve and collateral conductance, expressed as a fraction of normal maximal coronary conductance under conditions of maximal coronary vasodilation. For this particular relation, the conditions were an occluded LAD and a 60% area reduction of the LCx, with other details provided in the text. Reproduced with permission from Demer L, Gould KL, Kirkeeide, R, 1988. (31).

5 mL/min/g. The equation for conductance is the inverse of resistance:

$$c = \frac{1}{R} = \frac{flow}{pressure\ gradient}$$

In this case, for a pressure gradient of 90 mm Hg, normal coronary conductance would be about 5.5 mL/min/100 g/mm Hg at maximum flow. These values agree well with the experimentally observed value of 5.6 mL/min/100 g measured by Schaper et al. during adenosine-induced vasodilation (89).

In order to estimate the value of collateral conductance that would provide normal resting flow to the collateral-dependent bed, the special case of complete occlusion may be considered. For normal resting flow to the collateral-dependent bed, the sum of collateral resistance (R_c) and distal resistance, R_3, may be no greater than normal resistance. This condition requires that R_c not exceed four times the normal minimal vascular bed resistance (R_{min}), because normal resting vascular bed resistance is five time R_{min}. Normal resting flow is then maintained when the vascular bed is dilated to R_{min} in series with a collateral resistance of four times R_{min}. This value of R_c corresponds to a collateral conductance of one-fourth the maximal distal conductance, or a relative collateral conductance at 0.25.

Wusten et al (85) measured collateral conductance in acutely occluded coronary arteries of dogs. Relative collateral conductance was 0.06 in beagles, which have relatively well-developed native collaterals, and 0.02 in mongrel dogs having less developed native collaterals prior to occlusion. Schaper et al. (89) showed that with gradually occluded coronary arteries in dogs, relative collateral conductances were 0.05 and 0.08 initially. As the coronary arteries were gradually occluded, collateral conductance increased over several weeks to 0.25 at 4 weeks and 0.34 at 8 weeks. Maximum conductance of 0.37 was reached at 18 weeks. This physiologic range of collateral conductance is shown in Figure 14.4 (31).

For well-developed collaterals sufficient to provide normal resting perfusion distal to a complete occlusion, the extent of steal after administration of vasodilators increases with progressively severe stenosis of the supply artery, as shown in Figure 14.5 (31).

At one extreme or boundary condition, a collateral conductance of infinity, which is not a physiologic condition, corresponds to direct attachment of the dependent bed to the supply artery. In that hypothetical situation, the myocardial perfusion reserve (MPR) would be the same as the arterial coronary flow reserve (CFR) of the supply artery and conditions for steal would not occur, since the collateralized bed would, in effect, be attached to the supply artery and no longer fed through collaterals. However, even in dogs with long-term maximally developed collaterals, collateral conductance does not even remotely approach such high values. Clinically, in 1,100 PET studies, we have observed two patients with such highly developed collaterals that no dipyridamole perfusion defect was seen.

At the other extreme of the network model, a collateral conductance of zero corresponds to absence of collaterals. In that case, the value of MPR is the same as the arterial CFR for the occluded native coronary artery, that is, one, or no increase after dipyridamole. Therefore, in physiologic or

practical terms, an MPR of less than one indicates steal, with resting collateral flow present in proportion to the extent to which MPR falls below one after administration of vasodilators.

PREDICTIONS FROM THE NETWORK MODEL

According to our analysis, myocardial perfusion increases and MPR is above one due to antegrade arterial flow after administration of arteriolar vasodilators, with up to 94% area reduction of the native artery for a stenosis length twice the normal lumen diameter. Myocardial steal occurs with a fall in perfusion after administration of vasodilators and an MPR of less than one only with substantial resting collateral flow and a stenosis of the native artery exceeding 94% area reduction, a degree of severity that reduces forward antegrade resting flow and prevents any increased antegrade arterial flow. This conclusion agrees with clinical observations that collaterals are rarely seen with stenoses less than about 95% narrowing, even given the limitations of angiographic assessment of collateralization and stenosis severity.

Our model predicts that collateral development sufficient to provide a significant proportion of resting myocardial perfusion is usually associated with myocardial steal after potent coronary arteriolar vasodilators. The extent of collateral flow provided at rest is proportionally and directly related to the degree of steal after vasodilators. Finally, MPR of less than one indicates steal, and the extent to which MPR falls below one quantitatively reflects the degree of steal. We therefore consider myocardial perfusion reserve by PET as an experimental and clinical means for identifying collateral flow and/or stenotic proximal coronary arteries.

Several differences between coronary artery flow reserve and myocardial perfusion reserve deserve emphasis. MPR in the range of one to five parallels or is equal to arterial CFR

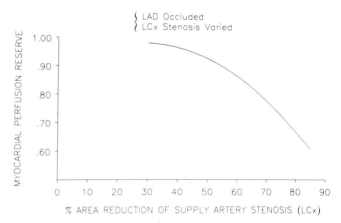

Fig. 14.5 Effect of supply artery stenosis on myocardial perfusion reserve of a well-collateralized LAD bed. For this simulation, collateral capacity was assumed sufficient to provide normal resting coronary flow, that is, a normal resting collateral conductance of 0.2 with an occluded LAD and progressive stenosis of the LCx coronary artery. See text for details. Reproduced with permission from Demer L, Gould KL, Kirkeeide R, 1988. (31).

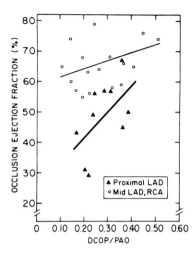

Fig. 14.6 Relation between distal coronary occlusion pressure/ aortic pressure ratio (DCOP/Pao), left ventricular ejection fraction during balloon inflation, and lesion location. LAD = left anterior descending; RCA = right coronary artery. Reproduced with permission from Rentrop KP, Thornton JC, Feit F, et al., 1988. (80).

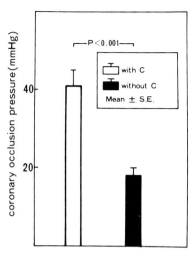

Fig. 14.8 Coronary occlusion pressure at 40 sec of balloon inflation in 8 patients with and 14 without collateral vessels (C). Reproduced with permission from Mizuno K, Horiuchi K, Matui H, et al., 1988. (82).

and reflects the effects of stenosis dimensions, aortic pressure, vascular tone, and so forth on maximum coronary flow. MPR of less than one quantitatively reflects collateral function and then does not equal or parallel arterial CFR. Arterial CFR of less than one does not occur except with dynamic worsening of stenoses or the collapsing stenosis phenomenon (84). Thus, myocardial perfusion reserve by PET, or microspheres, but not arterial coronary flow reserve by flowmeter, accounts for collateral function.

CLINICAL UTILITY OF ASSESSING COLLATERAL FLOW

Having described the mechanism and a clinical means of assessing collateral flow in humans, we come to a question about the utility of identifying collateralized myocardium. Well-developed collaterals clearly serve to protect myocardium and maintain ventricular function. Rentrop et al. (80)

have measured left ventricular ejection fraction during coronary occlusion of PTCA in patients with and without collaterals. Adequacy of collateral flow was quantified in terms of distal coronary back pressure with balloon occlusion expressed as a fraction of aortic pressure.

For proximal LAD stenoses there was a direct relation between ejection fraction and distal coronary pressure during balloon occlusion, Figure 14.6 (80). For more distal occlusions, the relation was weaker, as would be expected, and right coronary occlusion caused no fall in ejection fraction, as seen in Figure 14.7 (80).

Patients with good collaterals at arteriography had higher distal coronary pressure on balloon occlusion, Figure 14.8 (82), and maintained lactate extraction, as in Figure 14.9

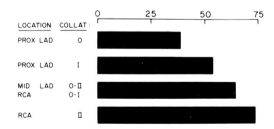

Fig. 14.7 Relation between collateral class and mean left ventricular ejection fraction during balloon inflation in the proximal left anterior descending (PROX LAD), mid-left anterior descending (MID LAD), or right coronary artery (RCA). Reproduced with permission from Rentrop KP, Thornton JC, Feit F, et al., 1988. (80).

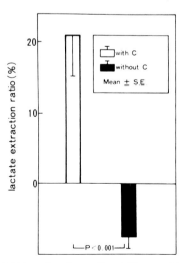

Fig. 14.9 Lactate extraction ratio at 40 sec of balloon inflation in 7 patients with and 12 without collateral vessels (C). Reproduced with permission from Mizuno K, Horiuchi K, Matui H, et al., 1988. (82).

(82), compared to patients without collaterals. Patients with good collaterals also maintained systolic and diastolic left ventricular pressures, and positive and negative dp/dt during balloon occlusion compared to patients without collaterals, illustrated in Figure 14.10 (82).

Consequently, the presence of well-collateralized myocardium provides some protection against necrosis. Figure 14.11 illustrates a clinical example. This patient was a 41-year-old man with a 10-year history of palpitations, which were worse with emotional stress, coffee, and considerable chronic anxiety. Four months previously he had a day of chest

soreness radiating to both arms, without recurrence. He had a normal rest ECG and mitral valve prolapse by exam and subsequent LV angiogram. He underwent a good thallium exercise tolerance test at another hospital, with a hypertensive response 140/84 increasing to 212/108 at maximum exercise with heart rate increasing from 96 to 160. He had no chest pain, nonspecific J-junction depression with upsloping ST segment, and an equivocal inferior stress thallium perfusion defect on one view but no other views. The thallium exercise tolerance test was interpreted as probably normal. His total cholesterol was 236 and HDL was 27.

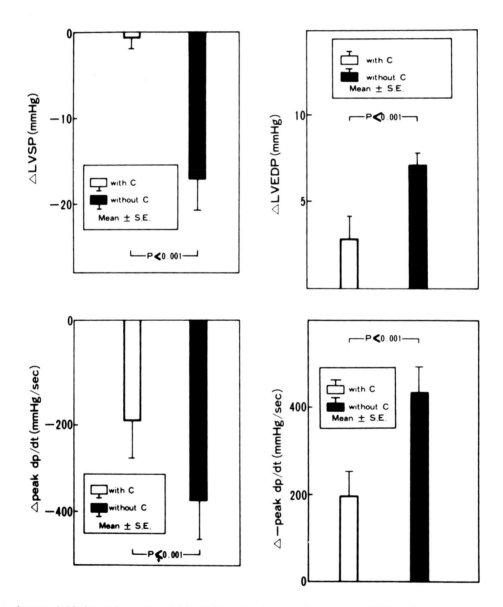

Fig. 14.10 The changes (△) in hemodynamic variables (left ventricular systolic pressure [LVSP], left ventricular end-diastolic pressure [LVEDP], maximal rate of rise of left ventricular pressure [peak dp/dt] and maximal rate of fall of left ventricular pressure [−peak dp/dt] during balloon inflation in 8 patients with and 14 without collateral vessels (C). Reproduced with permission from Mizuno K, Horiuchi K, Matui H, et al., 1988. (82).

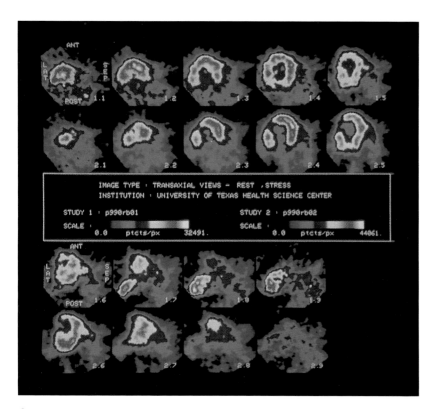

A

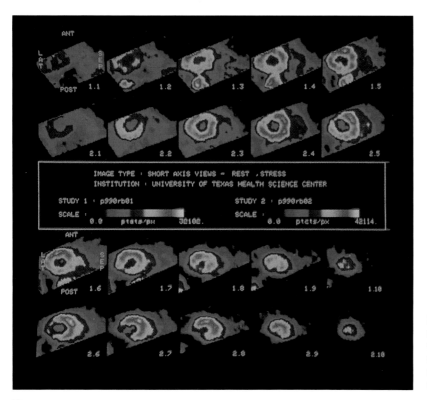

B

Fig. 14.11 PET study resulting in decision against mechanical intervention, due to well-developed collaterals to a single occluded artery with no other coronary arteries at risk. See text for details. (**A**) acquisition views; (**B**) short-axis views; (*continued*)

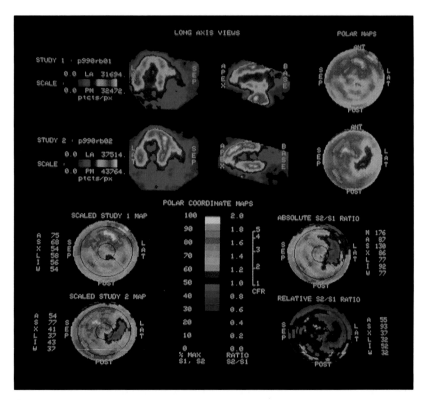

Fig. 14.11 (*continued*) (**C**) long-axis views and polar maps.

C

Due to his considerable anxiety, the patient requested a PET study, shown in Figure 14.11. The rest scan (S1) showed a small lateral non-transmural scar. The dipyridamole scan showed a severe defect beginning anteriolaterally at the base and spiraling laterally toward the apex, where it was inferiolateral. The absolute S2/S1 ratio image showed a fall in activity below resting levels after dipyridamole, indicating intense myocardial steal. This distribution is characteristic of an isolated Ramus Intermedius coronary artery, which by PET was interpreted as occluded and completely collateralized but with normal flow reserve of all other coronary arteries. Based on the PET scan, the patient had no evidence of myocardium at risk, since the involved artery was well collateralized and no other arteries were involved. Due to his young age and the moderately large size of myocardium, and to confirm a decision against mechanical intervention based on PET, coronary arteriography was done. The arteriogram confirmed the above findings, normal ventricular function, and supported the decision for medical therapy based on the PET scan alone.

15

Assessing Myocardial Infarction, Ischemia, and Viability

Distinguishing necrotic from viable myocardium is important for managing patients with acute myocardial infarction, particularly following thrombolysis therapy when revascularization or balloon angioplasty may be indicated if viable myocardium remains. The extent of myocardial infarction and/or viability depends on how it is measured. Thallium exercise perfusion imaging in the peri-infarction period is most commonly used for this purpose (96–103).

For example, Rozanski et al. (97) reported in 1981 that in 35 out of 43 patients (81%) with stress defects, redistribution on ^{201}Tl exercise tolerance tests (ETT) improved left ventricular wall motion after bypass surgery (Table 15.1) (97). However, 19% with reversible stress defects did not improve. Although most patients with fixed defects on ^{201}Tl ETT did not show improved wall motion, 4 of 29 did improve despite fixed defects. In 1989, Tamaki et al. (16,101) found that 8 of 23 myocardial segments (35%) with transient defects on thallium ETT single photon emission tomography (SPECT) did not improve LV function postoperatively; 14 of 33 patients with fixed defects (42%) improved LV function postoperatively (Table 15.2) (16).

In 1988, Cloninger et al. (99) reported that in 95 patients with their first suspected or documented myocardial infarction and incomplete redistribution on thallium ETT, 72 (76%) improved redistribution images and 24% did not improve after PTCA, as shown in Figure 15.1 (99). Of 16 patients with prior and acute suspected or documented myocardial infarction and incomplete redistribution, 8 improved redistribution images after PTCA and 8 did not. These reports suggest that identifying myocardial viability and postoperative improvement in LV function by stress thallium imaging is of limited predictive accuracy for improvement after mechanical intervention, and therefore is limited for assessing viability.

Of the many possible reasons for thallium ETT failing to predict viability, two possible explanations stand out. Either the imaging technology of thallium is inadequate or the basic concept of identifying necrosis by a fixed defect on thallium ETT is incorrect. With regard to the first alternative, exercise perfusion imaging on ^{13}N ammonia by PET improves prediction of postoperative improvement of LV function, but only modestly (16,101). In 14 of 48 segments with transient perfusion defects by PET (30%), there was no improved LV function postoperatively; 5 of 27 segments with fixed defects (19%) had improved LV function, despite fixed defect (Table 15.3) (16). Therefore, in the same investigational study, the

errors of exercise perfusion imaging for predicting viability and postoperative improvement in LV function decreased only modestly from 35%–42% for SPECT to 20%–30% by exercise perfusion PET imaging.

The errors of 20%–30% in predicting viability and postoperative improvement in postoperative LV function based on transient stress perfusion defects may be due in part to a problem with the basic concept of exercise perfusion imaging as a means of assessing viability.

Figure 15.2 shows conceptually a defect both on stress (left panel) and at redistribution or rest (right panel). Due to washout of thallium from the normal area on the 4-h scan, the relative severity of the defect appears to decrease as if redistribution had occurred, suggesting viability. However, the apparent partial redistribution may be due to washout of radionuclide from normal areas. Similarly, a rest PET perfusion scan will have a less severe-looking defect than the exercise PET perfusion scan, owing to greater uptake of radionuclide by normal myocardium. Therefore, apparent partial redistribution provides no information about viability in the area of the resting defect, since apparent lessening of defect severity may be due to washout of activity from the normal area, or lower resting flow as compared to flow in the exercise study.

Figure 15.3 illustrates that a partly reversible exercise perfusion defect identifies the area of limited flow reserve around a central injured area of myocardium (left panel). It does not provide data on how much viable myocardium is left in the area of the defect with potentially partial damage. Exercise stress perfusion imaging therefore provides a measure of the zone at risk having low flow reserve (right panel) but not of viability within the area of a fixed defect.

PET has been developed for identifying ischemic, viable, or necrotic/fibrotic myocardium by imaging metabolic analogues, especially FDG and the potassium analogue [82]Rb. Therefore, a brief review of myocardial metabolic imaging is necessary.

MYOCARDIAL METABOLIC IMAGING TO DETERMINE VIABILITY

Myocardial glucose metabolism is regulated primarily by serum fatty acid levels, particularly as affected by insulin levels, and oxygen availability (15) modified by catechols (104).

Table 15.1 Comparison of the Thallium-201 Redistribution Pattern with the Postoperative Wall Motion Response in 72 Asynergic Segments

		Preoperative thallium-201 redistribution pattern	
		Normal	Abnormal
Postoperative	Improved	35	4
wall motion	Not improved	8	25

Source: Adapted with permission from Rozanski A, Berman DS, Gray R, et al., 1981. Reference 97.

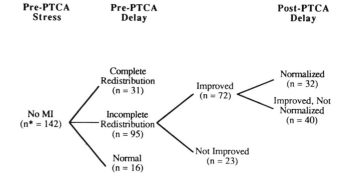

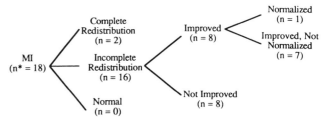

Fig. 15.1 Characterization of thallium-201 redistribution before percutaneous transluminal coronary angioplasty (PTCA) and the findings in subsequent 4-h delayed images after angioplasty in 142 studies in 124 patients without prior myocardial infarction (MI) and in 18 studies in 17 patients with prior infarction. *n = number of studies. Reproduced with permission from Cloninger KG, DePuey EG, Garcia EV, et al., 1988. (99).

After fasting, normal myocardium metabolizes primarily fatty acids and glucose metabolism is suppressed. In the presence of injured or ischemic but viable myocardial cells, lack of oxygen inhibits fatty acid oxidation, and myocardial metabolism is shifted toward anaerobic glycolysis of glucose. Accordingly, some relative measure of glucose metabolism under appropriate conditions indicates whether myocardium is normal, ischemic, viable, or necrotic.

The glucose analogue, ^{18}F-2-fluoro-2-deoxyglucose (FDG, half-life 110 min) is a positron radiotracer providing good PET images of the heart after intravenous injection. FDG parallels glucose in myocardial uptake, transport, and phosphorylation by hexokinase in the cell. However, the phosphorylated compound FDG-G-PO4 cannot be metabolized and is trapped in the cell in proportion to the uptake, phosphylation, and metabolism of exogenous glucose (15).

Table 15.2 Comparison of Preoperative Stress-Delayed ^{201}Tl Findings and Postoperative Wall Motion Response

		Preoperative stress-delayed ^{201}Tl findings		
		Transient defect	Persistent defect	Overall
Postoperative	Improved	15	14	29
wall motion	Not improved	8	19	27
	Overall	23	33	56

Source: Adapted with permission from Tamaki N, Yonekura Y, Yamashita K, et al., 1989. Reference 16.

Table 15.3 Comparison of Preoperative Rest-Stress ^{13}N Ammonia Findings and Postoperative Wall Motion Response

		Preoperative rest-stress [^{13}N] ammonia findings		
		Transient defect	Persistent defect	Overall
Posoperative	Improved	34	5	39
wall motion	Not improved	14	22	36
	Overall	48	27	75

Source: Adapted with permission from Tamaki N, Yonekura Y, Yamashita K, et al., 1989. Reference 16.

REVERSIBLE STRESS PERFUSION DEFECT

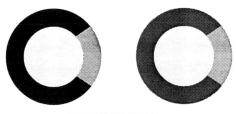

VIABLE OR SCAR

Fig. 15.2 Schematic of thallium washout from normal areas of an exercise image (left panel) resulting in relative redistribution on the 4-h delayed image (right panel), which is consistent with either scar or viable myocardium.

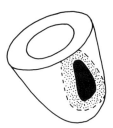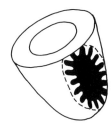

Fig. 15.3 Schematic of an enlarging or worsening defect with stress, compared to the central resting defect of a rest or redistribution thallium image. This partially reversible defect indicates the area of low flow reserve around a central resting defect but does not provide information on the viability (or necrosis) of myocardium within the resting defect.

Under conditions of oral glucose loading when fatty acid levels are depressed, normal and viable ischemic myocardium takes up FDG, but necrotic or fibrotic myocardium does not, thereby producing a negative image or defect in the FDG image where tissue is non-viable (17,18,23). Under fasting conditions, when myocardium metabolizes fatty acid and ketones, normal myocardial FDG uptake is suppressed. In this circumstance, viable ischemic tissue loses fatty acid metabolism and takes up FDG, reflecting anaerobic glycolysis, thereby producing a positive image of viable ischemic area but no uptake in normal or scar tissue (13–15,20–22).

PET PROTOCOL FOR ASSESSING VIABILITY AND NECROSIS OR ISCHEMIA BY FDG IMAGING

For the question of whether myocardium is viable or necrotic, we obtain FDG images after an oral *glucose load* when both normal and ischemic myocardium take up FDG but necrotic tissue does not. For the viability-infarct size protocol, non-fasted patients are given 50 g of oral glucola on arrival in the PET lab. Diabetic patients have their usual breakfast with insulin or oral hypoglycemic drugs in their usual doses. ECG and blood pressure are monitored and a transmission scan is obtained, as previously described. FDG, 10–15 mCi, is then

injected intravenously; data collection begins 45 min later and lasts for 20–30 min to collect 20 to 30 million counts per whole heart data set.

We use this protocol clinically to decide on interventions for chronic stable coronary artery disease, old myocardial infarction, or ischemic cardiomyopathy, or after acute myocardial infarction both with and without reperfusion by thrombolysis or PTCA. Since, under glucose-loaded conditions, ischemic viable and normal non-ischemic myocardium both take up FDG, perfusion imaging with ^{82}Rb or ^{13}N ammonia is carried out first to identify underperfused areas. Viable ischemic areas are then identified by a low flow area or defect on the perfusion image associated with FDG uptake, or no defect in that area on the FDG image, indicating metabolically active viable myocardium despite the low flow. Such low-flow, metabolically active areas of viable myocardium are therefore defined by a flow metabolism mismatch (perfusion defect, normal FDG). Necrotic myocardium is identified by defects on both perfusion and FDG scans, indicating low flow and *no* metabolic activity, a pattern referred to as a flow-metabolism match (perfusion defect, FDG defect) (15).

CLINICAL EXAMPLES OF FDG IMAGES

Figure 15.4 illustrates a 71-year-old man with heart failure felt to be inoperable by two cardiologists, owing to silent ischemic cardiomyopathy. The perfusion image (upper row) shows large defects of the entire inferior myocardium. The FDG image (lower row) indicates metabolically active viable myo-

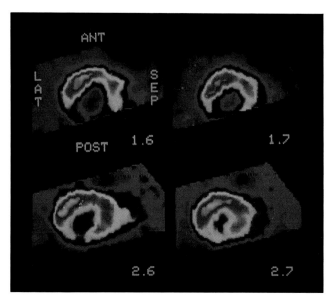

Fig. 15.4 71-year-old man with heart failure without angina pectoris or clinical infarction; the patient had three-vessel CAD and an ejection fraction of 35%–40%. The resting perfusion study with ^{13}N ammonia showed a large inferior perfusion defect (upper row) that took up FDG, indicating viable myocardium (lower row) except for a very small nontransmural infarcted area. On the basis of an extensive area of hypoperfused viable myocardium, bypass surgery was carried out.

cardium of most of the inferior myocardium. Accordingly, by-pass grafting was carried out.

Patients with underperfused, viable myocardium identified by FDG uptake (17) or by stress PET perfusion imaging alone (16,101) demonstrate improved LV function after bypass surgery. For patients having recent myocardial infarction, 75%–80% of patients and 50%–70% of myocardial segments have significant remaining viable myocardium (17,18,21,23), 85% of which demonstrate improved contractile function after reperfusion (Figure 15.5) (17). By thallium redistribution studies, approximately half of post-infarction patients have viable myocardium (18,102), with approximately 30% being classified as completed infarctions without viable myocardium when they have viable tissue by PET studies; therefore, based on the literature, perhaps up to 30% of patients with viable myocardium are missed by thallium imaging and do not undergo therapeutic intervention, (Figure 15.6 [102] and Table 15.4) (101). Therefore, this protocol is especially valuable for determining whether viable myocardium remains and whether a follow-up intervention is needed after thrombolysis.

Either the glucose-loaded or the fasting protocols, or both, are used for clinical purposes to decide on interventions after myocardial infarction either with or without reperfusion (glucose-loaded, viability protocol) or for assessing stenoses of equivocal severity (fasting, exercise ischemia protocol). Since, under glucose-loaded conditions, ischemic viable and normal non-ischemic myocardium both take up FDG, perfusion imaging at rest is carried out first to identify underperfused areas. Viable areas are then defined by a flow-metabolism mismatch (perfusion defect, normal FDG uptake) and non-viable areas as a flow-metabolism match (perfusion defect, FDG defect) (15).

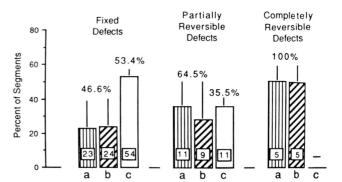

Fig. 15.6 Summary of the PET findings in the segments with fixed, partially reversible, and completely reversible thallium defects. Values in bars indicate number of segments; a = normal, b = ischemic, c = infarcted. Percentage of segments with evidence of metabolic viability is indicated by the summed values on the left for each thallium category, while the percentage of segments with infarction is indicated by the values on the right (above the stippled bars). Reproduced with permission from Brunken RC, Kottou S, Nienaber CA, et al., 1989. (102).

For the clinical question of whether viable myocardium is ischemic owing to a coronary artery stenosis, we carry out cardiac PET with FDG in the *fasting state* either with exercise, or at rest in the case of unstable angina, when ischemic viable myocardium traps FDG but necrotic and normal myocardium do not. In this protocol, a rest perfusion scan using ^{13}N ammonia is obtained. The patient then undergoes a standard Bruce treadmill exercise test with ECG monitoring. The perfusion tracer, ^{13}N ammonia, is injected intravenously at peak tolerated stress, which is maintained for 45–60 s more, and then a stress image is obtained. While the patient is at rest after stress is completed and stress perfusion images are obtained, FDG is injected, and 45 min later FDG imaging is begun to obtain the metabolic data.

The myocardial conversion to anaerobic glycolysis during ischemia caused by exercise stress persists for hours during the post-exercise resting conditions after the ischemia is over. Therefore, FDG is taken up in areas that were ischemic during stress, and a positive image of the ischemic area is obtained in retrospect. The complete sequence of images then includes resting perfusion, stress perfusion, and stress FDG. An area with a normal resting perfusion image but a stress perfusion defect that takes up FDG is metabolically ischemic, due to a severe flow-limiting stenosis. An area with a normal resting image, a stress perfusion defect, and no FDG uptake has a mild-to-moderate flow-limiting stenosis that is

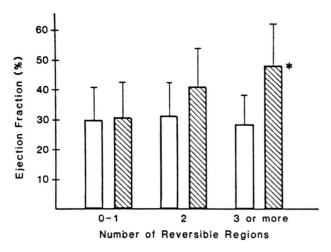

Fig. 15.5 Left ventricular ejection fraction according to number of regions of reversible dysfunction as predicted with PET criteria, before operation (open bar) and afterward (hatched bar). Bars represent means, and error bars equals 1 SD. Asterisk denotes a significant difference between preoperative and postoperative values (P < 0.05 by Student's t-test). Reproduced with permission from Tillisch J, Brunken R, Marshall R, et al., 1986. (17).

Table 15.4 Number of Segments with ^{201}Tl Perfusion Defect and ^{18}F Deoxyglucose (FDG) Uptake

	FDG(+)	FDG(−)	Total
Transient defect (group 1)	21	1	22
Persistent defect (group 2)	15	24	39
Total	36	25	61

Source: Adapted with permission from Tamaki N, Yonekura Y, Yamashita K, et al., 1988. Reference 101.

not severe enough to cause metabolic ischemia. An area with a rest perfusion defect, a comparable stress perfusion defect, and no FDG uptake is myocardial scar or necrosis.

LIMITATIONS OF FDG IMAGING

Since FDG imaging is currently considered clinically optimal (15) for assessing myocardial infarction and viability, it is important to emphasize the conditions in which it is applicable and those under which it is not reliable for assessing ischemia viability and necrosis. After *oral glucose loading* in chronic coronary artery disease and acute myocardial infarction, myocardial areas with a rest perfusion defect and *increased* FDG uptake after glucose loading (flow-metabolism mismatch) are viable and demonstrate improved LV function after revascularization (15,17). Areas with a perfusion defect and *low* FDG uptake after glucose loading (flow-metabolism match) identify necrotic or fibrotic myocardium showing no improvement after revascularization. *After fasting and exercise stress* in chronic coronary artery disease, FDG uptake identifies ischemic viable myocardium as a positive image with no uptake in normal or necrotic tissue (13–15,21,22).

However, there are several circumstances where myocardial FDG uptake is not consistent or predictable and therefore fails to differentiate necrotic from viable tissue (105). Normally perfused and contracting myocardium of *diabetic patients* may not take up FDG either with or without glucose loading, even after their usual dose of insulin and/or oral hypoglycemic agents. This failure of FDG uptake in diabetics after glucose loading may erroneously suggest necrosis when the myocardium is normal. In such instances, perfusion im-

aging or measures of cell membrane integrity discussed subsequently are the major guides to viability versus necrosis for intervention. Finally, one paper reports that even after glucose loading, one third or more of patients with acute myocardial infarction showing areas of FDG uptake fail to demonstrate improved function or metabolic viability after successful bypass surgery (95).

In the *fasting state at rest* in normal and diabetic subjects, FDG uptake either with or without evolving myocardial infarction is so variable as to be uninterpretable. Additionally, after fasting, at rest in the setting of acute evolving myocardial infarction, intense FDG uptake may occur in areas of myocardium that are necrotic, as documented by lack of FDG uptake after glucose loading, by left ventricular akinesis, and by arteriographic involvement of the corresponding coronary artery (Figure 15.7). A similar observation has been made in experimental animals, using cardiac autoradiography (106). For these patients, necrotic tissue erroneously appears viable, owing to intense FDG uptake. In our early experience, before recognizing these problems, two such patients had bypass surgery on the basis of intense FDG uptake in the occluded artery distribution after fasting, but demonstrated no recovery of function and remained in chronic heart failure post-operatively despite open bypass grafts. Therefore, we now do not carry out FDG imaging in the fasting, resting state in acute evolving myocardial infarction.

The mechanism for FDG uptake in recently infarcted myocardium is unclear. In experimental chronic cerebral infarction, elevated FDG uptake is observed in infarcted tissue in association with white blood cell phagocytosis of cellular debris (107), as illustrated in (Figure 15.8) (107). In areas with highly active phagocytosis, the intensity of FDG uptake in

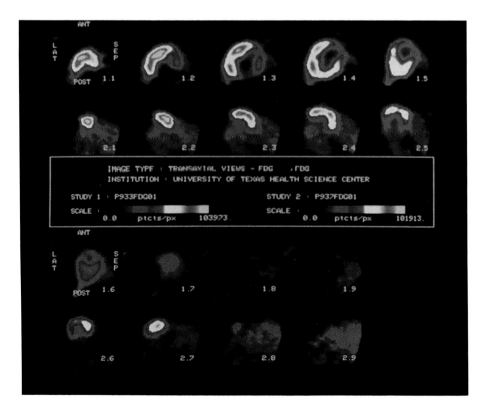

Fig. 15.7 Resting PET scans of FDG obtained after oral glucose loading, in upper of paired image rows (S1), and after fasting, in the lower row (S2). A severe defect in FDG uptake after glucose loading indicates necrotic myocardium. However, repeat study after fasting shows intense FDG uptake in this same area. Reproduced with permission from Gould KL, Haynie M, Hess MJ, et al. 1990. (148).

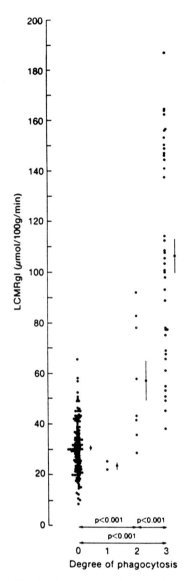

Fig. 15.8 Relationship between local cerebral glucose metabolic rate CMR$_{glc}$ (LCMR$_{glc}$) derived from the phagocytes and the degree of phagocytosis in tissue ipsilateral to the occlusion. The means ± SEM are indicated along with the differences between the groups. Grade 0, no observation of phagocytes; grade 1, a few phagocytes; grade 2, a moderate number of phagocytes; grade 3, a large number of phagocytes. Reproduced with permission from Komatsumoto S, Greenberg JH, Hickey WF, et al., 1989. (107).

chronic cerebral infarction may be many times higher than FDG uptake of normal brain. FDG uptake by white blood cell in myocardial infarction in acute short-term experiments (6 h) is insufficient (108) to explain these observations. However, longer-term experiments on white blood cell uptake of FDG in evolving myocardial infarction comparable to those observed for cerebral infarction, or comparable to our observations in man, have not been carried out. Consequently, FDG uptake in evolving myocardial infarction after fasting, which we observed, may be associated with phagocytic ac-

tivity of white blood cells, as found in cerebral infarction (107).

In these circumstances, where myocardial uptake of FDG is unpredictable or taken up in myocardium by unclear mechanisms perhaps unrelated to viability, the application of quantitative models for deriving absolute glucose utilization in g/mg/min is inappropriate. Even under usual circumstances, the usefulness of absolute measurements of myocardial flow (27,64–66) or glucose consumption in myocardium (105) or brain (67) does not appear necessary for patient studies, since most clinical reports showing the real benefits of FDG imaging use end points of relative FDG uptake or uptake relative to a perfusion tracer.

Finally, in contrast to chronically reduced resting flow to viable myocardium, reperfused myocardium during acute myocardial infarction makes interpretation of a perfusion-metabolism mismatch on FDG images quite complex. A defect on a perfusion image after reperfusion with a patent artery suggests a no-reflow phenomenon associated with necrosis and an FDG defect. Alternatively, perfusion may be normal or near normal, either with or without an FDG defect. In this case, a reverse mismatch may occur, with no perfusion defect associated with an FDG defect; the significance of such a case has not been documented. With reperfusion in myocardial infarction, the zone of myocardium at risk may not be readily defined by a resting perfusion defect, which is the basis for the perfusion-metabolism mismatch to define viable myocardium characteristic of chronic stable coronary artery disease. Since most of our patients had received thrombolysis therapy in this study, we avoided these problems by using relative FDG uptake compared to normal myocardium (after glucose loading) without reference to a metabolism/perfusion ratio.

PROTOCOL FOR ASSESSING MYOCARDIAL VIABILITY AND INFARCT SIZE BASED ON ^{82}RB KINETICS

Other aspects of cell behavior not dependent on perfusion or metabolic imaging are also markers of myocardial cell viability and/or necrosis. These include release of myocardial CPK enzymes or other cell components such as inosine (109,110), phosphate (111,112), or potassium (109–118), but such approaches do not regionally locate and size the area of infarction or viability. The leak of potassium from myocardial cells is an immediate early marker of impaired cell membrane function and necrosis that has been well documented by a substantial literature (109–118). Therefore, a quantitative imaging method utilizing a potassium analogue reflecting cell membrane function might be useful for assessing viability and infarct size.

The intracellular-extracellular potassium gradient is maintained by intact myocardial cell membranes, the characteristics of which have been well documented (113–120). Damaged cell membranes associated with myocardial necrosis leak potassium from cells (116–118) into interstitial space (114) and venous effluent (111–115). Figure 15.9 illustrates the rise in extracellular potassium with time after occlusion. This potassium loss is reversible on reperfusion up to the end of the plateau phase (114). Reperfusion after the plateau

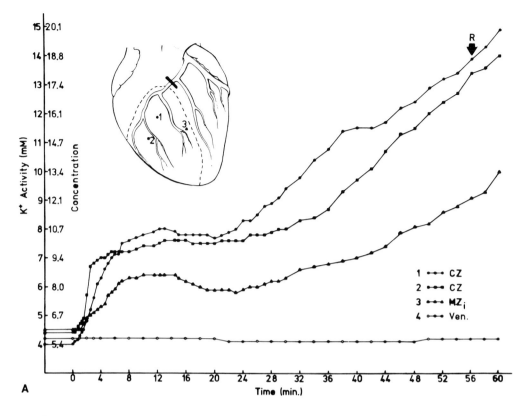

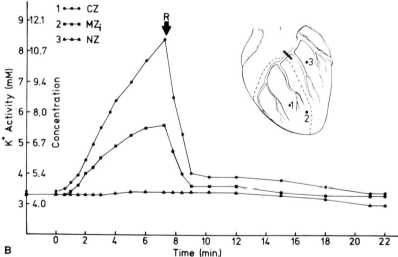

Fig. 15.9 (A) Time course of mid-myocardial extracellular K^+ activity (a_k^+) rise, recorded at two sites in the center of the ischemic zone (CZ) and inside margin of ischemic zone (MZ_1) during a 56-min occlusion. The a_k^+ rose more rapidly and to greater levels in the center of the ischemic zone than at the margin. The rate of a_k^+ rise slowed significantly and entered the plateau at all three sites 5–10 min after occlusion. Approximately 25 min after the occlusion, a second, slower rise in a_k^+ occurred at all three sites. This rise continued after release of the occlusion at 56 min (arrow R). The systemic a_k^+, measured by an intravenous probe (electrode 4), did not change during the entire occlusion period. Note especially the inhomogeneity in the a_k^+ rise in the center of the ischemic zone. **(B)** Normalization with earlier reperfusion. Reproduced with permission from Hill JL, Gettes LS, 1980. (114).

phase during the second rise of extracellular potassium does not reverse further potassium loss and cell necrosis. The extent of potassium loss from myocardial cells is directly and linearly related to CPK enzyme loss (115,117,118) reflecting extent of necrosis, Figure 15.10 (117). In addition to being a marker of necrosis, radioactive potassium, ^{43}K, has also been used for myocardial imaging (120–123).

Rubidium is a potassium analogue with a variety of medically useful radioactive forms, including ^{81}Rb, ^{82}Rb, ^{84}Rb, and ^{86}Rb. Myocardial cell membrane transport, trapping, and flow-extraction characteristics of potassium and rubidium parallel

each other (124–131). Figure 15.11 shows the close parallel between the kinetics of rubidium and potassium (131). Rubidium tracers have also been used for assessing perfusion in animals (37–39,126–140) and in man (1,4,12,19,28,141–147). For PET imaging, the strontium-82/rubidium-82 generator has been developed (35) and adapted for commercial production (36). Clinically, it is useful for qualitative infarct imaging (19) and has high sensitivity/specificity for diagnosis of coronary artery stenosis and its severity (1,4). Therefore, the behavior and kinetics of rubidium in myocardium are well established.

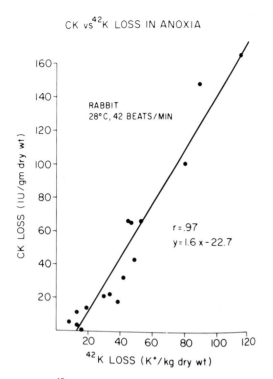

Fig. 15.10 Net ^{42}K loss after reoxygenation of isolated perfused rabbit septums after varying durations of anoxia. Longer periods of anoxia produced progressively increasing net potassium losses after reoxygenation. These losses are plotted against net CK loss as determined by analysis of effluent from hearts during 60 min after reoxygenation. Periods of anoxia of 10–20 min produced no significant net ^{42}K loss or CK loss. Thereafter, there was a linear relationship between the magnitude of the net potassium losses after reoxygenation and the net CK losses from the tissue. Reproduced with permission from Conrad GL, Rau EE, Shine KI, 1979. (117).

The basis for using ^{82}Rb in assessing viability and infarct size has also been demonstrated in animals (26). Upon delivery by coronary flow to myocardium, rubidium enters normal cells where it is trapped. However, if these cells are necrotic (TTC-negative) the delivered rubidium leaks or washes out of the cells. In dogs with myocardial infarction and reperfusion, myocardial rubidium washout measured by beta probes over the 120 to 240 s after intravenous injection identifies necrotic versus viable myocardium with high reliability and little overlap (26).

In corresponding clinical validation studies, we have shown that in patients with evolving myocardial infarction, cell membrane dysfunction, as evidenced by abnormal kinetics of the potassium analogue ^{82}Rb, parallels abnormal intracellular metabolism of the glucose analogue, FDG. This observation is important for an integrated understanding of how to identify viable versus necrotic myocardium in clinically applicable physiologic terms. An important associated demonstration was that the size of myocardial infarct showing a rubidium leak measured in man by PET equals the size of myocardial infarction showing abnormal glucose metabolism measured by FDG imaging (105,148).

The clinical protocol based on rubidium kinetics utilizes the same resting perfusion protocol described previously, with the exception that the image data is acquired in list mode. As illustrated in Figure 15.12 (148), the resting PET data collected in list mode is divided into an early phase image (first 15–110 s) and a late phase image (all data after 120 s). As described subsequently in detail, a new defect or worsening defect on the late image as compared to the early image indicates washout or failure to trap rubidium, and therefore necrosis. Residual myocardial trapping of rubidium on the late image within a defect, reflecting partial or limited washout, indicates some residual viable myocardium.

The basis for automated quantitation of infarct size by PET, based on kinetics of ^{82}Rb, is shown in Figure 15.13 (148). Viable myocardium traps rubidium with no washout from a

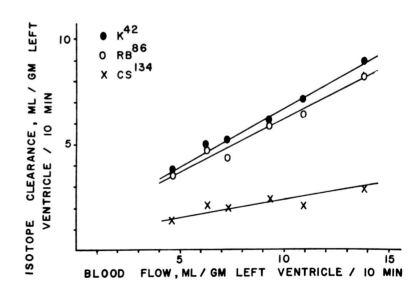

Fig. 15.11 The relationship between the rate of coronary blood flow and the simultaneous rates of my clearance of K^{42}, Rb^{86}, and Cs^{134} in dogs. Reproduced with permission from Love WD, Isihara Y, Lyon LD, et al., 1968. (131).

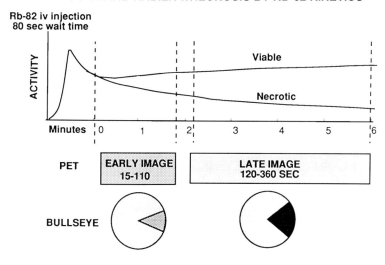

MYOCARDIAL VIABILITY/NECROSIS BY RB-82 KINETICS

Fig. 15.12 Schematic of the clinical protocol utilizing the kinetic changes of ^{82}Rb after intravenous injection for assessing myocardial viability. Reproduced with permission from Gould KL, Haynie M, Hess MJ, et al., 1990. (148).

region of interest on the time-activity curve (upper panel). Infarcted myocardium fails to retain rubidium, which washes out from cells after initial uptake (middle panel). A mix of infarcted and viable tissue in the field of view results in an intermediate level of washout proportional to the percent of viable or infarcted tissue. The activity in the late (S2) rubidium image relative to the early (S1) image therefore reflects the extent of washout and the proportion of viable or necrotic myocardium.

In order to avoid questionable assumptions of complex models, we use a simple measurement scheme to quantify rubidium washout, in which percent viable myocardium is equal to the ratio of activity in the late to the early image, corrected for background activity, written as % V = (S2-B)/(S1-B). By rearranging this simple expression, an equation is obtained (Fig. 15.13), (148) relating the late/early activity ratio (S2/S1) to percent viability, S2/S1 = % V + [B-B (%V)]/S1. For purposes of objective automated infarct sizing, we then defined necrotic myocardium as less than 50% viable tissue. An average value of 55% of maximum activity remains in severe perfusion defects (scar) on PET scans of rubidium, due to the combination of spillover, partial volume errors, positron range, and background activity. Average activity of normal myocardium is typically 85% of maximum activity on rubidium PET scans under resting conditions. Substituting these values into the equation of Figure 15.2 gives the relative S2/S1 threshold, 0.825, below which myocardium was defined as necrotic. Percent of the myocardium that was infarcted, as defined above, was then automatically determined from the polar map display of the relative S2/S1 ratio image as that percent of the relative S2/S1 polar map falling below the threshold of 0.825.

For assessing viability by ^{82}Rb, 40–50 mCi of ^{82}Rb is infused intravenously from a strontium-82/rubidium-82 generator (Squibb) over 30–60 s. The generator is eluted daily for calibration and for strontium breakthrough. For the example shown here, immediately after completion of rubidium imaging, 10 mCi of FDG was injected intravenously. Data col-

lection of the FDG images is started 45 min later and lasts 30 min, with acquisition of approximately 30 million counts per whole heart data set. Data collection of rubidium activity was begun in list mode at 80 s (defined as zero time of data col-

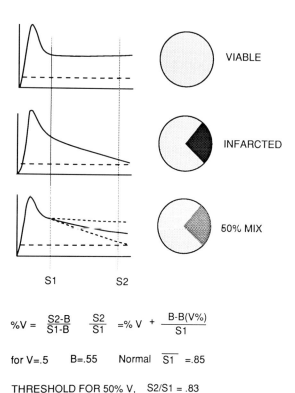

$$\%V = \frac{S2\text{-}B}{S1\text{-}B} \qquad \frac{S2}{S1} = \%\,V + \frac{B\text{-}B(V\%)}{S1}$$

for V=.5   B=.55   Normal $\overline{S1}$ =.85

THRESHOLD FOR 50% V,   S2/S1 = .83

Fig. 15.13 Basis for automated quantitation of infarct size by PET based on the kinetics of ^{82}Rb. Reproduced with permission from Gould KL, Haynie M, Hess MJ, et al., 1990. (148).

lection) after the beginning of [82]Rb infusion, to allow for blood pool clearance, and continued through 360 s. During the fixed 6-min data collection, typically 15 to 25 million counts were obtained. Early and late images were reconstructed using the first 15–110 s and 120–360 s of data, respectively. Each original nine-slice image set of early and late data were reformatted into true short-axis, true long-axis, and polar maps in paired side-by-side display, as previously reported (10). A relative ratio image of the late to early polar maps was also displayed as a ratio polar map (relative S2/S1) for quantitative analysis.

For the myocardial ischemia protocol, patients were fasted for 16 h before the study, and no glucola was given, the remainder of the protocol being the same as for the glucose-loaded, viability protocol. FDG images were processed into true short- and long-axis views and polar map displays in a paired, side-by-side comparison to the late rubidium images.

Since many of our patients had undergone reperfusion therapy for acute myocardial infarction, the concept of a perfusion-metabolism mismatch (perfusion defect, FDG uptake) to define viable myocardium or a perfusion-metabolism match (perfusion defect, FDG defect) to define necrotic myocardium was not clearly applicable. Accordingly, the size of the infarcted area on the FDG image is automatically determined as the percent of the FDG polar map display that was less than 55% of maximum FDG uptake in that polar map.

Figure 15.14 (148) shows early (S1) and late (S2) images after a single intravenous injection of generator-produced [82]Rb in a patient with an evolving acute inferior myocardial infarction in true short-axis views (panel A), and in horizontal and vertical long-axis views (panel B). The early images are shown in the upper row of each pair of image rows (study 1). The late images are in the lower row of each pair of image rows (study 2). The number after the decimal is the image plane for both study 1 and study 2. In the system of color coding, white indicates the highest activity, red next-highest, and yellow intermediate, with green and blue being lowest relative activity. In true short-axis views of panel A, the image planes are arranged from the AV ring at the upper left to the apex at the lower right. The anterior wall is at the top of each image, the free LV wall is on the left, and the septum is on the right of each tomograph. The open "C" in the basal short-axis views in the upper left images of panel 3A is due to the membranous septum of the left ventricular cavity, which is avascular and therefore appears as a defect but reflects normal anatomy.

Panel B of Figure 15.14 shows horizontal (left) and vertical (right) long-axis views of the heart. Early images are shown in the top row, with late images in the lower row of the top half of the figure. The horizontal long-axis views are oriented as if looking down from above. The vertical long-axis tomographs are oriented as if looking at the left side of the body cut head to toe. Anterior myocardium is at the top, inferior at the bottom, apex at the left, and the AV ring on the right.

Tomographic data is summarized in a polar display as if looking at the patient from the outside toward the apex of the left ventricle located in the center of the bullseye, with the outer rim of the bullseye corresponding to the AV ring. Polar displays on the left (lower half of figure) show the rela-

tive activity on a scale of 0 to 100%, with the early study being the upper (S1) and the late study being the lower (S2) of the polar maps on the left side of the panel. The lower right polar display, labeled relative S2/S1 ratio, shows the relative change in normalized activity of the late image divided by the relative distribution of normalized activity of the early image (relative instead of absolute values), on the scale of 0 to 2. It therefore quantifies the relative change in activity from early to late images. The upper right polar map, labeled absolute S2/S1 ratio, is used for comparing rest-stress images and has no meaning or use for comparing early-late images.

In Figure 15.14, the early rubidium image (S1) shows some perfusion to the inferior wall that washes out to leave a severe defect, indicating necrosis in this area. Letters and numbers beside each polar map show quantitative results. For regions of the heart, A is anterior, S is septal, X is apex, L is lateral, and I is inferior. The numbers beside the rubidium relative S2/S1 polar display of Figure 15.14B (lower right) indicate the percentage of the polar map below the 0.825 threshold. Quantitative measurements of infarct size for Figure 15.14B on the relative S2/S1 rubidium polar map (lower right) indicate that 10% of the heart demonstrated rubidium washout and therefore was necrotic, located inferiorly.

The numbers beside the FDG polar display (S2) of Figure 15.15 (148) are the percentage of the polar display below 55% of the maximum. The infarct size on the FDG image of Figure 15.4, shown beside the lower left (S2) polar map, indicates that 13% of the heart failed to take up glucose and was therefore necrotic, also inferiorly.

Figure 15.16 (148) correlates infarct size based on rubidium washout with automated sizing and with visual estimates on the polar display of the late/early rubidium ratio images, the first 36 patients studied with both [82]Rb and FDG after glucose loading. Figure 15.17 (148) correlates the visually estimated infarct size on rubidium and FDG images. However, to avoid possible observer bias, the automated infarct sizes by rubidium and FDG were also correlated, shown in Figure 15.18 (148). The patients with very large infarct areas had previous infarctions and severe ischemic cardiomyopathy, and were being considered for cardiac transplantation. For these very large infarct areas, the relation between infarct size by rubidium and FDG is less good, due primarily to probable overestimates by the FDG method, since some of the largest infarct sizes by FDG would appear to be incompatible with survival.

In one patient, with the smallest infarct by FDG, the late rubidium and FDG images appeared visually identical but the FDG activity in the infarct area was just above the 55% threshold for automated determination of size; therefore, the automated infarct size by FDG was smaller than the visual size of the infarct on both FDG and rubidium images.

Several patterns of rubidium washout on early-late rubidium images were observed, illustrated in Figure 15.19 and Figure 15.20. Washout types I through III reflect progressively larger and more severe infarctions (148). Type IV is a fixed severe defect without initial activity and therefore without washout, indicating old scar or necrosis, an occluded artery, and no collateral flow. All Type IV images had severe large infarct areas by FDG that corresponded to the rubidium images. For Type IV there is no rubidium washout, since there is no rubidium activity (or FDG) delivered into the infarct

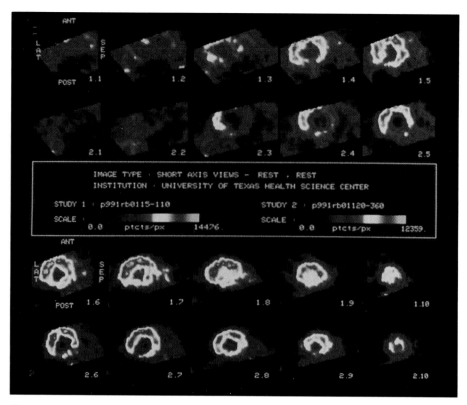

A

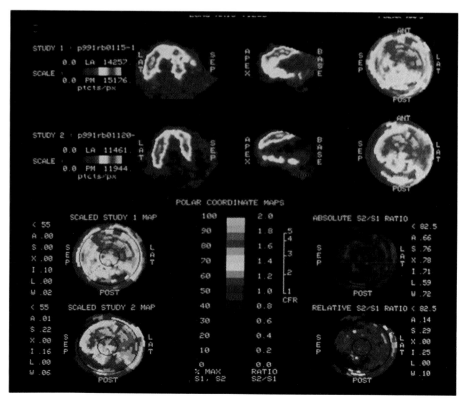

B

Fig. 15.14 Sequential rubidium images early (S1) and late (S2) after intravenous injection of a patient with an evolving acute inferior myocardial infarction. **(A)** short-axis views. **(B)** horizontal (left) and vertical (right) long-axis views. See text for details. Reproduced with permission from Gould KL, Haynie M, Hess MJ, et al., 1990. (148).

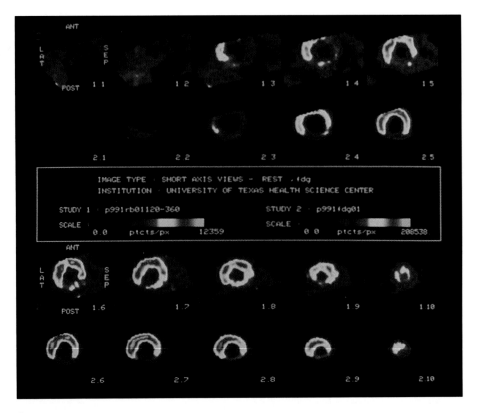

A

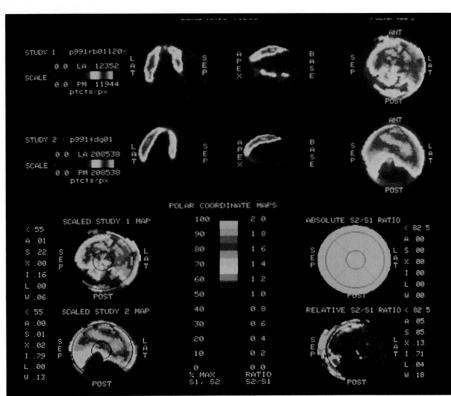

Fig. 15.15 Comparison of late rubidium images (S1) with FDG images (S2) of the same patient. **(A)** short-axis views. **(B)** long-axis views. See text for details. Reproduced with permission from Gould KL, Haynie M, Hess MJ, et al., 1990. (148).

B

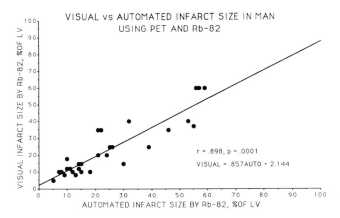

Fig. 15.16 Relation of infarct size based on rubidium images, by the automated threshold method and by visual estimates on the polar display of the late/early ratio images.

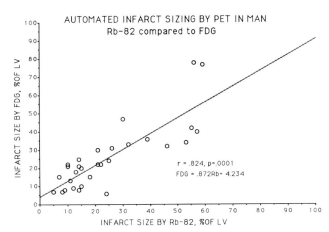

Fig. 15.18 Relation of infarct size by the automated threshold method, using rubidium and FDG images. Reproduced with permission from Gould KL, Haynie M, Hess MJ, et al., 1990. (148).

zone. The size of Type IV infarction was automatically determined as the percentage of the late rubidium polar map (S2) below 55% of maximum, comparable to the 55% threshold for the FDG polar map. For rubidium images of Type V pattern, the late images showed increased activity with relative S2/S1 ratio greater than 0.825, suggesting mostly viable myocardium with only small visual infarcts on both rubidium and FDG images. Of 36 rubidium studies, 9 were Type I, 12 were Type II, 9 were Type III, 2 were Type IV, and 4 were mixed, of which 1 showed Types I and II in different parts of the heart, and 3 were Type V in part of the heart with Types II, III, or IV in other parts.

Of the 36 patients with FDG and rubidium studies, there were six patients in whom there was no or little uptake of FDG by myocardium (Table 15.5) (145), the activity being entirely or primarily in blood pool in four patients. In the remaining two of these six patients, part of the normal myo-

cardium took up FDG but large areas of the left ventricle failed to take up FDG, despite normal contractile function on LV angiogram and normal resting flow (no perfusion defect) through non-infarct related, normal, or minimally narrowed coronary arteries. All six of these patients were diabetic, treated with insulin, oral hypoglycemic agents, or dietary regimens. Since these six FDG images were uninterpretable, they were excluded from the quantitative analysis comparing FDG to rubidium.

In three additional patients, FDG and rubidium images were markedly discordant, owing to defect size on FDG im-

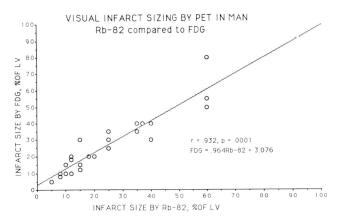

Fig. 15.17 Relation of visually estimated infarct size by rubidium and FDG imaging. Reproduced with permission from Gould KL, Haynie M, Hess MJ, et al., 1990. (148).

PATTERNS OF RB-82 WASHOUT

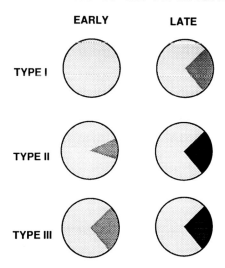

Fig. 15.19 Characteristic types of rubidium washout in acute evolving myocardial infarction.

PATTERNS OF RB-82 WASHOUT
(Continued)

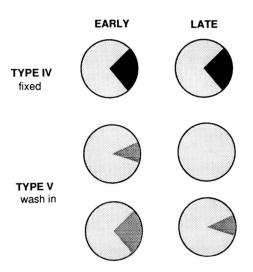

Fig. 15.20 Characteristic changes on early and late rubidium images having a fixed, severe defect (Type IV) or wash-in of rubidium (Type V), indicating delayed delivery associated with low flow and late trapping by viable myocardium.

Table 15.5A FDG vs. Rb Washout in Evolving MI

FDG failures, all diabetic	6
Blood pool only (4), no uptake in areas of normal flow and function (2)	
Visual discordance, FDG > Rb	3
Areas of normal flow, function but no FDG (3), also diabetic (2)	
Visual concurrence, FDG = Rb	27
Total with Rb and FDG	36

Table 15.5B FDG vs. Rb Washout in Evolving MI

After glucose loading for Dx necrosis		
No myocardial FDG uptake or erroneous regional failure of uptake	9/42	(21%)
After Fasting for Dx Ischemia, Viability		
Intense FDG uptake in areas of necrosis by FDG after glucose loading	6/6	(100%)
Visual concurrence Rb washout with adequate FDG studies	27/27	(100%)

ages being grossly larger visually and by automated sizing than on rubidium images; this large defect size on FDG images was caused by lack of FDG uptake in myocardial areas of normal contraction and normal perfusion by non-infarct related, normal, or mildly narrowed coronary arteries; two of these three patients were also diabetic. However, these three patients with aberrant absence of regional FDG uptake were included in the quantitative comparison of the FDG with rubidium for infarct sizing, since at least substantial parts of the myocardium took up glucose appropriately.

There was visual concurrence in location and visual size of the infarct area on rubidium and FDG images in 25 of 27 remaining patients, in whom FDG was normally taken up by normal areas of myocardium not involved in the infarction. In two of these 27 patients the essential visual interpretation was the same, but the infarct size on the FDG image was somewhat larger than by rubidium; both patients had no FDG uptake in small areas of normal contraction and perfusion by non-infarct related arteries. For the quantitative comparison of infarct size on rubidium with FDG images, only the 6 patients with unusable FDG images were excluded, leaving 30 of the 36 patients with paired FDG and rubidium studies, including those with some regional deficiency of FDG uptake despite normal contraction and perfusion through non-infarction-related arteries to those areas.

Thus, out of 43 patients with acute evolving myocardial infarction studied with FDG after glucose loading, 9, or 21%, had no myocardial uptake anywhere in the heart or had large areas of normal myocardium that did not take up glucose after glucose-loading, despite normal contraction and perfusion. Eight out of these nine were diabetic (148).

Of the seven patients studied with FDG after a 16-h fast, two failed to take up FDG anywhere in the heart, either after fasting or glucose loading. Five showed intense FDG uptake in areas of infarcted myocardium, as defined by (a) a severe defect or lack of FDG uptake on glucose-loaded images, in contrast to normal myocardium which did take up FDG; (b) akinesis on LV angiogram in the area of the defect on perfusion and glucose-loaded FDG images; or (c) arterial occlusion, severe stenosis, and/or intraluminal clot in the infarct-related artery by arteriography. Figure 15.7 illustrates the phenomenon of intense FDG uptake by recently infarcted myocardium (148). The upper of each pair of tomographic rows (S1) shows FDG images after glucose loading. The lower row of each pair (S2) shows FDG images after fasting. Under glucose-loaded conditions, the normal myocardium took up FDG but the infarct area failed to take up FDG, corresponding to an akinetic anterior wall and an occluded LAD at arteriography. After glucose loading, the normal myocardium took up FDG, with peak activity of 103,973 cts/pixel.

However, after fasting, this same area of necrosis took up FDG intensely, with a peak activity of 101,913 cts/pixel. Therefore, the intensity of FDG uptake in the necrotic area after fasting is not due to relative upscaling of image intensity referenced to suppressed FDG uptake in normal myocardium. Rather, it is due to intense FDG uptake in an area of infarcted myocardium that is so strong that it downscales relative intensity of the rest of the image.

Our results demonstrate that the size of infarcted myocardium defined by abnormal rubidium kinetics is comparable to the size of infarcted myocardium defined by lack of FDG uptake on PET images. They also indicate that in myocardial necrosis, the loss of cell membrane integrity as reflected by abnormal kinetics of the potassium analogue, [82]Rb, parallels loss of intracellular intermediary glucose metabolism as reflected by lack of FDG uptake. Our observations extend the well-described behavior of potassium as a marker of myocardial necrosis into clinical application for infarct sizing and relate it to more recent measures of viability based on metabolic imaging. Thus, myocardial necrosis or viability may be identified by measures of either glucose metabolism or cell membrane integrity.

STRESS PERFUSION IMAGING FOR ASSESSING MYOCARDIAL NECROSIS AND VIABILITY IN MAN

Several reports have defined myocardial viability in terms of stress perfusion defects that reverse with redistribution after thallium stress testing (96–100) or by separate rest stress imaging with ^{13}N ammonia by PET (16). The results suggest that PET is more accurate than ^{201}Tl for assessing viability (15,16,18,101,102). Patients with no viable myocardium by thallium stress-redistribution studies have viable myocardium by PET imaging of FDG; approximately 30% of patients classified as having completed infarctions without viable myocardium by thallium exercise testing have viable tissue by PET studies (18,102). Stress thallium imaging appears to overestimate extent of necrosis (15,16,18,99–103). Based on such comparisons now in the literature, PET imaging of FDG has been considered by many investigators in the field to be the optimal method for assessing myocardial viability, particularly in resting perfusion defects.

However, it may not be appropriate to compare reversible stress perfusion defects with resting metabolic abnormalities, since they provide different information. Stress perfusion defects not present at rest or redistribution indicate areas of limited coronary flow reserve that are measures of zones at risk, not viability per se. For severe stenoses that reduce resting flow, the defect severity on stress perfusion images may be more intense and/or larger than at rest, simply because adjacent areas with normal flow reserve have greater perfusion tracer activity associated with higher stress flow, unrelated to viability in the perfusion defect. Thus, reversible stress defects reflect flow capacity of normal myocardium around a resting defect but do not provide information on viability of myocardium within a resting perfusion defect.

With reperfusion, the definition of viability becomes more complex, since the zone at risk characteristically contains a mix of viable and necrotic tissue with a patent artery and adequate flow. In this case, stress-induced enlargement of a perfusion defect may indicate additional zones at risk, with low coronary flow reserve around the damaged area or limited flow capacity in the central damaged region due to edema or obliteration of vascular channels. However, it does not provide information on whether there is viable myocardium in the more central reperfused area of injury.

Current literature on assessing myocardial viability by metabolic imaging compared to stress perfusion imaging does

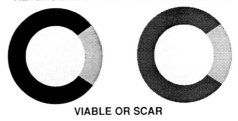

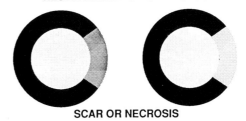

Fig. 15.21 Schematic comparing the changes on sequential stress-redistribution thallium images (upper) and early-late rubidium washout images (lower).

not clearly differentiate viability as proportion of "live" or "dead" myocardium in an injured area, distinct from the zone at risk of low coronary flow reserve indicated by a stress perfusion defect. The proportion of "live" or "dead" myocardium in an injured area, particularly with reperfusion, is indicated by rubidium kinetics reflecting membrane function, or by FDG uptake expressed as a relative percent of normal adjacent areas without reference to resting or stress perfusion. Figure 15.21 compares conceptually a stress defect that redistributes to rubidium washout. For stress thallium, the defect becomes less severe (redistributes), owing to washout of normal areas. The defect on serial [82]Rb images becomes worse with loss of [82]Rb trapping in the necrotic myocardium.

MYOCARDIAL ZONES AT RISK

Extent of myocardial necrosis and viability are related to degree of flow reduction and metabolic demands. Compared with a normal flow of 1 mL/min/g, necrosis usually occurs at 0.1 mL/min/g, but with greater metabolic demand it may occur at higher flows, for example, 0.3 mL/min/g. For a variety of other unclear reasons, myocardial necrosis is heterogenous for a given level of reduced flow, or the flow threshold separating injured viable from necrotic myocardium is variable, particularly for flow expressed as mL/min/g. By expressing flow or perfusion as a percent of normal in a specific heart, some of this threshold variability is reduced, since the normal flow levels reflect the normal supply demand for that heart.

Therefore, an approach for assessing myocardial viability is based on the observation that after 1 h of perfusion below 10%–20% of normal resting myocardial perfusion measured by microspheres, myocardium is largely necrotic (27,64–66).

By imaging the relative uptake of the perfusion tracer [82]Rb at rest, non-viable myocardium can be identified as distinct from viable myocardium and validated by comparison to TTC staining in dogs (27). However, background "noise" and spillover activity in PET scan defects using ^{13}N ammonia or [82]Rb may be 10%–50% of normal resting myocardial values. Therefore, the application of this approach by perfusion imaging requires operator-intense background and spillover corrections that make its routine application difficult. We are currently developing automated methods to solve this problem.

Referencing FDG uptake to a perfusion image for obtaining a perfusion-metabolism match (necrotic) or perfusion-metabolism mismatch (viable) pattern (15) is a way of defining a perfusion zone at risk under resting conditions, that is, a zone of low resting flow. However, reduction in resting myocardial perfusion occurs only with very severe coronary stenoses, where small degrees of luminal worsening due to platelet deposition or spasm may cause occlusion and thrombosis. Accordingly, such lesions tend to be unstable. Therefore stable, chronically reduced, resting antegrade flow is not common or a general enough occurrence to define reliably a zone at risk. Most coronary artery stenoses either occlude or have normal resting flow but reduced flow reserve.

In addition, the narrow range of flow from levels measurably reduced below normal to lower flows associated with progressive thrombosis and occlusion is difficult to assess within the "noise" level of PET images. Therefore, defining a zone at risk by rest perfusion imaging, and hence viability by a resting perfusion-metabolism mismatch, applies to a relatively small proportion of patients in the wide spectrum of coronary artery disease and may not be readily interpreted in acute evolving myocardial infarction and/or reperfusion.

Although the concept of a perfusion-metabolism mismatch is important and often predicts viable myocardium in resting defects, its general clinical applicability may be somewhat limited, owing to the difficulty of defining a perfusion zone at risk under resting conditions and/or after reperfusion. Consequently, we utilize FDG uptake and/or rubidium washout at rest not only with reference to resting perfusion but also as compared to dipyridamole defects, in order to evaluate completely the proportions of viable and necrotic myocardium mixed together in the resting defect as well as the zone at risk defined by limited flow reserve. For an objective, automated sizing of the infarction, a threshold proportion of predominantly viable or necrotic myocardium was defined in our studies for binary classification to compare abnormalities in FDG metabolism with abnormalities of rubidium kinetics by an objective method, as described earlier.

QUALIFICATIONS ON ASSESSING MYOCARDIAL VIABILITY

Metabolic imaging for myocardial viability is widely viewed as the best validated advantage of PET over thallium perfusion imaging (15). However, this claim is based on only two clinical reports involving a total of 39 patients in the world's literature (17,103), as shown in Table 15.6. The accuracy of FDG imaging for predicting improvement of poorly contracting LV segments after bypass surgery was 78% (103) to 85% (17), as compared to 65% (16) to 81% (97) for thallium.

The initial report on FDG in 17 patients indicates that 85% of hypokinetic segments taking up FDG improved function after bypass surgery (17). However, ejection fraction improved significantly only in those with three or more segments involved (Fig. 15.5). Data was not provided on the *percent of patients* with three or more viable regions that would warrant bypass surgery or the number of patients out of only 17 showing improved ejection fraction.

Table 15.3, from a study of rest-exercise PET using ^{13}N ammonia, shows that 34 of 48 segments with transient perfusion defects, or 71%, improved after bypass surgery. Of myocardial segments with transient reversible perfusion defects on thallium exercise imaging, Table 15.1 (97) and Table 15.2 (16) show that 65% (15/23) to 81% (35/43) improved after bypass surgery. Therefore, based on published literature, prediction of post-operative recovery in 78%–85% of LV segments taking up FDG may not be much better than improved post-operative function in 65%–81% of LV segments with reversible stress defects by thallium perfusion imaging. Fur-

Table 15.6 Comparison of Clinical Imaging Trials for Patient Management of Viable Myocardium

Diagnostic Test	Accuracy		Patients		Reference
	Pos	*Neg*			
Predicting improved postop	85%	92%	17	Tillisch	NEJM 314:884, 1986 (17)
LV wall motion by FDG	78%	78%	22	Tamaki	AJC 62:202, 1988 (103)
Predicting improved postop	81%	86%	25	Rozanski	Circ 64:936, 1981 (97)
LV wall motion by [201]Tl	65%	58%	31	Tamaki	JNM 30:1302, 1989 (16)
	86%	78%	26	Iskandrian	AJC 51:1312, 1983 (98)
	Sn	*Sp*			
Diagnosis of coronary artery	95%	100%	50	Gould	AJC 7:775, 1986 (1)
stenosis using [82]Rb with a	94%	95%	193	Demer	Circ 79:825, 1989 (4)
fast PET scanner or [13]NH$_3$	97%	100%	32	Schelbert	AJC 49:1197, 1982 (5)
	97%	100%	49	Yonekura	AHJ 113:645, 1987 (6)
	98%	93%	146	Williams	JNM 30:845, 1989 (177)

thermore, studies of LV segments do not reflect the proportion of patients with large enough viable areas to warrant interventions.

For comparative purposes, Table 15.6 also lists the major clinical imaging trials of PET, involving 470 patients, reporting a 95% or greater sensitivity and specificity for the diagnosis of coronary artery disease. The number of studies and relative improvement in diagnostic power supports the use of PET for perfusion imaging as much as or more than for identifying reversible wall motion abnormalities.

Recent abstract reports and data reviewed in this chapter suggest that FDG uptake may have significant limitations for routinely assessing viability clinically, owing to lack of uptake in viable myocardium in some patients and uptake by necrotic myocardium in others. Furthermore, in one study, 22% of LV segments with preoperative FDG uptake had no improvement in LV function after bypass surgery (Table 15.6), consistent with our observation that under fasting conditions necrotic myocardium may take up FDG. The literature has also not made a distinction between viability in a resting perfusion defect versus a reversible stress defect caused by limited flow reserve around the resting defect. Although this question is only now being studied, it is our clinical impression that by both FDG and rubidium washout criteria, substantial viable myocardium warranting PTCA or bypass surgery is not as commonly found in significant resting perfusion defects as previously reported, certainly not in 85%. Although FDG imaging detects more viable segments than thallium imaging, there is little evidence that it identifies more post-infarction patients needing mechanical intervention than does thallium imaging.

With stress or dipyridamole perfusion imaging, the visual intensity of the resting defect appears greater, owing to more activity delivered to normal myocardium around the resting defect. However, this apparent reversibility of the resting defect does not indicate viability or even a zone of reduced flow reserve around the resting defect. Only a larger or new defect after dipyridamole indicates a new zone at risk. Consequently, in our experience, the number of patients with enough viable myocardium in a resting defect after documented myocardial infarction to warrant mechanical intervention is considerably lower than the 85% suggested by previous literature on percent of LV segments showing improvement (17), and perhaps as low as 25%–35% of patients.

COMBINED ASSESSMENT OF MYOCARDIAL INFARCT SIZE, VIABILITY INFARCT SIZE, AND ZONE AT RISK

As a measurement conceptually separate from infarct size and viability, we define the area of reduced flow reserve or zone at risk by dipyridamole perfusion imaging (1,3,4) rather than rest perfusion imaging. Therefore, we conceptually use the term "viability" of myocardium in reference to a nontransmural, mixed, or incomplete infarction, as distinct and different from what is loosely termed in the literature as "viability" of areas with normal resting perfusion within a zone at risk, identified by reduced flow reserve and a stress perfusion defect due to a stenotic artery. Imaging analogues of cellular metabolism (FDG) or membrane function (rubidium)

identify viability and necrosis in a mixed or incomplete infarction either with or without a resting perfusion defect and with or without reperfusion. Dipyridamole or exercise stress perfusion imaging identifies zones of adequate resting flow but low flow reserve at risk of potential further extension of necrosis. Thus, in the literature, viability is loosely defined, depending on how it is measured.

Comparing metabolic versus stress perfusion imaging as reported in the literature (16,18,101–103) may therefore be inappropriate, since they provide independent, different information. A rest perfusion defect may enlarge laterally with stress because of reduced flow reserve caused by a proximal stenosis. The perfusion defect may also become more intense owing to increased radiotracer activity in surrounding areas of normal flow reserve. An enlarging and intensifying defect after stress therefore defines the zone at risk of low flow reserve due to a stenosis that is by definition "viable" myocardium. However, it does not provide information on viability of myocardium in the more central area of the defect that may be infarction or mixed infarction. Therefore, the conclusion that metabolic imaging by PET is better than stress thallium imaging for identifying viable myocardium may be inaccurate, because reversible stress thallium defects do not provide information about viability in a resting perfusion defect.

Complete analysis of such regions requires assessing viability of myocardium in the central infarcted or partially infarcted myocardium at rest, as well as the larger zones at risk around that region or in other parts of the heart with reduced flow reserve signifying proximal stenoses. Thus, complete clinical evaluation for a major intervention like bypass surgery or PTCA requires imaging coronary flow reserve and cell membrane integrity by the potassium analogue, ^{82}Rb, or cell metabolism by the glucose analogue, FDG.

PRACTICAL CONSIDERATIONS

Although FDG is well documented for assessing myocardial viability (15), it requires a cyclotron and takes approximately 3 h for the entire rest study, including the sequence of imaging ^{13}N ammonia for perfusion, the time for FDG uptake, and FDG imaging for metabolic activity. This 3-h period for one viability study limits the patient volume to approximately four per day, which may be below the minimum volume for economic break-even, depending on the clinical charge (149). Assessing myocardial viability with generator-produced ^{82}Rb at rest (without dipyridamole imaging) requires only 35 min to complete and therefore may be more practical from a clinical point of view.

For clinical applications, ^{82}Rb is well suited for assessing both viability/infarct size at rest and the zone at risk by dipyridamole perfusion imaging in a brief (1-h) single study. The use of dipyridamole in the peri-infarction period is safe and useful for risk stratification (150–156). A rubidium washout study for infarct size is carried out as part of a rest-dipyridamole sequence by collecting the *rest* data in list mode. Dipyridamole perfusion images using rubidium are then obtained. For the rest-dipyridamole comparison to define the zone at risk, all the list mode data is reconstructed into a single rest image and compared to the dipyridamole image. For the resting rubidium washout analysis to determine infarct size-viability, the rest data is divided into early and late rubidium images. The entire data set for infarct size-viability and rest-stress requires 1 h to acquire in our laboratory. The same sequence of viability and stress images with ^{13}N ammonia and FDG requires 4–5 h, owing to the longer data collection times for both these tracers, the longer time for decay of ^{13}N ammonia for rest-stress studies in sequence, and the longer uptake period of FDG.

Thus, using rubidium kinetics to evaluate myocardial viability may have several advantages. It does not require a cyclotron and its expense. The entire rest rubidium study takes significantly less time than for ^{13}N ammonia and FDG, thereby allowing the economy of higher patient volumes at reasonable cost (149). By combining viability measurements with dipyridamole stress using rubidium, complete information on the injured myocardium and on other zones at risk are obtained. Finally, it avoids the problems of inadequate FDG uptake in diabetics and variable patient responses to fasting or glucose loading.

Based on feasibility shown here, assessing cell membrane integrity with the potassium analogue, ^{82}Rb, appears useful for clinically evaluating myocardial viability and infarct size.

16

PET Compared to Other
Imaging Modalities

Although thallium treadmill testing and dipyridamole PET are both used for "stress" perfusion imaging, there are major differences between these two procedures. Single photon emission computed tomography (SPECT) is limited by lack of attenuation correction, depth-dependent changes in resolution, and limited sampling frequency. Of these, the lack of attenuation correction is the major problem, because attenuation of activity from the inferior wall of the heart and septum (in men) and anterior wall (in women) is dependent on highly variable body habitus and orientation of the heart in the chest. Therefore, assumed constant or "standardized" attenuation corrections are not useful but must be measured.

Figure 16.1 illustrates the importance of attenuation correction. A rest perfusion image with ^{13}N ammonia was reconstructed by standard PET techniques with attenuation correction (upper panel labeled S1). The lower of each image pair (labeled S2) was reconstructed from the same data without the attenuation correction. The S2 images are therefore ideal SPECT scans collected with 360° of spatial sampling and high radionuclide energy (511 keV), thereby minimizing attenuation losses compared to much lower energy thallium or technetium. The SPECT image from the same data without attenuation correction shows severe inferior and septal defects typical of false-positive defects associated with tissue attenuation on thallium SPECT scans. Therefore, the high number of false-positive SPECT scans, or low specificity, can be explained by lack of attenuation correction as illustrated in this example, which cannot be distinguished from a real perfusion defect.

The three-head SPECT scanner does not solve this problem but rather makes it worse. In the experience of investigators who have used PET, rotating, and three-headed SPECT systems, artifactual inferior defects appear to be as common or more common with the three-headed SPECT system than with standard SPECT (personal communication from M. Merhige, Buffalo, N.Y.). The reason is that the better sampling of the three-headed SPECT system shows more clearly the attenuation of phantoms from posterior wall and septum. As the imaging technology improves from planar to rotational SPECT to three-headed SPECT to complete-ring SPECT, attenuation correction becomes increasingly important. Even with PET, in our experience, as resolution and sampling frequency improve in more advanced PET scanners, attenuation

correction becomes more critical and more difficult to do accurately. There are a number of additional reasons for false-positive SPECT scans as recently reported (176).

The higher-energy technetium compounds for SPECT have been thought to decrease the problem of artifactual inferior and septal defects due to attenuation. However, in our experience, higher energy emission does not reduce this problem. The images in Figure 16.1 were obtained with 511-keV emission of a positron radionuclide. Without attenuation correction, there is an artifactual severe inferior and septal defect. Other technical details relating clinical diagnostic accuracy to scanner performance are described in more detail in Chapter 17.

Exercise stress does not increase coronary blood flow as much as intravenous dipyridamole or adenosine. Using PET to measure absolute coronary flow and coronary flow reserve, Schwaiger observed the normal increase in coronary flow with treadmill exercise to be 2.5 times baseline, compared to 4.1 times baseline for intravenous dipyridamole (pers. comm. from Marcus Schwaigert, MD). The stronger stimulus for increasing coronary flow (dipyridamole) increases its sensitivity and specificity for detecting and quantifying severity of coronary artery stenosis (1–4,9,45–50,56,57).

Figure 16.2A illustrates examples of normal exercise thallium scans with abnormal dipyridamole PET images confirmed by coronary arteriography. Figure 16.2B illustrates abnormal exercise thallium scans, with normal PET images corresponding to normal coronary arteriograms.

SENSITIVITY AND SPECIFICITY OF EXERCISE THALLIUM IMAGING AND DIPYRIDAMOLE PET

As presented in Table 16.1, the average sensitivity and specificity of thallium exercise testing in the last 2,877 cases published since 1983, weighted for number of cases, are 83% and 53%, respectively. Sensitivity and specificity of exercise thallium imaging is 80% to 90% in symptomatic patients in literature prior to 1983 (158–160). Studies since 1983 report sensitivity of 70% to 85% and specificity of 45% to 60% in both symptomatic (161–165) and asymptomatic (166,167) subjects, or those with atypical presentations (168), as sum-

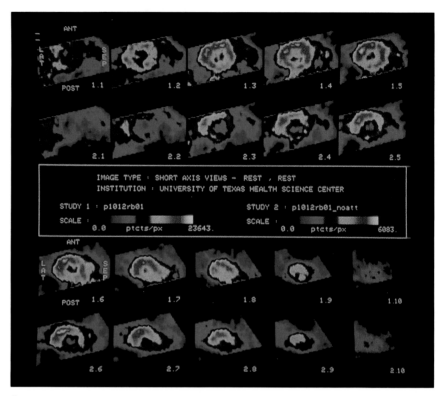

A

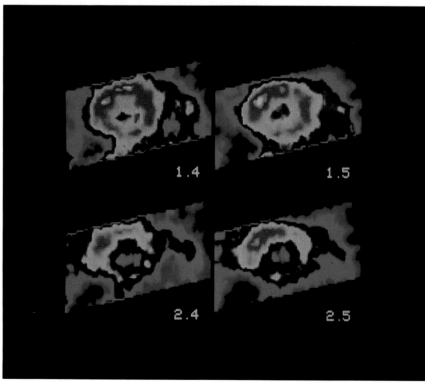

Fig. 16.1 Resting myocardial perfusion scan using ^{13}N ammonia with standard PET reconstruction, with attenuation correction (S1) and without attenuation correction (S2). Lack of attenuation correction causes a severe inferior defect that is artifactual and due to tissue attenuation in **(A)** short-axis views **(B)** magnified short axis, and **(C)** polar maps.

B

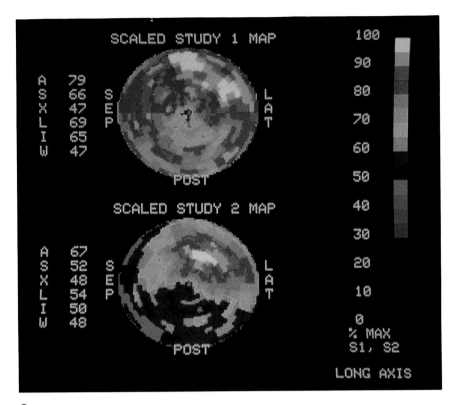

C

marized in Table 16.1. One explanation proposed for low specificity in recent reports is "referral bias"—that is, patients with negative thallium stress tests no longer undergo cardiac catheterization (162,164). The catheterized population in such a study would then be biased by this exclusion of normals, thereby skewing the population toward higher prevalence of disease. According to Bayes' theorem, as the

population is skewed toward greater prevalence of disease, the post-test probability of having no disease with a normal test and the observed apparent test specificity decrease in that population (60,169,170). The second argument made in support of this point of view is that the "normalcy rate" for exercise thallium SPECT is about 90% in uncathed patients having less than 5% probability of coronary artery disease by

Table 16.1 Comparison of Clinical Imaging Trials for Diagnosis of Coronary Artery Disease

Diagnostic Test	Accuracy		Patients	Reference	
	Sn	*Sp*			
Diagnosis of coronary artery	83%	47%	197	Van Train	JNM 27:17, 1986 (162)
disease by thallium stress	85%	52%	1,096	Ranhosky	Circ 78:II432, 1988 (163)
testing since 1983	95%	71%	210	DePasquale	Circ 77:316, 1988 (161)
	76%	49%	832	Schwartz	JACC 11:80A, 1988 (167)
	82%	62%	461	Iskandrian	JACC 14:1477, 1989 (164)
	94%	52%	81	Bungo	Chest 83:112, 1983 (168)
Average weighted for no. of cases	83%	53%			
	75%	67.5%	"corrected"	Diamond	JACC (in press) (157)
	65%	65%	"corrected"	Gould	JACC 14:1487, 1989 (170)
Diagnosis of coronary artery	95%	100%	50	Gould	AJC 7:775, 1986 (1)
stenosis using ^{82}Rb with a fast	94%	95%	193	Demer	Circ 79:825, 1989 (4)
PET scanner or $^{13}NH_3$	97%	100%	32	Schelbert	AJC 49:1197, 1982 (5)
	97%	100%	49	Yonekura	AHJ 113:645, 1987 (6)
	98%	93%	146	Williams	JNM 30:845, 1989 (177)

virtue of young age and no risk factors or family history (162,164).

The reported low specificity of 50% to 60% in recent literature is a fact that no one disputes (162–168). The explanation of this low specificity and therefore the diagnostic value of thallium stress testing depends on how one interprets this fact. Two alternative, opposing explanations are possible. In the first alternative, thallium stress testing has sufficiently low true specificity to make it of limited value in a population characterized by moderate prevalence of disease (10%–30%) and is therefore not economically or medically appropriate. In the second alternative explanation, thallium stress testing is so good that it excludes so many normals from cardiac catheterization in current study populations that the cath population of recent studies is now skewed toward high prevalence and low reported apparent specificity since normals are no longer being cathed; low specificity therefore results from referral bias.

However, we have demonstrated that the currently reported low specificity of 50% to 60% is unlikely to be due to referral bias (157,169,170). Accounting for referral bias by a sophisticated model, Diamond (157) estimated an average "corrected" sensitivity of thallium exercise testing of 67.5% and average "corrected" specificity of 75% (Table 16.1). His conclusion coincides remarkably well with the authors' estimates of 65% sensitivity and 65% specificity accounting for changing patterns of interpretation but without correction for referral bias (170); this estimate is discussed further below. Although referral bias is a valid concept, it cannot be invoked to explain away the poor sensitivity and specificity of thallium exercise testing. Diamond also concluded that (a) SPECT is not superior to planar thallium imaging in diagnostic accuracy; and (b) the use of low-risk groups to establish "normalcy" standards without comparison to coronary arteriography is not correct. In addition, a large recent study with a sensitivity of 76% and specificity of 49% was not biased by referral selection, because all 832 subjects, asymptomatic Air Force personnel, had coronary arteriograms (167) regardless of thallium exercise test results.

The study population with less than 5% probability of coronary artery disease upon which "normalcy rates" of thallium tests are calculated is characteristically a younger, more vigorous population selected to have few risk factors causing coronary artery disease. That younger population is also likely to have fewer causes for false-positive thallium stress tests as compared to an older group, where the risk of coronary artery disease is higher, as well as the risk of false-positive exercise tests due to differences in anatomy of the older, heavier person, including greater chest diameter, greater body mass and bone density, greater diaphragmatic and breast attenuation in the older person, and other factors that cause false-positive thallium images (164). Therefore, the "normalcy rate" for thallium testing from a young population with low probability of disease cannot be extrapolated to the study population at risk for coronary artery disease.

In previous reports (162,164), the uncathed low-risk normal group is used as if cathed to increase numbers of patients in the study and to show a favorable "normalcy rate" to offset low observed specificity, while simultaneously claiming this group to be uncathed in order to avoid the fact of low disease prevalence that disproves referral bias. Therefore, this low-

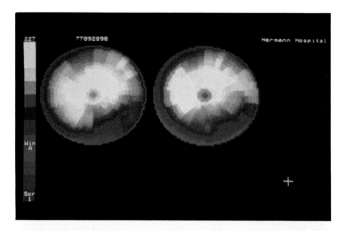

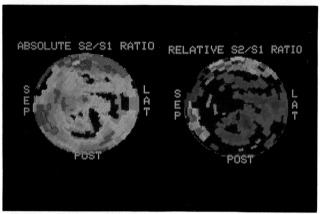

Fig. 16.2 (A) Normal thallium exercise test (upper panel) at rest (left image) and redistribution (right image) in an asymptomatic patient who had reduced flow reserve (lower panel, left image labeled ABS S2/S1 and relative changes rest to stress, right image labeled REL S2/S1) in anterior lateral, lateral and inferior areas confirmed at arteriography (see Case 4 and associated complete set of tomographic studies in Chapter 20, Fig. 20.4).

risk group treated as normal must be included in calculations of disease prevalence.

For example, in some reports, the calculation of disease prevalence in the study population incorrectly excluded the low-probability normal group, since these patients were not cathed but simultaneously were considered normal as if cathed in the overall complete study (162,164). Since the low-probability group is classified as normal in the study, the calculation of true prevalence of disease in the study population must include this group. As an additional example, Table 16.2 shows trends of prevalence and severity of disease from two sequential publications from one center in order to avoid institutional differences. In terms of single-, double-, or triple-vessel disease, the severity of disease decreased and the prevalence of disease fell in parallel with specificity from 1981 to 1986. Thus, referral bias with increasing prevalence of disease in the study population cannot explain low specificity, since actual current disease prevalence of 53% in this study population is lower than prevalence of 67% in earlier years and much lower than the prevalence of 90% that we

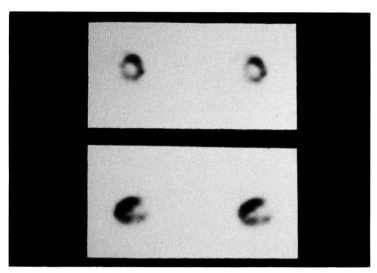

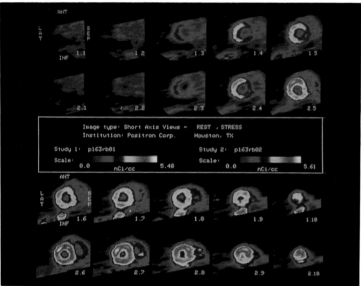

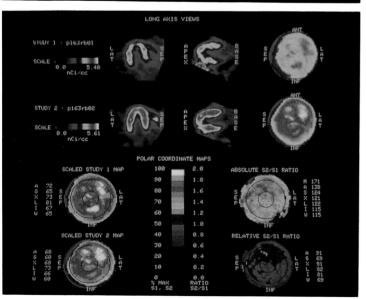

Fig. 16.2 (*continued*) **(B)** Abnormal thallium exercise test in short and long axis views (upper panel) with minimal redistribution. The corresponding short (middle panel) and long axis PET images (lower panel) were normal (images courtesy of Don Gordon, MD, Jacksonville PET Center, Florida).

Table 16-2 Changes in Disease Severity

| | Severity | | | Prevalence | | | |
| | | | | Significant CAD | | | |
Year	SVD	DVD	TVD	All Normals + CAD		Specificity	Sensitivity
1981	16%	24%	60%	45/67	(67%)	86%	91%
1986	25%	28%	47%	143/268	(53%)	47%	83%

Adapted with permission from Gould KL, 1989. Reference 171.

have shown is necessary to explain low specificity on this basis (170).

Why has current specificity of thallium stress testing decreased as compared to reported sensitivity and specificity in earlier literature? The study populations in these early studies consisted of patients undergoing cardiac catheterization on clinical grounds. Therefore, these early study populations had higher prevalence of disease, up to 85% (172), that was also more severe than current study populations, thereby causing more severe readily identifiable defects on scans. Conservative image interpretation in a population of high disease prevalence and severity will give reasonably good sensitivity and specificity, as reported in early literature. More recently, thallium stress testing has been applied to determine whether catheterization is indicated in the absence of a clear clinical diagnosis. Conservative image interpretation in a population of lower disease prevalence (30%–50%) or with milder disease, as recently reported, decreases sensitivity markedly (60,61). In order to maintain higher sensitivity, the reader then interprets images more aggressively by using lower diagnostic criterion levels (60), thereby keeping sensitivity high but at a cost of decreasing specificity.

As an illustration, consider disease prevalence to be 85% with 17 false-negative and 3 false-positive cases out of a study of 100 patients, 85% of whom have disease and 15 of whom are normal. Sensitivity, defined as true positives/true positives + false negatives, would be 80%. Specificity, defined as true negatives/true negatives + false positives, would also be 80%, comparable to early literature. If these same 17 false-negative and 3 false-positive cases were found in the same 100 subjects with 50% disease prevalence, the sensitivity would be 66% and the specificity 94%. In order to increase sensitivity the reader would interpret images with lower diagnostic criterion levels (more aggressively), thereby decreasing false negatives, but at a cost of increasing false positives. How far specificity falls depends on the relation between false positives and false negatives, which in turn depends on individual readers' "diagnostic criterion levels" (60).

Turner (60) has shown that at low diagnostic criterion levels, or aggressive image interpretation, specificity falls by more than 20% for every 10% gain in sensitivity, or the fraction of false positives increases more than 20% for each 10% decrease in false negatives, a 2-to-1 ratio. Therefore, as images were interpreted more aggressively in these 100 patients to decrease false negatives by 8 from 17 to 9, the false positives would increase by 16 from 3 to 20. Sensitivity in the lower-prevalence population would therefore be 82% and specificity 60%, as in current literature (Table 16.1). Therefore, recent literature showing the approximately same sensitivity but markedly lower specificity as compared to earlier literature can be explained by decreased disease prevalence

and severity in the study populations, combined with more aggressive image interpretation. As diagnostic criterion levels decrease (more aggressive interpretations) in current lower-prevalence study populations, the net information content of thallium stress testing is approximately 65% sensitivity and 65% specificity, which become skewed, as previously shown, to a sensitivity of 80% and specificity of 50% to 60% as reported in current literature (161–168) and explained by Figure 16.3.

Agreement on the accuracy of thallium stress testing has been published (157,169) and is summarized in Table 16.1 and by Figure 16.3.

This graph shows a true sensitivity and specificity of approximately 65% each. Due to the inverse relation between sensitivity and specificity, at a disease prevalence of 50%, if images were read in such a way as to give a sensitivity of 80%, then specificity would fall to 50%, consistent with published data. If images were read in such a way as to give higher specificity, then sensitivity would fall and cases would be missed. Therefore, the reported sensitivity and specificity vary, depending on how aggressively or conservatively ab-

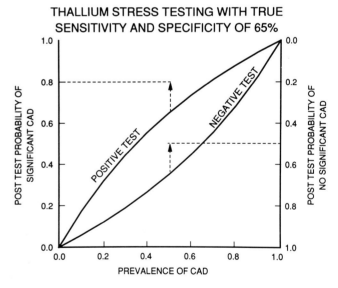

Fig. 16.3 For a disease prevalence of 50% and a true sensitivity and specificity of 65% each, interpreting stress thallium images more aggressively to increase post-test probability of disease for a positive test, or observed sensitivity, to 80% would cause the post-test probability of no disease for a normal test, or observed specificity, to fall to 50%, consistent with reported data. Reproduced with permission from Gould KL, 1989. (170).

normalities are called on exercise thallium scans. However, the net or combined sensitivity-specificity data content of thallium stress imaging corresponds to an approximate equivalent sensitivity and specificity of 65% each, consistent with Diamond's estimates (157). The pattern of reading images in most literature is to read more aggressively, thereby increasing sensitivity to 80% with the observed fall in specificity to 50%, as now reported.

DIRECT COMPARISON OF SPECT WITH PET

In a study population with a high prevalence (94%) of severe advanced CAD, the difference between PET and thallium SPECT is not apparent (175), because the disease is severe enough to cause high contrast between normal and abnormal areas of images. In addition, at a disease prevalence of 94%, the poor specificity of SPECT is not manifest because there are too few normals or those with less severe disease in the study population. The advantages of advanced PET technology are best observed for intermediate disease prevalence (< 60%) and/or moderate to less severe coronary artery disease, where the question of medical or mechanical intervention is unclear and thallium stress testing is most problematic. Table 16.1 compares reported sensitivity and specificity of thallium exercise testing and dipyridamole PET. In two other studies directly comparing PET and SPECT in appropriate populations (193,194,195), the diagnostic accuracy of PET was significantly higher than SPECT, despite inadequate counts (6 to 7 million counts per whole heart data set) in one study (195) and inappropriate PET software in the other (193,194). Using a faster scanner collecting adequate counts (30 to 50 million counts per whole heart data set) and optimized PET software, others have reported much higher sensitivity and specificity of 95% or higher (177), comparable to the first major study by the author (4). In an unpublished study of 40 patients with normal coronary arteriograms and normal dipyridamole PET scans, 18 had false positive thallium stress tests, for a specificity of 55% (pers. comm. from D. Gordon, Jacksonville, Fl.). Thus, although the extent of improved accuracy of PET over SPECT is dependent on the type of scanner, optimized software, and disease prevalence and severity in the study population, the diagnostic accuracy of PET is clearly superior to SPECT.

CLINICAL CONSEQUENCES OF POOR DIAGNOSTIC ACCURACY

For a sensitivity of 80% to 85% as most images are currently read, the 50% to 60% specificity of thallium testing has major medical and economic consequences. Using sensitivity and specificity of approximately 65% and 50%, respectively, for exercise electrocardiography and 80% and 60% for exercise thallium scintigraphy, as currently reported, the efficacy of conventional sequential testing for detecting coronary artery disease can be analyzed. In a population with 10%–15% prevalence of coronary disease, as would be expected in patients with positive risk factors (173,174), if the combination of a positive treadmill electrocardiogram followed by a confirm-

atory positive thallium scan were required for proceeding to catheterization, 48% of patients [1.0 − (.65)(.8)] with angiographically significant coronary artery disease would not be catheterized. If thallium testing were used in all patients instead of an initial EKG exercise test, *only 18% of the catheterized patients would be diagnosed as having disease* in a population with prevalence of disease of 10%, calculated as (0.8 × 10) ÷ (.8 × 10 + .4 × 90). Thus, low specificity of thallium stress testing as recently reported markedly reduces clinical utility of thallium stress testing in populations of lower prevalence, where a non-invasive test is most needed. Accordingly, Turner (60) concluded that (a) thallium stress testing is not adequate for screening patients for CAD, and (b) sensitivity and specificity would have to be approximately 95% for the test to be useful in screening, as reported for PET.

IMPACT OF ACCURATE NONINVASIVE DIAGNOSIS OF CORONARY ARTERY DISEASE

For a noninvasive test with 95% sensitivity and 95% specificity, as reported for PET (1,4–7,177) in a study population that was up to 40% asymptomatic, unnecessary cardiac catheterizations are largely avoided and severity of coronary artery disease is categorized non-invasively (1,4,12), thereby eliminating further unnecessary catheterizations in patients having mild disease detectable by PET and suitable for medical management. This greater accuracy of PET has major economic benefits by preventing unnecessary procedures due to false-positive or equivocal thallium stress tests that more than compensate for a somewhat higher cost per study than thallium stress testing, as well as providing improved medical management (149,171,178). The analysis of this economic benefit is given in Chapter 18.

RISK STRATIFICATION BY PERFUSION IMAGING

Prognostically, thallium stress testing predicts a probability risk of future events after myocardial infarction using either exercise stress (179) or dipyridamole (180). Exercise thallium imaging has also been used to predict future risk in ambulatory outpatients with angina pectoris (180–184). These studies emphasize the usefulness of physiologic or functional markers of coronary artery stenoses for long-term risk stratification, despite its limitations for detection and assessing severity of coronary artery disease. However, the probability of predicting a future event is a binary classification into high or low risk without basis or reference to anatomic disease, its location, or extent. Thus, this probability prediction is too vague and imprecise for current diagnostic decision-making regarding which coronary artery or arteries need what treatment (medical or mechanical) and when. Since thallium perfusion imaging provides some reasonable prediction of future events despite its inherent technical limitations, one might hypothesize that a more quantitative imaging technology, such as PET, providing quantitative regional data on both perfusion and metabolism, might give even better graded, quantitative prediction of future events involving specific myocardial regions or arteries. Consistent with this hypothesis, PET has been shown to be more accurate than thallium for identifying viable myocardium after infarction and predicting regionally improved LV function after bypass surgery (17). However, studies of risk stratification by PET have not been carried out.

Because of limited accuracy for diagnosis or prognosis in individual patients, Bayesian analysis has been applied to thallium imaging in order to improve its clinical usefulness. However, the judgement of a "hard-nosed" diagnostician who must face the consequences of life-and-death decisions has been succinctly summarized by Feinstein (185) as follows: "I know of no specific, constructive, practical diagnostic decision involving real-world patients, data and doctors, in which Bayesian methods have made a prominent contribution that could not have been achieved just as easily without Bayes' formula." This point has been analyzed by Turner (61), who concluded that thallium stress testing is not adequate for screening patients for CAD and that sensitivity and specificity would have to be approximately 95% for the test to be useful in screening, conclusions similar to those by Uhl (173). However, cardiac PET achieves this level of diagnostic accuracy.

COMPARISON TO CARDIAC MRI, FAST CT, SPECT, AND DSA

Some comparison to other high-technology imaging, particularly fast cine CT and NMR, is appropriate. All advanced imaging systems provide differing degrees of anatomic and functional information. At one extreme, optimal quantitative coronary arteriography gives anatomic resolution to within ± 0.1 mm, but no directly measured functional data on flow, viability, function, or metabolism. At the other extreme, positron imaging provides the greatest breadth and depth of functional information on perfusion and metabolism with lower anatomic resolution, which, however, at 5–6 mm for current positron cameras, is appropriate for the functional process being imaged. Fast cine CT and NMR lie between these extremes, as shown in Figure 16.4.

Relative maximum myocardial perfusion or regional perfusion reserve for assessing stenosis severity can be assessed by radionuclide imaging, echocardiography, nuclear magnetic resonance imaging, or computed tomographic scanning. The well-defined basic principles (3,50,56,57), regardless of imaging modality, are: (a) strong stimulus for increasing coronary flow, such as intravenous dipyridamole; (b) a method for monitoring relative regional perfusion changes at high-flow conditions to detect or quantify regional differences attributed to coronary arterial narrowing; and (c) whole heart three-dimensional imaging with adequate counts so that artifactual defects are not created or real defects missed because of inadequate counts, interplane undersampling, or changes in position of the heart in the field.

All of the above methods suffer from the failure of their "signal" or output information to increase in proportion to flow at the high flows necessary for non-invasive diagnostic imaging of myocardial perfusion. For fast computed tomography, intravenously injected perfusion tracers produce an input function that has a time duration greater than coronary

transit time (186), thereby causing the output signal to plateau as myocardial perfusion increases (187,188). Consequently, the density on CT images of myocardium does not increase proportionately as flow increases. As a result, regional abnormalities of maximum perfusion due to coronary disease cannot be identified reliably. Because this problem is a basic one regardless of the type of tracer, it also limits current echocardiographic measurements of perfusion after intravenous injection of microbubbles.

Although NMR provides some information on proton content and state, Paans et al. (189) have pointed out the limited signal intensity of NMR for cardiac metabolic or perfusion imaging. This limitation is a particular problem for imaging myocardial perfusion during high coronary flow conditions necessary for diagnosis of coronary artery disease. Since NMR signal intensity decreases markedly as flow velocity rises (190), the signal from such images enhanced by gadolinium also plateaus as coronary flow rises (191,192). Therefore, although there is a linear correlation between NMR signals (with intravascular gadolinium) and myocardial perfusion at coronary flow rates from resting down to ischemic conditions (191,192), at high flows necessary for identifying coronary artery disease, the NMR signal, even enhanced by gadolinium, does not increase appropriately. Consequently, significant regional differences in maximum myocardial perfusion due to coronary artery stenoses cannot be identified by NMR. It is, therefore, unsatisfactory for assessing coronary artery disease by perfusion imaging at high flows. Thus, NMR and fast cine CT are primarily suited for high-resolution anatomic imaging with limited capacity for non-invasive perfusion or metabolic imaging, whereas positron imaging has

THE INFORMATION SPECTRUM OF IMAGING TECHNOLOGIES

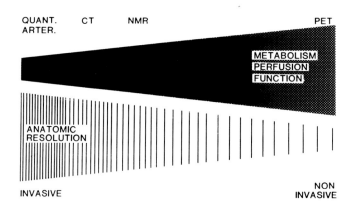

Fig. 16.4 Spectrum of anatomic and functional data from advanced imaging technology. The upper diagram indicates the spectrum of functional data, with PET most useful and high-resolution arteriography least useful for functional assessment. The lower diagram indicates the spectrum of anatomic data, with arteriography providing the maximal spatial resolution in terms of line pairs per mm. Computed tomography (CT) scanning and nuclear magnetic resonance (NMR) are intermediate between these extremes but fall toward the anatomic end of the imaging spectrum. Reproduced with permission from Gould KL, 1990. (205).

the reverse characteristic, with poorer anatomic resolution but more powerful perfusion or metabolic imaging. Perfusion radiotracer uptake also fails to increase proportionately as flow increases, because of falling myocardial extraction at high flows. When this problem is combined with the technical limitations of planar imaging or single proton emission computed tomography without attenuation correction, the resulting images do not accurately reflect regional maximum perfusion. Consequently, they are not quantitative, which probably explains their suboptimal diagnostic accuracy.

Myocardial uptake of positron radiotracers for PET perfusion imaging also fails to increase proportionately with flow. However, image reconstruction techniques in PET are better than those in single proton emission computed tomography because of coincidence counting and attenuation correction. Although limited by falling extraction of radiotracer at high flows, the signal from PET for following relative maximum perfusion is significantly better than other imaging modalities and is semi-quantitative, and the sensitivity and specificity is high. Figure 16.5 illustrates the limitations of various imaging modalities for assessing coronary flow reserve by various cardiac imaging technologies (205). It is not clear whether quantitative models can improve these results, although perfusion models considerably improve PET data toward the ideal.

Finally SPECT is frequently proposed as a less expensive tomographic substitute for positron imaging. However, the sensitivity and specificity of SPECT thallium perfusion imaging for the diagnosis of coronary artery disease remain limited at 70%–85% and 50%–60%, respectively, as previously discussed. In a study population with a high prevalence of advanced severe coronary artery disease, both PET and SPECT are likely to be positive, with comparable sensitivity and specificity. In a study population with a lower prevalence of disease that is also less severe, the differences between PET and SPECT become more apparent, as discussed earlier in this chapter.

Initial results of our direct comparison between PET and SPECT in an appropriate population with lower disease prevalence confirmed the currently reported sensitivity of 80%–85% and specificity of 50%–60% for thallium SPECT as being considerably below the 95–98% sensitivity reported for cardiac PET.

In our first 46 patients with both thallium exercise SPECT and dipyridamole PET for cases with a stenosis flow reserve of less than 3 by automated quantitative coronary arteriography, thallium scans were positive in 58%, whereas PET was positive in 95%. For milder disease with stenosis flow reserve of 3 to 4 by quantitative arteriography, PET identified 50% of cases and thallium stress imaging identified *none*. Thus, direct comparison of thallium exercise SPECT and PET confirm the superior imaging of the latter. Another report (175) directly comparing the two technologies studied a population with a disease prevalence of 94%, thereby virtually eliminating any assessment of relative specificity, which is quite low for SPECT in recent publications. Furthermore, no adequate assessment of quantitative severity of stenoses was made from arteriograms. Subsequent studies in more typical cardiology referral populations confirms the greater diagnostic accuracy of PET as compared to SPECT (193–195). Although

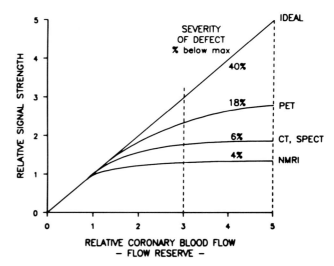

Fig. 16.5 Schematic showing the limits of various imaging modalities for detecting perfusion defects at high-flow states necessary in assessing coronary artery disease. Consider the example in which flow in a normally perfused segment of myocardium increases five-fold over testing levels versus a threefold increase in the distribution of a stenosed artery. Perfusion in the abnormal distribution is 40% below normal maximum [(5–3)/5 = 40%]. The proportional signal from each of several imaging modalities is shown as coronary flow increases. These signals do not increase in proportion to flow, for a variety of technical reasons. The data for positron imaging are better than for other modalities. However, uptake will always be limited by the nonlinear decrease in extraction of radiotracer as flow increases. The proportional change in signal with increasing flow is much worse for other imaging modalities. Reproduced with permission from Gould KL, 1990. (205).

newer technetium compounds appear somewhat better than ^{201}Tl for locating the involved artery, they are positive only with advanced disease, with no higher sensitivity and specificity than reported for thallium (165).

ARTERIAL CORONARY FLOW RESERVE BY DIGITAL SUBTRACTION ANGIOGRAPHY—INDICATOR DILUTION METHODS

Several investigators (196,197) have described an indicator-dilution method for determining arterial coronary flow or flow reserve by DSA techniques, recently validated experimentally by Nissen et al. (198). Sub-selective injections of an exact volume of contrast are made with an ECG-gated power injector at rest and after administration of a potent coronary arteriolar vasodilator, such as dipyridamole or intracoronary papaverine. A time-density curve is obtained from a region of interest over that coronary artery (not the myocardial bed) at rest and at a high flow state. With the same dose of contrast injected sub-selectively, the time-density curve during the high flow state is diluted by the greater volume of flow; the area under the time-density curve is therefore less during high flow than at rest in proportion to the increased flow.

The principle is shown in Figure 16.6 where the area under the arterial time-density curve decreases with increasing flow. The entire x-ray field may be processed and arterial coronary flow reserve determined for the whole artery, as described by Elion et al. (199). However, the method is highly sensitive to misregistration artifacts, owing to motion of the coronary arteries. Accordingly, for widespread routine clinical use in most cases, dual-energy DSA, as described by researchers at Mistretta's laboratory (200), might be necessary.

Other disadvantages are that standard cardiac catheter procedures must be altered to do sub-selective catheterization of each coronary artery, with separate, fixed-dose, ECG-gated power injection of each artery. Coronary arterial branching between the site of injection and the region of data sampling on the artery may invalidate the results. Drugs administered to produce high coronary flows, such as intracoronary papaverine, must be given with repeat power injection for each artery involved. For three-vessel disease, two sub-selective contrast injections would have to be given before and after papaverine administration in each of three arteries, for a total of six injections. Finally, even when measured properly, arterial coronary flow reserve reflects not only stenosis geometry but also ambient physiologic conditions. It may not, therefore, be sufficiently accurate for guiding PTCA. Although promising, this approach needs to be integrated into catheter laboratory procedures and validated clinically. An advantage is that it is not affected by, and is not invalidated by, significant collateral flow because it measures proximal coronary artery flow reserve.

CORONARY TRANSIT TIME METHODS

Vogel et al. (201,202) have developed an empirical method combining elements of transit time with myocardial bed density curves after fixed-dose contrast injections into the left main or right coronary artery (selective but not sub-selective injections). It is a hybrid approach, because the transit time theoretically reflects coronary arterial flow velocity, while the myocardial density curve reflects myocardial perfusion. The transit time as measured by DSA is a function of the intraluminal volume of the epicardial artery and capillary volume as well as time for passage of the contrast media through these two compartments. Peak myocardial density in Vogel's method was used to correct for changes in vascular volume after administration of vasodilators. However, the peak density is also affected by other factors, such as perfusion itself and collaterals. Vogel's approach is shown in Figure 16.7, where the area under the myocardial time-density curves increases with increasing flow after selective intracoronary contrast injection. This increased area under the time-density curve with increasing flow is the opposite of the arterial time-density curve, where the fixed dose of contrast media after sub-selective injection is diluted by higher flows, resulting in a decreased area under the arterial time-density curve. Vogel's hybrid technique has been confirmed in animals and applied clinically (201,202), but shows substantial variability as compared to flowmeter. It also requires altered catheter laboratory procedures, for example, ECG-triggered power in-

Arterial Coronary Flow Reserve by DSA

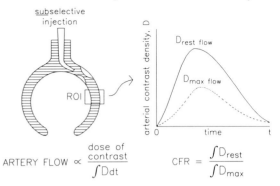

Fig. 16.6 Theory of determining arterial coronary flow reserve by DSA. See text for details. D, arterial contrast density; ROI, region of interest. Reproduced with permission from Demer L, Gould KL, Kirkeeide R, 1988. (31).

jections. Because of the effect of changing heart rate on the results, atrial pacing is also required. Finally, the method is purportedly not valid in the presence of collateral flow.

The basis for concluding that this method fails in the presence of collaterals is not clear. Theoretically, the area under the time-density curve of the myocardial bed supplied by antegrade arterial flow would increase regardless of whether collaterals were present. However, the area under the time-density curve of myocardium supplied by collaterals should fall below that at resting flows, thereby giving a perfusion reserve of less than one by this method. Since the researchers used an empirical approach in these studies, their results may not have appeared intuitively appropriate, because flow reserve measurements would have been less than one in the presence of significant collateral flow and therefore considered invalid. At present, DSA methods for measuring coronary flow reserve have not proved to be reproducible or accurate enough to be clinically useful (203).

Myocardial Perfusion Reserve by DSA

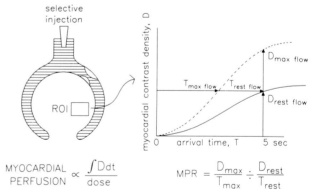

Fig. 16.7 Theory of determining myocardial perfusion reserve by DSA. D, myocardial contrast density; ROI, region of interest; T, arrival time. Reproduced with permission from Demer L, Gould KL, Kirkeeide R, 1988. (31).

From a clinical point of view, the specifications of a DSA system adequate for a cardiac catheter laboratory are not yet well defined. Certainly, such a system needs to have optimal image quality, adequate archiving and/or storage capability for high-volume turnover, and user-friendly operations. There remain significant questions about whether 512^2 or $1,024^2$ systems or dual-energy DSA are necessary for obtaining optimal quantitative data. Highly flexible systems will probably be necessary so that a choice can be made by the operator to select 512^2 at higher frame rates for left ventricular studies and $1,024^2$ at lower frame rates for quantitative coronary arteriography. Dual-energy DSA has the potential for major reductions in radiation dose to operator and patient during PTCA by allowing quantitation of stenosis severity while the balloon catheter is still in position, using more dilute contrast media through the guiding catheter. The rate, pressure, and number of balloon inflations could then be guided by precise quantitative measurements on-line without changing the catheters, thereby saving time and radiation dose and improving control of the procedure.

COMPARISON OF INVASIVELY DETERMINED ARTERIAL CORONARY FLOW RESERVE AND STENOSIS FLOW RESERVE

Because there are several techniques for assessing absolute arterial coronary flow reserve (CFR), it may be instructive to compare them. The Doppler technique (53) and the indicator dilution method described (198) provide direct measurements of arterial CFR as it is affected in any specific patient by stenosis geometry as well as by aortic pressure, vasomotor tone, hypertrophy (myocardial bed size), and response to the pharmacologic agent for inducing high flows in lieu of exercise stress. As a consequence of all these physiologic influences, the measurement of arterial CFR by these methods may vary considerably for a given patient or between patients, totally independent of equal stenosis severity. Therefore, these methods are not optimal for addressing the severity of the stenosis itself in adequately precise terms to guide clinical decisions prior to or during PTCA, thrombolysis, or other interventions in the catheter laboratory requiring reliable accuracy. Furthermore, they require changes in standard cardiac catheter procedures. However, they do provide a direct, approximate measure of arterial CFR; even well-developed collaterals do not affect these methods, but, on the other hand, cannot be assessed by them.

In isolated single-vessel disease, Pijls et al. (204) measured by DSA the relative transit time of a contrast bolus from the left main ostia to myocardial regions of interest in stenotic, as compared to adjacent normal, coronary arteries, under conditions of maximal coronary flow. This approach measures relative maximum flow or relative coronary flow reserve. For single-vessel disease, relative coronary flow reserve by this method correlated well with relative flow reserve by flowmeter. It is the invasive equivalent of relative maximum radionuclide distribution on a non-invasive dipyridamole perfusion image. Like radionuclide relative flow reserve, it provides a reasonable functional measure of stenosis severity at coronary arteriography. However, it will be subject to the same limitations as any measure of relative flow reserve for multivessel or "balanced" disease. It also requires an intracoronary power injection of contrast media and prolonged breath-holding to avoid motion artifacts. Although it may be difficult to implement for routine clinical studies, this approach provides important further verification of our concepts of relative and absolute coronary flow reserve.

In contrast to variability in absolute coronary flow reserve by flowmeter, Doppler catheter, or DSA due to physiologic variables, stenosis flow reserve (SFR) is derived from quantitative geometric analysis of a stenosis, accounting for all its dimensions at "standardized" conditions of perfusion pressure, response to vasodilator stimuli, and other physiologic variables, even when those conditions are not actually present in a given patient being studied. Consequently, measurement of SFR by this approach provides the adequate precision and standardized conditions for assessing the severity of the stenosis itself, without artifacts due to other physiologic variables. However, that measurement of SFR by quantitative geometric analysis may not equal the directly measured arterial CFR in that patient at that time, because the other physiologic variables for that patient may not be the same as those arbitrarily assumed for the standardized geometric analysis. Finally, direct measurements of arterial CFR indicate the adequacy of flow under stress for a given size of myocardial bed relative to coronary artery size, even with diffuse disease. However, they are affected by heart rate, vasomotor tone, hypertrophy, and so on, in the absence of coronary disease. SFR is not affected by varying physiologic conditions, since it utilizes "standard conditions." Again, however, SFR under these standardized conditions may not equal arterial flow reserve measured directly under other conditions.

The quantitative geometric approach requires only minimal change in current catheter laboratory procedures, that is, obtaining appropriate views and calibration images. It is suitable for either film-based analysis or DSA systems, thereby making it more applicable for widespread clinical use. Therefore, in our opinion, the optimal invasive method to assess stenosis severity suitable for routine clinical use in the cardiac catheter laboratory is the quantitative geometric approach.

Accuracy and Performance of the Positron Scanner

The technical performance characteristics of a positron scanner are intimately linked to its diagnostic and quantitative accuracy. Historically, the greatest emphasis of standard PET scanner design has been in-plane resolution. The importance of axial sampling, count rate capacity, and clinical, user-friendly software have not been recognized. The reason for this traditional design emphasis is that PET evolved as an esoteric, expensive, complex, neurologically oriented research tool. Past neurologic research using PET has required primarily high resolution to quantitatively measure metabolic (FDG) activity of brain. The radionuclide metabolic analogues for brain imaging have sufficiently long half-lives that adequate count content of images could be obtained by longer imaging time. Neither patient throughput nor high count rate capacity for adequate statistics with ultrashort half-life tracers was important. Axial sampling was not emphasized because measurements were made in-plane, and brain structures in under-sampled regions between image planes were not problematic because clinical questions were not addressed quantitatively.

With documentation of PET for accurate noninvasive cardiac applications using generator-produced [82]Rb, the design requirements of a PET scanner radically changed to incorporate count rate capacity, axial sampling and user-friendly clinical software, as discussed in this chapter. High resolution is not necessary for cardiac imaging, because the range of heart motion over 1–2 cm spreads myocardial activity over a spatial distribution much greater than the 5-mm resolution possible with PET. Furthermore, the parameters measured in the heart, flow and metabolism, are important over 1–2 cm areas of myocardium. Finer resolution is not clinically necessary. Therefore, we designed a camera that reconstructs images at 5-mm FWHM but has optimal axial sampling and count rate capacity. With this design we can choose in software to downgrade resolution to 7–10 mm FWHM, exchanging unnecessary resolution for improved statistical certainty, count rate capacity, and axial sampling. Accordingly, we elect to reconstruct cardiac images at 10-mm FWHM for cardiac studies and at 5 mm for brain studies.

With clinical application of PET to brain, particularly with [15]O tracers, the count rate capacity also becomes essential in order to obtain adequate counting statistics during the brief half-life of usable activity. For quantitatively sizing brain tumors in response to therapy, axial sampling also becomes critical, since the size of a 1–2 cm^3 tumor may vary by 100% depending on whether it falls within or between sample planes on two sequential studies using a conventional PET scanner design. Finally, the economic feasibility of clinical PET depends primarily on patient volume throughput (149), which is determined by count rate capacity. Therefore, we have developed the technology and concept that for clinical applications, the PET scan must have primarily high count rate capacity, good axial sampling, and clinical software with resolution adjusted to fit each application but playing a less important role than previously.

The three characteristics of positron scanners that are essential for routine clinical cardiac imaging with ultrashort-lived radionuclides, such as generator-produced [82]Rb, are outlined below.

AXIAL SAMPLING

The first characteristic is a scanner design with overlapping image planes, such that sampling is uniform between detector rings (55,206–209). If there is under-sampling between image planes, anatomic structures lying parallel to the imaging plane may show significant artifactual defects, or real defects may be missed, because of under-sampling between banks of detectors. Accordingly, a clinical camera must have significant overlap of the image planes to provide adequate sampling uniformly in the axial direction.

Our emphasis on the importance of high axial sampling for three-dimensional imaging of the heart and greater diagnostic accuracy has been confirmed by Senda et al. (206) in both phantoms and patient studies. They showed increased sensitivity of detecting myocardial perfusion defects by incorporating a second scan of the heart obtained by moving the patient along the Z axis by one-half the image plane separation. Specificity also improved, due to the finer axial sampling provided by the second interleaved scan, thereby avoiding artifactual false-positive results. Hoffman et al. (208) and Bendriem et al. (209) have also confirmed the necessity for fine axial sampling.

In our own clinical experience with three-dimensional imaging of the heart with the initial University of Texas prototype (1,4,55,207), even with close spacing of image planes (10.8 mm separation for 11-mm axial resolution), movement of the patient or detector and a second scan are required to achieve the necessary axial sampling for volumetric data recovery, even though axial sampling with early prototype design is enough to give good sensitivity/specificity (1,4) but with limited quantitation (4,12).

Axial indexing or movement of either patient or detectors creates several problems, especially with short-lived isotopes. Data are lost during the time required for the movement and acquisition of interleaved image planes, since they are acquired at a later time as a separate data collection and therefore contain different physiological data. For very short half-life radionuclides, such as ^{82}Rb and ^{15}O, a second scan cannot be obtained without injecting the radionuclides a second time, since during the time required to obtain adequate counts on the first scan, activity decays sufficiently to prevent acquisition of a second scan. These limitations hinder three-dimensional quantitation of the physiologic process with very short-lived radionuclides, unless a PET camera with high axial sampling is used.

To achieve this axial sampling, a staggered detector design has been developed and patented (207) as a unique solution that avoids moving the patient for an interleaved second scan. The POSICAM 6.5 BGO camera utilizes 1320 BGO scintillation crystals 8.5 × 20 × 30 mm in size. These crystals are viewed by 720 photomultiplier tubes (PMTs), which detect the scintillation light and convert it to electrical pulses. The detectors and PMTs are grouped in 120 modules, each with 11 crystals and 6 PMTs that are placed in a circle with a diameter of 78 cm. Each module of 11 crystals and 6 PMTs is light-tight and self-contained for rapid replacement by unscrewing two thumb wheel screws and removing two connectors.

The staggered detector design doubles the axial sampling and the number of slices, while reducing the slice separation to 5.125 mm. Every alternate detector in the circle of crystals is offset by one-half the detector position, axially. The offset produces axial sampling that is equivalent to manually moving the detectors by one-quarter of the detector length. The offset detectors create additional cross-coincidences and in-between slices to collect simultaneously 21 image planes from the six-ring system. The number of photomultiplier tubes is also reduced by sharing the light from 2 crystals with 1 PMT. Each module contains 11 crystals grouped with one row of 6 crystals adjacent to a row of 5 crystals.

The placement of PMTs and crystals is shown in Figure 17.1. The crystals are numbered 1 through 11 and the PMTs are labeled A through F. Light output from crystal 1 is collected mostly by PMT A, and similarly, the light output from crystal 3 is collected mostly by PMT B. The light from crystal 2 is shared equally between PMT A and PMT B. The output from the two PMTs can be described pictorially by a two-dimensional energy histogram showing the light intensity as contour lines, as in Figure 17.2. Identification of a crystal is made by the relative values and locations of the signals on the histogram. This positioning is achieved digitally, whereby the integrated output of the PMTs is digitized by a fast analog-to-digital converter (ADC). The crystal identification is achieved by a read-only lookup table in the detector-encoder circuit.

The detector design also allows shorter septa, which in turn allows a smaller, more compact mechanical gantry. The

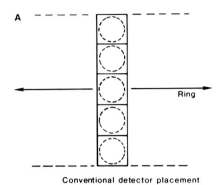

Conventional detector placement

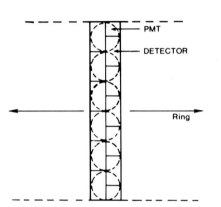

New method of placing detectors in POSICAM

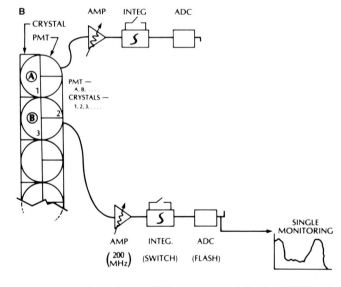

Fig. 17.1 (A) Crystals and PMT arrangement for the POSICAM detector module. **(B)** The crystals are numbered 1,2,3, . . . , and the PMTs are labeled A,B,. . . . Light output from crystal 1 is primarily detected by PMT A, while light output from crystal 2 is detected by PMTs and A and B equally. Reproduced with permission from Mullani NA, Gould KL, Hartz RK, et al., 1990. (207).

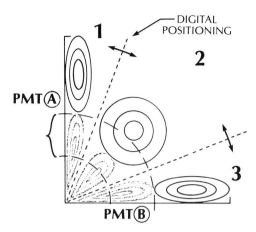

Fig. 17.2 Pictorial representation of a two-dimensional energy histogram from the light outputs of PMTs A and B. The contour lines show the relative value of the energy spectrum. The three photopeaks corresponding to the crystals 1, 2, and 3 are shown. Crystal decoding is achieved digitally with a look-up table in a read-only memory (ROM).

detector design uses conventional ¾" PMTs and a conservative 2:1 crystal-to-PMT positioning scheme in order to minimize specialized electronics and to simplify the encoding scheme for more stable operation. The system has been designed to accept a variety of different scintillators, including barium fluoride (BaF$_2$) (200) and standard bismuth germinate (BGO). This design has been implemented in the POSICAM 6.5 (Positron Corporation) having six rings of BGO detectors (five staggered rings) simultaneously producing 21 overlapping image planes (207).

The system for collecting light from 11 crystals to 6 PMTs is referred to as a 2:1 system because of two-to-one splitting of light for encoding. The actual ratio of crystal to PMTs is 11:6 for the module and 1320:720 for the whole system. The positioning accuracy of the 2:1 system, or any other shared crystal–PMT combination, depends on the number of light photons collected and the statistical quality of the signal from each PMT. Therefore, positioning accuracy will depend on the energy resolution of the scintillator, light collection from the scintillator to the PMT, and the total electronic integration time of the light output from the scintillator.

The 2:1 detector positioning is easily encoded and decoded, since there is a large difference in the signals between the two PMTs for the 3 crystal positions. The large separation of signals on the energy histogram allows a very short integration time in the discriminator circuit, thereby minimizing the dead-time losses and improving the speed of operation of the detector module. The large separation of the PMT outputs for crystal identification also permits greater variation of PMT performance without significantly affecting detector encoding accuracy. Minor changes in gain, which are inevitable in PMTs, do not require major corrective efforts, nor do they degrade the acquired data.

The staggered detector-PMT design (Fig. 17.1) and the energy histogram by which a decay event is located (Fig. 17.2)

use a short-event integration time which minimizes dead-time loss and increases camera "speed." This "speed," or capacity to faithfully record high coincident count rates, is essential to clinical performance, as discussed subsequently.

The upper panel of Figure 17.3 relates the staggered crystal design with a higher order of cross coincidence planes and finer axial sampling. The lower panel shows the standard crystal arrangement with fewer cross coincidence planes, resulting in a variation of sensitivity along the Z axis. Sensitivity along the Z axis in standard PET cameras varies from 2 to 1 or greater in adjacent slices, owing to interplane under-sampling. With higher-order cross coincidence planes, axial sensitivity is much more uniform, as shown by the sensitivity graphs of Figure 17.4. Figure 17.4 is a visual schematic of the variation in sensitivity with the staggered crystal design and with conventional detector arrangements. The lower panel shows a uniform axial and in-plane sensitivity with staggered crystals and higher orders of cross plane coincidences. The upper panel shows the variation in axial and in-plane sensitivity associated with standard camera designs having marked axial under-sampling.

The staggered crystal design provides up to four orders of cross coincidence planes, with maximum uniformity of axial sampling and maximum sensitivity. Standard positron cameras do not employ higher orders of axial cross coincidence planes, owing to larger septa, and therefore have greater variation in axial sensitivity, which may result in artifactual defects or poor quantitative data recovery.

The effect of inadequate axial sampling in both axial directions, and the partial volume errors caused by angulation

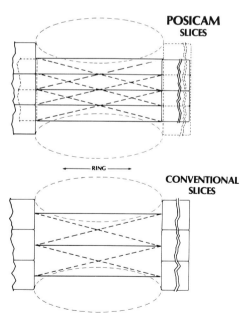

Fig. 17.3 Cross coincidence utilization of a conventional system as contrasted with a staggered detector cross coincidence utilization for POSICAM. The zero order lines are shown as solid lines, and the higher order cross coincidences are shown as dashed lines.

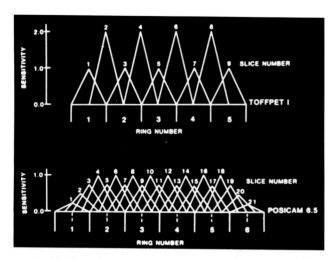

Fig. 17.4 Comparison of the slice sensitivity with conventional cross coincidence utilization as compared to POSICAM sensitivity, using zero to fourth-order cross coincidence crosses.

of an organ with respect to the imaged plane, can be simultaneously demonstrated by a special phantom (207). Several 1-cm thick fingers of radioactivity were placed in the field of view at angles of 0°, 30°, 45°, 60°, and 90° to the axial direction. These fingers of radioactivity simulating the myocardium at different positions were imaged with a single scan. The reconstructed images were displayed by creating long-axis slices through them, such that all the fingers of radioactivity were viewed. The drawing of the phantom is shown in Figure 17.5. This phantom has been designed to test quantitative accuracy of the recovery coefficients for volumetric imaging as a function of the object size and the angle of the involved plane.

Figure 17.6 shows the axial reconstruction of this phantom. Imaged by a standard camera without staggered crystals, for fingers of activity in the plane of the detectors, long-axis images show data dropout due to variation in axial sensitivity, even with our old prototype camera with a 50% overlap in sample planes, more than most other standard scanners but still inadequate. By moving the phantom axially one half-slice and acquiring a second interleaved image, these gaps disappear. Based on the experience with this initial scanner, we designed the current new scanner to provide uniform axial sensitivity with good axial sampling when tested with a more difficult phantom, shown in Figure 17.7. Long-axis tomographs in Figure 17.8 show no undersampled gaps.

Recovery of activity data is also determined by the partial volume problem that affects all positron tomography. However, in a camera with comparable resolution and sampling in the X, Y, and Z axes, this effect is minimized. For looking at relative distribution or changes, such as rest/stress, partial volume problems are similarly minimized. The greater sensitivity of PET for perfusion imaging in the diagnosis of coronary artery disease is due to technically better three-dimensional data recovery, as compared to standard planar or SPECT imaging. Three-dimensional volumetric quantitation of POSICAM was tested by scanning, with a single scan, sev-

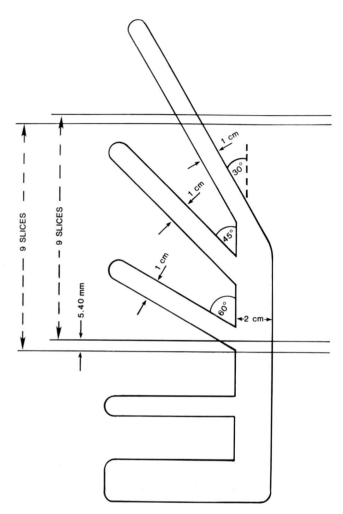

Fig. 17.5 Special finger phantom for evaluating partial volume and axial sampling of an object simulating the myocardium at different angles with respect to the imaged plane. The model "walls" of the "myocardium" are 1 cm thick and inclined at 0°, 30°, 45°, 60°, and 90°. Axial sampling and quantitation errors due to partial volume errors are demonstrated by taking coronal sections through the data.

eral spheres (207), which were 13, 16, 21, 24, 31, and 39 mm in diameter. The spheres were positioned in a circle of approximately 5-cm radius and placed in a 20-cm diameter, uniform distribution of attenuating medium, such as water. All the spheres were filled with the same concentration of radioactivity, and the phantom was scanned both at the center of the gantry and at a position 7 cm off-center to evaluate the capability of recovering three-dimensional activity from the spheres.

Profiles were drawn through the spheres in the reconstructed images, and the 50% points of the maximum in the profiles were used as edges of the spheres. Sagittal and coronal views were also obtained from all the slices to determine if artifacts were present, as a measure of the adequacy of three-dimensional imaging (Fig. 17.9). Regions of interest

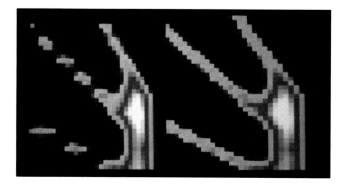

Fig. 17.6 Axial slices reconstructed of the phantom in Figure 17.5, using the first prototype University of Texas scanner in one data acquisition image (left) and with a second data acquisition image after moving the phantom one half-slice axially. There are under-sampled planes axially (left) that fill in with adequate axial sampling. These observations led to the staggered crystal design that provides adequate axial sampling in one data acquisition. Reproduced with permission from Gould KL, 1990. (205).

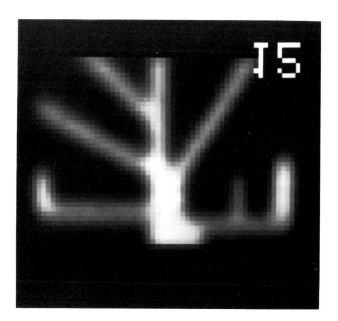

Fig. 17.8 Transaxial images obtained of the axial sampling phantom with the "myocardial walls" tilted at 0°, 30°, 45°, 60°, and 90° to the image plane, showing the uniform recovery of myocardial activity regardless of the tilt angle with respect to the image plane. Reproduced with permission from Mullani NA, Gould KL, Hartz RK, et al., 1990. (207).

were drawn over each sphere in each slice and three-dimensional count density was plotted against the known volume of the spheres, shown in Figure 17.10. This good correlation demonstrates the system's capability of recovering three-dimensional volumetric concentrations with a single scan. The true three-dimensionality of sampling by the staggered crystal design is demonstrated by reconstructing sagittal cut and measuring diameter of the spheres in radial and axial planes as compared to known diameters. There is excellent correlation for both axial and in-plane measurements (Fig. 17.11), which no other PET scanner currently in operation can duplicate (207).

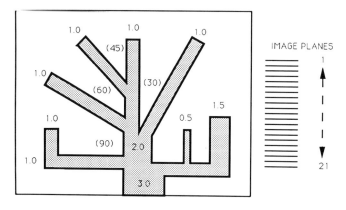

PARTIAL VOLUME PHANTOM

Fig. 17.7 The more advanced Mullani finger phantom for testing adequacy of axial sampling. Reproduced with permission from Mullani NA, Gould KL, Hartz RK, et al., in press. (207).

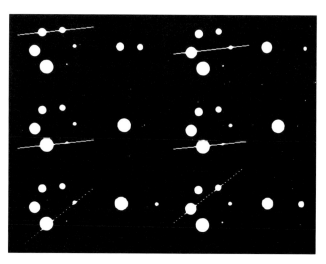

Fig. 17.9 Central image slices of the sphere phantom. The spheres are 13, 16, 21, 24, 31, and 39 mm in diameter, filled with equal concentrations of radioactivity, and surrounded by scattering medium in a 20-cm diameter phantom. Axial cuts (sagittal and coronal views) through the spheres are shown for different angles and spheres next to the transaxial image. The line through the spheres shows the plane of the axial cut, and the resulting image produced along this plane is shown to the right of the transaxial image. Reproduced with permission from Mullani NA, Gould KL, Hartz RK, et al., 1990. (207).

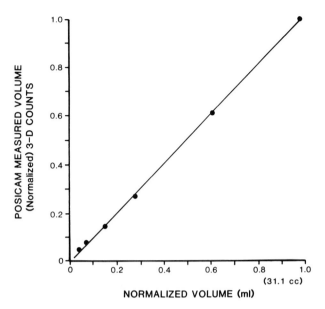

Fig. 17.10 Total counts measured in the three-dimensional region of interest encompassing the spheres are plotted against the known volumes of the sphere. The relationship is linear and quantitatively accurate. Reproduced with permission from Mullani NA, Gould KL, Hortz RK, et al., 1990. (207).

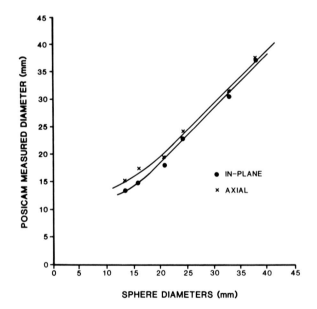

Fig. 17.11 Diameter of the spheres measured in-plane and in the axial direction, plotted against the known diameters of the spheres. Data was obtained from a single scan of the spheres' phantom. For the smallest sphere, PET slightly overestimated diameter, owing to spillover associated with partial volume errors inherent in all PET scanners. Reproduced with permission from Mullani NA, Gould KL, Hartz RK, et al., 1990. (207).

COUNT RATE CAPACITY

The second important characteristic of a medical positron camera is the capacity for accepting high count rates in order to obtain adequate counts during the short half-life of ^{82}Rb or ^{15}O (207,210–214), and particularly for obtaining adequate early (100-s duration) and late images for viability measurements based on rubidium washout. For example, our old prototype scanner acquires 15 to 25 million counts over 5 min for a whole-heart resting image of ^{82}Rb, including all slices, the minimum for diagnostic accuracy being 12 to 15 million. The determinants of count rate capacity for true coincident counts are complex. They include (a) the proportion of random coincidences dependent on the crystal type and coincidence window, (b) dead-time losses of front-end electronics related to detector light decay time and PMTs, and (c) dead-time losses of back-end electronics related to energy discrimination, address encoding, data transfer to memory, and computer architecture. Details of these important factors have been published (207).

The new staggered crystal scanner acquires 30 to 55 million counts over 5 min. Positron scanners based on the block design, with an 8:1 crystal-to-PMT ratio with its high dead-time losses, collect only 6 million counts over 5 min for a whole-heart image of ^{82}Rb. In our experience, this statistical content is frequently associated with artifacts and is unacceptable, since it is associated with a corresponding lower sensitivity and specificity (195) than reported with "fast" scanners acquiring higher counts per whole-heart data set (1,4,177). For 100-s images of rubidium washout, a block design scanner simply cannot acquire the data fast enough to produce usable 100-s images of rubidium washout for determining viability. Consequently, such cameras must use cyclotron-produced radionuclides, with their accompanying greater expense. Good image contrast provided by high counts, low dead-time losses, and good signal-to-noise ratio are required for high diagnostic accuracy, particularly for more moderate disease severity in lower prevalence populations, where non-invasive imaging is most needed.

CLINICAL SOFTWARE

The third characteristic essential for a clinical camera for routine clinical work is user-friendly, clinically oriented, automated, quantitative software for data analysis that has been developed and validated in clinical applications (30). For example, our display software for cardiac studies (10) utilizes automated normalization and three-dimensional rotational routines, side-by-side tomographic images of rest and stress in true long- and short-axis views, paired rest-stress polar map or three-dimensional topographic displays of relative and absolute coronary flow reserve and its changes, automated quantitation of severity and size of defects with statistical comparison to normals, automated sizing of infarcted versus viable areas, simple menu-driven clinical data entry, and visual interpretation routines, all elected by single push-button commands, as described previously (10).

The heart in the majority of patients moves left, anterior, and/or downward on the stress as compared to transmission and rest images. Such motion may produce incorrect attenuation, causing artifactual defects, particularly of the left inferior lateral free wall of the left ventricle. However, by software that superimposes the transmission and emission images, translation between the transmission, rest, or stress images can be recognized and images corrected, allowing accurate interpretation. The heavy technological support usually needed for PET can be eliminated by designing clinical software transparent to the user and validated for routine applications, with consequent reduction in costs of technical personnel. Currently, a nurse and technician carry out all of our studies using the rubidium generator, with physician time reduced to a minimum for patient management and safety.

For widespread routine cardiac practice, ease of use, patient throughput, and economy, a simple-to-use radionuclide source is essential, such as the ^{82}Rb generator, which does not require a cyclotron but allows all of the major aspects of cardiac imaging for clinical purposes described in previous chapters. However, ^{82}Rb imaging requires a scanner with the capacity for accepting the high count rates necessary to collect 15 to 25 million counts in the 5 min available before most radioactivity is gone. For 100-s serial images of ^{82}Rb washout for determining myocardial viability, this characteristic of the scanner is essential. Thus, the economics and extent to which PET is used clinically on a widespread basis for better diagnostic accuracy than is currently available depends in large part on the capacity of the camera for high count rate imaging with ^{82}Rb. The basic PET scanner design of the current largest x-ray equipment manufacturers was derived from neurologic applications before the importance of count rate capacity or cardiac applications with generator-produced radionuclides were recognized. For this reason, we developed the University of Texas PET scanner design to meet a clinical need not previously recognized.

ARTIFACTS IN PET IMAGE QUANTITATIVE DISPLAYS

For technically good PET images, there are several characteristic, recognizable artifacts that may occur in quantitative polar displays. They are related primarily to operator interaction and judgment in choosing long-axis and apex slices that define short axis data and polar displays. These problems are listed in Table 17.1 and illustrated in Figures 17.12 through 17.17.

As illustrated in Figure 17.12, incorrect orientation of the long axis in both horizontal and vertical planes will produce areas of no activity or defects on the short-axis views and hence on the polar display. If the long axis is not parallel to the true long axis of the heart, such that the short axis perpendicular to it is too basal or proximal (middle panel of Fig. 17.12), the polar display will show a crescentic edge defect

Table 17.1 Potential Errors in Automated PET Quantitation

Incorrect apex or basal slice
Incorrect long axis
Heart size smaller than field
Blood pool activity on early image
Polar display distorts anatomy

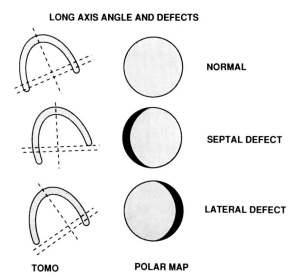

Fig. 17.12 Edge artifacts due to incorrect long-axis placement.

that is an artifact. Since the membranous septum normally causes a small septal defect, this artifact is an exaggeration of normal anatomy.

An incorrect long-axis orientation in the other direction causes an artifactual lateral defect on short-axis and polar displays, as in the lower panel of Figure 17.12. Incorrect long-axis orientation in the vertical plane will cause comparable crescentic proximal or basal defects of the anterior or inferior aspects of the short-axis and polar displays (not shown). We call these incorrect displays edge artifacts and exclude the outer or basal ring of data ($\frac{1}{2}$ cm) from quantitative analysis. For comparing rest-stress, stress-stress, early-late or perfusion-metabolism paired images, such edge artifacts may incorrectly suggest change or lack of change. However, these edge artifacts are readily recognized and corrected by redrawing the long axis orientation correctly and repeating the polar display analysis.

Figure 17.13 illustrates a similar artifact caused by choosing the apex slice incorrectly. The upper left panel shows a

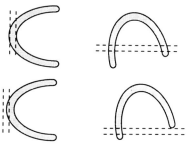

Fig. 17.13 Apical or basal artifacts due to incorrect choice of apical or basal slices.

HEART SMALLER THAN FIELD SIZE

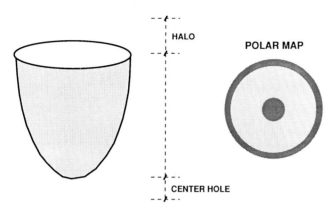

Fig. 17.14 Halo or apex artifacts due to heart being smaller than the field size.

correct apex choice. For a second comparative image in the lower left panel, the apex slice is too distal, thereby making an apical defect suggesting a stress perfusion defect as compared to rest, a washout defect on late as compared to early rubidium image, a stress defect as compared to the prior stress image, or a metabolic defect as compared to no perfusion defect in the prior paired image with a correctly chosen apical slice. Similarly, an incorrectly chosen basal slice (lower right) will suggest an abnormality compared to the prior study that is an artifact. We call this an apex or basal slice location artifact.

Both edge artifacts and apex location artifacts may occur together if the heart is substantially smaller than the depth or length of the scanner field size along the Z axis, as in Figure 17.14. Each short axis slice is fixed at 0.5 cm thick for a fixed number of short-axis planes defined by the detector construction necessary for Z axis sampling of the largest human hearts. This image field is therefore too big for small hearts, with the consequences that the polar display will always show a circumferential edge artifact or halo (Fig. 17.14) if the correct apex slice is chosen by the operator. The solution to this problem is to choose the correct apex slice and recognize

VISUAL DISTORTION BY POLAR DISPLAY

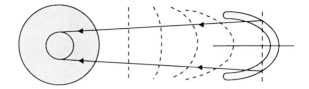

Fig. 17.16 Distortion of cardiac anatomy by conforming a three-dimensional bowl shape to a flat polar map.

the basal halo artifact for what it is without calling it an abnormality.

Figure 17.15 illustrates a minor artifact that affects primarily the quantitation of ^{82}Rb washout. The clearing blood pool on early-to-late ^{82}Rb images may be "seen" as washout by the automated program for determining infarct size by the area of washout. Blood pool washout then makes the automatically measured infarct size for the whole heart somewhat bigger than it actually is. The solution is to check the automated measure of infarct size by washout visually; by this means, observer judgment can estimate washout area within the LV wall.

Polar displays of three-dimensional data distort cardiac physical anatomy significantly, as in Figure 17.16. Since the three-dimensional data must be compressed at its center to fit onto a flat surface, the area of the apex on the polar display is smaller than in three-dimensional reality. Consequently, 38% of the myocardium is contained within the small central ring of the polar display, with the balance in quarters in the more basal areas, Figure 17.17. Although visually distorted, the automated quantitation of the heart beyond 2.5 standard deviation limits is correct, since it is derived from the original short-axis views. However, a defect that fills the inner small apical ring is in reality bigger than a defect occupying an

BLOOD POOL ON EARLY IMAGE

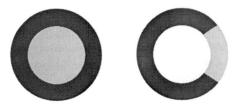

WASHOUT AREA TOO BIG (MINOR EFFECT)

Fig. 17.15 Artifact of excessive ^{82}Rb washout due to blood pool clearing.

PERCENT OF LV IN POLAR MAP AREAS

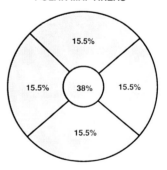

VISUAL DISTORTION QUANTITATION CORRECT

Fig. 17.17 Percent of cardiac image in the quadrants and apical circle of a polar display.

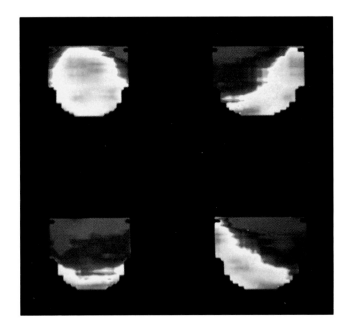

A

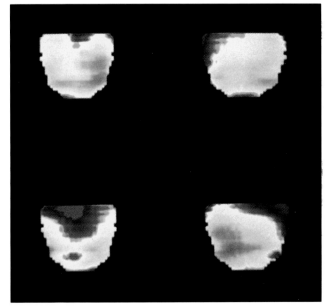

B

Fig. 17.18 Topographic display in anterior (upper left), posterior (lower left), septal (upper right), and lateral (lower right) views, which do not distort spatial proportions as do polar map displays. **(A)** Large myocardial infarction in inferior posterior, posterior lateral, and posterior septal myocardium, corresponding to an occluded dominant RCA by arteriography. **(B)** a small posterior, posterior lateral myocardial infarction corresponding to a small non-dominant RCA occlusion by arteriography. **(C)** a small anterio-apical myocardial infarction and a second separate posterior myocardial infarction corresponding to an occluded distal LAD and an occluded non-dominant RCA by arteriography. See Chapter 20 for clinical examples of three-dimensional topographic displays.

entire more basal quadrant. The automated analysis software will provide correct deficit size as percentage of the whole polar map; this may disagree with the visual impression of defect size at the apex compared to basal regions.

The solution to the visual distortion caused by polar displays is to utilize topographic displays shown in Figure 17.18, developed at our lab (55). This display provides visual images that correspond to automated quantitative defect size. Software for automated defect sizing and multi-view topographic display has been completed and is now being tested clinically. A series of clinical examples of 30 topographic displays are provided in Chapter 20.

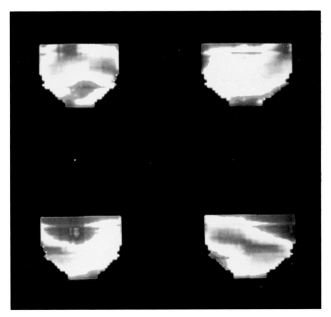

C

18

Economics of Cardiac PET

The introduction of new medical technology into widespread clinical use requires analysis of the benefits to patient care as compared to the costs of its introduction and application. The analysis is inherently inexact, for several reasons. It reduces subjective benefits of individual well-being to statistical or monetary equivalents for comparison to other technologies or to alternative approaches. In addition, for new technology there is no exact or controlled past record on which to base cost and benefit projections. However, for PET, there are extensive publications on the specific clinical advantages for cardiac imaging in large numbers of patients. The technology is also sufficiently advanced from the stage of university-based development to manufacturing that cost projections are reasonably accurate.

Translation of the subjective benefits for patients into cost equivalents for analytical purposes is always uncertain and at best only "reasonable." The benefit-cost equivalences for the current analysis are not intended to imply value judgments on other technologies, current medical practices, or the value of human well-being or life. Rather, this analysis is made because the current evolutionary stage of PET provides a unique opportunity to analyze, understand, and optimize the introduction of a major new medical technology for economical patient care.

This cost analysis for clinical PET of the heart using generator-produced ^{82}Rb and cyclotron-produced tracers is undertaken by approaching sequentially the clinical problem, current non-invasive radionuclide methods, PET, the cost of PET per study, and costs of PET versus thallium imaging or no intervention for evaluation of chest pain, of asymptomatic men at high risk for coronary artery disease and of myocardial viability after myocardial infarction or thrombolysis therapy. Finally, a comparative pro forma for cyclotron-produced radionuclides is also developed.

THE CLINICAL PROBLEM

Accurate non-invasive assessment of coronary artery stenosis and myocardial ischemia/viability in symptomatic or asymptomatic subjects remains a major medical problem for a number of reasons. Coronary heart disease continues to be the leading cause of death in most technologically advanced countries, responsible for one-third to one-half of all deaths between the ages of 35 and 64 years. Much of this heart disease is asymptomatic until some serious clinical event occurs, with 40% to 60% of patients having sudden death or myocardial infarction without prior symptoms (215–218). Up

to 13% of middle-aged men in the general population have coronary artery disease (219,220), most without symptoms. Silent ischemia is increasingly recognized in symptomatic and asymptomatic individuals (221,222) and has an unfavorable prognosis when observed in patients with recent unstable angina (223) or during exercise testing (224). Asymptomatic subjects with reversible defects by dipyridamole thallium testing have a very high cardiac event rate and mortality (225). However, risk factors of hypercholesterolemia, family history, hypertension, and smoking have a low sensitivity and specificity for identifying individuals who have significant coronary artery disease (173). Two thirds of healthy adult males, aged 40 to 55, who have highest cholesterol and blood pressure risk factors remain well over the subsequent 25 years (226).

Therefore, important questions are how to detect coronary artery disease and how to quantify it, particularly when atypical symptoms or absence of symptoms provide no clinical guide to severity or therapy that would prevent sudden death or myocardial infarction. Physiologic measures of stenosis severity, multidimensional anatomical quantitative analysis of stenoses, and/or metabolic measurements of myocardial ischemia thus become necessary to select patients for appropriate coronary procedures and to avoid unnecessary ones. With the availability of effective cholesterol-lowering drugs and radical risk factor modification, selection of patients for medical therapy also requires non-invasive evaluation to assess severity and progression/regression of coronary artery disease.

As thrombolysis for acute myocardial infarction has become widespread, identification of ischemic, viable myocardium is essential for deciding upon definitive follow-up procedures such as PTCA or bypass surgery. For a completed myocardial infarction without remaining viable tissue, further interventions are not indicated. For patients with substantial ischemic viable myocardium continuing at risk, PTCA or bypass surgery may be indicated. Therefore, a reliable method for identifying ischemic, viable myocardium and its extent would substantially reduce unnecessary procedures and select those patients for whom a follow-up procedure would be most beneficial.

COST PER PET STUDY USING ^{82}RB

In order to analyze the cost and therefore charges per PET study, a realistic pro forma is shown below, using the following assumptions:

1. A study for assessing myocardial perfusion consists of a rest image and a dipyridamole stress image.
2. The PET scanner price for complete turnkey operations is $2,400,000 with $461,000 down and a $1,939,000 loan at 12% interest.
3. Bad debt: 20%
4. Tax rate: 34%
5. Inflation: 6%
6. Charge per study: $1,200

The analysis is shown in Table 18.1 for a charge of $1,200 per study for the technical fee without a physician's professional fee, considered later. Bad debt refers to studies done for which incomplete payment or no payment is made. A steady state of 8 patients per day is assumed, based on experience with the first private clinical installations in Atlanta and Marietta, Georgia, and Jacksonville, Florida. Expenses include salaries for technical staff to operate the PET facility and a maintenance contract for the scanner beginning in the second year, the first year being covered by warranty. Costs of the ^{82}Rb generator are estimated to be $20,000 per month. Other entries are self-explanatory.

The internal rate of return on investment in the PET facility for an optimal case load of 8 patients per day at a charge of $1,200 each is 17%. This return is reasonable for the investment made relative to the risks of maintaining case load and collecting 80% or more of payments due. A fall in daily case load of only 2 patients, to 6 per day reduces the internal rate of return to 7%. A return of 7% is comparable to that from a bank savings account or certified deposit and is inadequate for the investment risk. For a charge of $1,200 per study, the break-even point is 5 patients per day, as shown in Figure 18.1. Therefore, the economy of clinical PET de-

Table 18.1 Pro forma for Clinical Cardiac PET with ^{82}Rb

Assumptions	Camera price:	$2,400,000	Amt down:	$461,000		
	Interest rate:	12.00%	Bad debt:	20.00%	Loan value:	$1,939,000
	Tax rate:	34.00%	Inflation:	6.00%	Price:	$1,200

PET Studies	Year 1	Year 2	Year 3	Year 4	Year 5
Daily average	4	6	8	8	8
Volume/year	1,040	1,560	2,080	2,080	2,080
Charge/study ($)	1,200	1,272	1,348	1,429	1,515
Revenue ($)	1,248,000	1,984,320	2,804,506	2,972,776	3,151,142
Less bad debt ($)	249,600	396,864	560,901	594,555	630,228
Net revenue ($)	998,400	1,587,456	2,243,604	2,378,221	2,520,914
Expenses ($)					
Technician	30,000	31,800	33,708	35,730	37,874
Nurse	30,000	31,800	33,708	35,730	37,874
Depreciation	480,000	480,000	480,000	480,000	480,000
Maintenance	0	254,400	254,400	254,400	254,400
Isotope (^{82}Rb)	240,000	254,400	269,664	285,844	302,994
Rent/overhead	20,000	21,200	22,472	23,820	25,250
Utilities	10,000	10,600	11,236	11,910	12,625
Admin/secr	50,000	53,000	56,180	59,551	63,124
Supplies	52,000	82,680	110,240	110,240	110,240
Crash cart	26,000	67,416	71,461	75,749	80,294
Total expenses ($)	938,000	1,287,296	1,343,069	1,372,975	1,404,675
EBIT*	60,400	300,160	900,536	1,005,246	1,116,239
Interest	216,476	178,288	135,257	86,768	32,130
EBT†	−156,076	121,872	765,279	918,478	1,084,109
Less taxes	−53,066	41,436	260,195	312,282	368,597
EAT‡	−103,010	80,436	505,084	606,195	715,512
Add back dep¶	461,000	461,000	461,000	461,000	461,000
After tax CF§	357,990	541,436	966,084	1,067,195	1,176,512

IRR** on investment of $2,400,000 at end of 5 yr 17%/year

* Earnings before interest and taxes.
† Earnings before taxes.
‡ Earnings after taxes.
§ Cash flow.
¶ Depreciation.
** Internal rate of return.

Source: Adapted with permission from Gould KL, Goldstein RA, Mullani NA, 1989. Reference 149.

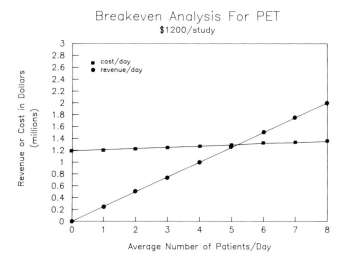

Breakeven Analysis For PET
$1200/study

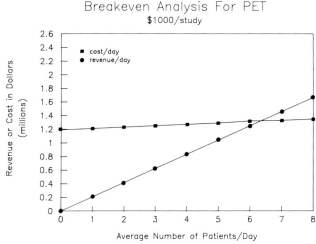

Breakeven Analysis For PET
$1000/study

Fig. 18.1 Break-even analysis for PET operations at $1,200 per cardiac study, including rest and stress images. Vertical axis shows revenue or cost in millions of dollars per year, and horizontal axis shows average number of patients studied per day. Break-even is approximately 5 patients per day. Reproduced with permission from Gould KL, Goldstein RA, Mullani NA, 1989. (149).

Fig. 18.2 Break-even analysis for PET operations at $1,000 per cardiac study, including rest and stress images. Vertical axis shows revenue or cost in millions of dollars per year, and horizontal axis shows average number of patients studied per day. Break-even is approximately 6.5 patients per day. Reproduced with permission from Gould KL, Goldstein RA, Mullani NA, 1989. (149).

pends on the number of studies per day, with the break-even being 5 per day, or 1,300 per year, at a technical fee of $1,200 per study.

A decrease in payment to $1,000 per study becomes borderline at 8 patients per day, with an internal rate of return of only 7%, again comparable to a bank savings account. At this charge per study, a decrease in case load to 6 per day results in an internal rate of return of −3%, a loss. As shown in Figure 18.2, the break-even point at a charge of $1,000 per study is approximately 6.5 cases per day, which is too close to the optimal capacity of 8 for predictably breaking even.

Based on this analysis, the technical charge for clinical PET with [82]Rb could be $1,200 per study with a case load of 6 to 8 studies per day. Fewer studies or lower charges are not economical. With a professional fee, the total cost would be $1,500 per study. The question then arises: What is the impact or societal cost/benefit relative to current thallium perfusion imaging, which is less costly per study but also has a lower diagnostic yield and therefore incurs real additional costs resulting from less accurate diagnosis?

ECONOMIC ANALYSIS OF PET FOR EVALUATING PATIENTS WITH CHEST PAIN

The following assumptions and analysis are hypothetical, for purposes of illustration, based on available data and/or conservative, reasonable estimates. No criticisms of standard current diagnostic or therapeutic practices or medical management are intended or implied. The purpose is to determine whether the greater diagnostic yield of PET compensates for its greater cost per study as compared to thallium exercise

testing, such that the overall costs of medical management based on PET imaging is comparable (or not) to that for thallium imaging for assessing patients with chest pain. Most of the assumptions for this analysis listed below are the same for both PET and thallium imaging. Assumptions that are different for these two technologies are based on literature references indicated.

Assumptions

1. Analysis is per 100 patients with chest pain, including atypical chest pain, where a reliable non-invasive test is most needed to prevent arteriography of normals.

2. Prevalence of significant coronary artery disease by coronary arteriography in this group is conservatively estimated at 25% (61,169).

3. Based on recent publications through 1988, sensitivity of stress thallium imaging ranges from 76% to 93% and is here assumed to be 85%; specificity ranges from 49% to 91% and is here assumed to be 60%, based on the largest, most recent reports, for false-positive results of 40% (161–168,173).

4. Cost of exercise thallium testing is $950 per study, including professional fee.

5. Sensitivity and specificity of PET is 95% or higher (1,4–6,177).

6. Cost of PET is $1,500 per study ($1,200 technical fee plus $300 physician's fee).

7. Coronary arteriography at a total cost of $6,000 per patient, including professional fees, is done in all patients with a positive non-invasive test.

8. Of those patients with significant coronary artery disease (CAD), 85% are treatable either by percutaneous transluminal coronary angioplasty (PTCA) or saphenous vein bypass grafting (SVBG).

9. Half of patients with treatable significant CAD by coronary arteriography have PTCA at a cost of $10,000 each and half have SVBG at a cost of $20,000 each.

Analysis of Cost of Medical Management Based on Exercise Thallium Imaging

1. Of 100 patients with chest pain, 25 have significant CAD and 75 do not, based on prevalence of 25%.

2. The total number of positive thallium tests is (25)(85%) + (40%)(75) = 21.3 + 30 = 51.3.

3. Therefore, 51.3 patients undergo coronary arteriography on the basis of a positive thallium test.

4. Of these 51.3 patients, 21.3 have significant CAD and 30 do not, as shown in step 2 above.

5. Of the 21.3 with CAD, 18 are treatable with interventions (85%), of whom 9 have SVBG and 9 have PTCA.

6. Of the 25 patients with CAD, (25)(15%) = 3.75 patients have normal exercise thallium tests, are not cathed, and therefore are "missed."

7. Total cost of medical management based on thallium imaging is

Thallium test:	100 × $950	= $95,000
Coronary arteriography	51.3 × $6,000	= $307,800
PTCA	9 × 10,000	= $90,000
SVBG	9 × 20,000	= $180,000
Total Cost		= $672,800

Analysis of Cost of Medical Management Based on PET Using ^{82}Rb

1. Total number of positive PET tests is (95%)(25) + (5%)(75) = 23.8 + 3.8 = 26.6

2. Therefore, 26.6 patients have coronary arteriography, based on PET.

3. Of these 26.6 patients, 23.8 have significant CAD and 3.8 do not, as shown in Step 1 above.

4. Of the 23.8 with CAD, 20.2 are treatable (85%), 10 by PTCA and 10 by SVBG.

5. Of the 25 patients with CAD, (25)(5%) = 1.25 patients have normal PET tests, are not cathed, and therefore are "missed".

6. Total cost of medical management based on PET is

PET	100 × $1,500	= $150,000
Coronary arteriography	26.6 × 6,000	= $159,600
PTCA	10 × 10,000	= $100,000
SVBG	10 × 20,000	= $200,000
Total Cost		= $609,600

These figures show that PET is comparable or less costly than thallium imaging for the diagnosis and management of patients with chest pain. The reason is that a large number of patients with positive stress thallium tests and normal coronary arteries undergo coronary arteriography, whereas these patients have normal PET scans and thereby avoid catheterization. In addition, for PET, 1.25 patients are "missed," versus 3.75 patients for thallium imaging.

For calculating the potential economic impact of the lower diagnostic yield with thallium imaging, the following additional assumptions and analysis for loss of wages/productivity were made.

1. Because it identifies mild (earlier) CAD, a normal PET study need not be repeated for 5 years, since this time period would likely be required for clinically severe coronary artery narrowing to develop from stenoses mild enough to produce no stress perfusion defect by PET.

2. Mortality of those individuals with severe CAD, missed and untreated, ranges from 6% to 25%, and is here assumed to be 7% per year (216,224,227,231). For the five-year period following a PET scan, the cumulative mortality in the missed patients is therefore 35%.

3. Yearly wages lost at $30,000 per year for 5 years is $150,000, and cost of mortality per deceased person is $5,000, for a total expense of $155,000 per deceased person.

4. For a mortality of 7% per year, over a 5-year period following diagnostic evaluation, the mortality is (35%)(3.75) = 1.31 deaths per 5 years in the "missed" cases after thallium testing versus (35%)(1.25) = .44 deaths per 5 years in the "missed" cases after PET. Medical management based on thallium imaging therefore theoretically incurs a mortality of 1.31/.44, or 3.0 times that for PET, with corresponding losses of wages and productivity and with costs of mortality.

5. Loss of wages and productivity over a 5-year period due to mortality in the "missed" are

Thallium	1.3 × $155,000	= $201,500
PET	0.44 × $155,000	= $68,200

6. The total combined cost of medical management of those patients diagnosed as having CAD and of wages lost due to mortality in the missed, untreated individuals over a 5-year period per 100 patients would be

	Medical costs	Lost productivity
Thallium	$672,800 + $201,500	= $874,302
PET	$609,600 + $68,200	= $677,802

Conclusions for Evaluating Chest Pain

Although the cost of cardiac PET with ^{82}Rb at $1,500 per study is higher than for thallium imaging at $950 per study, the greater diagnostic yield of PET theoretically results in lower overall costs of medical management compared to thallium imaging for evaluating patients with chest pain. These results are summarized in Tables 18.2 and 18.3.

ECONOMIC ANALYSIS OF EVALUATING ASYMPTOMATIC, HIGH-RISK MALES

Testing of asymptomatic individuals with risk factors for CAD has generally been considered inappropriate for several reasons. The limited diagnostic yield of current non-invasive

Table 18.2 Economic Analysis of PET for Dx/Rx Chest Pain

	Thallium	PET
Costs of tests (per 100)	$ 95,000	$150,000
Coronary arteriography	307,000	159,600
PTCA, SVBG	270,000	300,000
Total costs	$672,800	$609,600
Patients Dx/Rx	18	20

Source: Adapted with permission from Gould KL, Goldstein RA, Mullani NA, 1989. Reference 149.

testing does not provide good identification of normals and abnormals. For this limited diagnostic yield, cost of current non-invasive testing leading to large numbers of normal patients undergoing coronary arteriography is excessive, thereby making "screening" tests inappropriate. In the past, interventional therapy, especially bypass surgery, was also not appropriate for this group. Finally, this approach is considered "case-finding" by health insurance companies, which is viewed as increasing their costs.

However, technologies for accurate non-invasive diagnosis, mechanical intervention, and pharmacologic therapy have evolved sufficiently for us to reconsider the potential impact of this approach. For purposes of discussion, high-risk individuals are defined as males 45 to 65 years old with one or more risk factors of smoking, hypertension, hypercholesterolemia (or abnormal HDL/LDL ratios), and family history of CAD.

Assumptions

1. Analysis is per 100 patients with risk factors for CAD.
2. Prevalence of CAD in asymptomatic males 45–65 years old with one or more risk factors ranges from 15% to 35% (174,219,220), with disease that is anatomically severe ranging from 7% to 35% and here assumed to be 8% of patients with risk factor(s) (174).
3. Of the 8% of patients with risk factors who have severe CAD, mortality is 7% per year (216,224,227–231), as assumed previously, or 35% over 5 years.
4. Mean income in this risk factor group is $30,000 per year.

Table 18.3 Economic Analysis of PET for Dx/Rx Chest Pain

	Thallium	PET
Medical Dx/Rx (per 100)	$672,800	$609,600
Lost productivity over 5 yrs	201,500	68,200
Total cost	$874,302	$677,802
Mortality (persons per 5 yrs)	1.31	0.44

Source: Adapted with permission from Gould KL, Goldstein RA, Mullani NA, 1989. Reference 149.

Analysis of Productivity and Wages Lost Due to Premature Mortality from Unidentified CAD

1. Over 5 years, mortality in the group with 8% severe CAD is 8 × 35% = 2.8 per 100, for an incidence of 5.6/1,000/year, which is at the lower end of the range reported in the literature (216, 224, 227–231).
2. Loss of productivity over 5 years:

   2.8 × $30,000/year × 5 = $420,000
3. Cost of mortality: $5000 × 2.8 = $14,000
4. Total five-year cost in lost productivity with no diagnostic or therapeutic intervention = $434,000

Analysis of Costs for Identifying and Treating Asymptomatic High-Risk Males by PET

1. Cost of PET studies per 100 individuals is

   100 × $1,500 = $150,000
2. With a sensitivity of 95% for severe disease, in the group with 8% prevalence of severe disease, PET identifies (95%)(8) = 7.6 of these patients, and 0.4 are missed.
3. Cost of treatment at $30,000 each for coronary arteriography, PTCA, SVBG, and/or drugs is

   7.6 × $30,000 = $228,000
4. Treatment failure occurs in (10%)(7.6) or 0.76 persons exposed to a mortality of 7% per year, or 35% over 5 years, resulting in (0.76)(35%) or .266 deaths over 5 years. Productivity lost over 5 years is

   0.266 × $30,000 × 5 years = $39,900
5. Mortality in the 0.4 missed cases is 7% × 0.4 = .028 with associated lost productivity over 5 years of

   .028 × $30,000 × 5 = $3,200
6. Total cost of PET screening and treatment, including therapeutic failures, is:

PET	$150,000
Treatment	$228,000
Lost productivity, Rx failures	$39,900
Lost productivity, missed cases	$3200
Total	$421,100
7. Deaths over 5 years are 0.76 after PET screening and treatment, as compared to 2.8 per 100 individuals with no interventions.

Conclusions for Diagnosing and Treating Asymptomatic High-Risk Men

Identifying asymptomatic high-risk males by PET is theoretically comparable to or less costly than a policy of no testing or treatment, and results in lower mortality. These results are summarized in Tables 18.4 and 18.5.

Table 18.4 Economic Analysis of PET for ASx High-Risk Males

No Dx/Rx Intervention (over 5 yrs)	Lost Productivity
2.8 deaths × $30,000 × 5 years	$420,000
2.8 deaths × $5,000 mortality costs	14,000
Total cost no Dx or Rx	$434,000
PET Dx and Rx Intervention/5 yrs	Costs
PET studies	$150,000
PTCA, SVBG	228,000
Rx failure, lost productivity	39,900
Missed patients, lost productivity	3,200
Total cost PET Dx/Rx	$421,100

Source: Adapted with permission from Clin Cardiol, 1990. Reference 239.

Table 18.5 Economic Analysis of PET for ASx High-Risk Males

No Dx/Rx intervention (per 100 patients over 5 yrs)	
Loss of productivity + mortality cost	$434,000
Mortality (persons per 5 yrs)	2.8
PET Dx and Rx intervention (per 100 patients per 5 yrs)	
Cost of Dx/Rx + loss of productivity	$421,000
Mortality (persons per 5 yrs)	0.76

Source: Adapted with permission from Clin Cardiol, 1990. Reference 239.

ECONOMIC ANALYSIS OF EVALUATING POST-MI/THROMBOLYSIS PATIENTS FOR MYOCARDIAL VIABILITY

In the medical imaging field and in cardiology, identification of viable myocardium after acute myocardial infarction or after thrombolysis has often been considered the most important potential application of PET. Accordingly, the following analysis considers that point of view. However, the results of this analysis are surprising, raising potentially serious questions, as outlined below.

Additional Assumptions

1. For patients having recent myocardial infarction, 75% to 80% of patients and 50% to 68% of myocardial segments have significant remaining viable myocardium (17,18,21,23,102), 85% of which reportedly demonstrates improved contractile function after reperfusion (17). Here we assume conservatively that 50% of post-MI/thrombolysis patients have significant remaining viable myocardium, much lower than the 75% to 80% reported (17,18,21,23,102). Although this estimate may be too high, as discussed subsequently, it is used here as the best conservative estimate from the literature.

2. By thallium redistribution studies, only slightly over half of these patients, or approximately 30% of the total, have viable myocardium (18,102), with approximately 20% being classified as completed infarctions without viable myocardium when they have viable tissue by PET studies;

therefore, 20% of the patients with viable myocardium are missed by thallium imaging and do not undergo therapeutic intervention.

3. Of patients with viable myocardium remaining, 70% have coronary anatomy suitable for SVBG or PTCA. Of these, half are treated by PTCA and half by SVBG.

4. Of the patients with myocardial infarction with viable myocardium who are not identified (missed), mortality is 10% per year post-infarction, at the lower end of the reported range (216,227,230,231–237).

Cost Analysis of Medical Management Based on Thallium Rest/Redistribution Imaging

1. Cost of thallium imaging per 100 patients is 100 × $950 = $95,000.

2. The number of patients with viable myocardium by thallium imaging who are treatable by intervention is, from assumptions 2 and 3 assumption above, 30 × 70% = 21 patients, of whom half have PTCA and half have SVBG. Cost of intervention is

    PTCA   10.5 × $10,000 = $105,000
    SVBG   10.5 × $20,000 = $210,000

3. Therapy fails in 10% × 21 = 2.1, with a 10% × 2.1, or .21, mortality, causing loss in productivity over 5 years of .21 × $30,000 × 5 years = $31,500.

4. Of the 50 post-MI/thrombolysis patients with viable myocardium, 30 were identified by thallium imaging, with 20 missed. In those missed patients, the mortality is 10% per year, or 10% × 20 = 2.0, patients, with lost productivity over a 5-year period of 2 × $30,000/yr × 5 yr = $300,000.

5. Total costs of post-MI management based on thallium imaging: $741,500.

Cost Analysis of Medical Management Based on PET

1. Cost of PET imaging for 100 patients is 100 × $1,500 = $150,000.

2. The number of patients with viable myocardium suitable for intervention from the 1st and 3rd assumption above is 50 × 70% = 35 patients, of whom half have PTCA and half have SVBG, for a therapy cost of

    17.5 × $10,000 = $175,000
    17.5 × $20,000 = $350,000

3. Therapy fails in 10% × 35 = 3.5 cases, with a mortality of 10% × 3.5 or 0.35, causing loss of productivity over 5 years of 0.35 × $30,000 × 5 years = $52,500.

4. Total cost based on PET is

PET imaging	$150,000
PTCA + SVBG	$525,000
Lost, productivity, Rx failure	$52,500
Total	$727,500

Conclusion on Evaluating Patients for Myocardial Viability After Myocardial Infarction

At first glance this analysis suggests that the greater diagnostic yield of PET compensates for its greater cost as compared to thallium imaging for medical management of the post-MI patient. The overall cost of medical management based on PET would then be comparable or lower than for thallium imaging, as summarized in Table 18.6.

However, this conclusion has to be modified by several unanswered questions. In this analysis, based on published data, the apparent advantage of PET is in the identification by FDG imaging of more patients with viable myocardium than by thallium imaging. There are five potential problems with this supposition, as follows.

1. In the initial report on FDG (17), functional recovery of hypokinetic regions occurred in 85% of local LV regions, but the percent of patients with improved ejection fraction was not given. For transient rest-exercise defects on ^{13}N ammonia images, (16) 34 of 48 LV segments, or 71%, improved, as presented in Table 15.3. Thus, 71% to 85% of segments judged viable by PET showed postoperative recovery. In reports on thallium stress testing, shown in Tables 15.1 and 15.2, 65% (15/23) to 81% (35/43) of segments with transient thallium perfusion defects showed improvement after bypass surgery (16,97). Bonow et al. (238) have recently reported in an abstract that reversible perfusion defects on resting thallium images give comparable results to FDG imaging. Thus, PET may identify somewhat more regions than thallium imaging, owing to better resolution. However, since three or more regions need to improve in order for ejection fraction to increase postoperatively, PET may not identify more patients needing revascularization. There are no published data showing better patient outcome with viability by PET. Finally, in a recent report, a substantial number of patients showing myocardial FDG uptake after glucose loading demonstrate later loss of LV function and metabolic activity despite successful bypass surgery (95).

2. Recent preliminary data (105,106,148) suggest that FDG uptake may not be an optimal measure of viability. In up to 21% of patients, large areas of myocardium may fail to take up FDG despite normal perfusion and function. On the other hand, depending on the fasting/fed state, necrotic myocardium may take up FDG.

Table 18.6 Economic Analysis of PET for MI/Thrombolysis

	Thallium	PET
Cost of tests (per 100)	$ 95,000	$150,000
PTCA, SVBG	315,000	525,000
Rx failures, loss of productivity (over 5 yrs)	31,500	52,500
Misses, no Rx, loss of productivity (over 5 yrs)	300,000	0
Total costs	$741,500	$727,500
Mortality (persons per 5 yrs)	2	0.35

Source: Adapted with permission from Gould KL, 1989. Reference 171.

3. The literature has not distinguished between viability in a resting perfusion defect and a reversible stress defect caused by limited flow reserve around the resting defect, outlined by stress perfusion imaging. Although this problem is only now being studied, it is our clinical impression that by both FDG and rubidium washout imaging, substantial viable myocardium warranting an intervention is not as commonly found in a significant resting perfusion defect as previously reported. With stress or dipyridamole imaging, the visual intensity of the resting defect appears greater because of more activity delivered to normal myocardium around the resting defect. However, this apparent "reversibility" of the resting defect does not necessarily imply viability or even a zone of reduced flow reserve around the resting defect. Only a larger defect or new defect after dipyridamole indicates a new zone at risk. Consequently, in our experience the number of patients with enough viable myocardium in a resting defect after documented myocardial infarction to warrant mechanical intervention is considerably lower than the 85% suggested in the literature (17), being 30% to 50% of patients.

4. Based on Tables 18.2 through 18.6, the cost of intervening after myocardial infarction appears to be greater than the cost of identifying specific individuals with subclinical disease to be treated by rigorous risk factor management before myocardial infarction. The overall costs of medical care are least in Tables 18.4 and 18.5 for the asymptomatic patient, intermediate in Tables 18.2 and 18.3 for patients with angina pectoris, and greatest in Table 18.6 for patients after myocardial infarction. The clarity of the benefits and the differential between the approaches with and without PET are greatest for the lowest-cost approach to the asymptomatic subject and become increasingly unclear for the higher-cost approach based on assessing myocardial viability after myocardial infarction.

5. The economics of clinical PET become less favorable for the use of cyclotron-produced radionuclides. Table 18.7, A–D, shows a conservative pro forma analysis for a clinical cyclotron operation. The basic problem is that initial capital costs are twice that of a scanner using ^{82}Rb and patient throughput is reduced by half, owing to the longer time required for each study. The time required for each study is longer because cyclotron-produced tracers have a longer half-life, requiring a longer wait between rest-stress imaging and also longer imaging times. At the same dollar charge per procedure as for ^{82}Rb, financial break-even is not achieved, because adequate numbers of patients cannot be put through a cyclotron-based operation.

While assessing viability by PET has received the most intense attention by investigators in the imaging field and by cardiology, there are serious questions about this emphasis as the sole or major benefit of PET in cardiovascular medicine from scientific, clinical, and economic points of view. Based on our analysis and clinical experience to date, the greatest benefit of PET may be in identifying coronary artery disease accurately and non-invasively in order to avoid unnecessary procedures and to prevent progression or to cause regression by vigorous risk factor management. Assessing viability is an important additional benefit, particularly if obtained as an integral part of an economical, brief test using generator sources of radionuclides for accurately determining the presence, location, and severity of coronary artery stenoses throughout the coronary vascular tree.

OVERALL CONCLUSIONS ON THE ECONOMIC ANALYSIS OF CLINICAL CARDIAC PET WITH GENERATOR-PRODUCED ^{82}RB

Although the cost for PET with ^{82}Rb at $1,500 per study using current technology is higher than for ^{201}Tl at $950 per study, the greater diagnostic yield of PET results in comparable or lower overall medical management costs than no diagnostic tests/interventions, and comparable or lower overall costs than thallium imaging for evaluating patients with chest pain, asymptomatic high-risk males, and patients after acute myocardial infarction/thrombolysis for myocardial viability, as summarized in Table 18.2 through Table 18.7. If more realistic charges for thallium stress testing of $1,200 per study are used, the economy of PET becomes even greater.

Figure 18.3 shows the comparative diagnostic costs of PET, SPECT, and arteriography graphed as a function of disease prevalence (149,171,239). For this figure, sensitivity and specificity for SPECT were 80% and 50%, respectively, as published (161–168), and for PET they were 95% and 95%, respectively, as published (1,4–6,177). Cost of SPECT was $1,000 per study, including professional fees, and for PET using generator-produced ^{82}Rb it was $1,500. Each positive non-invasive test by both technologies was assumed to lead to arteriography, costing $6,000. If the cost of arteriography in false-positive tests is counted into the cost of identifying or ruling out disease, the overall cost of medical care based on thallium SPECT is higher than for PET, owing to the higher costs of definitive caths for the false-positive SPECT results. Figure 18.4 shows the direct costs of definitive arteriography

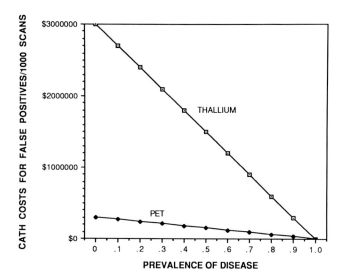

Fig. 18.4 Comparative costs of definitive coronary arteriography for false-positive results of the non-invasive tests as a function of disease prevalence. Reproduced with permission from Gould KL, 1989. (171).

for false-positive non-invasive tests, in order to emphasize this point (171).

Since PET also provides an approximate quantitative assessment of severity (1,4,12), it can potentially be used as a substitute for arteriography in patients with mild to moderate disease amenable to medical therapy. If one assumes that approximately 30% to 40% of patients undergoing coronary arteriography need a mechanical procedure (PTCA, bypass surgery), a large part of the balance of arteriograms not leading to a procedure because of less severe or no disease could be prevented by identifying those patients suitable for medical therapy by PET. As an illustration, this instance is shown by the lower line of Figure 18.3, where half of the arteriograms have been eliminated on the basis of PET results. Therefore, the use of the ^{82}Rb generator instead of a cyclotron for cardiac PET reduces the cost of PET imaging to a reasonable range for routine clinical use.

However, technologies for accurate non-invasive diagnosis, mechanical intervention, and pharmacologic therapy for reversal of CAD have evolved sufficiently to reconsider the potential impact of this approach. High-risk individuals may be defined as males 45 to 65 years old with two or more risk factors of smoking, hypertension, hypercholesterolemia (or abnormal HDL/LDL ratios), and/or family history of coronary artery disease. Identifying asymptomatic high-risk males by PET is theoretically comparable to or less costly than a policy of no testing or treatment, as previously shown, and would result in lower mortality.

With cyclotron-produced ^{13}N ammonia, a rest-exercise test or a rest-dipyridamole test takes 2 h, which limits the patient throughput to 4 or 5 per day. At the same time, the cost of a PET-cyclotron facility is twice that of a scanner used for cardiac studies with generator-produced ^{82}Rb. Table 18.7, A–B, shows a pro forma for a clinical cyclotron site operating at maximum capacity of 5 per day at $1,500 charge per study, which is $300 higher than the $1,200 charge for the ^{82}Rb rest-

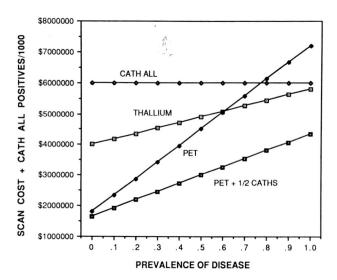

Fig. 18.3 Comparative costs of ^{201}Tl SPECT and PET with generator-produced ^{82}Rb as a function of disease prevalence. Reproduced with permission from Gould KL, 1989. (171).

Table 18.7A Pro Forma for General Hospital, Anywhere, USA

<table>
<tr><td colspan="4" align="center">Assumptions</td></tr>
<tr><td colspan="4">Equipment: POSICAM with cyclotron (no rubidium)
Transaction Type: Purchase</td></tr>
<tr><th>Category</th><th>Value</th><th>Category</th><th>Value</th></tr>
<tr><td>Number of Procedures per Day</td><td></td><td>Equipment Cost</td><td>$4,600,000</td></tr>
<tr><td>Year 1:</td><td>4</td><td>Down Payment</td><td>$920,000</td></tr>
<tr><td>Year 2:</td><td>5</td><td>Years Financed</td><td>5</td></tr>
<tr><td>Year 3:</td><td>5</td><td>Interest Rate</td><td>10.0%</td></tr>
<tr><td>Year 4:</td><td>5</td><td></td><td></td></tr>
<tr><td>Year 5:</td><td>5</td><td>Other Equipment Costs</td><td></td></tr>
<tr><td></td><td></td><td>ECG Monitor</td><td>$5,000</td></tr>
<tr><td>Imaging Days</td><td>250</td><td>Defribrillator</td><td>$2,500</td></tr>
<tr><td>Charge per Procedure</td><td>$1,500</td><td>Emergency Cart</td><td>$5,000</td></tr>
<tr><td></td><td></td><td>Rigging Expense</td><td>$0</td></tr>
<tr><td>Inflation Rate</td><td>4.0%</td><td>Other Equipment</td><td>$195,000</td></tr>
<tr><td>Bad Debt Rate</td><td>9.0%</td><td>Total Other Equipment</td><td>$207,500</td></tr>
<tr><td></td><td></td><td></td><td></td></tr>
<tr><td>Years to Depr. Equipment</td><td>5</td><td>Building Cost</td><td>$300,000</td></tr>
<tr><td>Years to Depr. Build/Improve</td><td>15</td><td>Down Payment</td><td>$30,000</td></tr>
<tr><td></td><td></td><td>Years Financed</td><td>7</td></tr>
<tr><td>Corporate Tax Rate</td><td>0</td><td>Interest Rate</td><td>12.0%</td></tr>
<tr><td></td><td></td><td>Improvement Cost</td><td>$0</td></tr>
<tr><td>Beginning Cash</td><td>$0</td><td>Down Payment</td><td>$0</td></tr>
<tr><td></td><td></td><td>Years Financed</td><td>0</td></tr>
<tr><td>Staffing</td><td></td><td>Interest Rate</td><td>0.0%</td></tr>
<tr><td>Number of Nuclear Physicians</td><td>0</td><td>Administrative Costs</td><td></td></tr>
<tr><td>Nuclear Physician Salary</td><td>$0</td><td>Service Contract</td><td>$415,000</td></tr>
<tr><td>Nuclear Physician Fee per
Procedure</td><td>$0</td><td>Consumables per Proc.</td><td>$50</td></tr>
<tr><td></td><td></td><td>Radiopharmaceuticals:</td><td></td></tr>
<tr><td>Number of Nuclear Technologists</td><td>1</td><td>Rubidium</td><td>$0</td></tr>
<tr><td>Nuclear Technologists Salary</td><td>$30,000</td><td>Cyclotron Isotopes</td><td>$20</td></tr>
<tr><td></td><td></td><td></td><td></td></tr>
<tr><td>Number of Registered Nurses</td><td>1</td><td>Rent</td><td>$0</td></tr>
<tr><td>Registered Nurse Salary</td><td>$36,000</td><td>Utilities</td><td>$10,000</td></tr>
<tr><td></td><td></td><td>Other Medical Supplies</td><td>$0</td></tr>
<tr><td>Number of Other Support Staff</td><td>1</td><td></td><td></td></tr>
<tr><td>Average Salary</td><td>$42,000</td><td>% of Cyclotron
Procedures</td><td>100%</td></tr>
<tr><td>Employee Benefit Rate</td><td>28.0%</td><td></td><td></td></tr>
</table>

Table 18.7B Operating Expenses and Forecasted Income Statement

Expenses	Year 1	Year 2	Year 3	Year 4	Year 5
Salaries	$ 108,000	$ 112,320	$ 116,813	$ 121,485	$ 126,345
Professional fees	0	0	0	0	0
Benefits	30,240	31,450	32,708	34,016	35,377
Equipment maintenance	0	415,000	431,600	448,864	466,819
Radiopharmaceuticals	20,000	26,000	27,040	28,122	29,246
Consumable supplies	50,000	65,000	67,600	70,304	73,116
Rent	0	0	0	0	0
Utilities	10,000	10,400	10,816	11,249	11,699
Medical supplies	0	0	0	0	0
Interest expense	383,066	313,529	237,690	153,909	61,355
Depreciation	981,500	981,500	981,500	981,500	981,500
Total expenses	$1,582,806	$1,955,199	$1,905,766	$1,849,449	$1,785,456

Table 18.7C

Number of Procedures	Year 1 1,000	Year 2 1,250	Year 3 1,250	Year 4 1,250	Year 5 1,250
Income: patient billing	$1,500,000	$1,950,000	$2,028,000	$2,109,120	$2,193,485
Less: bad debt	135,000	175,500	182,520	189,821	197,414
Gross income	1,365,000	1,774,500	1,845,480	1,919,299	1,996,071
Operating expenses	1,582,806	1,955,199	1,905,766	1,849,449	1,785,456
Net operating income	(217,806)	(180,699)	(60,286)	69,851	210,615
Cumulative net income	($217,806)	($398,504)	($458,791)	($388,940)	($178,325)
Break-even: number of procedures per day	4.67	5.54	5.17	4.81	4.44

Table 18.7D PET System: Forecasted Statement of Cash Flow and Rates of Return

	Year 1	Year 2	Year 3	Year 4	Year 5
Beginning cash	0	($841,028)	($764,487)	($643,371)	($475,900)
Net operating income	($217,806)	(180,699)	(60,286)	69,851	210,615
Add back: depreciation	981,500	981,500	981,500	981,500	981,500
Less: principal payment	654,723	724,259	800,099	883,879	976,433
Less: down payments	950,000	0	0	0	0
Total pre-tax cash flow	(841,028)	76,542	121,115	167,471	215,682
After-tax cash flow	(841,028)	76,542	121,115	167,471	215,682
Cash at end of year	($841,028)	($764,487)	($643,371)	($475,900)	($260,218)

dipyridamole study analyzed previously. Even with this higher charge per study, the break-even patient load is 5 patients per day, which is at the upper limit of daily patient throughput achievable using cyclotron-produced radionuclides. Consequently, the facility operates in deficit throughout 5 years without breaking even on an initial large capital investment.

With new technical improvements in the attenuation correction and image reconstruction now nearing completion, the time required for a rest-dipyridamole study is reduced to 40–45 min. The patient volume throughput then increases to 10 to 12 patients per day, thereby reducing cost per study to that for [201]Tl. Having tested the essential design characteristics for a clinical cardiac PET scanner in over 1,100 studies at the University of Texas and over 2,000 cases at private sites, we are now designing a scanner to reduce cost of the scanner by 30% to 40%. As these advances reach clinical availability, the cost of PET for even smaller patient volume could become comparable to that of thallium, and the difference between cost of a study using [82]Rb and one using cyclotron-produced radionuclides becomes even more marked.

CARDIAC PET IN NON-UNIVERSITY PRACTICE

Clinical cardiac PET utilizing the [82]Rb generator (1,4,19,28,35,36) is practical in non-university cardiologic practice (177,178,240). Since the first private practice PET study in March 1988, in Atlanta (177), over 2,000 patients have been studied in private practice sites. However, some qualifications are important to mention. Based on our experience in over 1,000 university-based clinical studies and the 2,000 private practice studies, it is necessary to utilize all tomographic views available for interpretation—the acquisition,

short-axis, long-axis, and polar map views—together. Short-axis views alone commonly fail to show abnormalities seen on long-axis views. For "balanced" three-vessel coronary artery disease, the polar map displays showing relative and absolute flow reserve of the whole heart demonstrate abnormalities more accurately than the tomographic views alone.

It is also our observation that processing PET data with software designed for SPECT imaging having different reconstruction filters, rotational algorithms, and so on, optimized for SPECT, are unsatisfactory for PET images. Although the diagnostic accuracy of PET data processed by SPECT software is better than by SPECT imaging (193,194), PET images processed with SPECT software are overly smoothed, with data displaced into neighboring pixels (blurring) by multi-step rotational schemes or excessive smoothing. Even with inappropriate software, the specificity of PET for diagnosis of CAD was higher than for SPECT (193,194), but the sensitivity in those studies was comparable to SPECT. The explanation is that suboptimal processing of PET data by SPECT software, in our experience, lowers diagnostic content in comparison to software specifically designed for PET reconstruction and display (10), with which higher diagnostic accuracy is obtained (1,4–6,177).

Another reason for lower sensitivity (or specificity) is inadequate total counts in the whole-heart image set. Six million counts per whole-heart image set, as reported with a block camera design having high dead-time losses (195), seriously compromises diagnostic content for short-lived tracers like [82]Rb or [15]O water. By comparison, for [82]Rb we acquire approximately 15 to 35 million counts per whole-heart data set and achieve a greater sensitivity and specificity. In count-poor studies, summing slices makes them look better but does not overcome the basic inaccuracy due to inadequate counts in the whole-heart data set. Therefore, high count rate capacity, good Z axis sampling without interplane under-sampling (207), and quantitative validated, clinical software (10) are important for achieving high sensitivity and specificity in clinical applications.

The question often arises as to whether imaging by PET is too sensitive for traditional cardiac practice, detecting coronary artery disease that causes no symptoms, whereas the traditional approach is to use medical or mechanical intervention only for symptoms of ischemia. However, the marker of ischemia then becomes the question. Are chest pain, electrocardiographic change, abnormalities of exercise thallium images, or stress abnormalities in left ventricular function specific and sensitive indicators of coronary artery disease?

As reviewed previously, the sensitivity and specificity of exercise thallium imaging are currently reported as 70%–80% and 50%–60%, respectively. Consequently, these endpoints are not reliable indicators of disease or are reliably positive only with advanced anatomic severity. In order to evaluate functional stenosis severity or its changes over the entire range from mild to severe narrowing, maximum perfusion abnormalities reflecting direct fluid-dynamic effects of arterial narrowing are necessary, regardless of metabolic ischemia. Because finding even mild coronary artery narrowing without ischemia now results in significant dietary and/or medical intervention, a way of reliably identifying and following such patients without ischemic endpoints becomes important.

There is growing evidence that specific mediators, thromboxane and serotonin, are responsible for chronic stable atherosclerosis changing to unstable syndromes of accelerating angina pectoris, myocardial infarction, and sudden death (241). Prevention of these acute syndromes by pharmacologic blockers combined with stringent cholesterol lowering to reverse coronary atherosclerosis could have further profound effects on management of coronary artery disease, particularly if diagnosis and evaluation of severity can be made non-invasively.

Positron emission tomography provides sufficiently accurate diagnosis and assessment of coronary stenosis severity and myocardial viability to be the basis for practicing optimal traditional cardiology based on the traditional symptoms-oriented approach using PET as an aid or substitute for diagnostic catheterization in many instances. It is particularly useful after thrombolysis during acute myocardial infarction for choosing between medical and mechanical intervention on the basis of remaining viable myocardium, arterial patency, and the extent of additional myocardium at risk.

However, its quantitative functional information, combined with current mechanical interventions, medical therapy to lower cholesterol for coronary artery disease reversal, and drugs to prevent unstable coronary syndromes are the basis for management of asymptomatic patients with silent coronary atherosclerosis at comparable or less cost to the patient and society than current approaches.

19

Radiation Burden, Facilities, and Regulatory Status

As shown in Table 19.1, the radiation burden to patients by positron tracers of ^{82}Rb, ^{13}N ammonia, and ^{18}F FDG are generally comparable to or lower than standard cardiac nuclear tracers such as ^{201}Tl, because the half-life of the positron tracers is short (242–252). Optimal clinical benefit with most appropriate choice of test, its safe application, and proper interpretation within the clinical context of a specific patient for a given radiation dose make positron imaging an optimal clinical tool with relatively low radiation burden to patient and staff.

PERSONNEL AND FACILITY REQUIREMENTS

Two types of facilities for cardiac PET are appropriate. The first is a positron camera utilizing generator-produced ^{82}Rb in the absence of a cyclotron. The second includes a cyclotron-radiochemistry complex. For clinical studies, both facilities would require a room approximately 15 ft by 15 ft for the camera, with an attached smaller space, 10 ft by 10 ft, as a computer room, control console, and reading center. Appropriate cardiac drugs and resuscitation equipment are required in the imaging room, including defibrillation and intubation facilities and emergency cardiac drugs. Since the stress provided for the screening test utilizes intravenous dipyridamole, appropriate ECG monitoring should be available. Physician supervision is necessary for carrying out these studies because of the infusion of vasoactive drugs comparable to exercise stress. On occasion, patients with coronary artery disease undergoing dipyridamole–hand grip stress develop angina pectoris, which requires reversal utilizing intravenous aminophylline. Aminophylline is effective in reversing the effects of dipyridamole quickly. Consequently, the test sequence may be well controlled. A physician trained and experienced in clinical cardiovascular medicine is essential for evaluating the patient during the test in order to determine whether this reversal step is necessary and for interpreting the results physiologically.

Available positron cameras have become sufficiently dedicated, with operational software transparent to the user, that a technician can carry out the procedure under the supervision of a physician. Physicians with expertise in physiologic cardiovascular imaging are the appropriate individuals for choosing the appropriate patients and the study to be done, and for carrying out the test protocol, for study interpretation, and for supervising the program. Such physicians may be cardiologists, internists, nuclear medicine physicians, or radiologists with knowledge of cardiovascular imaging, cardiovascular physiology, coronary arteriography, and clinical management of cardiac disease, particularly cardiac emergencies, resuscitation, arrhythmias, and cardiac arrest.

STATUS WITH REGULATORY AGENCIES

PET cameras are now commercially distributed as a Class II device registered with the Food and Drug Administration using Form 510K under FDA guidelines USDHHS Section 21CFR 807, Class II (Performance Standards), Premarket Notification for Medical Devices, under a grandfather clause for preexisting technology. The rubidium generator (Squibb) has been approved by the FDA for human use. Intravenous dipyridamole for stress perfusion imaging is currently being reviewed by the FDA, with approval expected soon.

Table 19.1 Radiation Burden of Positron Radionuclides*

| Radionuclide | References | Radiation Exposure (mrads/mCi) | | | |
		IV Dose (mCi)	Total Body	Heart	Target Organ
^{201}Tl	242–244	3	240	170	390 (bladder)
^{13}NH$_3$	242, 245	20	6	50	51 (bladder)
^{18}F-deoxyglucose	246–248	12	39	160	280 (bladder)
^{82}Rb	242, 249–251	45	2	11	71 (kidney)
H$_2$^{15}O	252	20	2	2	2 (intestines/testes)
C^{15}O	252	33	2	5	11 (lung)

* FDA guidelines for radiation burden: whole-body single dose, 3,000 mrems; whole-body annual dose, 5,000 mrems; other organs single dose, 5,000 mrems; other organs annual dose, 15,000 mrems.

20

Case Studies with PET

The unique information on cardiac pathophysiology provided by positron emission tomography (PET) may be illustrated by a series of case reports ranging from traditional, difficult management problems of advanced coronary artery disease to identifying and treating asymptomatic individuals. Several examples from PET centers in private practice are also shown to demonstrate routine PET in the private clinical setting. The cases are grouped into several categories of clinical problems as follows:

Diagnosis and assessing severity of coronary artery disease (cases 1–15) in asymptomatic individuals, for questionable or atypical chest pain, or in symptomatic patients in whom the extent and severity of disease is needed for decisions on medical treatment, coronary arteriography, percutaneous transluminal angioplasty (PTCA), or coronary bypass surgery.

Viability of myocardium in patients (cases 16–23) after myocardial infarction with or without thrombolysis in order to decide on mechanical or medical intervention.

Progression or regression of coronary atherosclerosis in individuals (cases 24–28) during medical management or after PTCA in order to detect restenosis, particularly in asymptomatic patients or those who do not have chest pain with ischemia.

Postcoronary bypass problems (cases 29–32), such as recurrent chest pain, particularly for complex cases of multiple PTCA and/or coronary bypasses in whom the specific artery causing angina pectoris or ischemia, needs to be identified for selective intervention and for routine follow-up in patients who do not have chest pain, despite documented ischemia.

The orientation of tomographs and polar map displays are described in Chapter 12, specifically Figures 12.5, 12.6, and 12.7. The information for each of these clinical images is included in the text for each case rather than in the legend. The PET images for some of the clinical examples have been presented in earlier chapters, specifically Figures 10.12, 12.8, 12.9, 12.10, 14.1, 14.11, 15.4, 15.7, 15.14, 15.15, and 16.1. Images of both generator-produced rubidium-82 and N-13 ammonia illustrate the comparability of these two radionuclides.

In selected examples, in addition to standard tomographs and polar maps, new three-dimensional (3D) topographic displays of cardiac PET are shown that do not distort the spatial size and shape of defects as occurs with polar map displays. These 3D topographic displays demonstrate the more accurate spatial quantitation and visualization of abnormalities compared to previously shown polar maps. Three-dimensional topographic maps of cardiac PET images are derived from short-axis data. Each panel of the topographic map views the left ventricle as if looking at the septum (upper row, first panel), at the anterior wall (upper row, second panel), at the left lateral wall (upper row, third panel), or the inferior wall (upper row, fourth panel). The dashed white line marks the upper limit of automated quantitative data, since the membranous septum often causes a normal defect at the atrioventricular (AV) ring. The black dashed lines delineate septal, anterior, lateral, and inferior quadrants with the lower dashed line delineating the apex. The colored scaling and automated quantitation, such as minimum activity values, mean activity in each quadrant, and percent of myocardium beyond 1.5, 2.0, and 2.5 standard deviations (SDs), are all the same as previously described for polar maps. The rest study is shown in the upper row (S1) and stress study in the lower row (S2). Similar displays are shown for the absolute S2/S1 ratio (ABS S2/S1, upper row) and for the relative change S2/S1 ratio (REL S2/S1, lower row).

Case 1: Severe "Balanced" Three-Vessel Coronary Artery Disease

A 61-year-old man presented with onset of severe angina pectoris approximately 10 years previously that limited normal low-level activity. Coronary arteriography at that time showed a 95% left anterior descending (LAD) stenosis, an 80% left circumflex stenosis, an 80% right coronary artery stenosis. The patient and his private physician declined coronary bypass surgery and undertook a strict dietary and exercise program. In order to follow his course noninvasively, rest–dipyridamole PET scans were carried out using rubidium-82 (Figure 12.8: A, acquisition view; B, short-axis; C, long-axis and polar maps; D, blackout of areas outside of 2.5 SDs from normal). The rest scan showed a mild, small apical defect suggesting a small apical scar. The dipyridamole scan showed severe defects of large size in the anterior, septal, apical, anterior lateral, lateral, posterior, and inferior myocardium. A small segment of inferior lateral myocardium demonstrated increased uptake of tracer indicating response to dipyridamole.

An extensive area, approximately one third of myocardium in anterior, apical, and inferior apical distributions, demonstrated decrease in activity during dipyridamole compared to rest, suggesting myocardial steal and collateralization. These results suggested progression of disease with probable occlusion of the LAD and right or left circumflex coronary arteries, commonly seen with such extensive resting collateral flow. Repeat coronary arteriography demonstrated complete occlusion of the proximal LAD and right coronary arteries, which were supplied extensively by collaterals from smaller proximal branches of these arteries, as well as from the left circumflex. Since the patient was clinically stable, with decreasing angina and increasing exercise tolerance, the patient continued to decline mechanical intervention but intensified his dietary control and exercise training. His total cholesterol decreased to approximately 100 with low-density lipoproteins (LDL) below 60 and high-density lipoproteins (HDL) of 47. Over the next 5 years, his exercise tolerance continued to improve dramatically with regression of the left circumflex coronary artery stenosis on follow-up arteriograms and more extensive collaterals to the occluded right and LAD coronary arteries.

Corresponding 3D topographic maps are shown in Figure 20.1A (rest, S1, upper row; dipyridamole, S2, lower row) and Figure 20.1B (absolute S2/S1 ratio, upper row; relative change S2/S1 ratio, lower row). These 3D displays clearly demonstrate severe septal, anterior, apical, and inferior septal defects with myocardial steal. There are less severe but definite reduction in coronary flow reserve of lateral myocardium. These findings are consistent with occluded, collateralized right and LAD coronary arteries and patent but stenotic left circumflex, as found at arteriography.

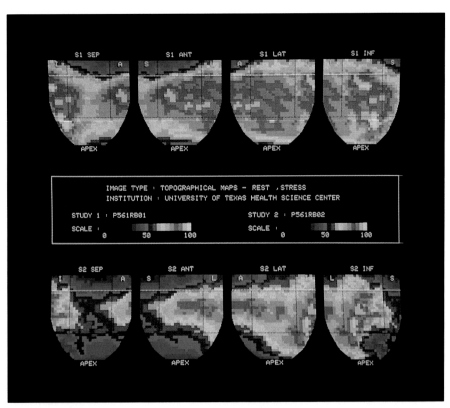

Fig. 20.1 Case 1.

A

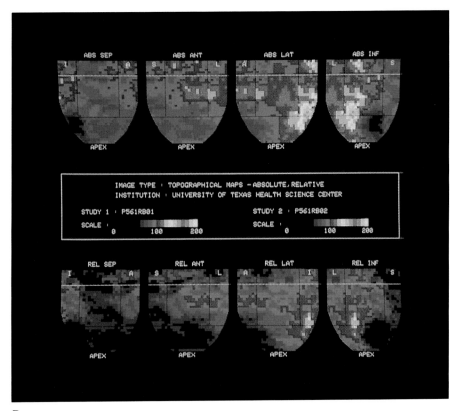

B

Case 2: Mild "Balanced" Three-Vessel Coronary Artery Disease

A 56-year-old man with familial hyperlipidemia was studied as part of a reversal protocol. Other risk factors included smoking and positive family history. The patient had no symptoms and previous thallium treadmill exercise testing was reported as normal. A rest–dipyridamole PET scan was carried out using rubidium-82 (Figure 12.9: A, acquisition view; B, short-axis; C, long-axis and polar maps). The rest image was normal. The dipyridamole image showed moderate defects of large size in the anterior, apical, inferior, and lateral myocardium consistent with moderate three-vessel coronary artery disease. Coronary arteriography confirmed these findings—with approximately 60% diameter stenosis of the mid-LAD, of the proximal left circumflex, and an obtuse marginal. The right coronary artery was a small nondominant vessel with diffuse disease. The patient was begun on a vigorous cholesterol-lowering program.

Corresponding 3D topographic maps are shown in Figure 20.2A where the rest scan is in the upper row (S1) and the dipyridamole scan in the lower row (S2), demonstrating mild septal, anterior, apical, lateral, and inferior defects. Figure 20.2B shows the absolute S2/S1 ratio (upper row) and relative change S2/S1 ratio (lower row), also showing reduced flow reserve.

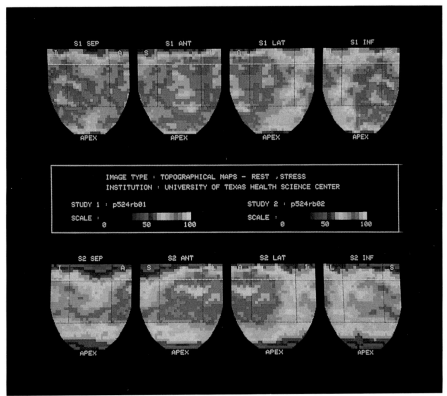

Fig. 20.2 Case 2.

A

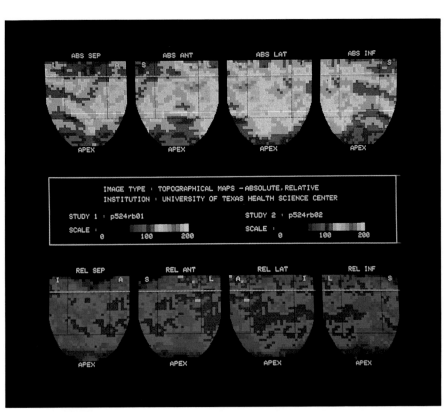

B

Case 3: Atypical Symptoms in a Young Man with Mitral Valve Prolapse

A 41-year-old man presented with long-standing chest pain, palpitations, and anxiety related to documented mitral valve prolapse by ECHO and clinical exam. He had been hospitalized on several occasions for chest pain with myocardial infarction ruled out by serial enzymes and electrocardiogram (ECG) follow-up. The patient also carried a diagnosis of a panic disorder and obsessive compulsive personality on psychiatric evaluation. Thallium exercise testing was interpreted as probably normal. Holter monitor showed minimal atrial and ventricular ectopic beats without significant arrhythmias. The patient's anxiety over his symptoms were associated with depression, sleep disturbance, poor appetite, 26-lb weight loss, hyperventilation, tremors, lightheadedness, and difficulty functioning at home and at work. Consequently, the patient requested a cardiac PET study.

Rest–dipyridamole PET scans were obtained using rubidium-82 (Figure 14.11: A, acquisition view; B, short-axis; C, long-axis and polar maps). The rest image was abnormal with a mild, small inferior lateral defect. The stress image showed a severe large perfusion defect spiraling from the anterior lateral myocardium around the lateral wall to the inferior lateral region and associated with painless ST changes on ECG during dipyridamole, disappearing with aminophylline. These results were interpreted as demonstrating an occluded intermedius ramus coronary artery that was well collateralized with no significant restrictions of flow reserve of the LAD, right, or left circumflex coronary arteries.

Due to the complexity of the management problem, coronary arteriography was carried out which confirmed an occlusion of a large intermedius ramus that was completely collateralized and was therefore not at risk of infarction. Other coronary arteries demonstrated no significant narrowing. Since the patient had no exertional angina pectoris, no chest pain during demonstrated steal by PET scan, and no myocardium at risk of infarction, it was concluded that he had both silent coronary artery disease and symptomatic mitral valve prolapse. Accordingly, he was reassured and medical treatment continued.

The corresponding 3D topographic maps are shown in Figure 20.3A (rest, S1, upper row; dipyridamole, S2, lower row) and 20.3B (absolute S2/S1 ratio, upper row; relative change S2/S1 ratio, lower row). These displays clearly demonstrate a severe defect on the dipyridamole scan spiraling from the anterior lateral myocardium, around the lateral wall, the inferior apex, typical of a ramus intermedius distribution. There is myocardial steal typically seen with an occluded collateralized artery.

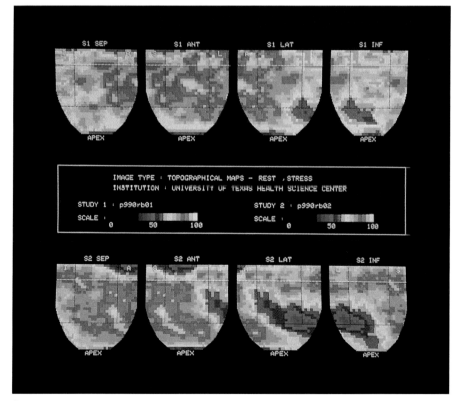

Fig. 20.3 Case 3.

A

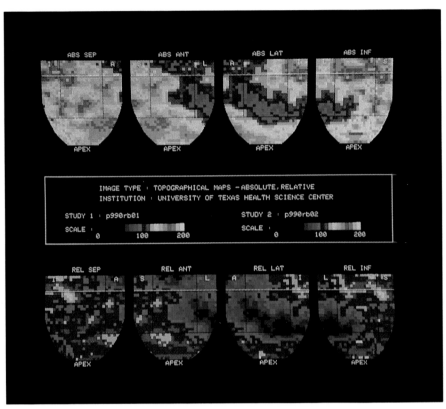

Fig. 20.3 Case 3 (*contd.*)

B

Case 4: Asymptomatic, Hypertensive Man with a Normal Thallium Stress Test

A 52-year-old man presented with no symptoms during regular distance jogging and was in good prior health except for chronic hypertension for which he was treated with diltiazem and captopril. A thallium treadmill test was normal (Figure 16.2A). Due to a personal interest in PET technology, he requested a PET scan under an approved study protocol, which was carried out with rubidium-82 at rest and after dipyridamole (Figure 20.4: A, acquisition view; B, short-axis; C, long-axis and polar maps). The rest scan was normal. The dipyridamole PET scan showed perfusion defects of the apex, anterolateral, posterolateral, and inferior myocardium. The absolute S2/S1 polar map most clearly showed reduced flow reserve of lateral and inferior myocardium, particularly compared to the normal thallium images (Figure 16.2A). In order to confirm these findings, coronary arteriography was carried out demonstrating an 85% stenosis of the first diagonal, and 80% stenosis of the first obtuse marginal, and two 75% stenoses of the right coronary artery. Due to severity of disease, three-vessel PTCA was successfully carried out.

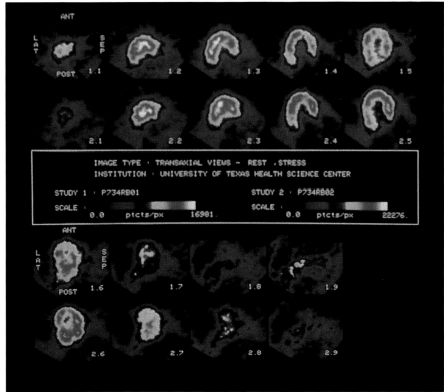

Fig. 20.4 Case 4.

A

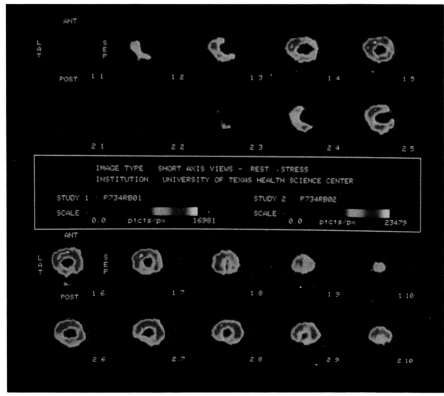

Fig. 20.4 Case 4 (*contd.*)

B

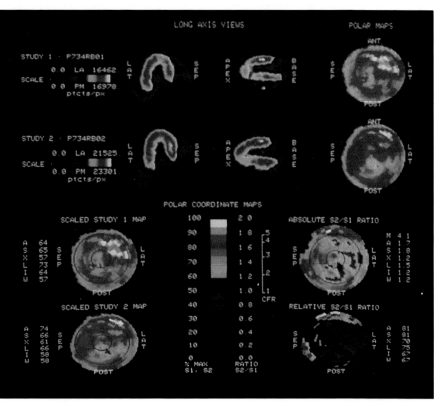

C

Case 5: Severe Silent Coronary Artery Disease with a Normal Thallium Exercise Treadmill Test

A 53-year-old man presented with a history of severe neck arthritis and 20 years of nonexertional, continuous resting chest wall pain that migrated throughout the anterior chest bilaterally, diagnosed as cervical nerve root compression. His risk factors included a history of elevated cholesterol to 240, and his father had a myocardial infarction at 69 years old. Thallium treadmill testing 1 year and 10 days prior to PET scan were both normal with good exertional effort, no chest pain, and no ST changes.

Because of an interest in medical technology, the patient requested a PET scan, which was carried out at rest and after dipyridamole using N-13 ammonia (Figure 20.5A). The rest image showed a mild, small apical defect, suggesting a small old, apical myocardial infarction despite absence of a clinical event. The dipyridamole image showed a large severe anterior and apical defect involving 29% of myocardium outside 2.5 SDs from normal. There were definite but less severe defects of the anterior septum and lateral wall. These results were interpreted as showing a severe mid-LAD stenosis, another more moderate LAD stenosis proximal to the first septal perforator, and a moderate stenosis of an artery to the lateral myocardial wall, probably a left circumflex stenosis.

Accordingly, he was scheduled for diagnostic catheterization and PTCA of three stenoses with surgical backup. Quantitative coronary arteriography confirmed a 72% diameter stenosis of the mid-LAD, a 56% diameter narrowing of the proximal LAD, and a 69% diameter stenosis of the mid-left circumflex. PTCA was carried out on these three lesions

without difficulty. During balloon inflation of the LAD, the patient had his first recognizable angina pectoris, characterized as a deep-squeezing substernal pain. On the next day he developed the same severe chest pain with ST elevations and on repeat arteriography demonstrated occlusion of the LAD which was successfully redilated. His hospital course was complicated by an upper gastrointestinal bleed responding to histamine blockers.

Ten days later, a repeat rest–dipyridamole PET scan demonstrated resolution of the previous perfusion defects. Approximately 3 months later, a repeat PET scan was again normal except for a small equivocal apical defect like that present on the first study; it did not become worse after dipyridamole (Figure 20.5B). The patient continued to do well until 4 weeks later when he had an episode of ventricular tachycardia during supervised exercise, without ST change or chest pain. Repeat rest–dipyridamole PET scan demonstrated recurrence of a moderate, large anterior apical defect suggesting restenosis (Figure 20.5C), confirmed by coronary arteriography. When offered repeat PTCA or coronary bypass surgery, the patient chose the latter which was successfuly carried out.

The 3D topographic displays for this series of PET scans at rest (S1, upper row) and after dipyridamole (S2, lower row) are shown prior to PTCA (Figure 20.5D), just after PTCA (Figure 20.5E), and late after PTCA (Figure 20.5F). The corresponding absolute S2/S1 ratio maps (upper row) nicely demonstrate the initial defect (Figure 20.5G), the normal scan after PTCA (Figure 20.5H), and restenosis but not as severe as initially (Figure 20.5I).

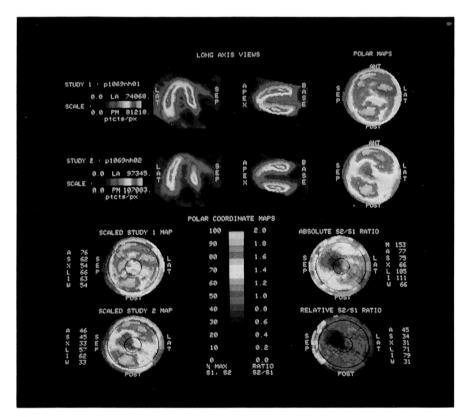

Fig. 20.5 Case 5 (20.5C, Reproduced with permission from reference 178).

A

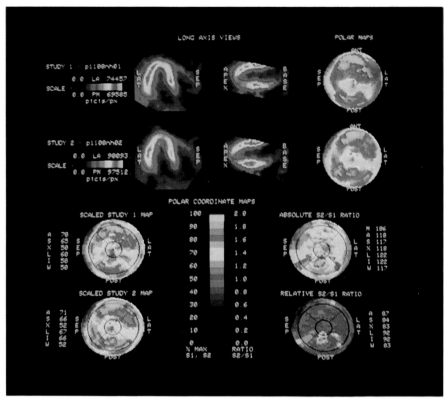

Fig. 20.5 Case 5 (*contd.*)

B

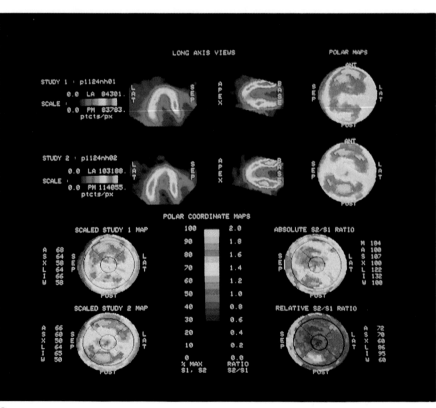

C

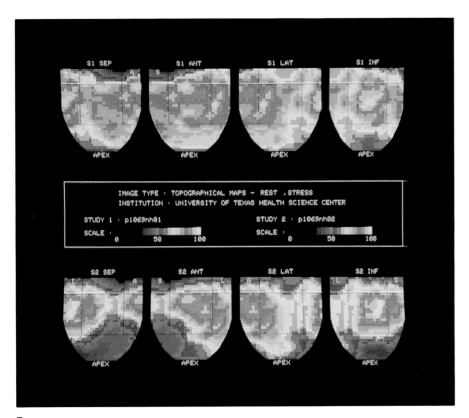

D

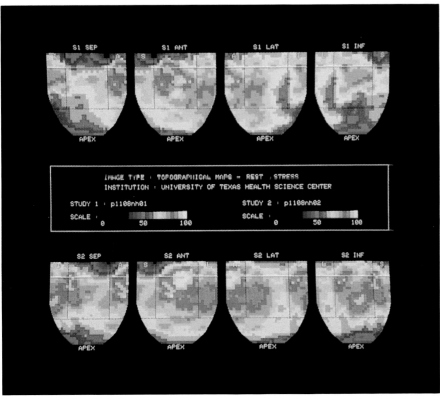

E

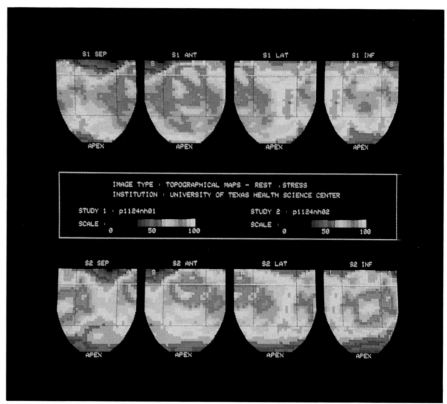

Fig. 20.5 Case 5 (*contd.*)

F

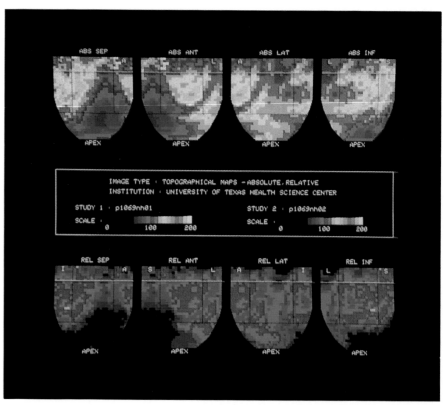

G

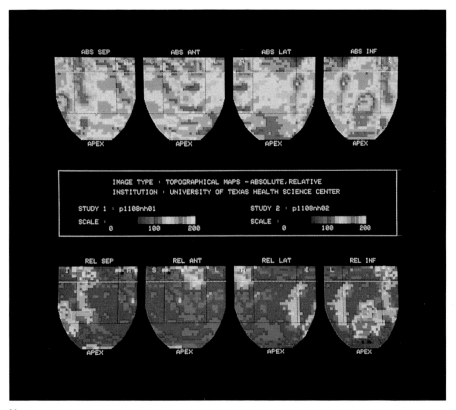

H

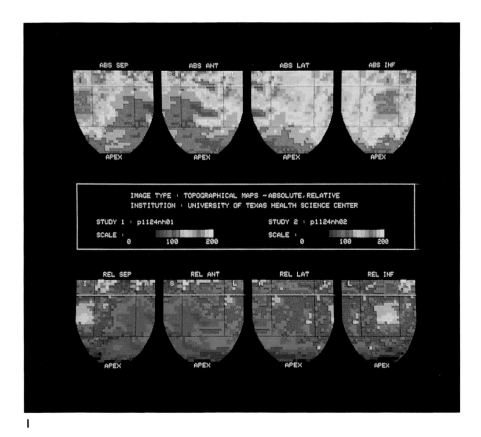

I

Case 6: Unexpected, Severe, Silent Coronary Atherosclerosis in a Young Jogger

A 31-year-old man, who has been a jogger for many years, recently noticed mild shortness of breath while running which he attributed to "getting old." He had no chest pain at any time. His coronary risk factors included a strong family history for coronary artery disease, familial hypercholesterolemia, and smoking for 7 years before quitting cigarettes and going on a low-fat diet 1 year prior to being seen at the PET center in Jacksonville, Florida. Although neither the patient nor the referring cardiologist suspected significant coronary artery disease, a routine screening PET study was carried out using rubidium-82 at rest and after dipyridamole handgrip (Figure 20.6: A, acquisition view; B, short-axis; C, long-axis and polar maps). The rest scan was normal, but the dipyridamole scan showed a large severe perfusion defect in the inferior, inferior septal, and inferolateral myocardium with a moderately severe defect of the anterior and apical myocardium. There was inferior myocardial steal indicated by a fall in activity during dipyridamole, consistent with extensive inferior collateralization. A total of 44% of the heart was outside 2.5 SDs of normal, involving anterior, septal, lateral, and inferior quadrants, indicating severe three-vessel disease.

Based on the PET scan, cardiac catheterization was carried out. It showed total occlusion of the right and subtotal occlusion of mid-marginal coronary arteries, significant left main disease, and moderate narrowing of the proximal LAD and first diagonal. Despite lack of symptoms, due to the extent and severity of disease, coronary bypass surgery was successfully carried out. Follow-up PET scan showed complete disappearance of the perfusion defects previously observed and relief of dyspnea on exertion.

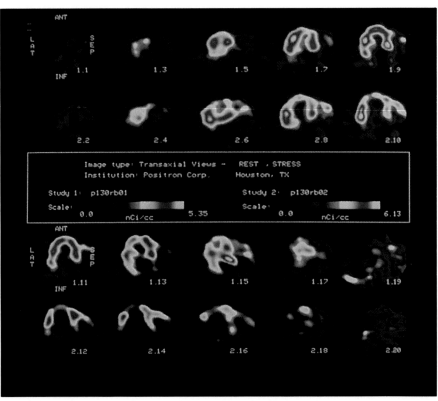

Fig. 20.6 Case 6. Reproduced with permission from reference 178.

A

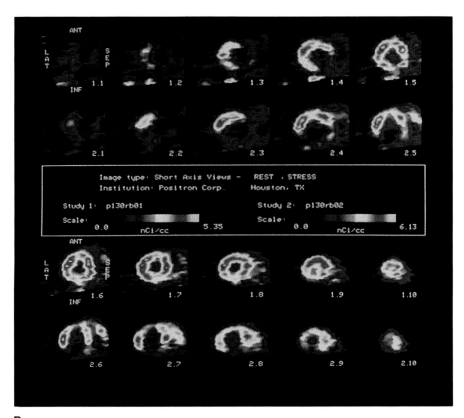

B

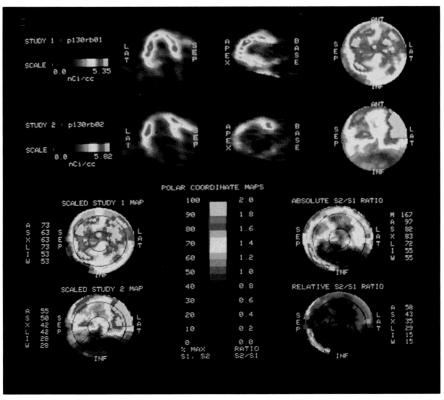

C

Case 7: Asymptomatic Mild Coronary Artery Stenosis with a Normal Thallium Exercise Stress Test

A 58-year-old executive had no history of heart disease, chest pain, palpitations, or other cardiovascular symptoms. He gave a history of a thallium treadmill test 2 years previously that showed no perfusion defects and no significant ST changes. The patient did not smoke, was not overweight, and walked 5 miles every morning. A routine screening cardiac PET scan was carried out with a rubidium-82 at rest and after dipyridamole handgrip (Figure 20.7: A, acquisition view; B, short-axis). The rest scan was normal. The dipyridamole PET scan showed a mild but definite lateral perfusion defect over a large area of lateral myocardium. The patient was advised of these results and wished to have confirmation by coronary arteriography. The arteriogram showed a moderately long 41% diameter stenosis of the left circumflex coronary artery, objectively measured by automated quantitative analysis. Accordingly, the patient was treated by a cholesterol-lowering diet with the potential addition of cholesterol-lowering drugs depending upon dietary reponse.

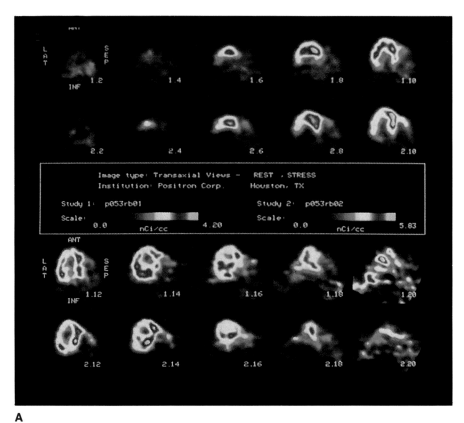

A

Fig. 20.7 Case 7 (20.7B, Reproduced with permission from reference 178).

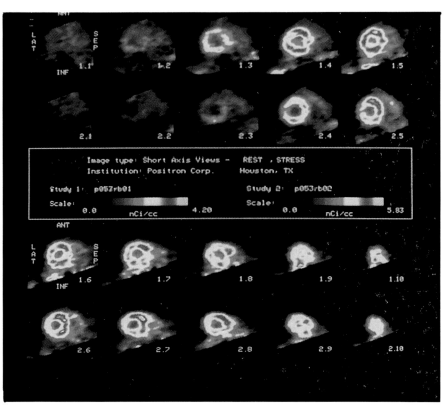

B

Case 8: Selection of Artery for PTCA by PET in a Patient with "Balanced" Multi-Vessel Disease Without a Normal Reference Artery

A 57-year-old man presented with 2 weeks of chest pressure leading to the diagnosis of myocardial infarction by ECG and enzyme changes. He was free of chest pain during the subsequent 4 weeks prior to being seen at the PET center in Jacksonville, Florida, until recent recurrant angina pectoris. Coronary risk factors included family history and smoking. Cardiac catheterization showed diffuse, moderate disease of the mid-LAD and proximal right coronary arteries with total occlusion of a dominant left circumflex coronary artery filling retrograde via collaterals. Since the patient had three-vessel disease with an occlusion of the left circumflex and a lateral nontransmural myocardial infarction, the referring cardiologist had no basis for locating the source of angina or for deciding upon medical therapy or mechanical intervention and if so, for which artery or all three arteries.

Accordingly, PET was carried out using rubidium-82 at rest and after dipyridamole handgrip (Figure 20.8A: A, short-axis view; B, long-axis and polar maps). The rest scan showed a small inferolateral defect, suggesting a small nontransmural infarcted area. The dipyridamole scan showed a large inferior and inferior lateral region of severely reduced coronary flow reserve, a fall in absolute activity below resting levels, indicating myocardial steal with collateralization of viable myocardium in the circumflex distribution. There was no clinically significant reduction of coronary flow reserve in the distribution of the LAD and right coronary arteries. Therefore, the patient underwent successful PTCA of his occluded left circumflex coronary artery based on the results of the PET scan with a relief of angina, thereby avoiding three-vessel bypass surgery.

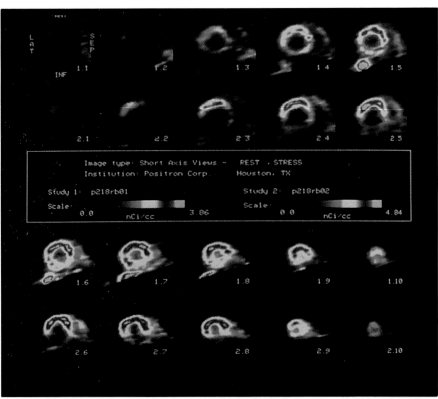

Fig. 20.8 Case 8 (20.8B, Reproduced with permission from reference 178).

A

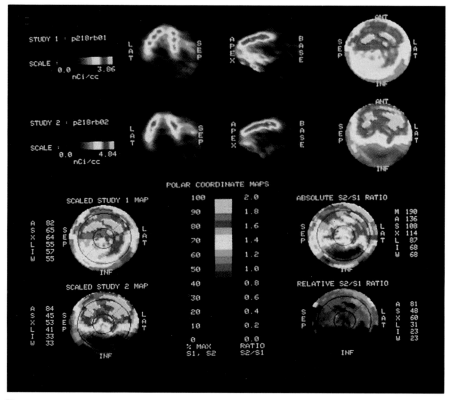

B

Case 9: Asymptomatic Man with Severe Coronary Artery Disease and Equivocal Exercise Tolerance Test

A 66-year-old man was asymptomatic with elevated cholesterol to 260 despite good adherence to a Pritikin diet for many years. He had a positive family history of heart disease and 2 years previously had an equivocal exercise tolerance test for which no further workup was recommended. The patient requested a PET scan which was carried out with N-13 ammonia at rest and after dipyridamole handgrip (Figure 20.9: A, acquisition view; B, short-axis; C, long-axis and polar maps). The resting image was normal. The dipyridamole image showed a severe mid-anterior and apical defect, a less severe septal defect, and a mild inferior defect. These findings suggested a moderate proximal LAD stenosis, a more severe mid-LAD narrowing, and a moderate right coronary artery narrowing. Coronary arteriography confirmed these findings with a 60% stenosis of the proximal LAD, subtotal occlusion of the mid-LAD, and a 75% narrowing of the proximal right coronary artery. Based on the severity and extent of disease, despite years of good dietary control, three-vessel PTCA was successfully carried out.

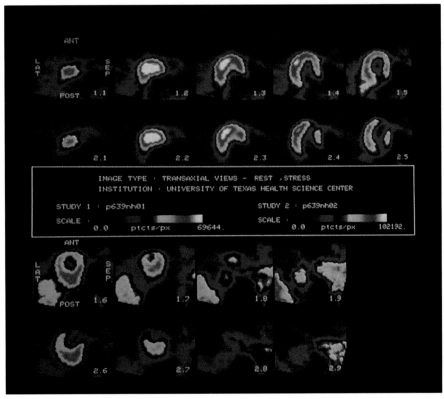

Fig. 20.9 Case 9.

A

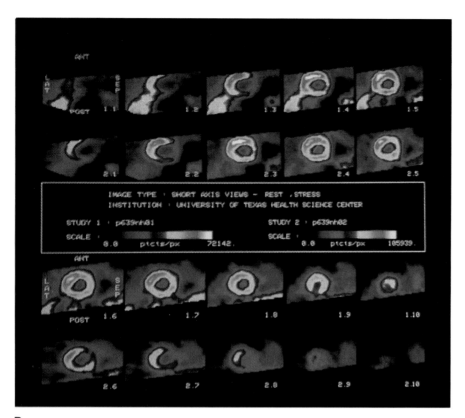

B

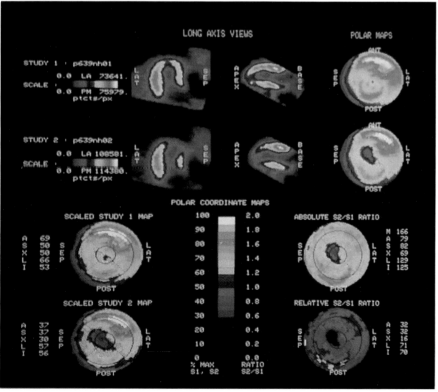

C

Case 10: Evaluation of Equivocal Chest Pain

A 77-year-old man presented with a history of an abdominal aortic aneurysm followed medically, and nonsurgical carotid artery disease without neurologic events or symptoms. One month prior to PET scan he had a brief episode of chest pain while walking briskly, associated with dryness in the back of his throat, but without recurrence. He had also noticed some increasing shortness of breath with exercise over the prior 3 weeks but without chest pain. He regularly walked 2 miles per day. He had a history of chronic hypertension for which he was treated with Vasotec and Cardizem with no history of myocardial infarction or cardiac events.

Rest–dipyridamole PET was carried out using N-13 ammonia (Figure 20.10: A, acquisition view; B, short-axis; C, long-axis and polar maps). The rest image showed a severe apical defect suggesting a resting apical scar. The dipyridamole image showed a moderately severe defect of the mid-anterior wall with enlargement of the severe apical defect; there were also large severe perfusion defects of the lateral, inferior, and inferior septal myocardium with a fall in activity below resting in the inferior lateral areas suggesting myocardial steal. After dipyridamole, the patient developed symptoms similar to that occurring 1 month prior to study and had inferior ST changes on ECG, both relieved with intravenous aminophylline.

These results were interpreted as showing an old apical myocardial infarction involving approximately 10% of the ventricle with large severe defects laterally and inferiorly, associated with myocardial steal indicating extensive collateralization usually seen with occluded arteries, probably the left circumflex, distal LAD, and posterior descending coronary arteries. Since the patient was relatively asymptomatic, he elected medical therapy with coronary vasodilators, cholesterol-lowering drugs, and diet.

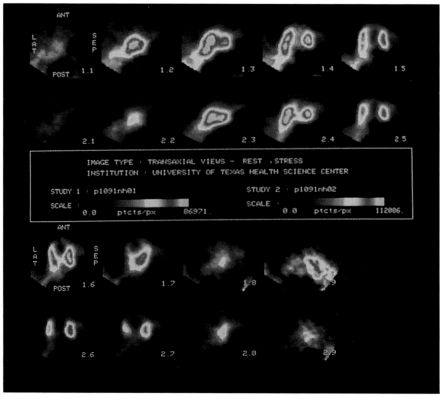

Fig. 20.10 Case 10.

A

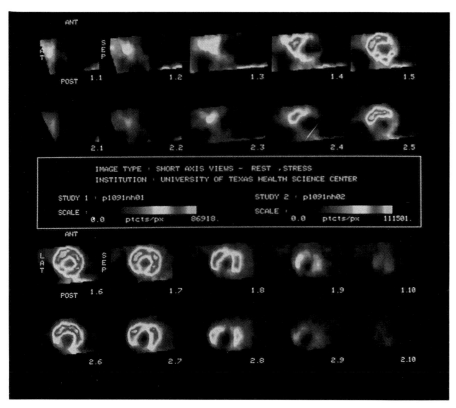

B

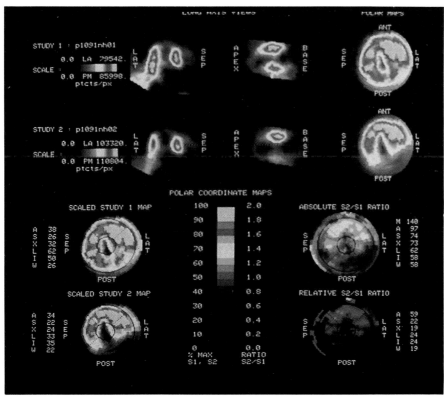

C

Case 11: Assessing Severity of Disease in a Man with Two Prior Myocardial Infarctions

A 66-year-old man presented with a history of two previous myocardial infarctions, the last occurring 1 year prior to his current PET study. He had a history of hypercholesterolemia, hypertension, and stable exertional angina. In order to evaluate extent of his disease, PET scans were obtained at rest and after dipyridamole handgrip using N-13 ammonia (Figure 20.11: A, acquisition view; B, short-axis; C, long-axis and polar maps). The resting PET scan showed a small, high posterior perfusion defect consistent with a nontransmural myocardial infarction. The stress image demonstrated a severe defect of the lateral and inferior myocardium with myocardial steal consistent with collateralization. There were mild anterior apical and inferior septal defects as well. These findings were interpreted as demonstrating three-vessel coronary artery disease with probable occlusion of an inferior coronary artery and substantial collaterals to the inferior area.

Coronary arteriography confirmed these findings, showing diffuse disease of the left circumflex with a 70% stenosis at the origin of an obtuse marginal. The right coronary artery was completely occluded with its bed supplied by collaterals from the diseased obtuse marginal. The LAD had diffuse plaquing without significant segmental narrowing and also supplied collaterals to the occluded right coronary bed. Since myocardium of the inferior wall was adequately collateralized, and the only artery with significant segmental narrowing was a marginal branch, the patient was treated with an aggressive cholesterol-lowering regimen rather than mechanical intervention.

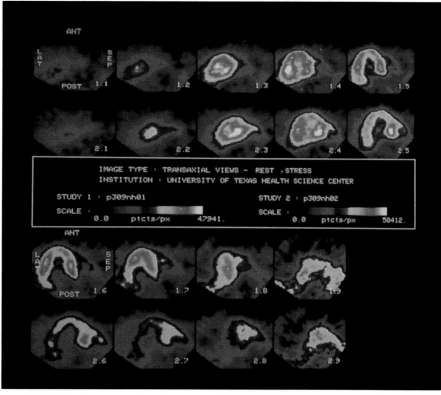

Fig. 20.11 Case 11.

A

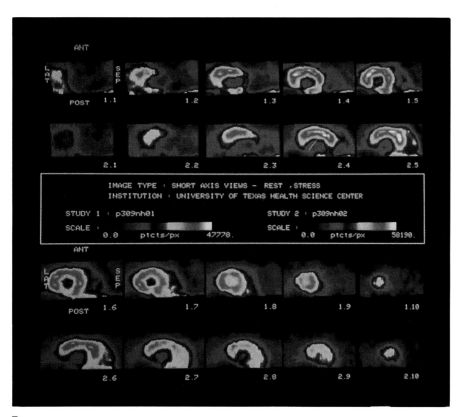

B

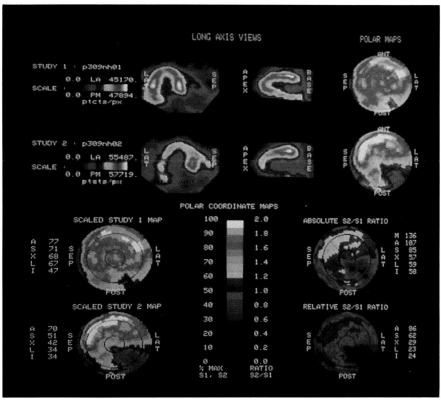

C

Case 12: Evaluating Severity of Symptomatic Coronary Artery Disease

A 68-year-old man with 3 years of stable exertional angina was referred for PET scan as part of a randomized study protocol of coronary artery disease reversal. Rest–dipyridamole PET was carried out using rubidium-82 (Figure 20.12: A, acquisition view; B, short-axis; C, long-axis and polar maps). The rest image demonstrated a moderate defect of medium size in the posterior septal and inferior myocardium. With dipyridamole, this defect became minimally larger and more intense, suggesting minimal viable myocardium in the border zones underperfused with stress. No other perfusion defects were present. Coronary arteriography demonstrated a dominant left circumflex with a severe narrowing at its junction and a posterior descending artery without other significant disease. Since the area supplied by this artery was fixed scar, and no other vessels were involved, medical therapy was maintained without mechanical intervention.

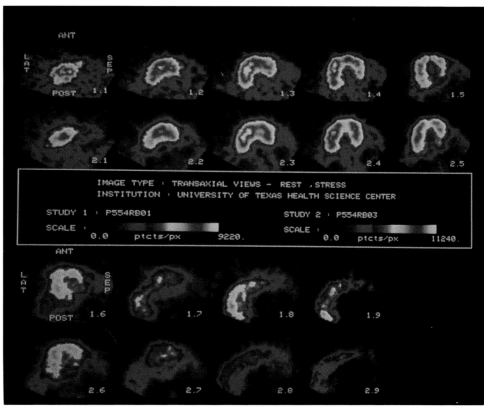

Fig. 20.12 Case 12.

A

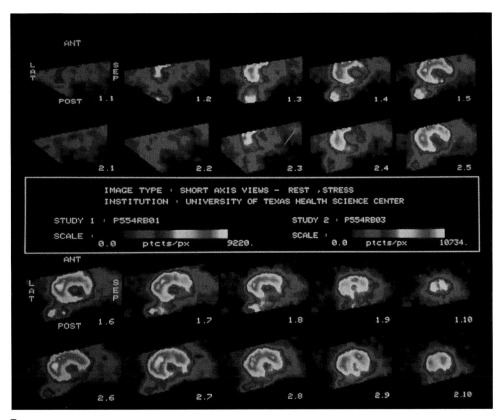

B

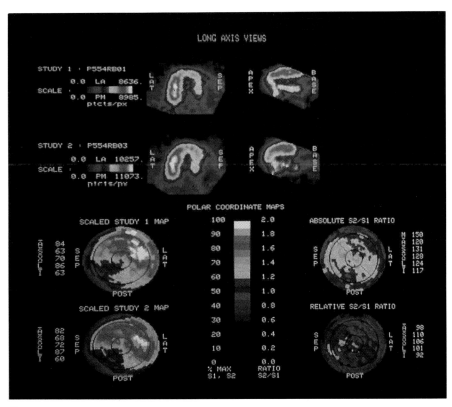

C

Case 13: Evaluating Severity of Stenoses in Progressive Angina Pectoris

A 52-year-old man presented with a history of myocardial infarction 4 years previously with residual exertional angina pectoris. Due to recent increasing angina, the patient had a thallium exercise treadmill test with mild left arm pain that did not require termination of exercise which was stopped due to fatigue. On what was considered a good effort, there were no ECG changes and the thallium perfusion images were normal (Figure 20.13E). The patient was referred for PET scan, carried out with N-13 ammonia and FDG at rest and with treadmill exercise after fasting (Figure 20.13: A, acquisition view; B, short-axis; C long-axis and polar map; D, magnified PET polar map to compare with thallium stress; E, thallium stress image (on left) and redistribution image (on right).

The rest perfusion PET image was normal. The exercise stress perfusion PET image showed a mild anterior, apical, and septal defect. The exercise stress FDG image did not demonstrate myocardial FDG uptake, thereby suggesting that metabolic ischemia was not present, since the perfusion defect was mild. Although the rest (S1) and dipyridamole images (S2) provide a correct diagnosis, the absolute S2/S1 and relative S2/S1 are good examples of scaling error and edge artifact caused by positioning the patient too far into the scanner thereby cutting off the proximal anterior base of the rest image. To confirm these findings as part of a study protocol, quantitative coronary arteriography was carried out that showed a proximal long tubular 46% diameter stenosis of the LAD coronary artery which wrapped around the apex to supply the inferior myocardium. In addition, there was a long proximal 47% diameter stenosis of the right coronary artery. Therefore, the patient was treated medically for probable spasm as a cause of his angina.

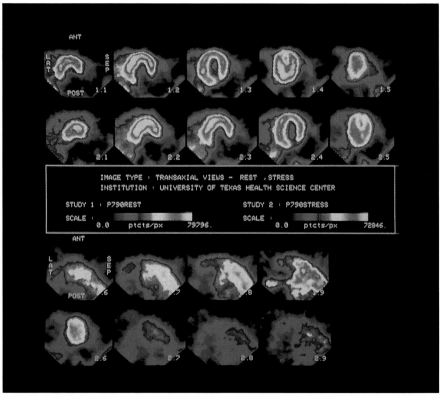

Fig. 20.13 Case 13.

A

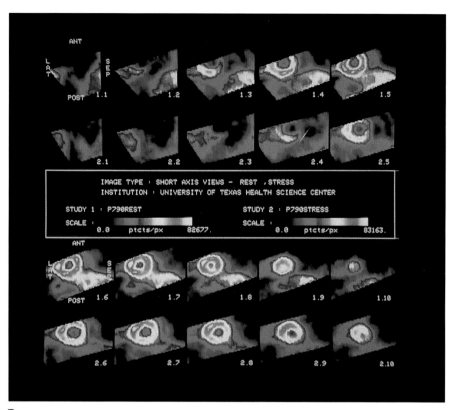

B

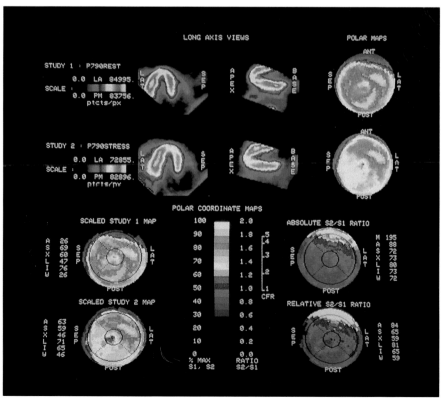

C

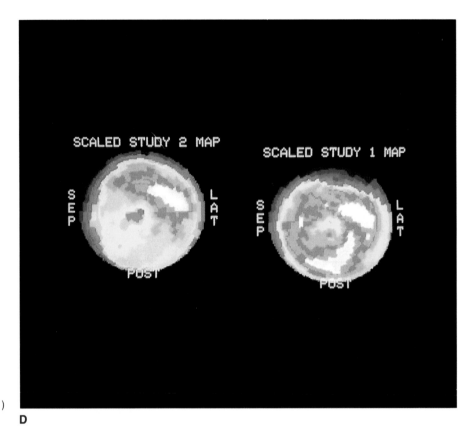

Fig. 20.13 Case 13 (*contd.*)

D

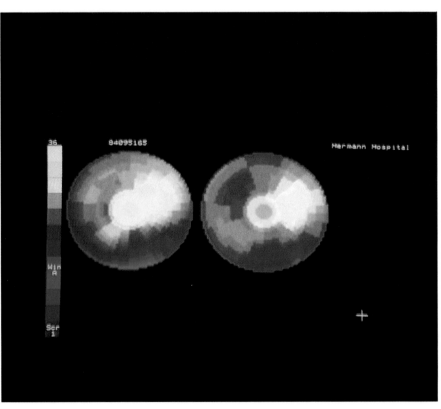

E

Case 14: Evaluating Severity of Stenoses in Known Silent Coronary Artery Disease

A 66-year-old man presented with a history of painless myocardial infarction 5 years previously with current symptoms of fatigue and dyspnea on exertion, worse with exercise stress. He was being treated with Cardizem and Tonocard for PVCs. He had four previous cardiac catheterizations, the last done 1 month prior to cardiac PET scan. The most recent coronary arteriogram demonstrated complete occlusion of the proximal LAD as noted previously, no segmental narrowing of the right coronary artery, and a complex stenosis of the proximal left circumflex, visually estimated to be 60% diameter narrowing by the referring cardiologist. Left ventricular angiography showed anterior basilar and posterior basilar contraction with an akinetic anterior myocardium and an estimated ejection fraction of 30%.

The patient was therefore referred for PET scanning to evaluate the significance of the left circumflex coronary artery. Rest–dipyridamole PET was carried out using N-13 ammonia (Figure 20.14: A, acquisition view; B, short-axis; C, long-axis and polar maps). The resting perfusion image showed a large severe defect of anterior, septal, and apical myocardium with lateral and inferior areas being normal. The dipyridamole image showed only minimal restriction of coronary flow reserve in the distribution of the left circumflex. Automated computer analysis of the previously obtained coronary arteriograms in the three views demonstrated stenoses of 42% to 47% diameter narrowing. Accordingly, bypass surgery or PTCA was not recommended. Due to symptoms of fatigue and dyspnea, Cardizem and Tonocard were discontinued and Procardia, Capoten, and digoxin started.

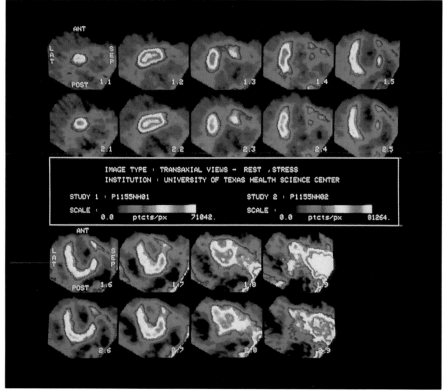

Fig. 20.14 Case 14.

A

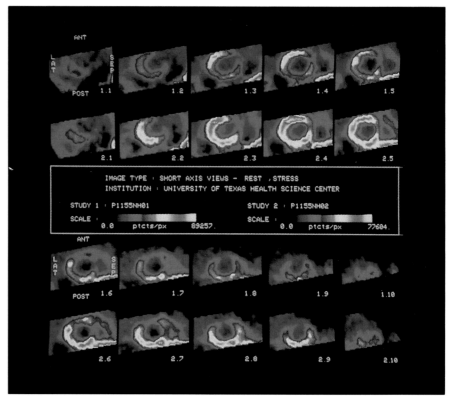

Fig. 20.14 Case 14 (*contd.*)

B

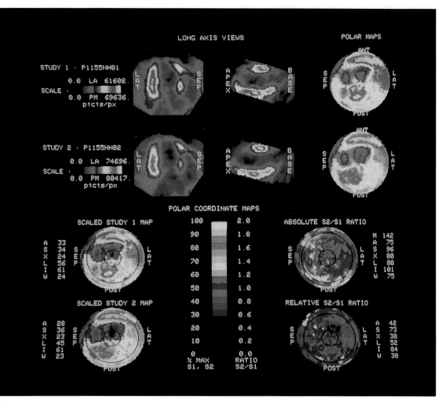

C

Case 15: Uniform Reduction of Coronary Flow Reserve in Hypertensive Heart Disease

A 35-year-old man presented with end-stage renal disease secondary to chronic severe hypertension of unknown etiology, undergoing evaluation for renal transplantation. He had no history of cardiovascular events or symptoms. Coronary arteriography and rest–dipyridamole PET scans with rubidium-82 were carried out as part of the renal transplant protocol. Rest–dipyridamole PET scans (Figure 20.15: A, acquisition view; B, short-axis; C, long-axis and polar maps) showed no regional perfusion defects. The absolute dipyridamole/rest ratio image showed uniform, homogenous depression of radionuclide uptake after dipyridamole. These results indicate a diffuse decrease in coronary flow reserve due to left ventricular hypertrophy and/or associated small vessel disease. Coronary arteriograms were normal. Left ventricular angiography showed global hypokinesis and a dilated left ventricle that was hypertrophied with marked left ventricular wall thickening.

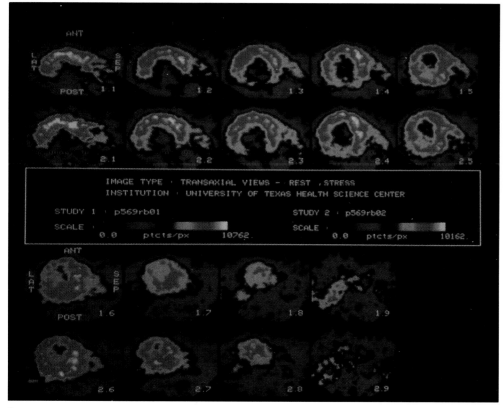

A

Fig. 20.15 Case 15 (20.15C, Reproduced with permission from reference 9).

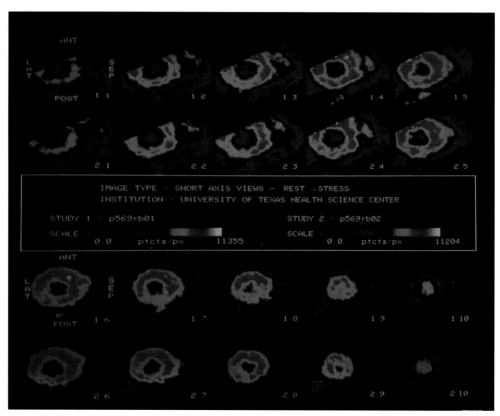

Fig. 20.15 Case 15 (*contd.*)

B

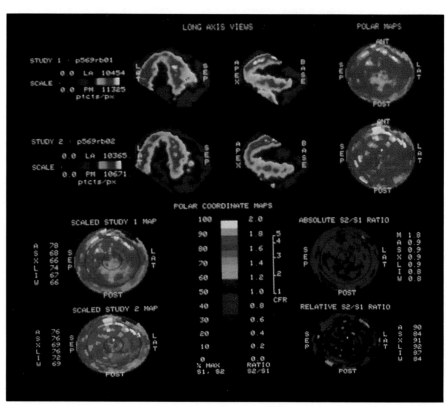

C

Case 16: Myocardial Viability in a Woman with Acute Myocardial Infarction

A 51-year-old woman with adult onset diabetes mellitus and hypertension was transferred from an outlying hospital with acute anterolateral myocardial infarction documented by loss of anterior R waves, ST elevation, T inversion, and creatine phosphokinase (CPK) increases to 677 mg/dL. During the first 2 days after acute myocardial infarction at that hospital, ECG showed evolving ST-T changes in standard leads II, III, aV_L, aV_F, and V_1 through V_5 without further enzyme rise.

Past medical history was remarkable for hypercholesterolemia, a strong family history of coronary artery disease, and heavy smoking. At admission, on day 3 after infarction, the patient was treated with intravenous nitroglycerin, heparin, and oral Lopressor. Serial CPKs showed no further increase and ECG remained stable. A gated blood pool scan showed an ejection fraction of 43% with anterior hypokinesis. Since the patient was transferred to University of Texas on the third day after her myocardial infarct, thrombolytic therapy was not instituted. The patient remained stable and on the ninth hospital day underwent submaximal thallium stress imaging, which showed a persistent apical and septal defect indicating myocardial necrosis.

In order to evaluate further the viability of her myocardium, serial, list mode, resting rubidium-82 images were obtained, as well as FDG scans after oral glucose loading. The early and late rubidium washout images are shown in Figure 20.16A. The early rubidium image (S1) showed moderate but reduced perfusion to the anteroapical wall indicating arterial patency but a high-grade stenosis of the mild-LAD. The late rubidium image (S2) demonstrated washout at the apex indicating necrotic myocardium. Mean activity in the apical and septal (distal) quadrants fall from S1 to S2 indicating washout. The distal anterior left ventricular wall retained rubidium indicating a substantial amount of viable myocardium remaining. Automated infarct size on the rubidium washout image (20.16AA) was 18% of the LV compared to 15% on the FDG image (20.16B, lower left polar map). As shown in Figure 20.16B, the late rubidium image (upper row, S1) matched the FDG image (lower row, S2), thereby confirming that approximately half of the distal anterior myocardium was viable with the remainder being necrotic, mostly at the apex. Figure 20.16C shows the 3D topographic maps of early (upper row, S1) and late (lower row, S2) rubidium images demonstrating apical washout and therefore necrosis; there was substantial anterior rubidium trapping by viable myocardium indicating viability.

Consequently, cardiac catheterization was carried out confirming a patent LAD with a high-grade stenosis in its midportion. In order to preserve the remaining viable myocardium, PTCA was successfully carried out at the time of diagnostic cath. After discharge, the patient did well with a follow-up scan at 3 months showing only a small apical scar, the anterior wall having normal flow and metabolism.

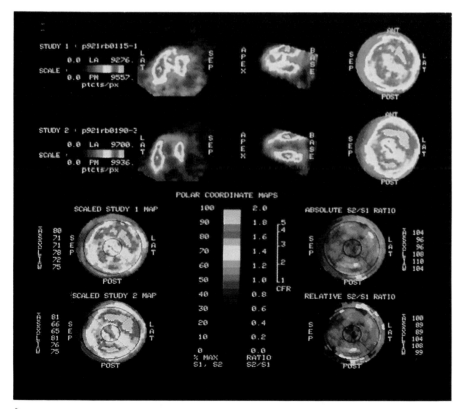
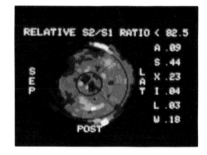

Fig. 20.16 Case 16. Reproduced with permission from reference 10.

A

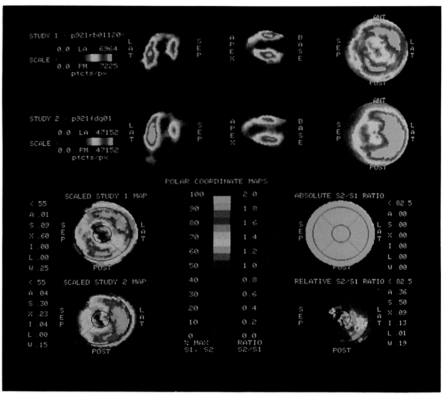

Fig. 20.16 Case 16 (*contd.*)

B

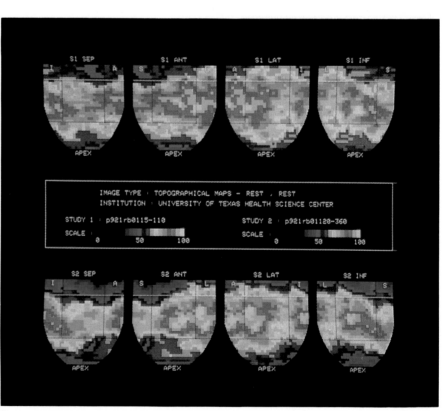

C

Case 17: Myocardial Necrosis/Viability in a Young Man with Recent Myocardial Infarction

A 38-year-old man had an inferior myocardial infarction 2 weeks previously associated with chest pain but symptom-free after the acute event. He was referred for evaluation of remaining viability and the question of whether other coronary arteries were involved.

PET scanning was carried out at rest and after dipyridamole with rubidium-82, and FDG imaging was obtained at rest after oral glucose loading. The early rest perfusion image (upper row, S1) showed a mild small defect that washed out on the late rubidium image (lower row, S2), revealing a moderately severe inferior posterior defect consistent with predominantly necrosis and only modest remaining viable muscle (Figure 15.14A). The late rubidium image (upper row, S1, Figure 15.14B) matched the FDG scan after glucose loading (lower row, S2) in showing a severe inferior defect and therefore necrosis. The dipyridamole scan showed a severe inferior defect in the area of infarct but no other restriction in coronary flow reserve (Figure 20.17: A, acquisition view; B, short-axis; C, long-axis and polar maps). These results were interpreted as showing predominantly necrosis in the inferior myocardium with no other arteries significantly involved. Therefore, medical therapy was recommended with these findings confirmed by coronary arteriography according to a necrosis/viability protocol.

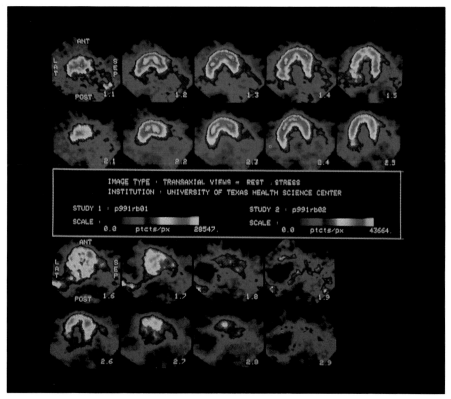

Fig. 20.17 Case 17.

A

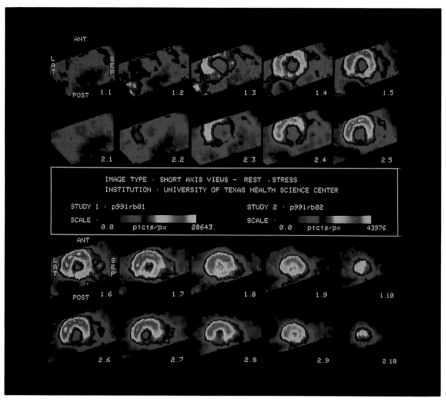

Fig. 20.17 Case 17 (*contd.*)

B

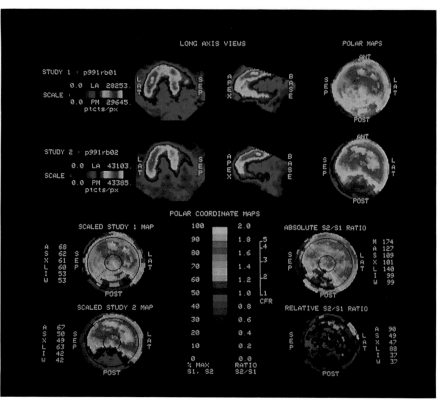

C

Case 18: Myocardial Viability after Thrombolysis for Acute Myocardial Infarction

A 74-year-old man with an anterior myocardial infarction 1 month prior to PET scanning. At the time he received intravenous streptokinase within 3 to 4 hours of onset of chest pain. Since the acute event, he had mild substernal chest discomfort on occasion but denied "real" chest pain. The ECG showed anterior septal Q waves with elevated ST segments and deep T inversion. He was referred for PET scanning in order to evaluate myocardial viability and the status of his other coronary arteries.

Rest–dipyridamole PET scans were carried out using rubidium-82 with rest perfusion images obtained in list mode. Resting FDG images were obtained after glucose loading. The rest perfusion images showed a severe resting defect of the anterior wall and apex, suggesting anterior and apical myocardial infarction. The stress perfusion image demonstrated an increase in severity and size of the anterior defect that extended into the septum with enlargement and severity of the apical defect as well (Figure 20.18: A, acquisition view; B,

short-axis; C, long-axis and polar maps). No other areas of myocardium had reduced flow reserve. Early–late rubidium-82 images showed a severe central defect that washed out at the borders (Figure 20.18D). The late rubidium-82 scan (Figure 20.18E, upper row, S1) matched the resting FDG image (Figure 20.18E, lower row, S2) showing defects of the middle to distal anterior myocardium and apex consistent with myocardial infarction.

Quantitative analysis showed that approximately 10% of the heart was infarcted with an additional stress defect or area at risk of 23% of the myocardium.

Based on these PET findings indicating completed central infarcted myocardium but a reasonably large surrounding zone at additional risk, diagnostic coronary arteriography and balloon angioplasty were carried out at a single cardiac catheterization. There was subtotal stenosis of the proximal LAD coronary artery that was successfully dilated, and a 30% diameter stenosis of a dominant left circumflex coronary artery that was not instrumented.

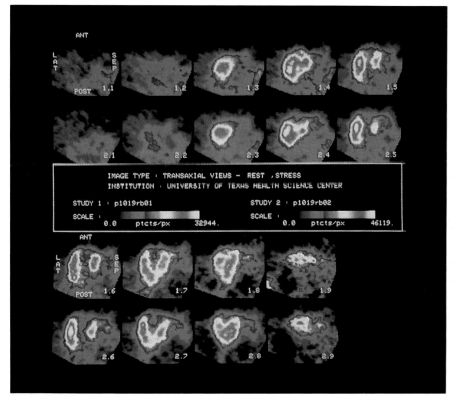

Fig. 20.18 Case 18.

A

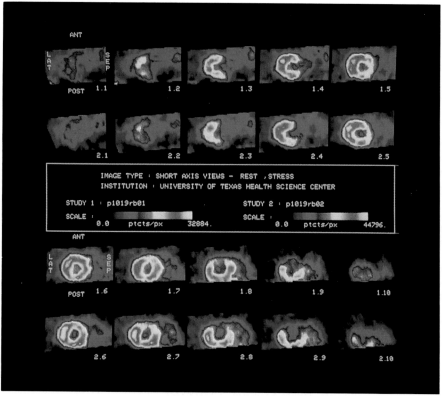

Fig. 20.18 Case 18 (*contd.*)

B

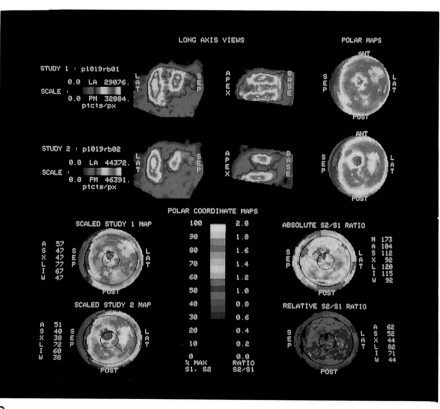

C

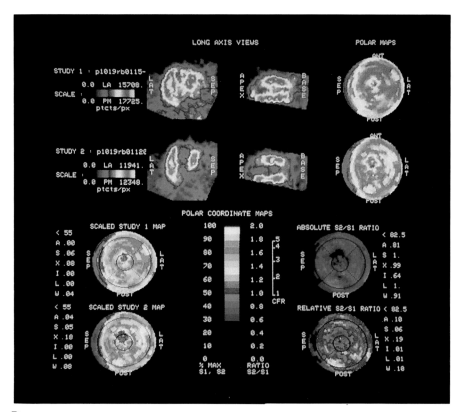

D

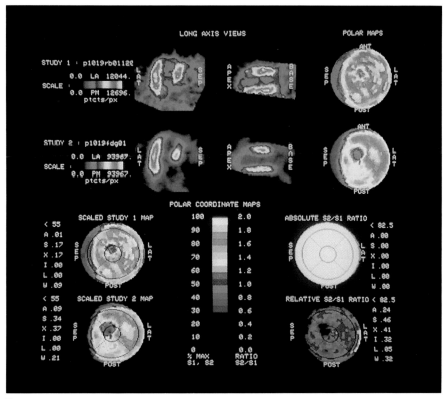

E

Case 19: Myocardial Viability of an Old Myocardial Infarction Due to Lupus Vasculitis

A 36-year-old man had severe lupus erythematosus associated with vasculitis since age 12. One year prior to PET scan he had an inferior acute myocardial infarction with a subsequent ejection fraction of 33% and right ventricular dilation. Coronary arteriography demonstrated total occlusion of the right coronary artery with diffuse disease of the LAD. Left ventricular angiogram showed an akinetic inferior wall.

The patient was referred for PET scanning to evaluate viability of the inferior wall and significance of the diffuse disease of the LAD. Rest–dipyridamole PET was carried out using rubidium-82, and resting FDG images were obtained after oral glucose loading. The rest perfusion image demonstrated a severe large defect of the inferior septal and inferior myocardium that did not change with dipyridamole, suggesting fixed scar (Figure 20.19: A, short-axis view; B, long-axis and polar maps). Early–late rubidium-82 images showed an initial severe defect that washed out to be even more severe (Figure 20.19C). The late rubidium-82 image (Figure 20.19D, upper row, S1) matched the FDG image having an identical defect (Figure 20.19D, lower row, S2) confirming a fixed scar. There was no reduction of coronary flow reserve in the distribution of the LAD. Consequently, the patient was continued on medical therapy without mechanical intervention.

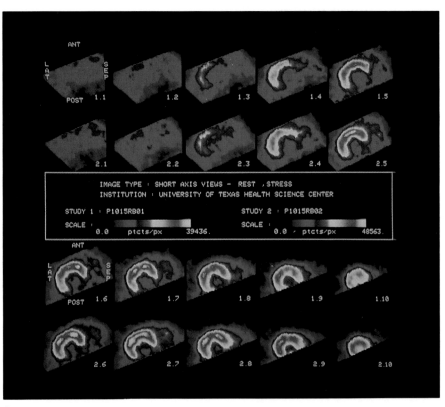

Fig. 20.19 Case 19.

A

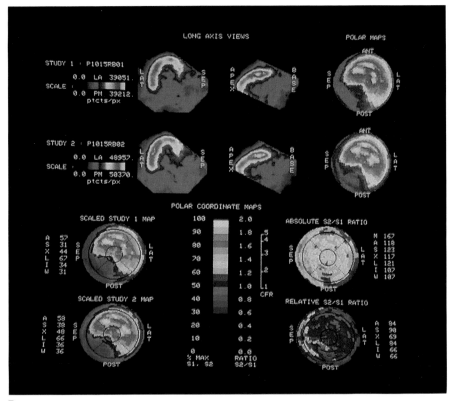

B

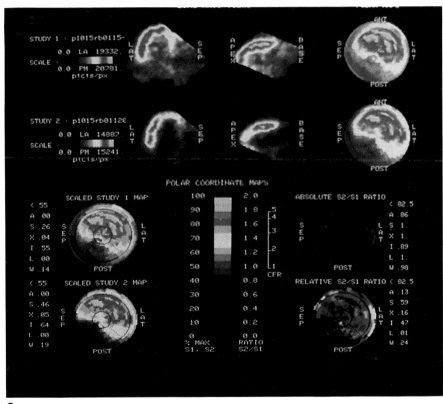

C

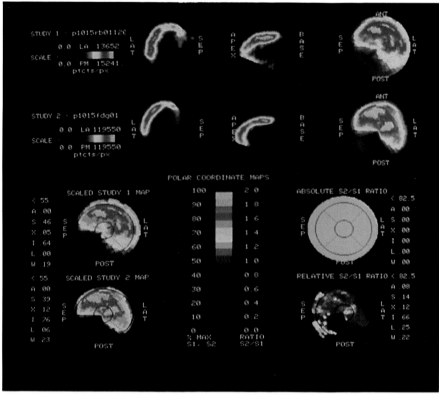

Fig. 20.19 Case 19 (*contd.*)

D

Case 20: Myocardial Viability in Remote Myocardial Infarction

A 63-year-old man presented with a history of myocardial infarction 4 months previously. Coronary arteriography demonstrated a severe proximal stenoses of the LAD, proximal left circumflex, and diffuse disease of the right coronary artery. The patient had a history of hypertension, hypercholesterolemia, and a positive family history of coronary artery disease. Resting ECG showed Q waves in the anterior precordial leads with persisting ST elevation and T inversion. The patient was referred for PET scanning in order to evaluate myocardial viability.

Resting list-mode PET was carried out with rubidium-82 and FDG imaging after glucose loading. The rubidium study showed a moderately severe defect on the early phase image of the anterior wall and apex with some washout of radiotracer (Figure 20.20: A, acquisition view; B, short-axis). The anterior septum also demonstrated some washout. Inferior and inferior lateral myocardium had normal perfusion on the early image but also demonstrated some washout. However, in all of these areas there was significant residual trapping of rubidium that indicated considerable remaining viable myocardium. These findings were interpreted as showing moderate nontransmural myocardial necrosis or scar of anterior, inferior, and inferior lateral regions. The late rubidium-82 image (upper row, S1) matched the FDG image (lower row, S2; Figure 20.20: C, acquisition view; D, short-axis view). The cumulative infarct size by PET was approximately 20% with an ejection fraction of 45% and global hypokinesis. Since there appeared to be remaining viable myocardium with some retention of rubidium trapping, and impaired ventricular function, coronary arteriography was carried out which showed subtotal occlusion of the proximal LAD, subtotal occlusion of a proximal obtuse marginal, and an 80% stenosis of the left circumflex artery, corresponding to regions of PET abnormalities. Coronary bypass surgery was recommended but the patient elected to defer.

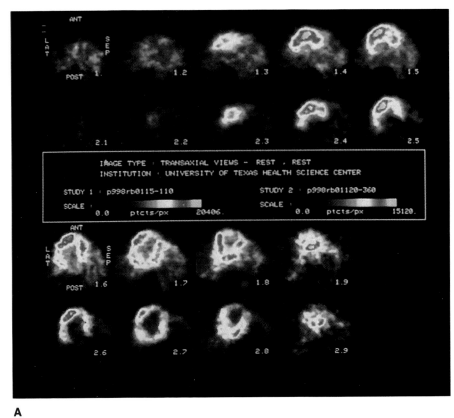

Fig. 20.20 Case 20.

A

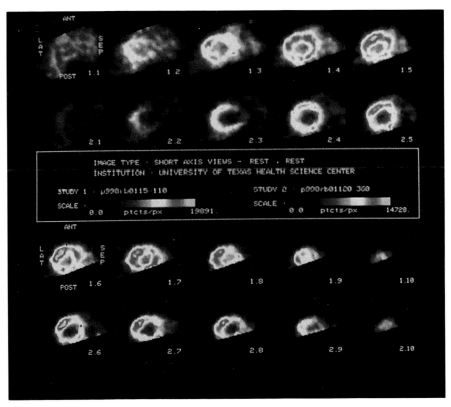

B

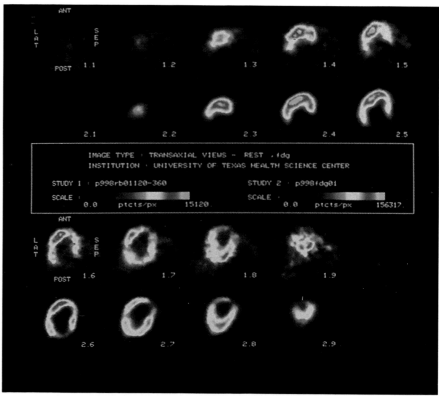

Fig. 20.20 Case 20 (*contd.*)

C

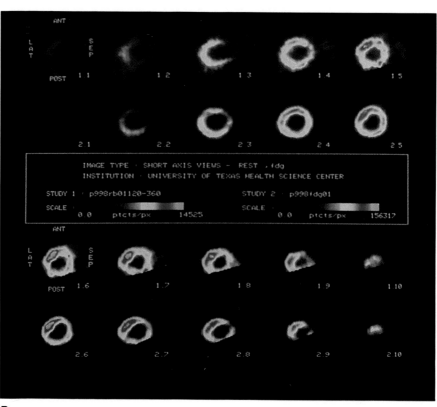

D

Case 21: Myocardial Viability in a Young Man with Myocardial Infarction and a Patent, Stenotic Infarct-Related Artery

A 28-year-old man had an acute inferior myocardial infarction 4 weeks previously and had received TPA 3 hours after the onset of pain. Coronary arteriography demonstrated a severe proximal stenosis of a large dominant left circumflex. Thallium exercise testing showed a large, fixed inferior lateral defect. Left ventricular angiogram showed inferior hypokinesis with an ejection fraction of 50%. The patient had an elevated cholesterol to 310 and a strong family history of heart disease with an uncle dying of myocardial infarction at age 31. In order to evaluate myocardial viability, rest PET scans were obtained using N-13 ammonia (upper row, S1) and FDG after oral glucose loading (lower row, S2; Figure 20.21: A, acquisition view; B, short-axis; C, long-axis and polar maps). The rest perfusion image demonstrated a severe inferior, inferior septal, and nontransmural, inferior lateral defect. The rest FDG image demonstrated a correspondingly severe defect of inferior and inferior septal areas but the inferior lateral myocardium in the distribution of the left circumflex artery was metabolically active, taking up FDG. Approximately 11% of the left ventricle was infarcted, and approximately 20% of the left ventricle was underperfused with viable myocardium indicated by FDG uptake. Quantitative arteriographic analysis demonstrated a 75% diameter stenosis of a large dominant circumflex. Accordingly, PTCA was carried out and the patient was put on a vigorous cholesterol-lowering regimen.

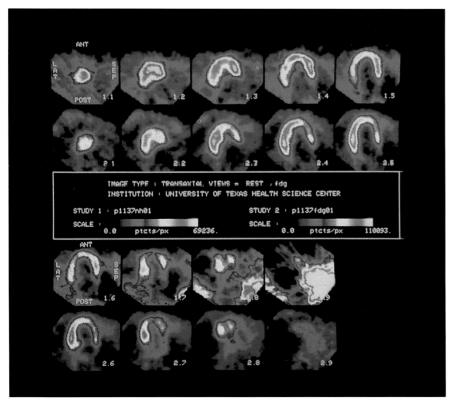

Fig. 20.21 Case 21.

A

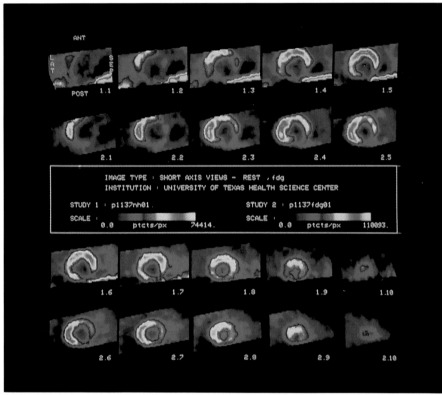

Fig. 20.21 Case 21 (*contd.*)

B

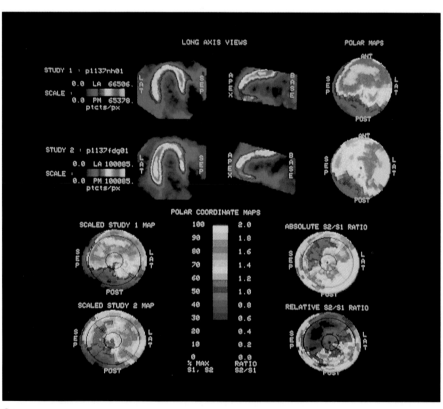

C

Case 22: Myocardial Viability in a Woman with an Acute Myocardial Infarction

A 58-year-old woman was admitted for chest pain 1 week prior to PET scanning, with Q waves in her anterior precordial leads, ST elevation, and T inversions suggesting acute myocardial infarction, confirmed by enzyme rise. Resting PET scans were obtained using rubidium-82 and FDG after oral glucose loading. The early rest perfusion image (upper row, S1) showed a severe defect that washed out to become a more severe large defect of the anterior myocardium and apex (lower row, S2) (Figure 20.22A). These images were interpreted as showing necrosis of the distal anterior wall and apex but with considerable viable myocardium in the proximal septum and anterior wall. The late rubidium-82 image (upper row, S1, Figure 20.22B) matched the FDG image (lower row, S2), which confirmed these findings. Coronary arteriography showed subtotal occlusion of the proximal LAD with collaterals from the right coronary filling the distal LAD bed. Left ventriculography demonstrated anterior and anterior lateral hypokinesis with apical dyskinesis and an ejection fraction of 35%. Due to the presence of substantial proximal myocardium that was viable but at risk, bypass surgery was carried out to the LAD coronary artery.

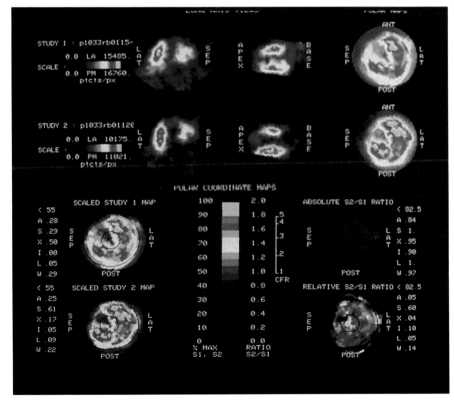

Fig. 20.22 Case 22.

A

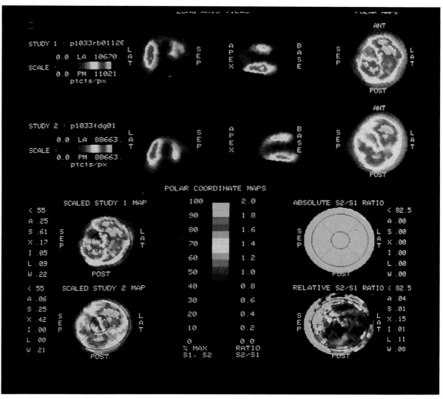

Fig. 20.22 Case 22 (*contd.*)

B

Case 23: Myocardial Viability in Severe Silent Coronary Artery Disease

A 72-year-old man presented with no previous chest pain, history of myocardial infarction, or events that might be interpreted as myocardial infarction. He had been a diabetic on insulin for 15 years. He recently developed congestive heart failure with fatigue and dyspnea on exertion for which he was treated with diuretics, digoxin, and nitrates. He also had a history of hypertension, and his father had a myocardial infarction in his fourth decade. He had a thallium exercise test interpreted as showing extensive fixed scar. Coronary arteriography demonstrated approximately 60% stenoses of the proximal LAD, 60% stenoses of the proximal left circumflex, and a small nondominant normal right coronary artery. His left ventricular angiogram showed severe regional contractile abnormalities with apical akinesis, global hypokinesis, and an ejection fraction of 40%. He obtained opinions from two different cardiologists who advised him that his heart was too damaged for bypass surgery and recommended medical therapy or cardiac transplantation. Therefore, he requested a PET scan and third opinion.

Myocardial perfusion imaging was carried out at rest and after dipyridamole using N-13 ammonia (Figure 20.23: A, acquisition view; B, short-axis; C, long-axis and polar maps). Resting FDG imaging was carried out after oral glucose load-ing. The resting perfusion images (upper row, S1, Figure 20.23A–E) showed a large defect in the inferior myocardium compared to a minimal defect on the FDG study (lower row, S2, Figure 20.23D,E) indicating underperfused viable myocardium. The stress perfusion image demonstrated severe large defects throughout the entire heart indicating severe three-vessel disease that restricted coronary flow reserve to extensive areas of viable myocardium (Figure 20.23A–C, lower row, S2). The patient had no chest pain during dipyridamole but had 5 mm of ST change on ECG, resolving with intravenous aminophylline and three nitroglycerine tablets over the next 10 minutes.

These results indicated a small nontransmural inferolateral myocardial infarction with severe restriction of coronary flow reserve to the entire remainder of the heart that was all viable and underperfused with stress. A magnified polar map (Figure 20.23E) and short-axis views (Figure 15.4) highlight the large inferior perfusion defect, a relatively mild FDG defect, and viable myocardium throughout most of the heart. Accordingly, due to extent of severe perfusion defects in large areas of viable myocardium, bypass surgery was recommended for silent ischemic cardiomyopathy. The patient then obtained an opinion from a fourth cardiologist who, after reviewing the arteriograms and PET scans, also recommended bypass surgery which was successfully carried out.

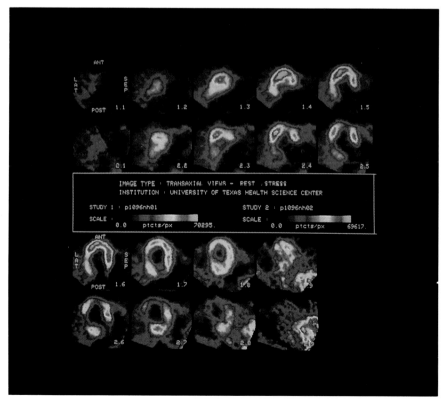

Fig. 20.23 Case 23.

A

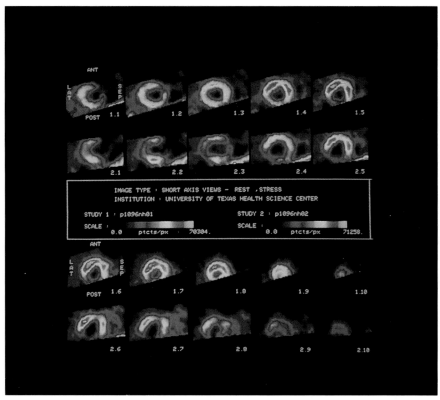

Fig. 20.23 Case 23 (*contd.*)

B

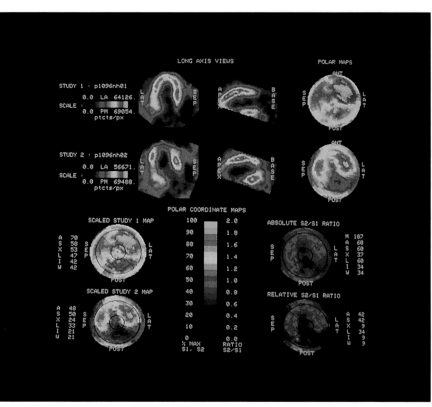

C

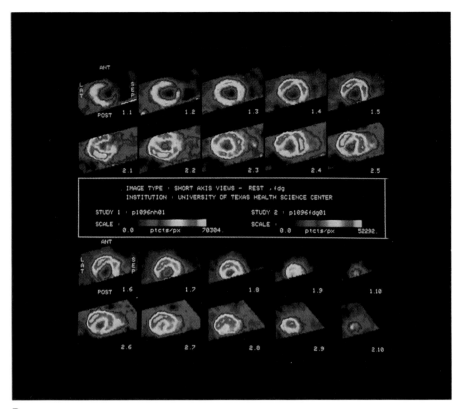

D

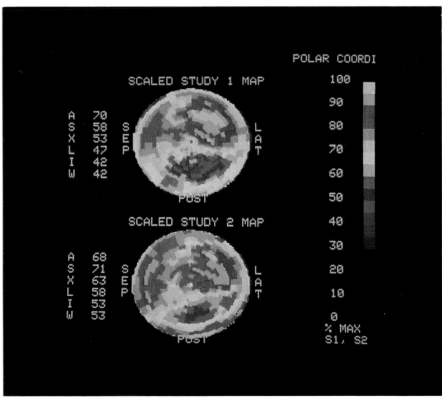

E

Case 24

A 61-year-old man had a previous inferior myocardial infarction, sudden death with successful resuscitation, and recurrent inducable ventricular tachycardia controlled on Mexitil, Procardia, Inderal, and aspirin. He never had chest pain or other symptoms and had no physical limitations. Coronary arteriography showed an occluded right coronary artery filling distally through collaterals, an occluded diagonal, a 50% diameter stenosis of the obtuse marginal, a 50% diameter stenosis of the proximal LAD, and no segmental narrowing of the left circumflex coronary arteries. Rest exercise perfusion studies were carried out using N-13 ammonia. Both scans showed a fixed inferior defect without perfusion abnormalities anterior or laterally (not shown).

Since the patient had never had angina pectoris as an endpoint for following his disease, a routine follow-up PET scan was obtained 6 months later without change in his clinical status. The repeat study was a rest–exercise perfusion and metabolic study using N-13 ammonia and FDG under fasting conditions. The rest scan was unchanged from the previous study showing inferior scar. Comparison of the first exercise scan (upper row, S1) to the follow-up exercise scan (lower row, S2) showed a new moderate mid-anterior wall perfusion defect and a severe lateral perfusion defect not previously present (Figure 12.10A). The exercise FDG scan showed intense uptake laterally corresponding to the more severe perfusion defect indicating metabolic ischemia (Figure 12.10B). There was no FDG uptake associated with the more moderate mid-anterior defect, indicating a restriction in coronary flow reserve not associated with metabolic ischemia. The routine follow-up PET scans therefore demonstrated moderate progression of the mid-LAD lesion and appearance of a new, severe left circumflex stenosis not present previously.

Repeat coronary arteriography confirmed progression of the mid-LAD stenosis from 50% to 70%. The left circumflex which previously had not demonstrated significant localized narrowing had developed a 90% stenosis in its proximal portion. Consequently, as a result of these findings, the patient was sent to bypass surgery, since symptoms were an inadequate guide to progression of his disease.

The corresponding 3D topographic maps are shown in Figure 20.24A comparing the first exercise perfusion study (upper row, S1) to the second exercise perfusion study (lower row, S2). There is marked worsening of the stress defects on the lateral view and mild worsening on the anterior view. Figure 20.24B compares the 3D follow-up exercise perfusion study (upper row, S1) to the exercise FDG study (lower row, S2), showing intense FDG uptake in the lateral wall corresponding to the stress perfusion defect.

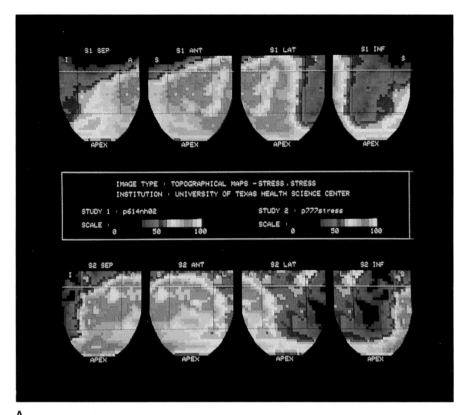

A

Fig. 20.24 Case 24 (Reproduced with permission from reference 10).

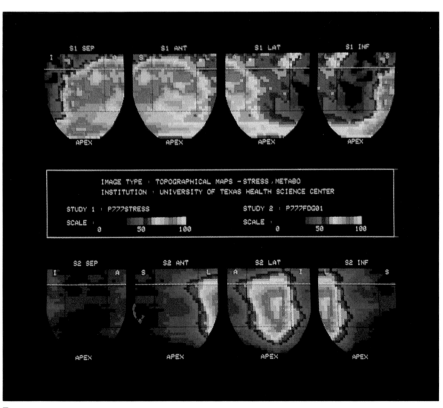

B

Case 25: Progression/Regression of Coronary Artery Stenosis During a Coronary Artery Disease Regression Protocol

A 49-year-old man with no symptoms had an abnormal exercise tolerance test and thallium perfusion defects without exertional angina pectoris. He had no history of a clinical event or myocardial infarction. Coronary arteriography showed extensive three-vessel disease with a subtotal occlusion of the mid-LAD, a 65% diameter stenosis of the left circumflex, and an occluded right coronary artery. There was extensive collateralization from the left circumflex and from multiple small proximal arteries to the distal beds of the LAD and right coronary arteries. Left ventricular angiogram showed distal anterior apical akinesis and inferior hypokinesis with ejection fraction of 49%.

Rest–dipyridamole PET scans were carried out with rubidium-82 (Figure 20.25: A, acquisition view; b, short-axis; C, long-axis and polar maps). The rest image was abnormal with defects in the anterior, apical, posterior lateral, posterior, and inferior myocardium. The dipyridamole image showed a large severe inferior and apical defect and moderately severe defects of septal, anterior, and lateral myocardium. A fall in inferior activity during dipyridamole suggested myocardial steal reflecting collateralization to viable inferior myocardium.

Comparisons of the initial dipyridamole scan (upper row, S1) to that after 2 years of a reversal protocol (lower row, S2) demonstrated marked improvement of the inferior perfusion defect (Figure 20.25: D, acquisition views; E, long-axis and polar maps), corresponding to regression of the left circumflex coronary artery stenosis on serial arteriograms. The anterior perfusion defect remained unchanged corresponding to an anterior apical scar and persisting subtotal occlusion of the mid-LAD coronary artery. The corresponding 3D topographic maps for the initial rest (upper row, S1) and dipyridamole (lower row, S2) study are shown in Figure 20.25F. The initial dipyridamole (upper row, S1) compared to the follow-up dipyridamole (lower row, S2) is shown in Figure 20.25G; the improved perfusion on the inferior posterior view (lower row, fourth image) is apparent.

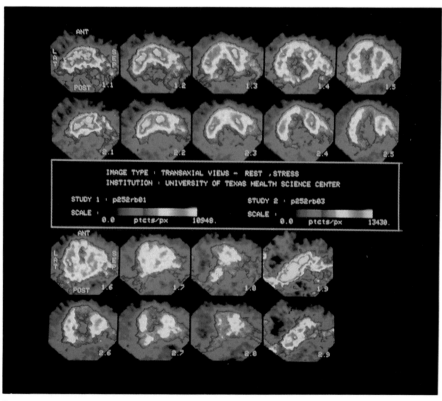

Fig. 20.25 Case 25.

A

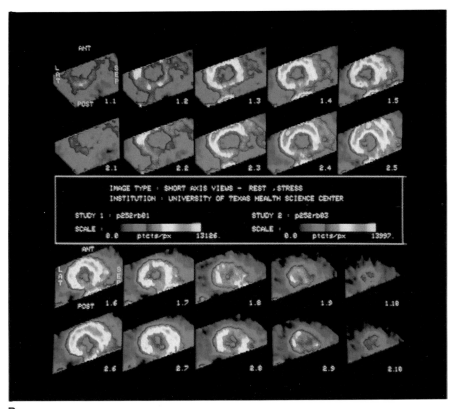

B

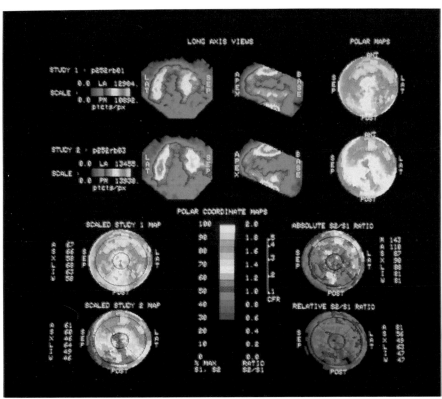

C

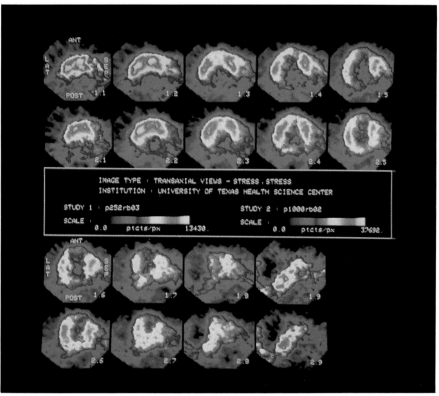

Fig. 20.25 Case 25 (*contd.*)

D

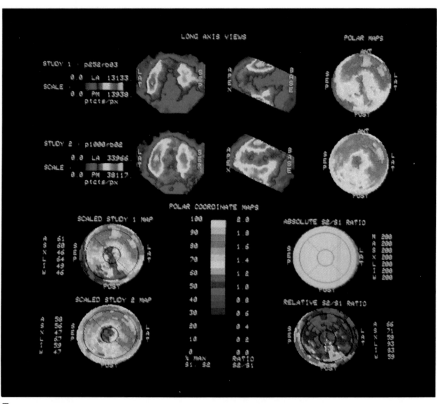

E

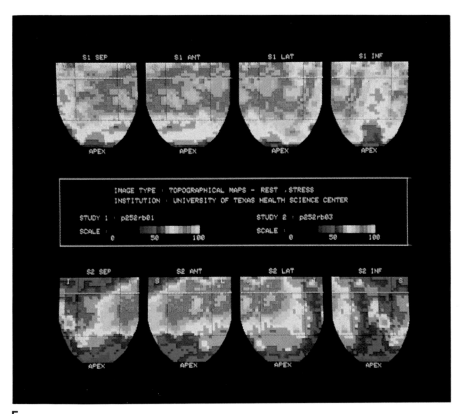

F

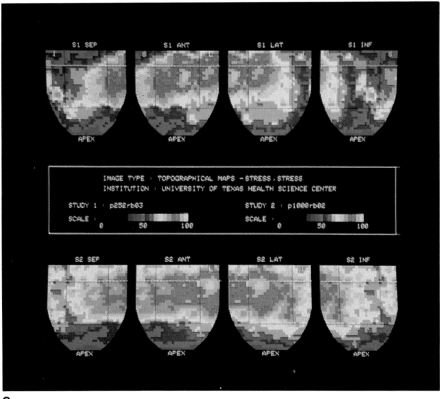

G

Case 26: Progression of Coronary Artery Disease of a Patient on a Randomized Control Treatment Protocol

A 58-year-old man had coronary arteriography 1 year previously for increasing angina pectoris due to known coronary artery disease over the previous 10 years. Arteriogram at that time showed proximal occlusions of the left circumflex and distal right coronary arteries with extensive collateralization of the posterior and lateral walls. There were two serial stenoses of the LAD and comparable mild stenosis of the first large diagonal and ramus intermedius arteries. Left ventricular size and global function were normal with mild hypokinesis of the posterior basal left ventricle.

As part of a protocol, resting and dipyridamole PET scans were obtained using N-13 ammonia. On the initial study, the rest image showed a mild small inferior posterior-basal defect, which became mildly worse and somewhat larger on dipyridamole, extending to the lateral wall. Eighteen months later, repeat rest–dipyridamole PET scans showed progression in severity of the perfusion defects. Comparison of initial (upper row, S1) and follow-up (lower row, S2) dipyridamole scans showed worsening severity over a larger area of the inferior myocardium with the appearance of mild perfusion

defects of the apex and septum not present previously (Figure 20.26: A, short-axis view; B, long-axis and polar maps). These results were interpreted as showing progression of LAD disease and associated further impairment of collateral flow to the inferior myocardium during dipyridamole. Quantitative coronary arteriography confirmed progression of diffuse disease of the proximal two thirds of the right coronary artery with 57% diameter stenosis at the narrowest part. Stenoses of the diagonal and ramus arteries also progressed while the LAD stenoses regressed. Corresponding 3D topographic maps are shown in Figure 20.26C comparing the initial dipyridamole (upper row, S1) with the follow-up dipyridamole study (lower row, S2). There is progression of impaired flow reserve on septal, anterior, lateral, and inferior views.

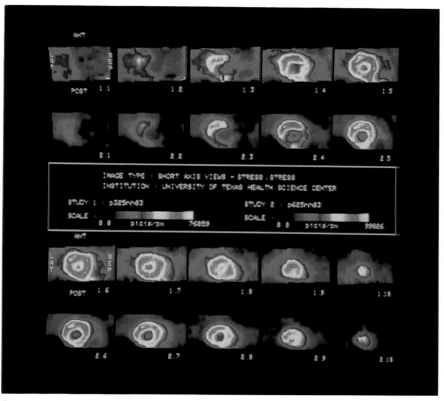

Fig. 20.26 Case 26.

A

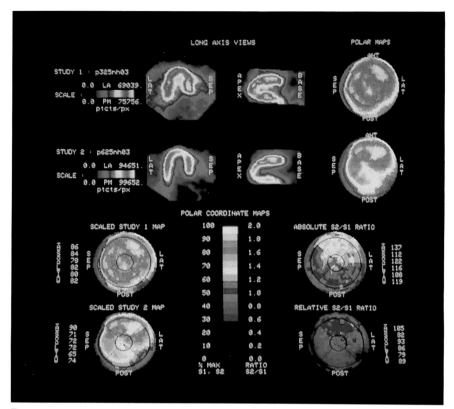

B

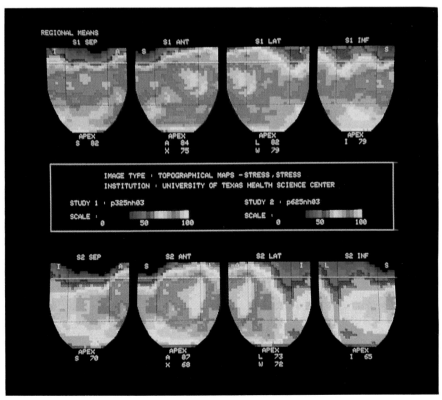

C

Case 27: Regression of Coronary Artery Disease on a Reversal Protocol

A 66-year-old man presented with stable exertional angina pectoris entering a coronary artery disease reversal protocol. Quantitative coronary arteriography showed an occluded right coronary artery, a 51% stenosis of the LAD, a 49% stenosis of the first diagonal. Initial rest–dipyridamole PET scans were carried out using N-13 ammonia. The rest scan showed a moderately severe defect of the inferior myocardium which became much larger and more severe on the dipyridamole image and extended to the apex (Figure 20.27: A, acquisition views; B, short-axis; C, long-axis and polar maps). In addition, there were less severe defects of the anterior and lateral myocardium. These findings coincided with stenosis on the arteriogram.

After 1 year on a vigorous reversal protocol, comparison of the initial (upper row, S1) and follow-up (lower row, S2) dipyridamole scans showed that anterior septal and lateral defects were less severe and the inferior defect had improved markedly (Figure 20.27D). These findings corresponded to regression of corresponding stenoses by arteriography and opening of the occluded right coronary artery on the second arteriogram. The corresponding 3D topographic maps are shown in Figure 20.27E comparing the initial (upper row, S1) to the follow-up (lower row, S2) dipyridamole scans. The inferior posterior view shows particularly well the improved perfusion due to opening of the right coronary artery.

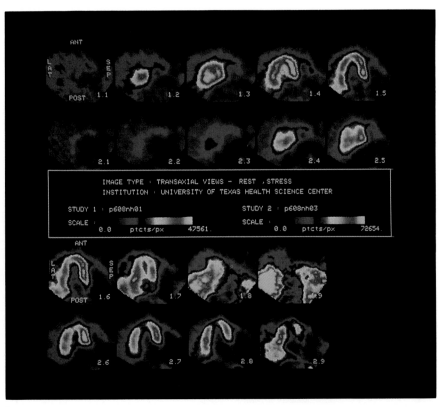

Fig. 20.27 Case 27.

A

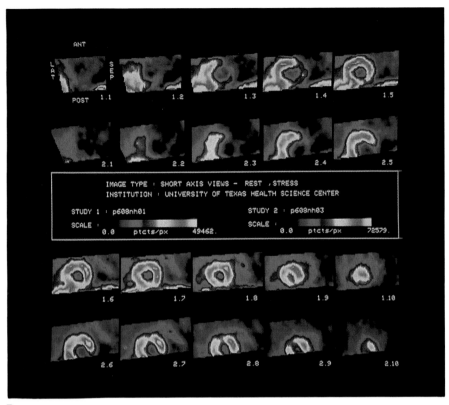

B

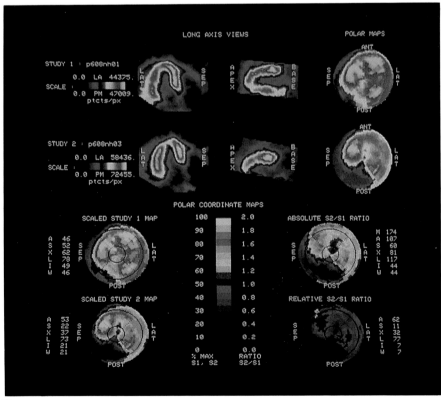

C

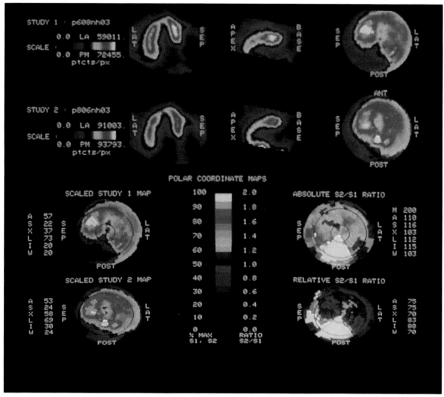

Fig. 20.27 Case 27 (*contd.*)

D

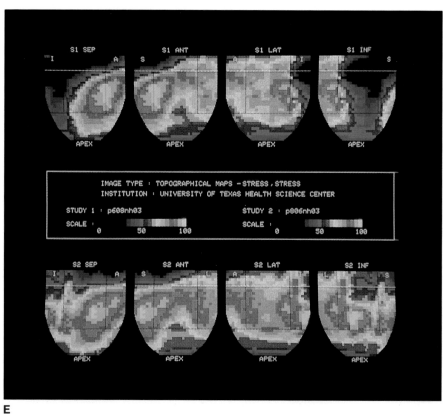

E

Case 28: Progression of Coronary Artery Disease to Painless Ischemia Requiring Bypass Surgery

A 65-year-old man presented without significant previous medical history, had good exercise tolerance, adhered to a good diet, and actively worked out until he had an early morning anterior myocardial infarction 1 year prior to his first PET scan. It was confirmed by ECG and enzyme rises but with minimal chest pain. He had coronary arteriography and PTCA of the LAD and obtuse marginal coronary arteries. Subsequent thallium exercise testing was interpreted as normal until 1 year later when repeat thallium exercise testing showed painless ST depression.

Repeat coronary arteriography demonstrated a tight restenosis of the obtuse marginal and mild narrowing of the right coronary and LAD. Rest and treadmill exercise PET images were obtained using N-13 ammonia and FDG under fasting conditions. The resting perfusion image showed a small apical defect (upper row, S1) and the stress image (lower row, S2) showed a perfusion defect in the anterior lateral myocardium (Figure 20.28A) associated with FDG uptake (FDG not shown), indicating metabolic ischemia with chest pain during exercise. Repeat PTCA of the obtuse marginal was carried out, and a follow-up PET scan was normal with disappearance of the anterior lateral stress perfusion defect and absence of FDG uptake during treadmill stress under fasting conditions (not shown). One year later, a repeat rest–exercise PET scan showed no significant change or progression of perfusion defects with only a minimal fixed defect at the apex (not shown).

Another year later, routine repeat rest–exercise PET showed a normal resting image (upper row, S1) but severe mid-anterior, anterior lateral, inferior lateral defect, and a moderate septal defect (Figure 20.28B). Direct comparison of the previous normal exercise stress study (upper row, S1, Figure 20.28C) compared to the following exercise study (lower panel, S2, Figure 20.28C) showed progression to severe perfusion defects over a large area of anterior, septal, apical, and lateral myocardium not present on the normal previous scan. Compared to the exercise perfusion defect (upper row, S1, Figure 20.28D), the corresponding stress FDG image under fasting conditions showed intense myocardial uptake over the anterior lateral segment in the region of the exercise perfusion defect, suggesting painless metabolic ischemia (lower row, S2). The patient also had painless 2.9-mm ST change on ECG during exercise that had not been present on previous treadmill tests.

Repeat coronary arteriography demonstrated progression of disease in the LAD and right coronary arteries with occlusion of the obtuse marginal on which two PTCA procedures had been previously carried out. Consequently, with painless progressive disease and a third restenosis (occlusion), the patient elected to have coronary bypass surgery.

The 3D topographic map in Figure 20.28E compares the normal exercise perfusion image after PTCA (upper panel, S1) to the follow-up exercise perfusion image showing progression of disease (lower panel, S2) in the septum, inferior, and apical areas.

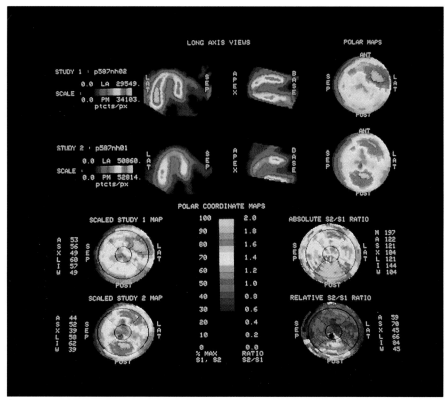

Fig. 20.28 Case 28.

A

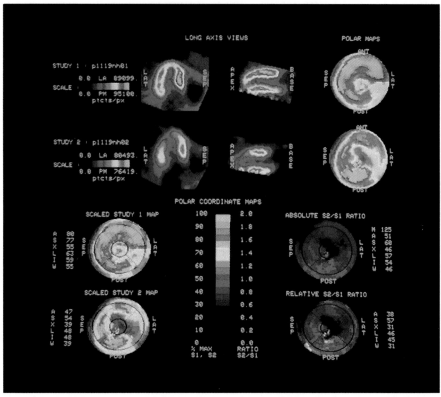

Fig. 20.28 Case 28 (*contd.*)

B

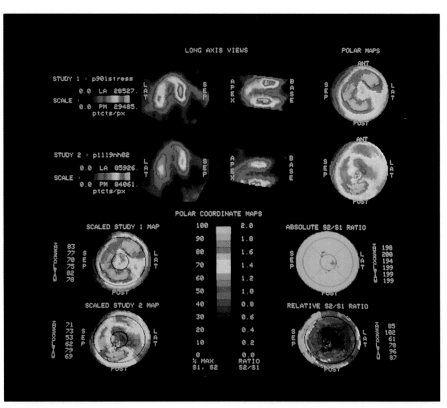

C

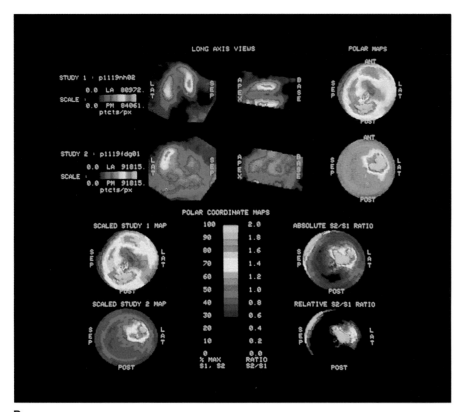

D

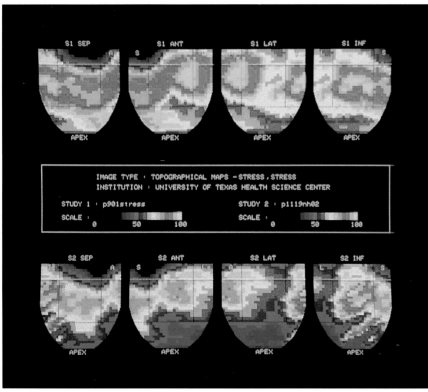

E

Case 29: Diagnostic Problem After Coronary Bypass Surgery

A slender 57-year-old woman presented with a history 4 months previously of neck pain and arrhythmias leading to coronary arteriography and bypass grafts to the right and diagonal coronary arteries with an internal mammary artery (IMA) implant to the LAD. Two months later, her symptoms recurred leading to repeat coronary arteriography that demonstrated an open IMA graft but with an anastomotic stenosis, a patent right bypass graft, and a patent graft to a small diagonal artery to a very small myocardial bed. Arteriograms of the native vessels showed an occluded right coronary artery, an 85% stenosis of the mid-LAD, an occluded small diagonal, and a 40% left circumflex narrowing. Over the 3 weeks prior to PET scan, the patient had recurrent arrhythmias, resting neck, and left arm pain when she was even 1 hour late with her medications. She requested evaluation by PET scanning for the status of her grafts and suitability of her myocardium for a potential repeat procedure. Her total cholesterol was 164, HDL 40, and LDL 105 on no cholesterol-lowering medications.

Rest–dipyridamole PET was carried out using N-13 ammonia (Figure 20.29: A, acquisition views; B, short-axis; C, long-axis and polar maps). Resting FDG images were obtained after glucose loading. The rest perfusion image (upper row, S1, Figure 20.29A–C) and the rest FDG image were both normal (FDG not shown), indicating no myocardial scar. The stress perfusion image (lower row, S1) had severe defects of the mid-anterior wall and apex with a mild septal defect, cumulatively involving 20% of myocardium. There was no impairment of coronary flow reserve laterally. Accordingly, a revision of her internal mammary artery anastomosis was successfully accomplished with relief of symptoms and return to full activity.

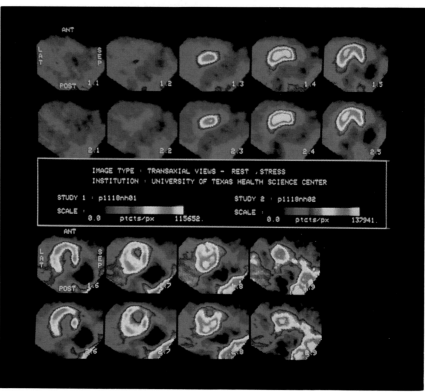

Fig. 20.29 Case 29.

A

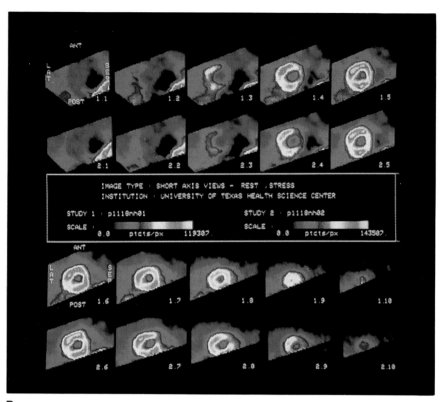

B

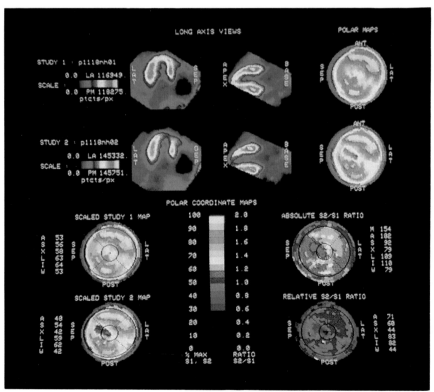

C

Case 30: Fatigue and Chest Pain After Coronary Bypass Surgery

A 55-year-old man presented with long-standing hypertension, a stable ascending thoracic aortic aneurysm, and a history of an IMA implant to the LAD for a 95% proximal LAD stenosis. The left circumflex and right coronary arteries were normal. Postoperatively, the patient had several different types of pain, including incisional chest pain, costochondral point tenderness, and reflex esophagitis with a known hiatal hernia. He subsequently developed a new type of chest pain unrelated to exercise, increased with stress, worse in cold weather while walking, and associated with marked increase in fatigue that prevented him from carrying out a full-time medical practice. Accordingly, he requested a PET scan in order to evaluate the status of his IMA-LAD implant. Rest–dipyridamole PET was carried out using N-13 ammonia (Figure 20.30A: A, acquisition views; B, short-axis; C, long-axis and polar maps). Rest images were normal, and dipyridamole images showed no restriction of coronary flow reserve in the LAD distribution. Accordingly, efforts were focused on changing his multiple antihypertensive medications to eliminate iatrogenic causes of fatigue without undergoing repeat arteriography.

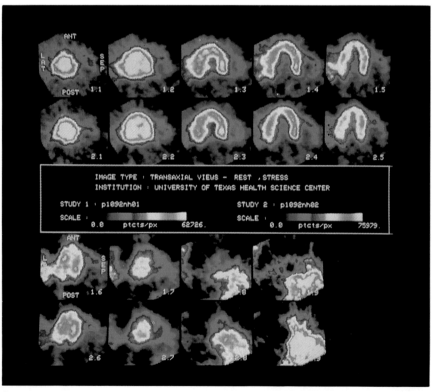

Fig. 20.30 Case 30.

A

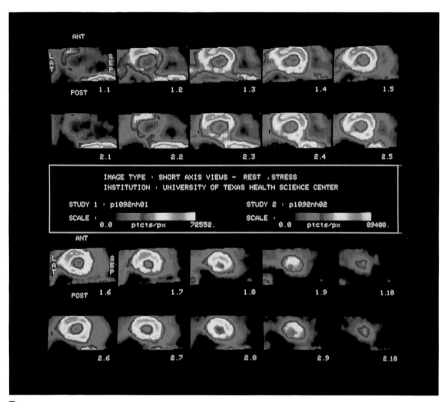

B

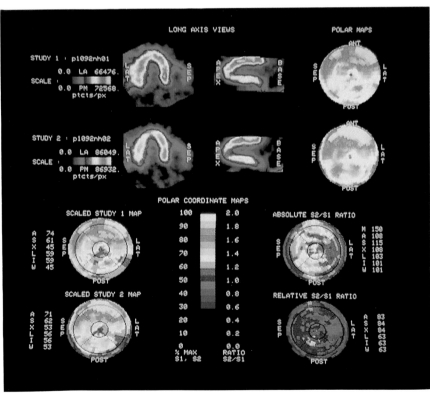

C

Case 31: Recurrent Chest Pain After Bypass Grafting and PTCA with Complex Disease of Native Circulation, Grafts, and Collaterals

A 67-year-old man had saphenous vein bypass grafts to the LAD, ramus intermedius, obtuse marginal, and the right coronary arteries 6 years previously. He did well postoperatively until 5 years later when he had recurrent chest pain relieved by PTCA of the LAD graft. Six months later angina recurred and was relieved again by repeat PTCA of the LAD graft. At that catheterization (second postoperative PTCA), his right and left circumflex coronary arteries were totally occluded, the proximal LAD had a 60% to 70% diameter stenosis, the first septal perforator had a 70% stenosis at its origin, and the obtuse marginal had a 70% to 80% stenosis. All grafts were patent but the right bypass graft had a 75% diameter mid-stenosis and the bypass graft to the LAD had a severe stenosis at its origin, both of which were successfully opened by a third PTCA. The grafts to the ramus intermedius and the obtuse marginal coronary arteries were patent without significant narrowing. The occluded left circumflex coronary artery filled retrogradely via the obtuse marginal, which, however, had a 70% to 80% diameter stenosis proximal to the insertion of the bypass graft.

After his third graft PTCA, he was asymptomatic until 2 weeks prior to his current admission when he had a non-Q wave myocardial infarction and postinfarction angina. A postinfarction thallium exercise test showed 3-mm ST depression of the inferior leads and an anterior–apical reversible defect. Accordingly, he was transferred from an out-of-state hospital to the University of Texas for further evaluation.

His past medical history was significant for hypertension, diabetes controlled with diet, peptic ulcer disease, and peripheral arterial disease with claudication and bilateral femoral popliteal bypasses previously. Physical examination and laboratory findings did not contribute further information.

Cardiac PET was carried out using rubidium-82 at rest and after dipyridamole (Figure 20.31: A, acquisition view; B, short-axis; C, long-axis and polar maps). In addition, after oral glucose loading, a PET scan was also obtained of FDG at rest in order to determine myocardial viability in comparison to rubidium-82 kinetics. The dipyridamole scan showed large severe perfusion defects of the septum, anterior lateral (diagonal distribution), and inferior lateral wall (ramus intermedius distribution) with a fall in absolute activity indicating myocardial steal and collateralization of both the septum and anterior lateral area. Although a relative perfusion defect was not apparent in the anterior wall and inferior myocardium, absolute coronary flow reserve to these areas was somewhat reduced suggesting diffuse, "balanced" coronary artery or graft disease but with more severe restriction to the septum and lateral wall.

These PET findings were interpreted as indicating open grafts to the LAD, right coronary artery, and either the ramus intermedius or obtuse marginal arteries. There was mild compromise in flow reserve of the LAD graft, severe disease of the septal perforator, and occlusion of one of the lateral grafts, either the ramus intermedius or obtuse marginal arteries associated with the inferior lateral nontransmural infarction. There was also myocardial steal and collateralization of the septal and lateral areas.

The early (upper row, S1) and late (lower row, S2) resting rubidium scans (Figure 20.31D) showed an initial mild inferior lateral defect which washed out somewhat on the late image indicating a small area of nonviable myocardium inferior laterally. The late rubidium-82 scan (upper row, S1) matched the FDG scan (lower row, S2), which confirmed a small lateral infarct (Figure 20.31E).

Thus, the PET studies indicated severe LAD disease proximal to an open but mildly compromised LAD graft and occlusion of a graft to the lateral wall with a small infarct and a large area of viable, collateralized, reversibly ischemic myocardium of septum and lateral wall. As a consequence of these PET findings, a tentative decision was made for more intense medical therapy without mechanical intervention because the proximal LAD and the occluded graft to the lateral wall were well-collateralized and not readily approachable by PTCA or surgery without endangering other grafts which were open by PET.

Repeat cardiac catheterization confirmed these findings. Coronary anatomy was as before in addition to a recurrent 60% proximal stenosis of the LAD graft and an occluded graft to the obtuse marginal, with extensive collaterals to both septum and anterolateral wall as predicted by PET. Since both the septum and lateral wall showed the most severe stress defects, these collateralized sites were considered the source of angina but appeared unlikely to infarct due to collateralization beyond already occluded or severely narrowed arteries. Therefore, more vigorous medical management was undertaken by increasing diltiazem and Isordil to maximally tolerated doses with continuation of aspirin and Lopressor. The patient's pain resolved and he was discharged without undergoing another mechanical intervention at the time. The corresponding 3D topographic maps show perfusion at rest (upper row, S1) and after dipyridamole (lower row, S2) with severe septal and lateral defects characteristic of proximal LAD disease with an open, more distal LAD graft (Figure 20.31F).

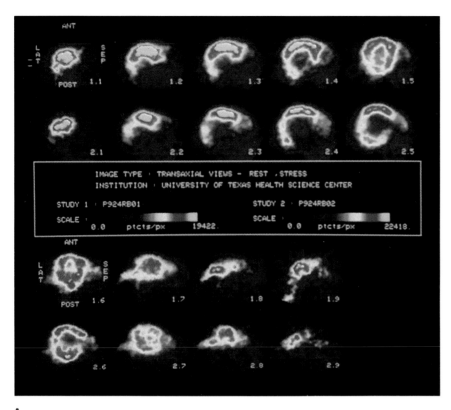

A

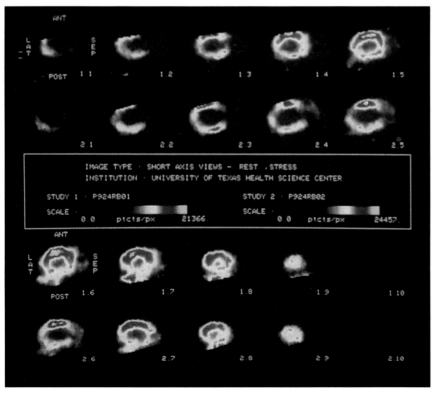

Fig. 20.31 Case 31 (20.31B and C, Reproduced with permission from reference 178).

B

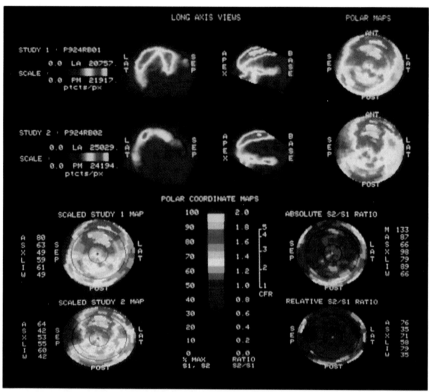

Fig. 20.31 Case 31 (*contd.*)

C

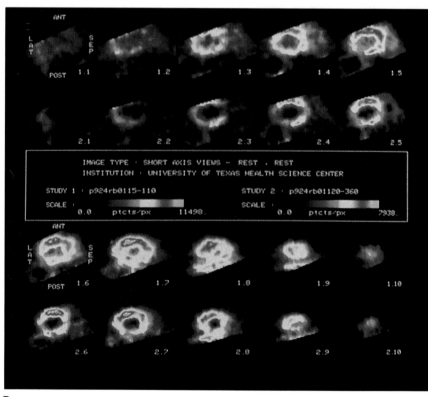

D

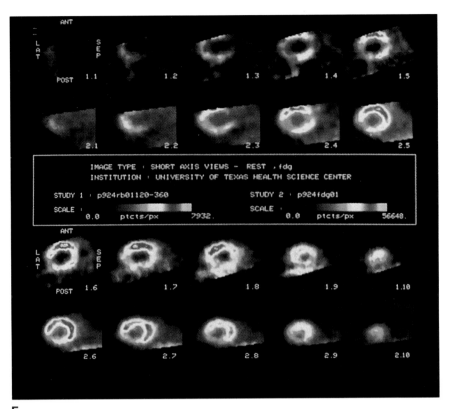

E

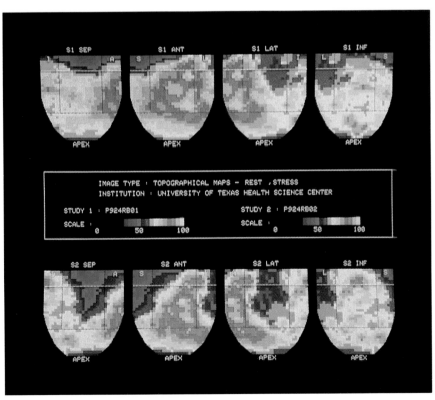

F

Case 32: Recurrent Angina Pectoris 8 Years After Coronary Bypass Surgery

A 60-year-old woman presented with an IMA implant to the LAD for a proximal tight LAD stenosis 8 years previously. She had been asymptomatic until 6 weeks previously when she developed angina with walking. Repeat coronary arteriography showed a patent internal mammary graft to the LAD and a moderately severe right coronary artery stenosis estimated to be 50% to 75% narrowed. The LAD proximal to the IMA graft was severely diseased and involved a large septal perforator. The patient was referred for PET scanning in order to determine whether the right coronary artery was severe enough to cause her angina.

Rest–dipyridamole PET imaging was carried out using N-13 ammonia (Figure 20.32: A, acquisition view; B, short-axis; C, long-axis and polar maps). The rest image was normal. The dipyridamole image showed a defect of the anterior septum associated with angina and ST changes in the precordial chest leads, all relieved with aminophylline. There was no evidence of an inferior perfusion defect. These scans indicated that the source of her angina was from the septal perforator and not from the right coronary artery. Since a mechanical approach to this isolated septal perforator was difficult and might jeopardize the distal LAD, more vigorous medical therapy was recommended.

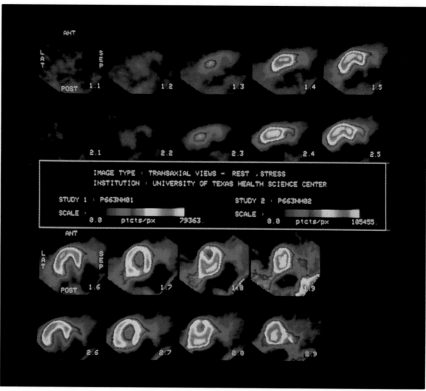

Fig. 20.32 Case 32.

A

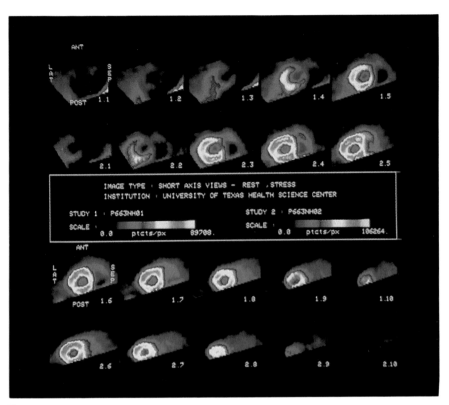

B

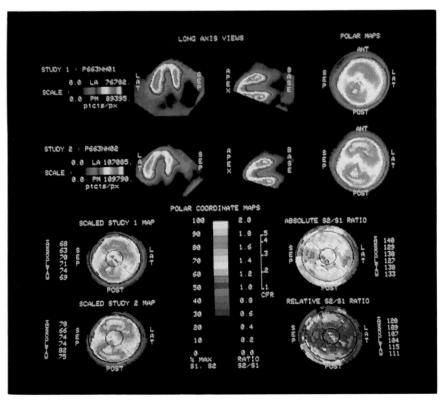

C

References for Chapters 11–20

1. Gould KL, Goldstein RA, Mullani NA, Kirkeeide R, Wong G, Smalling R, Fuentes F, Nishikawa A, Mathews W. Non-invasive assessment of coronary stenoses by myocardial perfusion imaging during pharmacologic coronary vasodilation. VIII. Clinical feasibility of positron cardiac imaging without a cyclotron using generator-produced rubidium-82. J Am Coll Cardiol 7:775–89, 1986.
2. Kirkeeide RL, Gould KL, Parsel L. Assessment of coronary stenoses by myocardial perfusion imaging during pharmacologic coronary vasodilation. VII. Validation of coronary flow reserve as a single integrated functional measure of stenosis severity reflecting all its geometric dimensions. J Am Coll Cardiol 7:103–13, 1986.
3. Gould KL. Identifying and measuring severity of coronary artery stenosis. Quantitative coronary arteriography and positron emission tomography. Circulation 68:237–45, 1988.
4. Demer LL, Gould KL, Goldstein RA, Kirkeeide RL, Mullani NA, Smalling RW, Nishikawa A, Merhige ME. Assessment of coronary artery disease severity by positron emission tomography. Comparison with quantitative arteriography in 193 patients. Circulation 79:825–35, 1989.
5. Schelbert HR, Wisenberg G, Phelps ME, Gould KL, Eberhard H, Hoffman EJ, Gormesm A, Kuhl DE. Non-invasive assessment of coronary stenosis by myocardial imaging during pharmacologic coronary vasodilation. VI. Detection of coronary artery disease in man with intravenous N-13 ammonia and positron computed tomography. Am J Cardiol 49:1197–207, 1982.
6. Yonekura Y, Tamaki N, Senda M, Nohara R, Kambara H, Konishi Y, Koide H, Kureshi SA, Saji H, Ban T, Kawai C, Torizuka K. Detection of coronary artery disease with ^{13}N-ammonia and high-resolution positron-emission computed tomography. Am Heart J 113:645–54, 1987.
7. Selwyn AP, Allan RM, L'Abbate AL, Horlock P, Camici P, Clark J, O'Brien HA, Grant PM. Relation between regional myocardial uptake of rubidium-82 and perfusion: absolute reduction of cation uptake in ischemia. Am J Cardiol 50:112–21, 1982.
8. Deanfield JE, Shea MJ, Wilson RA, Horlock P, de Landsheere CM, Selwyn AP. Direct effects of smoking on the heart: silent ischemic disturbances of coronary flow. Am J Cardiol 57:1005–09, 1986.
9. Gould KL, Kirkeeide R, Buchi M. Coronary flow reserve as a physiologic measure of stenosis severity. Part I. Relative and absolute coronary flow reserve during changing aortic pressure. Part II. Determination from arteriographic stenosis dimensions under standardized conditions. J Am Coll Cardiol 15:459–74, 1990.
10. Hicks K, Ganti G, Mullani N, Gould KL. Automated quantitation of 3D cardiac PET for routine clinical use. J Nucl Med 30:1787–97, 1989.
11. Gould KL. Percent coronary stenosis: Battered gold standard, pernicious relic, or clinical practicality? J Am Coll Cardiol 11:886–88, 1988.
12. Goldstein RA, Kirkeeide R, Demer L, Merhige M, Nishikawa A, Smalling RW, Mullani NA, Gould KL. Relations between geometric dimensions of coronary artery stenoses and myocardial perfusion reserve in man. J Clin Invest 79:1473–78, 1987.
13. Camici P, Araujo LI, Spinks T, Lammertsma AA, Kaski JC, Shea MJ, Selwyn AP, Jones T, Maseri A. Increased uptake of 18 F-fluorodeoxyglucose in postischemic myocardium of patients with exercise-induced angina. Circulation 74:281–92, 1986.
14. Grover-McKay M, Schelbert HR, Schwaiger M, Sochor H, Guzy PM, Krivokapich J, Child JS, Phelps ME. Identification of impaired metabolic reserve by atrial pacing in patients with significant coronary artery stenosis. Circulation 74:281–92, 1986.
15. Schelbert HR, Buxton D. Insights into coronary artery disease gained from metabolic imaging. Circulation 78:496–505, 1988.
16. Tamaki N, Yonekura Y, Yamashita K, Senda M, Saji H, Konishi Y, Hirata K, Ban T, Konishi J. Value of rest-stress myocardial positron tomography using Nitrogen-13 ammonia for the preoperative prediction of reversible asynergy. J Nucl Med 30:1302–10, 1989.
17. Tillisch J, Brunken R, Marshall R, Schwaiger M, Mandelkern M, Phelps M, Schelbert H. Reversibility of cardiac wall-motion abnormalities predicted by positron tomography. N Engl J Med 314:884–88, 1986.
18. Brunken K, Schwaiger M, Grover-McKay M, Phelps M, Tillisch J, Schelbert H. Positron emission tomography detects tissue metabolic activity in myocardial segments with persistent thallium perfusion defects. J Am Coll Cardiol 10:557–67, 1987.
19. Goldstein RA, Mullani NA, Wong WH, Hartz RK, Hicks CH, Fuentes F, Smalling RW, Gould KL. Positron imaging of myocardial infarction with rubidium-82. J Nucl Med 27:1824–29, 1986.
20. Geltman EM, Biello D, Welch MJ, Ter-Pogossian MM, Roberts R, Sobel BE. Characterization of transmural myocardial infarction by positron-emission tomography. Circulation 65:747–55, 1982.
21. Schwaiger M, Brunken R, Grover-McKay M, Krivokapich J, Child J, Tillisch JH, Phelps ME, Schelbert HR. Regional myocardial metabolism in patients with acute myocardial infarction assessed by positron emission tomography. J Am Coll Cardiol 8:800–08, 1986.
22. Marshal RC, Tillisch JH, Phelps ME, Huang SC, Carson R, Henze E, Schelbert HR. Identification and differentiation of resting myocardial ischemia and infarction in man with positron computed tomography, ^{18}F-labeled fluorodeoxyglucose and N-13 ammonia. Circulation 67:766–78, 1983.
23. Brunken R, Tillisch J, Schwaiger M, Child JS, Marshall R, Mandelkern M, Phelps ME, Schelbert HR. Regional perfusion, glucose metabolism, and wall motion in patients with chronic electrocardiographic Q wave infarctions: evidence for persistence of viable tissue in some infarct regions by positron emission tomography. Circulation 73:951–63, 1986.
24. Sobel BE, Geltman EM, Tiefenbrunn AJ, Jaffee AS, Spadaro JJ, Ter-Pogossian MM, Collen D, Ludbrook PA. Improvement of regional myocardial metabolism after coronary thrombolysis induced with tissue-type plasminogen activator or streptokinase. Circulation 69:983–90, 1984.
25. Ter-Pogossian MM, Klein MS, Markham J, Roberts R, Sobel BE. Regional assessment of myocardial metabolic integrity in vivo by positron-emission tomography with ^{11}C-labeled palmitate. Circulation 61:242–55, 1980.
26. Goldstein RA. Kinetics of rubidium-82 after coronary occlusion and reperfusion. J Clin Invest 75:1131–37, 1985.
27. Garza D, Sease DR, Merhige ME, Hicks K, Mullani N, Gould KL. Non-invasive identification of viable versus infarcted myocardium by automated three-dimensional cardiac positron emission tomography with generator produced rubidium-82. J Nucl Med 30:865, 1989 (abstract).
28. Goldstein RA, Kirkeeide R, Smalling RW, Nishikawa A, Demer L, Merhige M, Mullani NA, Gould KL. Changes in myocardial perfusion reserve after PTCA: Non-invasive assessment with positron tomography. J Nucl Med 28:1262–67, 1987.
29. Demer LL, Kirkeeide RL, Haynie MP, Wallschlaeger EA, Holmes RL, Elson BM, Ornish DM, Gould KL. Feasibility of following pro-

gression/regression of coronary artery stenosis by positron emission tomography during dipyridamole-hand grip stress. Circulation 76:IV-4, 1987.

30. Demer LL, Goldstein R, Mullani N, Kirkeeide R, Smalling R, Nishikawa A, Fuentes F, Gould KL. Coronary steal by non-invasive PET identifies collateralized myocardium. J Nucl Med 27:977, 1986 (abstract).

31. Demer L, Gould KL, Kirkeeide R. Assessing stenosis severity: coronary flow reserve, collateral function, quantitative coronary arteriography, positron imaging, and digital subtraction angiography. A Review and Analysis. Prog CV Dis 30:307–22, 1988.

32. Gould KL. Coronary steal—Is it clinically important? Chest 96:227–29, 1989.

33. Gould KL, Buchi M, Kirkeeide RL, Ornish D, Stein E, Brand R. Reversal of coronary artery stenosis with cholesterol lowering in man followed by arteriography and positron emission tomography. J Nucl Med 30:345, 1989 (abstract).

34. Ornish DM, Scherwitz LW, Brown SE, Billings JH, Armstrong WT, Ports TA, McLanahan SM, Kirkeeide RL, Brand RJ, Gould KL. Can lifestyle changes reverse atherosclerosis? Lancet 336:129–133, 1990.

35. Yano Y, Cahoon JL, Budinger TF. A precision flow-controlled Rb-82 generator for bolus or constant-infusion studies of the heart and brain. J Nucl Med 22:1006–10, 1981.

36. Neirinckx RD, Kronauge JF, Gennaro GP. Evaluation of inorganic absorbents for rubidium-82 generator: I.Hydrous SnO_2. J Nucl Med 24:898–906, 1982.

37. Mullani NA, Gould KL. First pass regional blood flow measurements with external detectors. J Nucl Med 24:577–81, 1983.

38. Mullani NA, Goldstein RA, Gould KL, Fisher DJ, Marani SK, O'Brien HA. Myocardial perfusion with rubidium-82. I. Measurement of extraction fraction and flow with external detectors. J Nucl Med 24:898–906, 1983.

39. Goldstein RA, Mullani NA, Fisher D, Marani S, Gould KL, O'Brien HA. Myocardial perfusion with rubidium-82. II. The effects of metabolic and pharmacologic interventions. J Nucl Med 24:907–15, 1983.

40. Schelbert HR, Phelps ME, Huang SC, MacDonald NS, Hansen H, Selin C, Kuhl DE. N-13 ammonia as an indicator of myocardial blood flow. Circulation 63:1259–72, 1981.

41. Schelbert HR, Phelps ME, Hoffman EJ, Huang SC, Selin CE. Regional myocardial perfusion assessed with N-13 labeled ammonia and positron emission computerized axial tomography. Am J Cardiol 43:209–18, 1979.

42. Yoshida K, Endo M, Himi T, Kagaya A, Masuda Y, Inagalsi Y, Fukuda H, Iinuma T, Yamasaki T, Firkuda N, Tateno Y. Measurement of regional myocardial blood flow in hypertrophic cardiomyopathy: Application of the first pass flow model using N-13 ammonia and PET. Am J Physiol Imaging 4:97–104, 1987.

43. Bergmann SR, Fox KAA, Rand AL, McElvany KD, Welch MJ, Markham J, Sobel BE. Quantification of regional myocardial blood flow in vivo with $H_2{}^{15}O$. Circulation 70:724–33, 1984.

44. Iida H, Kanno I, Takahashi A, Miura S, Murakami M, Takahashi K, Ono Y, Shishido F, Inugami A, Tomura N, Higano S, Fujita H, Sasaki H, Nakamichi H, Mizusawa S, Kondo Y, Uemura K. Measurement of absolute myocardial blood flow with $H_2{}^{15}O$ and dynamic positron-emission tomography. Circulation 78:104–15, 1988.

45. Gould KL, Lipscomb K, Hamilton GW. A physiologic basis for assessing critical coronary stenosis: instantaneous flow response and regional distribution during coronary hyperemia as measures of coronary flow reserve. Am J Cardiol 33:87–94, 1974.

46. Gould KL. Noninvasive assessment of coronary stenoses by myocardial imaging during coronary vasodilation. I. Physiologic principles and experimental validation. Am J Cardiol 41:267–78, 1978.

47. Gould KL, Westcott JR, Hamilton GW. Noninvasive assessment of coronary stenoses by myocardial imaging during coronary vasodilation. II. Clinical methodology and feasibility. Am J Cardiol 41:279–87, 1978.

48. Albro PC, Gould KL, Westcott RJ, Hamilton GW, Ritchie JL, Williams DL. Noninvasive assessment of coronary stenoses by myocardial imaging during pharmacologic coronary vasodilation. III. Clinical trial. Am J Cardiol 42:751–60, 1978.

49. Gould KL, Kelley KO, Bolson EL. Experimental validation of quantitative coronary arteriography for determining pressure-flow characteristics of coronary stenosis. Circulation 66:930–37, 1982.

50. Gould KL. Quantification of coronary artery stenosis in vivo. Circ Res 57:341–53, 1985.

51. Brown BG, Bolson E, Frimer M, Dodge HT. Quantitative coronary arteriography: Estimation of dimensions, hemodynamic resistance, and atheroma mass of coronary artery lesions using the arteriogram and digital computation. Circulation 55:329–37, 1977.

52. Marcus ML, Skorton DJ, Johnson MR, Collins SM, Harrison DG, Kerber RE. Visual estimates of percent diameter coronary stenosis: "A battered gold standard." J Am Coll Cardiol 41:882–85, 1988.

53. White CW, Wright CB, Doty DB, Hiratza LF, Eastham CL, Harrison DG, Marcus ML. Does visual interpretation of the coronary arteriogram predict the physiologic importance of a coronary stenosis? N Engl J Med 310:819–24, 1984.

54. Marcus ML, Harrison DG, White CW, McPherson DD, Wilson RF, Kerber RE. Assessing the physiologic significance of coronary obstructions in patients: Importance of diffuse undetected atherosclerosis. Prog CV Dis 31:39–56, 1988.

55. Kehtarnavaz N, DeFigueiredo RJP. A novel surface reconstruction and display method for cardiac PET imaging. IEEE Trans Med Imaging 3:108–15, 1984.

56. Gould KL. Assessment of coronary stenoses by myocardial perfusion imaging during pharmacologic coronary vasodilatation. IV. Limits of stenosis detection by idealized, experimental, cross-sectional myocardial imaging. Am J Cardiol 42:761–68, 1978.

57. Gould KL. The Coronary Circulation. From Positron Emission Tomography and Autoradiography: Principles and Applications for Brain and Heart, ed. Phelps M, Mazziotta J, Schelbert H. New York: Raven Press, 1986.

58. Shelton ME, Green MA, Mathias CJ, Welch MJ, Bergmann SR. Kinetics of copper PTSM in isolated hearts: a novel tracer for measuring blood flow with PET. J Nucl Med 30:1843–47, 1989.

59. Fujibayashi Y, Matsumoto K, Yonekura Y, Konishi J, Yakoyama A. A new zinc-62/copper 62 generator as a copper 62 source for PET radiopharmaceuticals. J Nucl Med 30:1838–42, 1989.

60. Turner DA. An intuitive approach to receiver operating characteristic curve analysis. J Nucl Med 19:213–20, 1978.

61. Turner DA, Battle WE, Deshmukh H, Colandrea MA, Snyder GJ, Fordham EW, Messer JV. The predictive value of myocardial perfusion scintigraphy after stress in patients without previous myocardial infarction. J Nucl Med 19:249–55, 1978.

62. Massof R, Emmel T. Criterion-free, parameter-free, distribution-independent index of diagnostic test performance. Applied Optics 26:1395–408, 1987.

63. Hlatky MA, Mark DB, Harrell FE, Lee KL, Califf RM, Pryor DB. Rethinking sensitivity and specificity. Am J Cardiol 59:1195–98, 1987.

64. Nicklas JM, Monsur JC, Pillai KM, Schork MA, Gallagher KP. Heterogeneity in ischemic myocardial blood flow: Determination of thresholds for tissue viability. Circulation 78 (suppl. II):644, 1988.

65. Hearse DJ, Crome R, Yellos DM, Wyse R. Metabolic and flow correlates of myocardial ischemia. Cardiovas Res 17:452–58, 1983.

66. Guth BD, Martin JF, Heusch G, Ross J, Jr. Regional myocardial blood flow, function and metabolism using phosphorus-31 nuclear magnetic resonance spectroscopy during ischemia and reperfusion in dogs. J Am Coll Cardiol 10:673–81, 1987.

67. Dichiro G, Brooks RA. PET quantitation: blessing and curse. J Nucl Med 29:1603–04, 1988.

68. Gould KL, Mullani N, Wong WH, Goldstein RA. Positron Emission Tomography. Chapter 13 in Cardiac Imaging and Image Processing, ed. Collins SM, Skorton DJ. New York: McGraw Hill, 1986.

69. Kochsiek K, Cott LA, Tauchert M, Neubaur J, Larbig D. Measurement of coronary blood flow in various hemodynamic conditions using the Argon technique. In Coronary Heart Disease (International Symposium in Frankfurt), ed. Kaltebach M, Lichtlen P. Stuttgart: Georg Thieme Verlag, 1971.

70. Wilcken DEL, Paoloni JH, Elkens E. Evidence for intravenous dipyridamole producing a coronary steal effect in the ischemic myocardium. Aust NZ J Med 1:8–14, 1971.

71. Wendt VE, Sundermeyer SF, Denbakker PB, Biag RS. The relationship between coronary blood flow, myocardial oxygen consumption and cardiac work as influenced by Persantine. Am J Cardiol 68:183–223, 1973.

72. Tauchert M. Koronarreserve und maximaler Saurstoffverbrauch des menschlichen Herzens. Basic Res Cardiol 68:183–223, 1973.

73. Tavazzi L, Previtali M, Salerno JA, Chimienti M, Ray M, Medici A, Specchia G, Bobba P. Dipyridamole test in angina pectoris: diagnostic value and pathophysiological implications. Cardiology 69:34–41, 1982.

74. Brown BG, Josephson MA, Peterson RB, Pierce CD, Wong W, Hecht HS, Bolson H, Dodge HT. Intravenous dipyridamole with isometric handgrip for near maximal acute increase in coronary flow in patients with CAD. Am J Cardiol 48:1077–85, 1981.

75. Shah A, Schelbert HR, Schwaiger M, Henze E, Hansen H, Selin C, Huang SC. Measurement of regional myocardial blood flow with N-13 ammonia and positron emission tomography in intact dogs. J Am Coll Cardiol 5:92–100, 1985.

76. Rossen JD, Simonetti I, Marcus ML, Winniford MD. Coronary dilation with standard dose dipyridamole and dipyridamole combined with handgrip. Circulation 79:566–72, 1989.

77. Schaper W, Gunter G, Winkler B, Schaper J. The collateral circulation of the heart. Prog CV Dis 31:57–77, 1988.

78. Flameng W, Wusten B, Schapler W. On the distribution of myocardial blood flow. II. Effects of arterial stenosis and vasodilation. Basic Res Cardiol 69:435–46, 1974.

79. Demer LL, Gould KL, Goldstein R, Kirkeeide R. Non-invasive assessment of coronary steal in man by PET perfusion imaging. J Nucl Med 31:259–270, 1990.

80. Rentrop KP, Thornton JC, Feit F, Van Buskirk M. Determinants and protective potential of coronary arterial collateral as assessed by an angioplasty model. Am J Cardiol 61:677–84, 1988.

81. Chambers CE, Brown KA. Dipyridamole-induced ST segment depression during thallium-201 imaging in patients with coronary artery disease; angiographic and hemodynamic determinants. J Am Coll Cardiol 12:37–41, 1988.

82. Mizuno K, Horiuchi K, Matui H, Miyamoto A, Arakawa K, Shibuya T, Kurita A, Nakamura H. Role of coronary collateral vessels during transient coronary occlusion during angioplasty assessed by hemodynamic, electrocardiographic and metabolic changes. J Am Coll Cardiol 12:624–28, 1988.

83. Meerdink DJ, Okada RD, Leppo JA. The effect of dipyridamole on transmural bloodflow gradients. Chest 96:400–05, 1989.

84. Gould KL. Collapsing coronary stenosis—A Starling Resistor. Internatl J Cardiol 2:39–42, 1982.

85. Wusten B, Flameng W, Schaper W. The distribution of myocardial flow. Part I: Effects of experimental coronary occlusion. Basic Res Cardiol 69(4):422–34, 1974.

86. Schaper W. The Pathophysiology of Myocardial Perfusion. Amsterdam: Elsevier North Holland Biomed, 1979.

87. Schaper W, Lewi P, Flameng W, Gijgon L. Myocardial steal produced by coronary vasodilation in chronic coronary artery occlusion. Basic Res Cardiol 68:3–20, 1973.

88. Flameng W, Wusten B, Winkler B, et al. Influence of perfusion pressure and heart rate on local myocardial flow in the colla-

89. teralized heart with chronic coronary occlusion. Am Heart J 89:51–59, 1975.

89. Schaper W, Flameng W, Winkler B, Wusten B, Turschmann W, Neugebauer G, Carl M, Pasyk S. Quantification of collateral resistance in acute and chronic experimental coronary occlusion in the dog. Circ Res 39:371–77, 1976.

90. Becker LC. Effect of nitroglycerine and dipyridamole on regional left ventricular blood flow during coronary artery occlusion. J Clin Invest 52:28–36, 1976.

91. Becker LC. Conditions for vasodilator induced coronary steal in experimental myocardial ischemia. Circulation 57:1103–10, 1978.

92. Wyatt D, Lee J, Downey JM. Determination of coronary collateral flow by a load line analysis. Circ Res 50:663–70, 1983.

93. Patterson RE, Kirk ES. Coronary steal mechanisms in dogs with one vessel occlusion and other arteries normal. Circulation 67:1009–15, 1983.

94. Chilian WM, Eastham CL, Marcus ML. Microvascular distribution of coronary vascular resistance in the beating left ventricle. Am J Physiol 20:779–88, 1986.

95. Pierard LA, DeLandsheere CM, Berthe C, Rigo P, Kulbertus HE. Identification of viable myocardium by echocardiography during dobutamine infusion in patients with myocardial infarction after thrombolytic therapy: Comparison with PET. J Amer Coll Cardiol 15:1021–31, 1990.

96. Bodenheimer MM, Banka VS, Fooshee C, Hermann GA, Helfant RH. Relationship between regional myocardial perfusion and the presence, severity and reversibility of asynergy in patients with coronary heart disease. Circulation 58:789–878, 1978.

97. Rozanski A, Berman DS, Gray R, Levy R, Raymond M, Maddahi J, Pantaleo N, Waxman A, Swan JHC, Matloff J. Use of thallium-201 redistribution scintigraphy in the preoperative differentiation of reversible and nonreversible myocardial asynergy. Circulation 64:936–44, 1981.

98. Iskandrian AS, Hakki A-H, Kane SA, Goel IP, Mudth ED, Segal BL. Rest and redistribution thallium-201 myocardial scintigraphy to predict improvement in left ventricular function after coronary arterial bypass grafting. Am J Cardiol 51:1312–16, 1983.

99. Cloninger KG, DePuey EG, Garcia EV, Roubin GS, Robbins WL, Nody A, DePasquale EE, Berger HJ. Incomplete redistribution in delayed thallium-201 single photon emission computed tomographic (SPECT) images: an overestimation of myocardial scarring. J Am Coll Cardiol 12:955–63, 1988.

100. Galli M, Bencivelli W, Pardo NF, Tavazzi L. Underestimation of residual ischemia by 201-thallium scintigraphy after myocardial infarction. Chest 94:876–78, 1988.

101. Tamaki N, Yonekura Y, Yamashita K, Senda M, Saji H, Hashimoto T, Fudo T, Kambara H, Kawai C, Bon T, Konishi J. Relation of left ventricular perfusion and wall motion with metabolic activity in persistent defects on ^{201}Tl tomography in healed myocardial infarction. Am J Cardiol 62:202–08, 1988.

102. Brunken RC, Kottou S, Nienaber CA, Schwaiger M, Ratib OM, Phelps ME, Schelbert HR. PET detection of viable tissue in myocardial segments with persistent defects at Tl-201 SPECT. Radiology 172:65–73, 1989.

103. Tamaki N, Yonekura Y, Yamashita K, Saji H, Magata Y, Senda M, Konishi Y, Hirata K, Ban T, Konishi J. Positron emission tomography using fluorine-18 deoxyglucose in evaluation of coronary artery bypass grafting. Am J Cardiol 64:860–65, 1989.

104. Merhige ME, Ekas RD, Mossberg K, Taegtmeyer HT, Gould KL. Catechol stimulation, substrate competition and myocardial glucose uptake in conscious dogs assessed with positron emission tomography. Circ Res 61:124–29, 1987.

105. Sease D, Garza D, Merhige ME, Gould KL. Does myocardial uptake of F-18-Fluoro-deoxy-glucose by positron emission tomography reliably indicate myocardial viability in acute myocardial infarction? Circulation 80:II-378, 1989. Scientific Meeting, 1989, accepted for presentation.

106. Bianco JA, Bakanauskas J, Carlson M, Jones S, Moring A, Alpert JS, Klassen V. Augmented uptake of 2-C-14-D-deoxyglucose in reversibly-injured myocardium. European J Nucl Med 13:557–62, 1988.

107. Komatsumoto S, Greenberg JH, Hickey WF, Reivich M. Local cerebral glucose utilization in chronic middle cerebral artery occlusion in the cat. J Cerebr Blood Flow Metabol 9:535–47, 1989.

108. Wijns W, Jacque AM, Leners N, Ferrant A, Keyeux A, Rahier J, Cogneau M, Michel C, Bol A, Robert A, Pouleur H, Charlier A, Beckers C. Accumulation of polymorphonuclear leukocytes in reperfused ischemic canine myocardium: relation with tissue viability assessed by Fluorine-18-2-Deoxyglucose uptake. J Nucl Med 29:1826–32, 1988.

109. De Jong JW, Goldstein S. Changes in coronary venous inosine concentration and myocardial wall thickening during regional ischemia in the pig. Circ Res 35:111–16, 1974.

110. De Jong JW, Verdouw PD, Remme WJ. Myocardial nucleoside and carbohydrate metabolism and hemodynamics during partial occlusion and reperfusion of pig coronary artery. J Molecul Cellular Cardiol 9:297–312, 1977.

111. Owen P, Thomas M, Young V, Opie L. Comparison between metabolic changes in local venous and coronary sinus blood after acute experimental coronary arterial occlusion. Am J Cardiol 25:562–70, 1970.

112. Opie LH, Thomas M, Owen P, Shulman G. Increased coronary venous inorganic phosphate concentrations during experimental myocardial ischemia. Am J Cardiol 30:503–13, 1972.

113. Case RB, Nasser MG, Crampton RS. Biochemical aspects of early myocardial ischemia. Am J Cardiol 24:766–75, 1969.

114. Hill JL, Gettes LS. Effect of acute coronary artery occlusion on local myocardial extracellular K+ activity in swine. Circulation 61:768–77, 1980.

115. Shine KI. Ionic events in ischemia and anoxia. Am J Pathol 102:256–61, 1981.

116. Nakaya H, Kimura S, Kanno M. Intracellular K+ and Na+ activities under hypoxia, acidosis, and no glucose in dog hearts. Am J Physiol 249:H1078–85, 1985.

117. Conrad GL, Rau EE, Shine KI. Creatine kinase release, potassium-42 content and mechanical performance in anoxic rabbit myocardium. J Clin Invest 64:155–61, 1979.

118. Johnson RN, Sammel, NL, Norris RM. Depletion of myocardial creatine kinase, lactate dehydrogenase, myoglobin and K+ after coronary artery ligation in dogs. Cardiovas Res 15:529–37, 1981.

119. Tancredi RG, Yipintsoi T, Bassingthwaighte JB. Capillary and cell wall permeability to potassium in isolated dog hearts. Am J Physiol 229:537–44, 1975.

120. Poe ND. Comparative myocardial uptake and clearance characteristics of potassium and cesium. J Nucl Med 7:557–60, 1972.

121. Ishii Y, MacIntyre WJ, Pritchard WH. Measurement of total myocardial blood flow in dogs with 43K and the scintillation camera. Circ Res 33:113–22, 1973.

122. Prokop EK, Strauss HW, Shaw J, Pitt B, Wagner HN. Comparison of regional myocardial perfusion determined by ionic potassium-43 to that determined by microspheres. Circulation 50:978–84, 1974.

123. Zaret BL, Strauss HW, Martin ND, Wells HP, Flamm MD. Noninvasive regional myocardial perfusion with radioactive potassium. Study of patients at rest, with exercise and during angina pectoris. N Engl J Med 288:809–12, 1973.

124. Ziegler WH, Goresky CA. Kinetics of rubidium uptake in the working dog heart. Circ Res 29:208–220, 1971.

125. Sheehan RM, Renkin EM. Capillary, interstitial, and cell membrane barriers to blood-tissue transport of potassium and rubidium in mammalian skeletal muscle. Circ Res 30:588–607, 1972.

126. Yipintsoi T, Dobbs WA, Scanlon PD, Knopp TJ, Bassingthwaighte JB. Regional distribution of diffusible tracers and carbonized microspheres in the left ventricle of isolated dog hearts. Circ Res 33:573–87, 1973.

127. Holman BL, Eldh P, Adams DF, Han MH, Poggenburg JK, Adelstein SJ. Evaluation of myocardial perfusion after intracoronary injection of radiopotassium. J Nucl Med 14:274–78, 1973.

128. Schelbert HR, Ashburn WL, Chauncey DM, Halpern SE. Comparative myocardial uptake of intravenously administered radionuclides. J Nucl Med 15:1092–100, 1974.

129. Nishiyama H, Sodd VJ, Adolph RJ, Saenger EL, Lewis JT, Gabel M. Intercomparison of myocardial imaging agents: 201Tl, 129Cs, 43K, and 81Rb. J Nucl Med 17:880–89, 1976.

130. Selwyn AP, Allan RM, L'Abbate A, Horlock P, Camici P, Clark J, O'Brien HA, Grant PM. Relation between regional myocardial uptake of rubidium-82 and perfusion: absolute reduction of cation uptake in ischemia. Am J Cardiol 50:112–21, 1982.

131. Love WD, Ishihara Y, Lyon LD, Smith RO. Differences in the relationships between coronary blood flow and myocardial clearance of isotopes of potassium rubidium, and cesium. Am Heart J 76:353–55, 1968.

132. Love WD. Isotope clearance and myocardial blood flow. Am Heart J 67:579–82, 1964.

133. Bing RJ, Bennish A, Bluemchen G, Cohen A, Gallagher JP, Zaleski EJ. The determination of coronary flow equivalent with coincidence counting technic. Circulation 29:833–46, 1964.

134. Moir TW. Measurement of coronary blood flow in dogs with normal and abnormal myocardial oxygenation and function. Circ Res 14:695–99, 1966.

135. McHenry PL, Knoebel SB. Measurement of coronary blood flow by coincidence counting and a bolus of 84RbCl. J Appl Physiol 22:495–500, 1967.

136. Mymin D, Sharma GP. Total and effective coronary blood flow in coronary and non-coronary heart disease. J Clin Invest 53:363–73, 1974.

137. Becker L, Ferreira R, Thomas M. Comparison of 86Rb and microsphere estimates of left ventricular bloodflow distribution. J Nucl Med 15:969–73, 1974.

138. Knoebel SB, Lowe DK, Lovelace DE, Friedman JI. Myocardial blood flow as measured by fractional uptake of Rubidium-84 and microspheres. J Nucl Med 19:1020–26, 1978.

139. Downey HF, Bashour FA, Parker PE, Bashour CA, Rutherford CS. Myocardial and total body extractions of radiorubidium in anesthetized dogs. J Appl Physiol 38:31–32, 1975.

140. Cohen MV. Quantitation of collateral and ischemic flows with microspheres and diffusible indicator. Am J Physiol 234:487–95, 1978.

141. Cohen A, Zaleski EJ, Luebs ED, Bing RJ. The use of positron emitter in the determination of coronary blood flow in man. J Nucl Med 6:651–66, 1965.

142. Cohen A, Gallagher JP, Luebs ED, Varga Z, Yamanaka J, Zaleski EJ, Bluemchen G, Bing RJ. The quantitative determination of coronary flow with a positron emitter (Rubidium-84). Circulation 32:636–49, 1965.

143. Donato L, Bartolomei G, Federighi G, Torreggiani G. Measurement of coronary blood flow by external counting with radioactive rubidium. Circulation 33:708–18, 1966.

144. Cohen A, Zaleski EJ, Baleiron H, Stock TB, Chiba C, Bing RJ. Measurement of coronary blood flow using rubidium84 and the coincidence counting method. Am J Cardiol 19:556–62, 1967.

145. Cowan C, Duran PVM, Corsini G, Goldschlager N, Bing RJ. The effects of nitroglycerin on myocardial blood flow in man. Am J Cardiol 24:154–60, 1969.

146. Knoebel SB, Elliott WC, McHenry PL, Ross E. Myocardial blood flow in coronary artery disease. Correlation with severity of disease and treadmill exercise response. Am J Cardiol 27:51–58, 1971.

147. Lurie AJ, Salel AF, Berman DS, DeNardo GL, Hurley EJ, Mason DT. Determination of improved myocardial perfusion after aortocoronary bypass surgery by exercise rubidium-81 scintigraphy. Circulation 54 (suppl. III):20–23, 1976.

148. Gould KL, Haynie M, Hess MJ, Yoshida K, Mullani N, Smalling RW. Myocardial metabolism of fluorodeoxyglucose compared to

cell membrane integrity for the potassium analogue Rb-82 for assessing viability and infarct size in man by PET. J Nucl Med (In press).

149. Gould KL, Goldstein RA, Mullani NA. Economic analysis of clinical positron emission tomography of the heart with rubidium-82. J Nucl Med 30:707–17, 1989.

150. Leppo JA, O'Brien J, Rothendler JA, Getchell JD, Lee VW. Dipyridamole-thallium-201 scintigraphy in the prediction of future cardiac events after acute myocardial infarction. N Engl J Med 310:1014–18, 1984.

151. Pirelli S, Inglese E, Suppa M, Corrada E, Campolo L. Dipyridamole-thallium-201 scintigraphy in the early postinfarction period. (Safety and accuracy in predicting the extent of coronary disease and future recurrence of angina in patients suffering from their first myocardial infarction.) European Heart J 9:1324–31, 1988.

152. Younis LT, Byers S, Shaw L, Barth G, Goodgold H, Chaitman BR. Prognostic value of intravenous dipyridamole thallium scintigraphy after an acute myocardial ischemic event. Am J Cardiol 64:161–66, 1989.

153. Bolognese L, Sarasso G, Aralda D, Bongo AS, Rossi L, Rossi P. High dose dipyridamole echocardiography early after uncomplicated acute myocardial infarction: correlation with exercise testing and coronary angiography. J Am Coll Cardiol 14:357–63, 1989.

154. Schofer J, Spielmann R, Sheehan FH, Lampe M, Schluter M, Mathey DG. Lack of correlation after reperfusion between ventricular function and infarct size estimated by thallium single-photon emission computed tomography. Internatl J Cardiac Imaging 3:203–08, 1989.

155. Nienaber CA, Spielmann RP, Salge D, Clausen A, Montz R, Bleifeld W. Quantitative spatial assessment of postinfarction myocardial ischemia by dipyridamole [201]thallium SPECT imaging. Zeitschrift für Kardiologie 75:536–41, 1986.

156. Casanova R, Patroncini A, Pirazzini L, Jacopi F, Capacci PF, Zarabini GE, Maresta A. Thallium scintigraphy and two-dimensional echocardiography after dipyridamole infusion in early post-infarction period. G Ital Cardiol 19:287–94, 1989.

157. Diamond GA. Suspect specificity. J Am Coll Cardiol (in press).

158. Ritchie JL, Trobaugh GB, Hamilton GW, Gould KL, Narahara KA, Murray JA, Williams DL. Myocardial imaging with thallium-201 at rest and during exercise. Comparison with coronary arteriography and resting and stress electrocardiography. Circulation 56:66–78, 1977.

159. Ritchie JL, Zaret BL, Strauss HW, Pitt B, Berman DS, Schelbert HR, Ashburn WL, Berger HJ, Hamilton GW. Myocardial imaging with thallium-201: a multicenter study in patients with angina pectoris or acute myocardial infarction. Am J Cardiol 42:345–50, 1978.

160. Maddahi J, Garcia EV, Berman DS, Waxman A, Swan HJC, Forrester J. Improved non-invasive assessment of coronary artery disease by quantitative analysis of regional stress myocardial distribution and washout of thallium-201. Circulation 64:924–35, 1981.

161. DePasquale EE, Nody AC, DePuey EG, Garcia EV, Pilcher G, Bredlau C, Roubin G, Gober A, Gruentzig A, D'Amato P, Berger H. Quantitative rotational thallium-201 tomography for identifying and localizing coronary artery disease. Circulation 77:316–27, 1987.

162. Van Train KF, Berman DS, Garcia EV, Berger HJ, Sands MJ, Friedman JD, Freeman MR, Pryzlak M, Ashburn WL, Norris SL, Green AM, Maddahi J. Quantitative analysis of stress thallium-201 myocardial scintigrams: a multicenter trial. J Nucl Med 27:17–25, 1986.

163. Ranhosky A, Gerlag DM. Quantitative interpretation provides no advantage over qualitative interpretation in intravenous dipyridamole thallium imaging. Circulation 78 (suppl. II):432, 1988.

164. Iskandrian AS, Heo J, Kong B, Lyons E. Effect of exercise level on ability of thallium-201 tomographic imaging in detecting coronary artery disease: analysis of 461 patients. J Am Coll Cardiol 14:1477–86, 1989.

165. Kahn JK, McGhie I, Akers MS, Sills NM, Faber TL, Kulkarni PV, Willerson JT, Corbett JR. Quantitative rotational tomography with ^{201}Tl and [99m]Tc 2-methoxy-isobutyl-isonitrile. A direct comparison in normal individuals and patients with coronary artery disease. Circulation 79:1282–93, 1989.

166. Nolewajka AJ, Kostuk WJ, Howard J, Rechnitzer PA, Cunningham DA. 201-thallium stress myocardial imaging: an evaluation of fifty-eight asymptomatic males. Clin Cardiol 4:134–38, 1981.

167. Schwartz RS, Jackson WG, Celio PV, Hickman JR. Exercise thallium-201 scintigraphy for detecting coronary artery disease in asymptomatic young men. J Am Coll Cardiol 11:80A, 1988.

168. Bungo MW, Leland OS. Discordance of exercise thallium testing with coronary arteriography in patients with atypical presentations. Chest 83:112–16, 1983.

169. Gould KL. Agreement on the accuracy of thallium stress testing. J Am Coll Cardiol (in press).

170. Gould KL. How accurate is thallium exercise testing? J Am Coll Cardiol 14:1487–90, 1989.

171. Gould KL. Goals, gold standards and accuracy of non-invasive myocardial perfusion imaging for identifying and assessing severity of coronary artery disease. Current Opinion Cardiol 4:834–44, 1989.

172. Hor G, Kanemoto N. Tl-201 myocardial scintigraphy: current status in coronary artery disease, results of sensitivity/specificity in 3092 patients and clinical recommendations. J Nucl Med 20:136–47, 1981.

173. Uhl GS, Froelicher V. Screening for asymptomatic coronary artery disease. J Am Coll Cardiol 1:946–55, 1983.

174. Houck PD. Epidemiology of total cholesterol to HDL ratio in 11,669 Air Force personnel and coronary artery anatomy in 305 healthy aviators. J Am Coll Cardiol 11:222A, 1988.

175. Tamaki N, Yonekura Y, Senda M, Yamashita K, Koide H, Saji H, Hashimoto T, Fudo T, Kambara H, Kawai C, Konishi J. Value and limitation of stress thallium-201 single photon emission computed tomography: comparison with nitrogen-13 ammonia positron tomography. J Nucl Med 29:1181–88, 1988.

176. Friedman J, Van Train K, Maddahi J, Rozanski A, Prigent F, Bietendorf J, Waxman A, Berman D. "Upward Creep" of the heart: a frequent source of false positive reversible defects during thallium-201 stress-redistribution SPECT. J Nucl Med 30:1718–22, 1989.

177. Williams BR, Jansen DE, Wong LF, Fiedotin AF, Knopf WD, Toporoff SJ. Positron emission tomography for the diagnosis of coronary artery disease: a non-university experience and correlation with coronary angiography. J Nucl Med 30:845, 1989 (abstract).

178. Gould KL, Gordon DG. PET and Clinical Cardiology. In Progress in Cardiology, vol 3/1, ed. Zipes DP, Rowlands DJ. Philadelphia: Lea & Febiger, 1990.

179. Iskandrian AS, Hakki AH, Kane-Marsch S. Prognostic implications of exercise thallium-201 scintigraphy in patients with suspected or known coronary artery disease. Am Heart J 110:135–43, 1985.

180. Pirelli S, Inglese E, Suppa M, Corrada E, Campolo L. Dipyridamole-thallium 201 scintigraphy in the early postinfarction period. (Safety and accuracy in predicting the extent of coronary disease and future recurrence of angina in patients suffering from their first myocardial infarction). European Heart J 9:1324–31, 1988.

181. Wackers FJ, Russo DS, Russo D, Clements JP. Prognostic significance of normal quantitative planar thallium-201 stress scintigraphy in patients with chest pain. J Am Coll Cardiol 6:27–30, 1985.

182. Brown KA, Boucher CA, Okada RD, Guiney TE, Newell JB, Strauss HW, Pohost GM. Prognostic value of exercise thallium-201 imaging in patients presenting for evaluation of chest pain. J Am Coll Cardiol 1:994–1001, 1983.

183. Ladenheim ML, Pollock BH, Rozanski A, Berman DS, Stanitoff

HM, Forrester JS, Diamond GA. Extent and severity of myocardial hypoperfusion as predictors of prognosis in patients with suspected coronary artery disease. J Am Coll Cardiol 7:464–71, 1986.

184. Kaul S, Finkelstein DM, Homma S, Leavitt M, Okada RD, Boucher CA. Superiority of quantitative exercise thallium-201 variables in determining long-term prognosis in ambulatory patients with chest pain: a comparison with cardiac catheterization. J Am Coll Cardiol 12:25–34, 1988.

185. Feinstein AR. The haze of Bayes, the aerial palaces of decision analysis, and the computerized Ouija board. Clin Pharmacol Ther 21:482–95, 1979.

186. Weiss RM, Shonka M, Chang W, Marcus ML. Coronary transit kinetics may hinder accurate measurement of perfusion with ultrafast computed tomography. J Am Coll Cardiol 11:226A, 1988 (abstract).

187. Rumberger JA, Feiring AJ, Lipton MJ, Higgins CB, Ell SR, Marcus ML. Use of ultrafast computed tomography to quantitate regional myocardial perfusion: a preliminary report. J Am Coll Cardiol 9:59–69, 1987.

188. Wolfkiel CJ, Ferguson JL, Chomka EV, Labin IN, Tenzer ML, Brundage BH. Myocardial blood flow determined by ultrafast computed tomography. Circulation 74 (suppl II):122, 1986 (abstract).

189. Paans AJM, Vaalburg W, Woldring MG. A comparison of the sensitivity of PET and NMR for in vivo quantitative metabolic imaging. European J Nucl Med 11:73–75, 1985.

190. Kaufman L, Crooks L, Sheldon P, Hricak H, Herfkens R, Bank W. The potential impact of nuclear magnetic resonance imaging on cardiovascular diagnosis. Circulation 67:251–57, 1983.

191. Johnston DL, Lui P, Brady T, Lauffer R, Weeden V, Okada RD. Gadolinium-DTPA as a myocardial perfusion agent during magnetic resonance imaging: Potential applications and limitations. J Am Coll Cardiol 5:476, 1985 (abstract).

192. Miller DD, Holmbang G, Gill JB, Dragotakes D, Kontor HL, Okada RD, Brady TJ. Detection of coronary stenoses by continuous paramagnetic contrast infusion during dipyridamole-induced hyperemia: the nuclear magnetic resonance imaging "stress test." Circulation 74 (suppl II):319, 1986 (abstract).

193. Marwick TH, Go RT, MacIntyre WJ, Underwood DA, Rehm PJ, King J, Beachler A, Saha G. Disparities between myocardial perfusion imaging using Rb-82 PET and Tl-201 SPECT after dipyridamole stress. J Nucl Med 20:861, 1989 (abstract).

194. Go RT, Marwick TH, MacIntyre WJ, Rehn PK, Underwood DA, Saha GB, Simpfendorfer CC. Initial results of comparative rubidium-82 and thallium-201 myocardial perfusion imaging in diagnosis of CAD. J Nucl Med 30:759, 1989 (abstract).

195. Kalus ME, Stewart RE, Gacioch GM, Squicciarini SA, Hutchins GD, Kuhl DE, Schwaiger M. Comparison of Rb-82 PET and Tl-201 SPECT for the detection of regional coronary artery disease. J Nucl Med 30:829, 1989 (abstract).

196. Rutishauser W, Simon H, Stucky JP, Schad N, Noseda G, Wellauer J. Evaluation of roentgen cinedensitometry for flow measurement in models and in the intact circulation. Circulation 36:951–63, 1967.

197. Bursch J, Johs R, Kirbach H, et al. Accuracy of videodensitometric flow measurement. In Roentgen-Cine-Videodensitometry, ed. Heintzen PH. Stuttgart: Thieme, 1971, pp 119–32.

198. Nissen SE, Elion JL, Booth DC, Evans J, DeMaria AN. Value and limitations of computer analysis of digital subtraction angiography in the assessment of coronary flow reserve. Circulation 73:562–71, 1986.

199. Elion JL, Nissen SE, DeMaria AN. Visual representation of coronary hyperemic reserve: methodology and evaluation. Circulation 72:III-263, 1985.

200. Molloi S, Peppler WW, Zarnstorff WC, Fotts JD, Miller WE, Taggort E, Van Lysel MS, Lee C, Cusma JT, Besozzi MM, Mistretta CA. Dual-energy rotational digital angiography for motion-immune cardiac imaging. Circulation 72:III-263, 1985.

201. Vogel RA. The radiographic assessment of coronary blood flow parameters. Circulation 72:460–65, 1985.

202. Hodgson JM, LeGrand V, Bates ER, Mancini GBJ, Averon FM, O'Neill WW, Simon SB, Beauman GJ, LeFree MT, Vogel RA. Validation in dogs of a rapid digital angiographic technique to mea-

sure relative coronary blood flow during routine cardiac catheterization. Am J Cardiol 55:188–93, 1985.

203. Zijlstra F, Fioretti P, Reiber JHC, Serruys PW. Which cineangiographically assessed anatomic variable correlates best with functional measurements of stenosis severity?: a comparison of quantitative analysis of the coronary cineangiogram with measured coronary flow reserve and exercise/redistribution thallium-201 scintigraphy. J Am Coll Cardiol 12:686–91, 1988.

204. Pijls N, Uijen G, Hoevelaken A, Arts T, Aengevaeren W, Bos H, Fast J, Leeuwen K, Van der Werf T. Mean transit time for assessment of myocardial perfusion by videodensitometry. Circulation 81:1331–40, 1990.

205. Gould KL. Experience with Clinical Positron Imaging of the Heart. In Nuclear Cardiovascular Imaging, ed. Guiberteau MJ. New York: Churchill Livingstone, 1990.

206. Senda M, Yonekura Y, Tamaki N, Tanaka Y, Komori M, Minato K, Konishi Y, Torizuka K. Axial resolution and the value of interpolating scan in multislice positron computed tomography. IEEE Trans Med Imaging, vol MI-4, 1:44–51, March 1985.

207. Mullani NA, Gould KL, Hartz RK, Hitchens RE, Wong GH, Bristow D, Adler S, Philippe E, Bendriem B, Sanders M, Gibbs B. Design and performance of Posicam 6.5 BGO Positron Camera. J Nucl Med (in press).

208. Raylman RR, Hutchins GD, Schwaiger M, Paradise AH. The effect of axial sampling and motion on three-dimensional quantification of myocardial defects with positron emission tomography. J Nucl Med 30:892, 1989.

209. Bendriem B, Dewey SL, Schlyer DJ. Dependence of the recovery coefficient on axial sampling in multislice positron emission tomography. J Nucl Med 30:892, 1989.

210. Wong WH, Mullani NA, Wardworth G, Hartz RK, Bristow D. Characteristics of small barium fluoride (BaF$_2$) scintillator for high intrinsic resolution time-of-flight positron emission tomography. IEEE Trans Nucl Sci, NS-31, 1:381–86, 1984.

211. Mullani NA, Gaeta J, Yerian K, Wong WH, Hartz RK, Phillipe EA, Bristow D, Gould KL. Dynamic imaging with high resolution time-of-flight PET camera - TOFPET I. IEEE Trans Nucl Sci, NS-31, 1:609–613, 1984.

212. Wong WH, Mullani NA, Phillipe EA, Hartz R, Gould KL. Image improvement and design optimization of the Time-of-Flight PET. J Nucl Med 24:52–60, 1983.

213. Mullani N, Wong W, Hartz R, Philippe E, Yerian K. Sensitivity improvement of TOFPET by the utilization of the interslice coincidence. IEEE Trans Nucl Sci, NS-29, 1:479–83, 1982.

214. Mullani NA, Ficke DC, Hartz R, Markham J, Wong WH. System design of fast PET scanners utilizing time-of-flight. IEEE Trans Nucl Sci, NS-28, 1:104–08, 1981.

215. Midwall J, Ambrose J, Pichard A, Abedin Z, Herman MV. Angina pectoris before and after myocardial infarction. Chest 81:681–86, 1982.

216. Reunanen A, Aromaa A, Pyorala K, Punsar S, Maatela J, Knekt P. The Social Insurance Institution's coronary heart disease study: baseline data and 5-year mortality experience. Acta Med Scand suppl 673:67–81, 1983.

217. Kannel WB, Abbott RD. Incidence and prognosis of unrecognized myocardial infarction. An update on the Framingham Study. N Engl J Med 311:1144–47, 1984.

218. Lown B. Sudden cardiac death: The major challenge confronting contemporary cardiology. Am J Cardiol 43:313–28, 1979.

219. Olofsson BO, Bjerle P, Aberg T, Osterman G, Jacobsson KA. Prevalence of coronary artery disease in patients with valvular heart disease. Acta Med Scand 218:365–71, 1985.

220. Langou RA, Huang EK, Kelley MJ, Cohen LS. Predictive accuracy of coronary artery calcification and abnormal exercise test for coronary artery disease in asymptomatic men. Circulation 62:1196–203, 1980.

221. Campbell S, Barry J, Rebecca GS, et al. Active transient myocardial ischemia during daily life in asymptomatic patients with positive exercise tests and coronary artery disease. Am J Cardiol 57:1010–16, 1986.

222. Resnekov L. Silent myocardial ischemia: therapeutic implications. Am J Med 79:30–34, 1985.

223. Gottlieb SO, Weisfeldt ML, Ouyang P, Mellits ED, Gerstenblith G.

Silent ischemia as a marker for early unfavorable outcomes in patients with unstable angina. N Engl J Med 314:1214–19, 1986.

224. Callaham P, Dubach P, Klein J, Risch M, Froelicher V. Prognostic significance of silent myocardial ischemia discovered during exercise testing. J Am Coll Cardiol 11:24A, 1988.

225. Younis LT, Byers S, Shaw L, Barth G, Goodgold H, Chaitman BR. Prognostic importance of silent myocardial ischemia detected by intravenous dipyridamole thallium myocardial imaging in asymptomatic patients with coronary artery disease. J Am Coll Cardiol 14:1635–41, 1989.

226. Oliver MF. Strategies for preventing and screening for coronary heart disease. Brit Heart J 54:1–5, 1985.

227. Madsen JK. Ischaemic heart disease and prodromes of sudden cardiac death. Brit Heart J 54:27–32, 1985.

228. Cohn PF. Silent myocardial ischemia: classification, prevalence, and prognosis. Am J Med 79 (suppl 3A):2–6, 1985.

229. Cohn PF. Silent myocardial ischemia: present status. Mod Con CV Dis 56(1):1–4, 1987.

230. Ringqvist I, Fisher LD, Mock M, et al. Prognostic value of angiographic indices of coronary artery disease from the coronary artery surgery study (CASS). J Clin Invest 71:1854–66, 1983.

231. Oberman A, Jones WB, Riley CP, Reeves JT, Sheffield LT, Turner ME. Natural history of coronary artery disease. Bull NY Acad Med 48:1109–25, 1972.

232. Smalling RW, Fuentes F, Matthews MW, Freund GC, Hicks CH, Reduto LA, Walker WE, Sterling RP, Gould KL. Sustained improvement in left ventricular function and mortality by intracoronary streptokinase administration during evolving myocardial infarction. Circulation 68:131–38, 1983.

233. Thanavoro S, Kleiger RE, Province MA, Hubert JW, Miller JP, Krone RJ, Oliver GC. Effect of infarct location on the in-hospital prognosis of patients with first transmural myocardial infarction. Circulation 66:742–47, 1982.

234. European Cooperative Study Group for streptokinase treatment in acute myocardial infarction: Streptokinase in acute myocardial infarction. N Engl J Med 301:797–802, 1979.

235. Howland JS, Vaillant HW. Long term survival of 224 patients with myocardial infarction treated in a community hospital. J Family Prac 10:979–83, 1980.

236. Pell S, D'Alonzo CA. Immediate mortality and five year survival of employed men with a first myocardial infarction. N Engl J Med 270:915–22, 1964.

237. Juergens JL, Edwards JE, Anchor RW, Burchell HB. Prognosis of patients surviving first clinically diagnosed myocardial infarction. Arch Intern Med 105:134–40, 1960.

238. Bonow RO, Bacharach SL, Cuocolo A, Dilsizian V. Myocardial viability in coronary artery disease and left ventricular dys-

function: thallium-201 reinjection vs fluorodeoxyglucose. Circulation 80 (suppl. II):377, 1989 (abstract).

239. Gould KL, Mulloni N, Williams B. PET, PTCA and economic priorities. Clin Cardiol 13:153–84, 1990.

240. Lyle FM, Gordon DG. The importance of timing with Rb-82 PET imaging of the heart. J Nucl Med 30:871, 1989 (abstract).

241. Willerson JT, Golino P, Eidt J, Campbell WB, Buja LM. Specific platelet mediators and unstable coronary artery lesions. Experimental evidence and potential clinical implications. Circulation 80:198–205, 1989.

242. Ter-Pogossian MM, Klein MS, Markham J, Roberts R, Sobel BE. Regional assessment of myocardial metabolic integrity in vivo by positron-emission tomography with ^{11}C-labeled palmitate. Circulation 61:242–55, 1980.

243. Atkins HL, Budinger TF, Lebowitz E, Ansari AN, Greene MW, Fairchild RG, Ellis KJ. Thallium-201 for medical use. Part 3. Human distribution and physical imaging properties. J Nucl Med 18:133–40, 1977.

244. Feller PA, Sodd VJ. Dosimetry of four heart-imaging radionuclides: ^{43}K, ^{81}Rb, ^{129}Cs, and ^{201}Tl. J Nucl Med 16:1070–75, 1975.

245. Lockwood AH. Absorbed doses of radiation after an intravenous injection of N-13 ammonia in man: concise communication. J Nucl Med 21:276–78, 1980.

246. Jones SC, Alava A, Christman O, Montanez I, Wolf AP, Revich M. The radiation dosimetry of 2-[F-18]Fluoro-2-Deoxy-D-Glucose in man. J Nucl Med 23:613–17, 1982.

247. Smith T. The radiation dosimetry of 2-[F-18]Fluoro-2-Deoxy-D-Glucose in man. J Nucl Med 24:447, 1983.

248. Reivich M, Kuhl D, Wolf A, Greenberg J, Phelps M, Ido T, Casella V, Fowler J, Hoffman E, Alavi A, Som P, Sokoloff L. The [^{18}F] fluorodeoxyglucose method for the measurement of local cerebral glucose utilization in man. Circ Res 44:127–37, 1979.

249. Kearfott KJ. Radiation absorbed dose estimates for positron emission tomography (PET): K-38, Rb-81, Rb-82, and Cs-130. J Nucl Med 23:1128–32, 1982.

250. Budinger TF, Rolio D. Physics and Instrumentation. Prog CV Dis 20:19–53, 1977.

251. Squibb Diagnostics, Directions for Cardiogen-82 (Rubidium-82), 1990.

252. Kearfott KJ. Absorbed dose estimates for positron emission tomography (PET): C^{15}O, ^{11}CO, and CO^{15}O. J Nucl Med 23:1031–37, 1982.

253. Gould KL. Positron Emission Tomography For Heart Disease: Clinical Update, ed. Braunwald E. Heart Disease: A Textbook of Cardiovascular Medicine. 3rd Edition. 10 Update. WB Saunders, 1990.

Index

Note: Numbers in **boldface** refer to figure
    numbers; numbers in *italics* refer to
    table numbers; numbers in roman
    face refer to page numbers.

A

Adrenergic sympathetic system, beta and
    alpha receptors, *10*
Alpha-blockade, and myocardial oxygen
    consumption, **11**
Alpha receptors, adrenergic sympathetic
    system, *10*
13-ammonia
    compared to 82-rubidium as
        radionuclide, 147, **148**
    diagnostic applications
        wall motion, *180*
Angina pectoris
    case studies, 258, 306
    predictive value of, 1
Angiography. *See* Arteriogram; Coronary
        arteriography; Digital subtraction
        angiography
Angioplasty (PTCA)
    pre- and post-, **180**
    trends, 1, **2**
Arterial input function, **167**
Arterial pressure
    analysis, 23–24
    left ventricular
        accuracy of measurement, **25**
        harmonic analysis of, **25**
        patterns of recordings, **26**
        time changing, 24–26
        zero reference for, 24
Arteriogram
    automated quantitative analysis, 109–119
    diameter measurement
        software, 97–98
        true vs. measured, **99**
    vs. direct measurement, **118**
    economics of, **224**
    edge detection, **99**
        software, 97
    limitations of, 119
    magnification correction, **100**
    vs. PET imaging, **203**
    stenosis assessment by, **84**, 115–116,
        118, 124–125
    See also Coronary arteriography
Artery, size, **89**
Attenuation correction, PET image, **197**
Automated analysis
    coronary flow reserve, 109–119
    fluid-dynamic analysis, 102–104
    myocardial infarction quantitation, **191**

stenosis geometry, **96**
Autoregulation, 12–13
    perfusion pressure vs. coronary blood
        flow, **13**
Axial sampling (PET), 207–212
    evaluation of, by phantom, 211–212
        finger phantom, **211**
        sphere phantom, **212**

B

Beta receptors, adrenergic sympathetic
    system, *10*
Blood flow
    myocardium
        collateral function and, **174**
        model of, 167–168
    See also Coronary blood flow
Body position, and blood pressure, **23**
Border recognition, software for, 97
Breakeven analysis, PET use, **219**
Bypass surgery. *See* Coronary bypass
    surgery

C

Cardiomyopathy, dilated, 142
Cardiovascular therapy, goals, 2
Case studies, positron emission
    tomography, 231–307
Catheter-manometer systems
    frequency responses of, 26–28, **27**
        clinical implications, 27–28
    pressure gradient measurements, **20**
    slow and fast, 27
    testing of, **26**
Catheterization
    arterial, **18**
    cardiac
        trends, 1, **2**
    diagnostic
        vs. PET testing, 3
    distal coronary
        experimental analysis, in vivo, 17–18
Chest pain, equivocal, 252
Cholesterol level
    drug intervention, 1
    and ischemic heart disease, 121
    and mortality, **123**, *124*
CLAS Trial, 1, *125*
Cohn et al. Angiographic Study, *124*
Collateral function
    assessing, 175–178
        by ejection fraction, **175**
        by PET, 169–178, **177**
        proximal vs. distal, **175**
    flow reserve, 112

and hemodynamic variables, **176**
    lactate extraction ratio, **176**
    model of, **173**
    myocardial blood flow, **174**
    network analysis, 170–171
        assumptions, 173
        predictions, 175
        results, 173–175
    occlusion pressure, **176**
    pressure loss
        with vasodilation, 172
    resistance, 171–172
    vasodilatory reserve, 172–173
Coronary arteriography
    catheterization, 3
    experimental procedure, 19–20
        methodology, 19
    extent of use, 2
    geometric dimensions, 95
        automated analysis, **96**
        reproducibility and accuracy of, *95*, 95
    in vivo, 17–28
    observer variability, 102, **103**, *103*, **104**
    phantom measurements of, 101, *102*
    quantitative analysis of, 3, 93–106
        generation system for, 96–97, **98**, 102
        vs. PET, *132*, **133**
    tomographic images, **149**
    at vasodilation, 20
Coronary artery, vasodilation,
    compensatory, in response to
    proximal coronary stenosis, 35–37
Coronary artery disease
    asymptomatic, 239, 261, 281
        case study, 250
    diagnosis
        noninvasive, 141
        by perfusion imaging, **144**
    and hypercholesterolemia, *134*
    progression of
        case study, 290
    progression/regression
        case study, 286
        measuring, *132*, **133**
        two-study display, **156**
    regression of
        case study, 292
    symptomatic
        case study, 256
    three-vessel
        case studies, 232–233, 233
Coronary artery stenosis
    assessment
        anatomic-geometric, 93–95
        by PET, 141–142
    asymptomatic, 1
        case study, 246

319

Coronary artery stenosis [cont.]
  and blood flow, **32**
    resistance, **33**
    at rest, **31,** 79–81
  changes in
    and flow reserve, 112–113
    measuring, 132
  collapsing
    experimental observations, 74
    fluid dynamics of, 74
    pressure-flow characteristics, 65–78
  compliant
    changing severity of, **76**
    fluid dynamics of, 74–78, **75, 76**
  diagnosis, 2–3
  diameter measurement
    arteriogram, 97–98
  drift
    Doppler analysis, **23**
  experimental analysis, in vivo, 17–28
    acute experiments, 18
    distal coronary catheter implantation,
      17–18
    postoperative course, 18
    proximal coronary catheter
      implantation, 17
    surgical chronic instrumentation, 17
  and flow reserve, 3, 81–83, 87, 112–113
  and flow velocity
    phasic patterns in, **43**
    pressure gradient with, **47**
  flowfield and energy distribution, **105**
  fluid-dynamic analysis
    from automated dimensional
      measurements, 102–104
    gradient-velocity relation and, **50**
  and perfusion reserve, **174**
  pressure drop-flow of, 105–106
  and pressure flow, 47–51
    fluid-dynamic analysis, 41–51
    phasic form, 44–45
  pressure gradient across, 82–83
    against other variables, **34, 36,** 87
  progression/regression, **127, 128**
  reversal of, 1
    baseline severity and, **130**
    clinical regimen, 134
    major trials, 124–125
    by risk factor modification, 121–134,
      123, **130,** *133*
  sequential
    coronary flow reserve, 81–82
    distal vs. proximal, **38**
    pressure-flow characteristics, 37–38
    slope of regression lines, **38**
  severity of
    defined, 33–35
    flow reserve and, **117**
    and hydraulic coefficients, *51*
  trials
    intervention, 123–124
    prevention, 121
  and vascular bed
    hemodynamic interactions, 31–39
  See also Stenosis geometry; stenosis
    percent
Coronary atherosclerosis
  incidence, 1
  silent, 1
    case study, 244
  See also Coronary artery stenosis
Coronary blood flow

change, **59**
compression
  subendocardium vs. subepicardium, *9*
factors influencing, 9–10
flowfield and energy distribution, **105**
fluid dynamic analysis, 41–51, 74–78, **75,**
  76, 102–104
gradient-flow relation and, **57**
during hyperemia, **37**
maximal
  stimulus for, 79, **80**
model of, **82**
and myocardial oxygen consumption, *9*
and perfusion pressure, **111**
and perfusion resistance, **81**
physiology, 7–14
pressure gradient and, **32**
regulation of, 10–11, *10*
  neural subsystems, *10*
resistance in, **33**
stenosis and
  at rest, **31,** 79–81
stenotic vs. nonstenotic artery, **32**
and tracer extraction, 165–167
  flowmeter measurement, **166**
  rubidium vs. microsphere injection,
    166
volume
  after vasodilation, **59**
Coronary bypass surgery
  case studies, 298, 300, 302
  trends, 2
Coronary circulation. *See* Coronary blood
    flow
Coronary constrictors, construction of, 20–
    21
Coronary Drug Project, *123*
Coronary flow reserve, 79–89
  absolute, **85**
    variability of, *86*
  absolute and relative, 83–86
    clinical application, limitations, 87–88
  as complementary measures, 87
  assessment
    by arteriograms, 109–119, **118**
    by DSA, 204–206, **205**
    by imaging techniques, **204**
    by invasive techniques, 206
    by PET, **158,** 164–165, **164**
  clinical relevance, 88–89, 118–119
  collateral flow, 112
  dynamic stenoses, 112–113
  experimental validation, 113
    by flowmeter measurement, 114–115,
      115, 117
    by quantitative coronary arteriography,
      113–114, **114, 117**
  flow model, 164–165, **164**
  and perfusion pressure, **83**
  PET defect
    visually scored, **158**
  physiological variables, 112
  and pressure gradient
    with stenosis, 82–83
  at prior exercise EKG, 89
  relative, **85, 86**
    arteriographic, 115–116, **118**
    directly measured, **115**
    and stenosis pressure gradient, 87
    variability of 86–87, *86*
  standardized conditions, 112

measured and assumed standardized
    variables, 113
  steal and, **171**
  stenosis and
    quantitative analysis of, 3
    sequential stenosis, 81–82, **81**
    severity of, **117**
  and stenosis percent, **80**
    arteriographic measurement, **84**
    Doppler catheter measurement, **84**
    during phenylephrine and
      nitroprusside infusion, **85**
    theoretical basis, 109–111, **110**
  variability of
    under different physiologic conditions,
      116–117
  and vascular bed
    size of, 113
Coronary flow velocity
  in compliant stenosis, **77**
  phasic patterns, **43**
  and pressure gradient, **60**
    baseline **45, 46**
    Doppler flow velocity transducer data
      analysis, **22**
    at rest, **44**
    with stenosis, **47**
    after vasodilation, **60**
    Starling resistor analysis, **68**
Coronary heart disease
  deaths, 1
  incidence, 1–3, *199*
  reversal
    life-style change and, 1, 3
  risk factors for, 1
Coronary microcirculation, 8–9
  myocardial, *9*
Coronary positron emission tomography.
    See Positron emission tomography
Coronary steal
  collateral network model, 170–171
  and flow reserve, **171**
  imaging, 142
  PET, **170, 171**
Cost-benefit analysis
  arteriogram, **224**
  PET, 217–227, *221, 223*
    breakeven analysis, **219**
    clinical implications, 217
    cost per study, 217–219, *218*
    vs. other testing methods, 219–220,
      224–226, **224**
    82-rubidium method, 220
    thallium exercise testing, 220, 224–226
CT scanning, fast cine, compared to other
    testing methods, 202

D

Deaths, heart disease, 1
Diagnostic tests
  accuracy, 198–202
  asymptomatic individuals, 220–222, *222*
  invasive, 2–3
  noninvasive, 2–3, 141
Diet, strict, *134*
Digital subtraction angiography (DSA)
  compared to other testing methods, 202
  coronary flow reserve
    assessment by, 204–206, **205**
    coronary transit time method, 205–206,
      205

Dipyridamole, in PET imaging, 167
Doppler flow velocity transducer
    calibration, **21**
    data analysis, 22–23
        body position and pressure, **23**
        coronary flow velocity and pressure
            gradient, **22**
        stenosis drift, **23**
    manufacture, 21–22
Doppler studies, coronary flow reserve, **84**
Drug intervention
    vs. mechanical intervention, 1, **2**
    for serum cholesterol reduction, 1

E

Economics. See Cost-benefit analysis
Edge detection, in arteriogram, **99**
Ejection fraction, collateral function, **175**
Electrocardiogram, prior exercise, **89**
Endothelium, 11–12
    dysfunctional, **12**
    intact function, **12**
Exercise testing. See Thallium exercise
    testing
Experimental studies
    by arteriography, 19–20
    by flowmeter measurement
        coronary flow reserve, 114–115, **115,**
        117
    by quantitative coronary arteriography
        coronary flow reserve, 113–114, **114,**
        117
    by Starling resistor, 68–74
    in vivo, 17–28
        acute experiments, 18
        distal coronary catheter implantation,
            17–18
        postoperative course, 18
        pressure-flow analysis, 17–28
        proximal coronary catheter
            implantation, 17
        surgical chronic instrumentation, 17

F

FATS trial (Brown), 1
FDG imaging
    clinical examples, 181–183
    compared with 82-rubidium images, **190**
    after fasting, **183**
    limitations of, 183–184
    for myocardium assessment, 181–183,
        181
    with phagocytosis, **184**
    washout, *192*
Finger phantom
    axial sampling evaluation by, **211**
    axial slice reconstruction by, **211**
    Mullani, **211, 212**
Finnish Mental Hospital Study, *122*
Flow reserve. See Coronary flow reserve
Flowmeter measurement
    coronary blood flow, **166**
    coronary flow reserve
        experimental, 114–115, **115, 117**
        correlation with perfusion imaging, **144**
Fluid dynamics
    analysis, 45–47
    basic principles, 41–42
    classical vs. Starling resistor dynamics,
        67, *72, 73*

Food and Drug Administration regulatory
    status, PET scanner, 229
Framingham Heart Study, **122**

G

Gradient-flow relation
    and coronary blood flow, **57**
    predicted vs. measured, 56–58, **56, 58,**
        58
    after vasodilation, **56**
Gradient-velocity relation
    and degree of stenosis, **50**
    measured vs. predicted, **50**
    vasodilation and, **48, 49**

H

Handgrip, with dipyridamole, 167
Helsinki Heart Study, *121*
Helsinki University Prospective
    Angiographic Study, *124*
Hemodynamics
    collateral function and, **176**
    with stenosis
        and distal coronary vascular bed, 31–
            39
        stenosis geometry, *55*
Hypercholesterolemia
    with CAD, *134*
    without CAD *134*
Hyperemia
    and coronary pressure flow, *35*
    reactive, 13–14
        coronary flow during, **37**
        schematic diagram, **13**
Hypertension
    asymptomatic, 237
    case studies, 237, 263

I

Imaging
    accuracy of diagnosis, 2–3
    artifacts in, 214–216, **214,** *214,* **215**
    with attenuation correction, **197**
    clinical examples and explanation, 147–
        157
    comparison of methods, **190**
    of coronary functions
        flow reserve, **204**
        left ventricular function, 142
        steal, 142, **170, 171**
    early and late, **189**
    quantitative, 214–216
    three-dimensional restructuring
        algorithm, 144–145
    tomograms, **140**
    washout, **191, 192,** *192,* **193**
In vivo
    coronary arteriography, 17–28
    fluid dynamics analysis, 45–47
Intervention
    risk assessment, 2–3
    symptom-based, 3
    trials, 123–124
Intra-stenotic distending pressure, **75**
Invasive techniques, diagnostic, 2–3, 206
Ischemic heart disease
    cholesterol level and, 121
    See also Myocardial ischemia

J

Jordan spheres, volume measurement by,
    212

K

Kuo et al. Angiographic Study, *124*

L

Lactate extraction ratio, collateral function
    and, **176**
Left ventricular
    arterial pressure
        harmonic analysis of, **25**
        patterns of recordings, **26**
    function
        imaging by PET, 142
Leiden Intervention Study, *124*
Life, prolongation and quality of, 2
Life-style, change, 1, 3
LifeStyle Heart Trial, 1
    quantitative coronary arteriography in,
        125–131, **126, 127**
    stenosis shape
        clinical implications, 131
        risk factors and, 132
        significance of changes, 131
    study patients, 125
Lupus vasculitis, case study, 272

M

Magnetic resonance imaging, compared to
    other testing methods, 202
Magnification correction, arteriogram, **100**
Mechanical intervention
    drug intervention vs., 1, **2**
    goals, 2
    thrombolytic therapy vs., **2,** *2*
    trends, 1–2
Metabolism, of myocardium, 7–8
Mitral valve prolapse, case study, 235
Mortality
    cholesterol level and, **123,** *124*
    risk factor modification and, *123*
    See also Deaths
Mullani finger phantom, **211, 212**
Multi-vessel disease, case study, 248
Multiple Risk Factor Intervention Trial
    Research Group, *122*
Myocardial infarction
    case studies, 254, 265, 267, 269, 274, 277,
        279, 284
    due to lupus vasculitis
        case study, 272
    incidence, 1
    infarct size
        and myocardial viability, 195
    PET assessment of, 142, 179–196
    quantitation of
        automated threshold method, **191**
        by 82-rubidium kinetics, **187, 191**
        visual estimates, **191**
Myocardial ischemia
    case study, 295
    PET assessment of, 142, 179–196
    silent, 1
Myocardial viability
    assessment, 222–223
        by FDG imaging, 181–183, **181**
        by perfusion imaging, **193**

Myocardial viability [cont.]
    by PET, 179–196, **182,** 222–223
    by potassium activity, **185**
    by 82-rubidium kinetics, 184–193, **187**
    by thallium imaging, 194–196, *194,* 222
    and infarct size, 195
    perfusion defect and, **181**
    zones at risk, 193–194
Myocardium
    blood flow, **174**
        microcirculation, *9*
        model of, 167–168
    defects
        reversibility of, **182,** *182*
    metabolism, 7–8
    oxygen consumption, *8*
        coronary blood flow and, **9**
        effect of alpha-blockade, **11**
    oxygen extraction, *8*
    salvage
        risk assessment, 2
    tracer uptake, **165, 168**
    viability. *See* Myocardial viability

N

Nash et al. Angiographic Study, *124*
National Cholesterol Education Program, **122**
Neural subsystems, and coronary blood flow regulation, *10*
NHLBI Type II Coronary Intervention Study, *124*
Nitroprusside
    effects on various measurements, **116**
    infusion, and coronary flow reserve, **85**
Noninvasive techniques, diagnostic, 2–3, 141

O

Occlusion pressure, collateral function, **176**
Oslo Study, *122*
Oxygen consumption, myocardial, *8, 11*

P

Percutaneous transluminal coronary angioplasty. *See* Angioplasty
Perfusion defect
    measuring, **133**
    and myocardium viability, **181**
    and redistribution pattern, **181**
Perfusion imaging, 143–158
    applications
        coronary artery disease, **144**
        myocardial viability, 193
    clinical
        procedure, 143–144
        radionuclides used, 146–147
    display and user interaction, 146
    flowmeter measurement correlation, **144**
    limitations of, **145**
    quantitation of, 159–168
        multiple-compartment model, 163–164
        one-compartment model, 159–160
        principles, 159
        two-compartment model, 162–163
    risk stratification by, 202

ROI statistics
    error analysis, 146
    sensitivity and specificity of, 157–158
    statistical analysis of abnormalities, 145–146
Perfusion pressure
    coronary blood flow and, **13,** 81, **111**
    decreased, related to stenosis, 37
    flow reserve and, **83**
    resistance
        coronary blood flow and, **81**
Perfusion reserve, vascular bed, **174**
PET. *See* Positron emission tomography
Phagocytosis, FDG imaging with, **184**
Phantom
    in arteriography, 101, *102*
    for axial sampling, 211–212
Phenylephrine
    effects on various measurements, **116**
    infusion, and coronary flow reserve, **85**
POSICAM detector
    detector arrangement, **209, 210**
    photomultiplier tubes
        crystal arrangement, **208**
        light output, **209**
    volume measurement by, **213**
Positron emission tomography (PET)
    applications, 169–178, **177**
        coronary artery stenosis, 141–142
        flow reserve, **158,** 164–165, **164**
        measuring stenosis changes, 132
        myocardial infarction, 142, 179–196
        myocardial ischemia, 142, 179–196
        myocardial viability, 179–196, **182,** 222–223
        rest and stress studies, 145, **151**
        steal, **170, 171**
        three-vessel disease, **153**
    basic principles, 139–142, **140**
    case studies, 231–307
    clinical summary, 141–142
    compared to other testing methods, 3, 197–206, *198,* 219–220, 224–226, **224**
        arteriography, 3, **203**
        catheterization, 3
        QCA, *132,* **133**
    diagnostic accuracy, 200–202
        clinical consequences, 202
        sensitivity and specificity, 198–200
    economics of, 217–227, *221, 223*
        breakeven analysis, **219**
        clinical implications, 217
        cost per study, 217–219, *218*
        vs. other testing methods, 219–220, 224–226, **224**
    facilities
        construction cost, *225*
        operating expenses and income, *225, 226*
        personnel requirements, 229
        university and private sites, 226–227
    FDG imaging. *See* FDG imaging
    handgrip with dipyridamole in, 167
    image
        artifacts in, 214–216, **214,** *214,* **215**
        with attenuation correction, **197**
        clinical examples and explanation, 147–157
        quantitative, 145, 214–216
        three-dimensional restructuring algorithm, 144–145
    perfusion imaging. *See* Perfusion imaging

quantitative analysis, *155*
scanner, **141**
    axial sampling, 207–212
    count rate capacity, 212–213
    FDA regulatory status, 229
    performance and accuracy, 207–216
    software design, 213
Potassium
    activity, **185**
    loss
        after reoxygenation, **186**
    and rubidium
        parallels, **186**
Predictive value, of symptoms, 1
Premature death, wages and productivity losses, 221–222, *221, 222*
Pressure drop-flow, of coronary artery stenosis, 105–106
Pressure flow
    analysis, 20
        experimental, in vivo, 17–28
        limitations of, 38–39
    fluid-dynamics, 41–51
    at high flow conditions
        with stenosis, 47–51
    during hyperemia, with stenosis, *35*
    measured vs. predicted, *73*
    phasic
        analysis of data, at rest, 42–44
        changes with progressive stenosis, 44–45
        and stenosis geometry, 53–63
    of stenoses
        collapsing, 65–78
        sequential, 37–38
        after vasodilators, *51*
Pressure gradient
    and coronary blood flow, **32**
    and flow reserve, 82–83
    and flow velocity, **47**
        baseline, **45**
        in compliant stenosis, **77**
        at rest, **44**
        vasodilation, **60**
    measurements, 20
        catheter-manometer systems, **20**
    across stenosis
        against other variables, **34, 36**
        viscous friction and exit separation contributing to, **54,** *55*
Pressure gradient-flow velocity relation, 61–62
    and absolute gradient/flow
        stenosis percent against, **34**
    pressure gradient-volume flow relation vs., 58–61
Pressure gradient-volume flow relation, 62–63
    and artery size, **89**
    vs. pressure gradient-flow velocity relation, 58–61
    velocity equations, **61**

Q

Quantitative coronary arteriography (QCA)
    applications, *132,* **133**
        coronary flow reserve, 113–114, **114,** **117**
        perfusion defect, **133**
    in LifeStyle Heart Trial, 125–131, **126,** **127**

R

Radionuclide
in perfusion imaging, 146–147
radiation dose, 229
82-rubidium vs. 13-ammonia, 147, **148**
Redistribution pattern
perfusion defect and, **181**
pre- and post-PCTA, **180**
Regional activity, PET imaging, 145
Reoxygenation, potassium loss after, **186**
Resistance
collateral function, 171–172
coronary blood flow
stenosis and, **33**
Rest (at)
coronary arteriography, 19–20
pressure-flow analysis, 20
Rest and stress
PET studies, 145
tomographic images, **151**
Risk assessment
of intervention, 2–3
by perfusion imaging, 202
Risk factors
asymptomatic individuals, 220–222, *222*
treating, 221
for coronary heart disease, 1
modification of
adherence and, **130**
and disease reversal, 1, 121–134, *133*
in LifeStyle Heart Trial, 132
and mortality, *123*
82-rubidium
applications, **187, 191**
myocardial viability, 184–193, **187**
compared to 13-ammonia as
radionuclide, 147, **148**
economics of use, 220
images
early and late, **189**
and FDG images, compared, **190**
washout, **191, 192,** *192,* **193**
vs. microsphere injection, **166**
and potassium, parallels, **186**

S

Scanner, PET. *See* Positron emission
tomography
Serum cholesterol. *See* Cholesterol level
Software
arteriography, 97–98
PET, 213
Sphere phantom, axial slices of, **212**
Starling resistor
experimental observations, 68–74
review of, 65–66
theory of measurements, 66–68
Steal. *See* Coronary steal
Stenosis, coronary artery. *See* Coronary
artery stenosis

Stenosis geometry
changes, *55*
LifeStyle Heart Trial, 131
after vasodilation, **54,** *55*
hemodynamic effects, *55*
pressure flow and, 53–63
risk factors and, 132
Stenosis percent
arteriographic measurement, **84**
change
control vs. treated group, *128,* **129**
mild severity, *129*
severe, *129*
control vs. treated group, **128**
coronary flow reserve and, **80, 84, 85**
diameter measurement accuracy, **97**
Doppler catheter measurement, **84**
observer variability of estimates, **94**
by observer group, **94**
as to specific arteries, **94**
against other variables, **34, 36**
visual estimates of, 3
Stockholm IHB Secondary Prevention Study,
123
Subendocardium, blood flow, *9*
Subepicardium, blood flow, *9*
Symptoms, predictive value of, 1

T

Thallium imaging
applications, 194–196, *194, 222*
wall motion, *180*
compared to other testing methods, 197–
202, *198*
diagnostic accuracy, 200–202
clinical consequences, 202
sensitivity and specificity, 198–200,
200
economics of, 220, 224–226
false normal, **198**
limitations, 2
Three-vessel disease, balanced, **153**
Thrombolytic therapy
vs. mechanical intervention, 2, **2**
trends, 1
Tomograms, **140**
coronary arteriography, **149**
cross-sectional, **149**
orientation of, **150**
Tracer
extraction of, 160, 165–167
flowmeter measurement, **166**
rubidium vs. microsphere injection, **166**
myocardial uptake, **165**
deficit, **168**
non-extracted, 160
time-activity curves, **160**
partially extracted, 161–162
time-activity curves, **161**

totally extracted, 161
time-activity curves, **161**
trapped, **162, 163**
Trials, CAS, 121–125
intervention, 123–124
prevention, 121
reversal, 124–125

V

Vascular bed
collateral function, 172–173
flow reserve, 113
hemodynamic interactions
stenosis and, 31–39
perfusion reserve
stenosis and, **174**
Vasodilation
arteriography at, 20
and blood flow volume, **59**
and collateral function, 172–173
distal coronary, 35–37
and gradient-flow relation, **56**
and gradient-velocity relation, **48, 49**
and pressure flow, *51*
pressure-flow analysis at, 20
and pressure gradient, coronary
volume flow, and flow velocity, **60**
stenosis geometry changes after, **54,** *55*
Viscous friction, and pressure gradient, **54,**
55
Visual estimates
coronary flow reserve, **158**
myocardial infarction, **191**
stenosis percent, 3
Volume measurement
Jordan spheres, **212**
POSICAM detector, **213**

W

Wadsworth Veterans Administration
Hospital Study, *123*
Wages and productivity losses, premature
death, 221–222, *221, 222*
Wall motion
ammonia-13 findings, *180*
preoperative vs. postoperative, *180*
thallium-201 redistribution pattern, *180*
Washout
FDG imaging, *192*
82-rubidium imaging, **191, 192,** *192,* **193**
World Health Organization Collaborative
Group, *122*
World Health Organization Study, *122*

X

X-ray imaging system, calibration of, 98–
101, **101**